New Techniques in Surgery Series

Jamal J. Hoballah • Alan B. Lumsden
Editors

Vascular Surgery

John Lumley and Nadey Hakim
Series Editors

Springer

Editors
Jamal J. Hoballah, M.D.
Division of Vascular Surgery
Department of Surgery
American University of Beirut
Medical Center
Beirut, Lebanon

Division of Vascular Surgery
Department of Surgery
University of Iowa Hospitals
and Clinics, Iowa City
IA, USA

Alan B. Lumsden, M.D.
Department of Cardiovascular Surgery
The Methodist Hospital
Houston
TX, USA

Series Editors
John Lumley, M.S., FRCS
Surgical Professorial Unit
University of London
St. Bartholomew's Hospital
London, UK

Nadey Hakim, KCSJ, M.D., Ph.D.,
FRCS, FRCSI, FACS, FICS
Max Thorek Professor of Surgery
West London Renal and Transplant Centre
Imperial College Healthcare NHS Trust
London, UK

ISBN 978-1-4471-6852-2 ISBN 978-1-4471-2912-7 (eBook)
DOI 10.1007/978-1-4471-2912-7
Springer London Heidelberg New York Dordrecht

Printed on acid-free paper

Springer is part of Springer Science+Business Media (www.springer.com)

Preface

The management of vascular disease continues to rapidly evolve, embracing endovascular and minimally invasive technology. Within this rapid change of pace, techniques that withstood the test of time will continue to serve as the foundation for newer methods that promise comparable or improved outcomes in a less invasive manner.

New Techniques in Surgery Series, Vascular Surgery, is intended to address new developments in the management of vascular disease that have been or are being developed to address the challenges facing the current techniques and technology. These include new developments to improve what is currently being done or techniques that address the challenges facing the existing technology.

In aortic surgery, new techniques continue to push the envelope in endovascular repair. Innovative techniques have been developed to deal with short-necked or juxtarenal aneurysms. Chimneys were devised to deal with short necks without resorting to fenestrated grafts. Surgeon-modified fenestrated and branched grafts have been improvised to deal with the lack of standard off-the-shelf fenestrated grafts. Techniques to deal with iliac aneurysms while preserving pelvic perfusion were created to further expand the utilization of endovascular repair. Comfort and expertise in endovascular techniques and the availability of off-the shelf endografts have allowed the surgeon to offer this technique in ruptured aortic and thoracic aneurysms. To further expand the endovascular techniques, hybrid procedures have been developed to deal with complex thoracic aneurysms, and aneurysms involving the arch vessels can now also be treated by endovascular methods. Laparoscopic and robotic surgery have also been explored as options to treat aortic pathology in a less invasive manner when endovascular repair is not possible, or as an alternative to endovascular repair. Similar exciting advances have been developed in all aspects of vascular disease, including occlusive disease, venous disease, dialysis access, and thoracic outlet syndrome.

To address these evolving techniques, the editors recruited experts and recognized authors to share with the reader their experience and the state-of-the-art management of vascular disease. This book is not meant to replace the traditional vascular textbook; it is intended to be a valuable reference to the practicing vascular surgeon on the newest current advancements in vascular surgery. This book is meant to expose vascular surgeons to currently developing techniques that are likely to become, in the near future, standard practice in the management of routine and complex vascular pathology.

Acknowledgments

We are grateful to our families, students, residents, and coworkers, notably Dr. Mel Sharafuddin and Dr. Joseph Naoum for their support towards the preparation of this volume.

The editors wish to thank the staff at Springer, notably Sarah Cody, Daniel Dominguez, and Srinath Raju for their efforts and editorial assistance to bring this volume to fruition.

Contents

Contributors

Parth B. Amin M.D. Division of Vascular Surgery, Department of Surgery, University of Iowa Hospitals and Clinics, Iowa City, IA, USA

Javier E. Anaya-Ayala, M.D. Department of Cardiovascular Surgery, Methodist DeBakey Heart and Vascular Center, The Methodist Hospital, Houston, TX, USA

Mohammad Bashir, M.D. Cardiothoracic Surgery, University of Iowa Hospitals and Clinics, Iowa City, IA, USA

Jonathan Bath, M.B.B.S. Division of Vascular Surgery, University of Pittsburgh Medical Center, Pittsburgh, PA, USA

Carlos F Bechara, M.D., M.S. Division of Vascular Surgery and Endovascular Therapy, Michael E. DeBakey Department of Surgery, Baylor College of Medicine and the Michael E. DeBakey VA Medical Center, Houston, TX, USA

Jean Bismuth, M.D. Department of Cardiovascular Surgery, Methodist DeBakey Heart & Vascular Center, The Methodist Hospital, Houston, TX, USA

Rabih A. Chaer, M.D. Division of Vascular Surgery, University of Pittsburgh Medical Center, Pittsburgh, PA, USA

Jae-Sung Cho, M.D. Division of Vascular Surgery, University of Pittsburgh Medical Center, Pittsburgh, PA, USA

R. Clement Darling, M.D. The Vascular Group PLLC, The Institute for Vascular Health and Disease, Albany Medical Center Hospital, The Center for Vascular Awareness, Inc, Albany, NY, USA

Hossam F. El-Sayed, M.D., Ph.D., RVT Division of Vascular Surgery, Department of Cardiovascular Surgery, Weil Cornell Medical College, The Methodist Hospital, Houston, TX, USA

Mark A. Farber, M.D., FACS Department of Surgery and Radiology, UNC Aortic Center, University of North Carolina Health Car, Chapel Hill, NC, USA

Javairiah Fatima Department of Surgery, Mayo Clinic, Rochester, MN, USA

Mark G. Davies, M.D., Ph.D., M.B.A. Department of Cardiovascular Surgery, Methodist DeBakey Heart and Vascular Center, The Methodist Hospital, Houston, TX, USA

Joss Dean Fernandez, M.D. Cardiothoracic Surgery, University of Iowa Hospitals and Clinics, Iowa City, IA, USA

Sidney M. Glazer, M.D., FACS Department of Surgery, University of California, Irvine, Orange, CA, USA

Jafar Golzarian, M.D. Department of Radiology, University of Minnesota, Minneapolis, MN, USA

M. Hamady, MBChB, FRCR Consultant Interventional Radiologist, Imperial College, St Mary's Campus, London, UK

Heitham T. Hassoun, M.D., FACS Department of Cardiovascular Surgery, Methodist DeBakey Heart and Vascular Center, The Methodist Hospital Physician Organization, Houston, TX, USA

Jamal J. Hoballah, M.D. Division of Vascular Surgery, Department of Surgery, American University of Beirut Medical Center, Beirut, Lebanon

Division of Vascular Surgery, Department of Surgery, University of Iowa Hospitals and Clinics, Iowa City, IA, USA

Mark Iannettoni, M.D. Cardiothoracic Surgery, University of Iowa Hospitals and Clinics, Iowa City, IA, USA

Nyla Ismail, Ph.D. Department of Cardiovascular Surgery, Methodist DeBakey Heart and Vascular Center, The Methodist Hospital Research Institute, The Methodist Hospital, Houston, TX, USA

William C. Jennings, M.D., FACS Department of Surgery, University of Oklahoma College of Medicine, Tulsa, OK, USA

Viviane Kazan, M.D. Division of Vascular and Endovascular Surgery, Department of Surgery, University of Toledo Medical Center, Toledo, OH, USA

Panos Kougias, M.D. Department of Surgery, Baylor College of Medicine, Houston, TX, USA

Alan B. Lumsden, M.D. Department of Cardiovascular Surgery, The Methodist Hospital, Houston, TX, USA

Joseph E. Maakaron Department of Internal Medicine, American University of Beirut Medical Center, Beirut, Lebanon

Michel S. Makaroun, M.D. Division of Vascular Surgery, University of Pittsburgh Medical Center, Pittsburgh, PA, USA

Manish Mehta, M.D., MPH The Vascular Group PLLC, The Institute for Vascular Health and Disease, Albany Medical Center Hospital, The Center for Vascular Awareness, Inc, Albany, NY, USA

Andrew Misselt, M.D. Department of Radiology, University of Minnesota, Minneapolis, MN, USA

Munier Nazzal, M.D., FRCS, FACS Division of Vascular and Endovascular Surgery, Department of Surgery, University of Toledo Medical Center, Toledo, OH, USA

Joseph J. Naoum, M.D., FACS Division of Vascular Surgery, Weill-Cornell Medical College, The Methodist Hospital, Houston, TX, USA

Rachael M. Nicholson, M.D. Division of Vascular Surgery, Department of Surgery, University of Iowa Hospitals and Clinics, Iowa City, IA, USA

Gustavo S. Oderich, M.D., FACS Division of Vascular and Endovascular Surgery, Gonda Vascular Center, Mayo Clinic Medical College, Rochester, MN, USA

Zaher K. Otrock Department of Pathology and Laboratory Medicine, University of Beirut Medical Center, Beirut, Lebanon

Heather P. Park, M.D. Department of Surgery, University of North Carolina Health Care, Chapel Hill, NC, USA

Vikas A. Pandey Imperial Vascular Unit, St. Mary's Hospital, London, UK

Kalpaj Parekh, M.D. Cardiothoracic Surgery, University of Iowa Hospitals and Clinics, Iowa City, IA, USA

Philip S.K. Paty, M.D. The Vascular Group PLLC, The Institute for Vascular Health and Disease, Albany Medical Center Hospital, The Center for Vascular Awareness, Inc, Albany, NY, USA

Eric K. Peden, M.D. Department of Cardiovascular Surgery, Methodist DeBakey Heart and Vascular Center, The Methodist Hospital Research Institute, The Methodist Hospital, Houston, TX, USA

George Pisimisis, M.D. Division of Vascular Surgery and Endovascular Therapy, Michael E. DeBakey Department of Surgery, Baylor College of Medicine and the Michael E. DeBakey VA Medical Center, Houston, TX, USA

Jihane Abou Rahal Department of Internal Medicine, American University of Beirut Medical Center, Beirut, Lebanon

Basel Ramlawi, M.D. Department of Cardiovascular Surgery, The Methodist Hospital, Houston, TX, USA

Michael J. Reardon, M.D., FACC, FACS The Methodist DeBakey Heart and Vascular Center, Weill Medical College of Cornell University, Houston, TX, USA

Department of Cardiovascular Surgery, The Methodist Hospital, Houston, TX, USA

Joseph J. RicottaII M.D., M.S., FACS Division of Vascular Surgery and Endovascular Therapy, Emory University School of Medicine, Atlanta, GA, USA

Sean P. Roddy, M.D. The Vascular Group PLLC, The Institute for Vascular Health and Disease, Albany Medical Center Hospital, The Center for Vascular Awareness, Inc, Albany, NY, USA

Melhem J. Sharafuddin, M.D. Division of Vascular Surgery, Department of Surgery, University of Iowa Hospitals and Clinics, Iowa City, IA, USA

Ali Taher Department of Internal Medicine, American University of Beirut Medical Center, Beirut, Lebanon

Nikolaos Tsilimparis, M.D. Division of Vascular Surgery and Endovascular Therapy, Emory University School of Medicine, Atlanta, GA, USA

Daynene Vykoukal, Ph.D. Department of Cardiovascular Surgery, Methodist DeBakey Heart and Vascular Center, The Methodist Hospital, Houston, TX, USA

Laura E. White, M.D. Department of Surgery, Methodist DeBakey Heart and Vascular Center, The Methodist Hospital, Houston, TX, USA

Part I

Aneurysmal Disease

Infrarenal Aortic Aneurysms: New Technologies

1

Laura E. White and Heitham T. Hassoun

Abstract

Nearly two decades after the first successful endovascular aortic repair (EVAR), steady advancements in device technology, deployment techniques, and imaging capabilities have allowed this treatment modality to replace traditional open aortic repair as the treatment of choice for patients undergoing elective abdominal aortic aneurysm (AAA) repair. EVAR now accounts for greater than half of all AAA repairs; however, certain challenges to EVAR remain including anatomic limitations and graft durability. These limitations are now being addressed with new technology and deployment modalities. Surveillance and surgical repair remain the primary focus of therapy for AAA, and this chapter aims to discuss developments in disease surveillance, interventional techniques, and the evolution of endograft devices for EVAR.

Keywords

Abdominal aortic aneurysm • Endovascular aortic repair • Aneurysm Stent graft • Endograft • Aneurysm surveillance

L.E. White, M.D.
Department of Surgery,
Methodist DeBakey Heart and Vascular Center,
The Methodist Hospital,
Houston, TX, USA

H.T. Hassoun, M.D., FACS (✉)
Department of Surgery, Johns Hopkins University School of Medicine, Johns Hopkins Medicine International,
1300 Thames St., Suite 200, MD 21231,
Baltimore, Maryland, USA

Department of Cardiovascular Surgery,
Methodist DeBakey Heart and Vascular Center,
The Methodist Hospital Physician Organization,
6550 Fannin Street, SM 1401, Houston, TX 77030, USA
e-mail: hhassoun@tmhs.org

Introduction

Abdominal aortic aneurysms (AAA) affect approximately 5 % of men and 1 % of women over the age of 60 years, and multiple epidemiological studies indicate that the incidence is increasing despite improved medical management of certain risk factors [1]. Weakening of the aortic wall due to systemic and local pathology combined with a genetic predisposition results in progressive wall stress and aneurysm dilation. Most AAAs remain asymptomatic and undetected, and unfortunately without intervention, rupture may occur [2]. In the

J.J. Hoballah, A.B. Lumsden (eds.), *Vascular Surgery*, New Techniques in Surgery Series,
DOI 10.1007/978-1-4471-2912-7_1, © Springer-Verlag London 2012

Table 1.1 Open vs EVAR: randomized trials

Endpoint	DREAM [6, 10]	EVAR-1 [7, 8]	OVER [9]
N	345	1,082	881
30-day mortality (%)			
Open	4.6	4.7	2.3
EVAR	1.2*	1.7*	0.2*
Secondary intervention Rate (%)			
Open	N/A	1.7	9.2
EVAR		5.1*	10.4
Long term survival (%)			
Open	69.9	54	90.2 %
EVAR	68.9 (mean 6.4 years)	54 (at 8 years)	93 % (mean 1.8 years)

*$P < 0.05$, *N* patients evaluated, *DREAM* Dutch Randomized Endovascular Aneurysm Management trial, *EVAR-1* United Kingdom Endovascular Aneurysm Repair trial, *OVER* Open Versus Endovascular Repair trial (Veterans Affairs Cooperative Study Group)

USA, AAAs are estimated as the tenth most common cause of mortality and are responsible for approximately 2 % of all deaths [3].

Since the first open AAA repair nearly 60 years ago, surveillance and surgical repair of AAAs remain the mainstay of therapy, with maximum aneurysm diameter between 5 and 5.5 cm the accepted threshold for repair in average risk patients [4]. It has been nearly two decades since Parodi and colleagues pioneered the first successful endovascular aortic aneurysm repair (EVAR) in humans, and with steady advances in device technology, deployment techniques, and imaging capabilities, this treatment modality has now replaced open aortic repair as the treatment of choice for patients undergoing elective AAA repair [5]. This evolution has been buoyed by large, randomized controlled trials that compared morbidity and mortality rates for EVAR vs. open AAA repair and demonstrated superior outcomes for EVAR (Table 1.1) [6–10].

EVAR now accounts for more than half of all AAA repairs, and despite the favorable clinical outcomes and patient demand for this less invasive approach to AAA repair, certain challenges to EVAR including anatomic limitations and graft durability remain and limit its potential applicability to some patients [11]. These limitations are now being addressed with new technology and deployment techniques. This chapter aims to discuss recent advances in the diagnosis and management of AAAs including developments in diagnosis and surveillance, EVAR devices and techniques, and medical management of AAAs.

Latest Developments in Diagnosis and Screening

Indications for open aortic repair were originally derived from the calculated risk of rupture rates based on aneurysm diameter, and this remains the mainstay of diagnosis and treatment algorithms for AAA. In a review published by the Society for Vascular Surgery, compiled data from multiple studies demonstrates very little risk of rupture for AAAs less than 5 cm in diameter. Once an AAA grows beyond 5.5 cm, however, the increase in annual rupture risk rises exponentially to 9.4 % [12, 13]. Therefore, current practice mandates elective repair for all symptomatic aneurysms and AAAs greater than 5.5 cm in diameter [4].

Aneurysm Screening and Imaging

Ultrasonography (US) is the preferred diagnostic technique for screening of AAAs as it detects the presence of an aneurysm at low cost with sensitivity and specificity approaching 100 % [14, 15]. Computed tomography (CT) surpasses US in reproducibility but its use for routine screening and surveillance should be limited due to radiation exposure and expense [16]. While serial CT scanning of AAAs has demonstrated a marginal shortening in proximal neck length and a small increase in neck diameter as the aneurysm grows during surveillance [17–19], early screening with CT instead of US fails to capture more patients anatomically suitable for EVAR. Therefore, many centers forgo CT evaluation until the aneurysm size approaches the indications for repair, and CT should be primarily used as an imaging modality for preoperative planning to evaluate the morphology of the AAA, iliofemoral access characteristics, device sizing, and also to detect anomalous or unusual arterial anatomy.

Asymptomatic patients who should be screened for AAA include those with risk factors including increasing age, male gender, white race, long history of smoking, personal or family history of AAA or other vascular aneurysms, hypertension, atherosclerotic disease, and hypercholesterolemia [4, 20]. Frequency of surveillance for patients with AAA depends on aneurysm size, with 12-month intervals for AAA 3.5–4.4 cm in diameter and 6-month intervals for AAA 4.5–5.4 cm in diameter [21]. These recommendations are based primarily on findings from the UK Small Aneurysm Trial which also showed that growth rate was greatest among smokers, lowest in patients with a lower ankle-brachial index and diabetes, and was unaffected by lipids and blood pressure. A recent European meta-analysis has demonstrated a significant decrease in aneurysm-related mortality and a 50 % reduction in the number of emergency operations for ruptured AAA after 3–5 years of US screening [22]. Additionally, a multicenter study in the United Kingdom by Kim et al. found sustained cost-effectiveness and improved survival rates in male patients participating in a 7-year US screening program [23]. Recognizing these developments, the USA implemented the Screening Abdominal Aortic Aneurysms Very Efficiently (SAAAVE) Act in 2007, which provides Medicare coverage of screening US for men 65–75 years of age who have ever smoked or men and women who have a family history of AAA [24].

Repair of Small AAA

Whether patients benefit from prophylactic repair of smaller aneurysms (i.e., 4–5 cm range) has been an area of much debate. Two randomized prospective clinical trials, the United States Aneurysm Detection and Management Study (ADAM) and the United Kingdom Small Aneurysm Trial (UKSAT), have determined surveillance alone every 3 or 6 months for AAA 4.0–5.4 cm in diameter is as effective as elective open surgical repair in reducing mortality risk. Most patients, however, did eventually require intervention as demonstrated by a 10-year follow-up report in which 74 % of patients from the surveillance cohort had undergone surgical repair [12, 25–28].

Despite the lack of evidence to support early open repair of small AAA, an endovascular approach may offer additional benefits. Smaller AAAs may be more anatomically amenable to EVAR, and in fact, studies have shown AAAs less than 5.5 cm in diameter have longer infrarenal necks, less angulation, less tortuosity, and longer iliac landing zones than larger aneurysms [18, 29]. In a prospective clinical series of 206 patients, Arko et al. found no significant difference in proximal neck diameter, but that larger aneurysms (>6 cm) had 27 % shorter and 15 % more angulated proximal necks than smaller aneurysms (<5 cm) [30]. Furthermore, two randomized clinical trials were initiated to evaluate EVAR outcomes vs. surveillance for small AAAs: (1) the European-based Comparison of Surveillance vs. Aortic Endografting for Small Aneurysm Repair (CAESAR) trial and (2) the United States' Positive Impact of Endovascular Options for Treating Aneurysm Early (PIVOTAL) trial [31–33].

The CAESAR trial enrolled 360 (of a planned 740) patients before the trial ended prematurely due to lack of funding and delay in patient enrollment. There was no difference in mortality between EVAR and surveillance at 3 years, but a surprising 58.2 % of patients required repair even at this short surveillance interval [34]. The PIVOTAL trial results demonstrated that in the 728 (of a planned 1,050) patients with AAA (4–5 cm) randomized to receive EVAR vs. ultrasound surveillance, mortality did not differ (4.1 % in each group) at a mean follow-up of 20 months. Aneurysm-related death and time to rupture were negligible (0.6 %) in both groups, and this led to the early discontinuation of enrollment in the study. The patients in the surveillance arm underwent a rigorous schedule of ultrasound or CT scan every 6 months, and nearly one third of this group subsequently underwent repair [33]. The number of patients in this study who "crossed over" from the surveillance to the treatment arm is consistent with the other large randomized controlled trials comparing early vs. late repair, with crossover rates ranging from 27 to 60 % [35].

Most of the surveillance patients in PIVOTAL who crossed over to intervention did so due to an enlarging aneurysm [33]. However, 11 % cited anxiety as the primary reason for pursuing treatment. Other studies have documented much higher rates: in the ADAM and UKSAT trials, as many as 26 and 23 % of patients requested early treatment due to "symptoms" or "increased anxiety," respectively [35]. The role that quality of life measures play in appropriate treatment selection remains an area of investigation. In summary, current recommendations provided by the Society for Vascular Surgery state that for aneurysms in the range of 4.0–5.4 cm, surveillance followed by selective repair is recommended for older males with significant comorbidities; some young healthy patients, particularly women, may see benefit from early repair between 5.0 and 5.4 cm [4]. Future long-term data on these patients should help elucidate the benefit vs. risk ratio for small aneurysm EVAR.

Development in EVAR Devices

Stent grafts are classified based on body characteristics (i.e., tube vs. bifurcated, unibody vs. modular), means of deployment (i.e., self-expanding vs. balloon-inflated), and mode of fixation (i.e., active vs. passive). They are produced from a combination of stainless steel, cobalt chromium, or nickel alloys with a durable graft material such as Dacron or PTFE [36]. The ideal aortic stent graft is hemostatic, user-friendly, and contains a low-profile delivery system which is flexible when maneuvering yet rigid enough to resist kinking. The graft material must be thin to facilitate a lower profile yet maintain low porosity and demonstrate strength and durability. Finally, the metal frame supporting the graft must provide a high column strength and durability, maintain resistance to external compression, corrosion and fatigue, and importantly, be radiopaque [37].

Current FDA-Approved Devices

The aforementioned requirements, combined with the stringent scrutiny of the Food and Drug Administration, have led to only 6 of 16 devices developed in the past two decades achieving approval, one of which was taken off the market in March 2001 [38]. Current Food and Drug Administration (FDA)-approved EVAR devices and their characteristics are listed in Table 1.2. Due to potential problems with distal attachment site failure, all current devices are bifurcated endografts which allow for distal attachment at the level of the iliac arteries. Unibody bifurcated grafts (i.e., the Powerlink, Endologix, Irvine, CA) are placed as a whole, requiring subsequent retraction of the second iliac limb via contralateral access. Modular bifurcated grafts are composed of a main body with a short contralateral limb and provide customized intraoperative deployment [39].

The AneuRx (Medtronic, Santa Rosa, CA) bifurcated, modular stent graft is composed of a nitinol frame and polyester graft material and contains no barbs or hooks for main body attachment. Bilateral femoral or iliac access is required for the main body and contralateral limb through a 21-French (F) and 16–19-F catheter, respectively. The device is currently in its sixth generation and has the largest cumulative clinical experience, with greater than 80,000 endoprostheses deployed worldwide as of 2010. Though the Aneuryx device has certain favorable characteristics such as the potential to treat the smallest aortic diameter, concerns for a higher risk of device migration remains due to the lack of an active proximal fixation mechanism [39]. The Talent (Medtronic, Santa Rosa, CA) abdominal stent graft is a modular, bifurcated stent of similar material that was designed to treat a larger range of aortic and iliac diameters, extending its indications to include AAA with aortic necks from 18 to 32 mm and iliac arteries from 7 to 22 mm in diameter. Long-term follow-up data of the most recent generation Talent graft demonstrates comparable results to other stent grafts, and its use in AAA with short necks (10–15 mm) has provided encouraging results at 5-year follow-up [40, 41].

Table 1.2 Current FDA approved EVAR devices

	AneuRx	Excluder	Zenith	Powerlink	Talent
Manufacturer	Medtronic (California, USA)	WL Gore and Associates (Arizona, USA)	Cook (Indiana, USA)	Endologix (California, USA)	Medtronic (California, USA)
FDA device approval	Sept. 1999	Nov. 2002	May 2003	Oct. 2004	Apr. 2008
Stent material	Nitinol	Nitinol	Stainless steel	Cobalt chromium alloy	Nitinol
Graft material	Polyester	PTFE[a]	Polyester	PTFE	Polyester
Proximal fixation	Infrarenal	Infrarenal	Suprarenal	Infrarenal	Infrarenal
Proximal fixation mechanism	Radial force and column strength	Anchors and radial forces	Hooks and suprarenal stent	Anchors on bifurcation	Radial force and column strength
Modularity	Modular bifurcated	Modular bifurcated	Modular bifurcated	Bifurcated unibody	Modular bifurcated
Main body size (mm)	D 20–28, L 135 and 165	D 23–31, L 120, 140, 160, 180	D 22-36[b], L 82, 96, 111, 125, 140	D 22-34[c], L 120, 135, 140, 155, 175	D 22–36, L 140, 155, 170
Iliac limb size (mm)	D 12–24, L 85, 115, 135	D 12–20, L 100, 120, 140	D 8–24, L 37, 54, 71, 88, 105, 122	D 13–25, L 55, 65, 70, 88	D 8–24, L 75, 95, 105
Delivery sheath size (F)					
Main body	19, 21	18	18, 20, 22	19, 21	22, 24
Contralateral limb	16–19	12	14, 16	9	20, 18
Conversion device	No	No	Yes	No	Yes

D diameter, *L* length
[a]Polytetra-fluoroethylene
[b]For 36 mm diameter length includes 95, 113, 131, 149 mm
[c]The 34 mm device is a separate component

The Excluder (W.L. Gore, Flagstaff, AZ) graft is also a bifurcated, modular stent graft composed of a nitinol frame and PTFE graft material with active fixation facilitated by anchoring barbs. Delivery of the main body and contralateral limbs is made through 18-F and 12-F sheaths for the standard diameter grafts. A significant advantage of this device is its relatively low profile, flexibility, and uncomplicated deployment system. The first-generation Excluder graft has been implicated in a substantial percentage of patients demonstrating aneurysm growth; however, later modifications of the graft with addition of a lower permeability membrane has demonstrated success in arresting AAA expansion and facilitating AAA sac regression [39, 42]. Furthermore, the latest version of this device (C3 delivery system) incorporates a unique feature for added deployment control which allows the surgeon/interventionalist to partially deploy and reposition the device. This feature may prove to revise EVAR techniques altogether and certainly will expand the anatomic inclusion criteria for most operators.

The Zenith Flex (Cook Inc., Bloomington, IN) endoprosthesis provides suprarenal fixation with an uncovered proximal stent and fixation barbs and is available in a wide range of sizes. Due to its ferromagnetic exoskeleton, this stent is unsafe for magnetic resonance (MR) imaging. Deployment is staged, with partial deployment of the main body preceding the barbed suprarenal fixation stent, and is completed with contralateral iliac limb followed by full release of the main body. Additional steps include removal of the top cap, adding the ipsilateral iliac limb, and inflating the balloon to secure sealing. The Zenith Flex provides flexibility with suprarenal fixation to abrogate stent migration and for the potential treatment of AAAs with shorter necks. The Powerlink device has been available since 2004 and is a unibody, bifurcated, self-expanding stent graft with infrarenal and suprarenal extensions available. Its deployment from a distal to proximal fashion, with fixation of the aortic bifurcation preceding suprarenal fixation, has the potential to prevent device migration and subsequent endoleak. Graft migration rates vary from 4.2 to 7 % and limb occlusion rates ranged from 1 to 2 %, with improvement once primary deployment at the aortic bifurcation was implemented [43–45]. A distinct advantage is the low-profile (9F) contralateral limb.

While all FDA-approved devices have unique features, little significant difference in EVAR outcomes, including endoleak, device migration, and graft occlusion rates, have been definitively determined [46]. The following section describes newer technology currently pending FDA approval in the USA but that may be available in Europe and elsewhere. These devices are considered "next-generation" devices aimed at expanding the anatomic inclusion criteria for EVAR.

Next-Generation Devices: Expanding the Anatomic Inclusion Criteria

EVAR requires certain aortoiliac anatomic criteria for adequate aneurysm exclusion and prevention of complications. On-label use of current FDA-approved devices would limit EVAR anatomical inclusion criteria to AAAs with a 10–15-mm infrarenal neck length, aortic diameter ≤32 mm, angulation <60°, and 7-mm iliac access diameter [4]. Mounting experience with the current devices, recognized need to expand therapy, and patient demand for this less invasive approach to AAA repair have driven industry to develop novel "next-generation" devices that either improve on the current prototypes or expand the anatomic inclusion criteria (Fig. 1.1). The most frequent anatomic features limiting potential EVAR are short and angulated proximal aortic necks [47]. The Anaconda (Vascutek, Terumo, Inchinnan, Scotland) and Aorfix (Lombard Medical, Oxfordshire, UK) stent grafts are designed to address AAAs with hostile neck anatomy, and both are currently in phase II US clinical trials.

The Anaconda is a unique tri-modular, repositionable stent graft composed of woven polyester with multiple independent ring stents that provide device flexibility. The main body size ranges from 19.5 to 34 mm for treatment of AAA from 16 to 32 mm in diameter. The Anaconda graft can be employed in AAAs with highly angulated proximal necks due to a saddle shape of the proximal stents: the apex of the convexity lies anteriorly-posteriorly and the concavity lies laterally. Fixation relies on the radial forces of two overlapping proximal components and four pairs of hooks, and during the implantation phase, the stents spread and flatten, moving proximally, therefore requiring adequate distance from the takeoff of the renal arteries. Two-year follow-up in patients with the Anaconda graft has shown no correlation of clinical or technical success or survival with degree of angulation of the proximal necks and no incidences of graft migration. Rates of proximal endoleak remain relatively high at up to 14 % [48–50].

Introduced in Europe in 2004, the Aorfix stent graft is a bifurcated or aorto-uni-iliac device developed with increased flexibility in order to acquire greater seal in proximal necks angulated greater than 45°. Four double hooks at the proximal end enhance fixation, and during deployment, pushrods maintain positioning of the proximal end of the graft and upon completion, the stent graft has a "fish-mouth" shape. Initial midterm results in a few small trials from Europe have demonstrated acceptable results in hostile

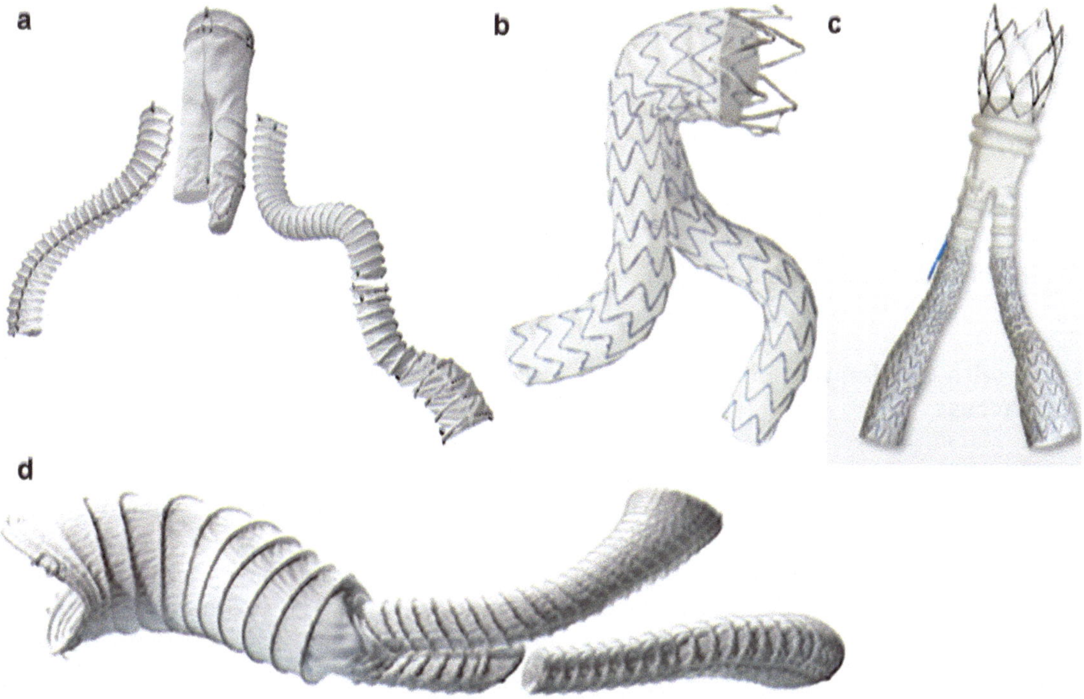

Fig. 1.1 Next-generation devices. (**a**) The Anaconda (Vascutek, Terumo, Inchinnan, Scotland); (**b**) the Endurant (Medtronic, Santa Rosa, CA); (**c**) the Ovation (TriVascular, Santa Rosa, CA); (**d**) the Aorfix (Lombard Medical, Oxfordshire, UK)

neck anatomy, and results from the larger US PIVOTAL trial are pending [51, 52].

Iliac artery anatomy must facilitate passage of the stent graft delivery system, and iliac tortuosity, calcification, and size are all potential limitations to EVAR. Even with adequate preoperative imaging and planning, 8–15 % of patients have iliac anatomy unsuitable for EVAR [53, 54]. Women and patients of Asian ancestry represent two particularly problematic populations for iliofemoral access [4, 55, 56]. Two novel devices that have a reduced profile to address access challenges, while maintaining characteristics of durability and flexibility, are the Endurant (Medtronic, Santa Rosa, CA) and Ovation (TriVascular, Santa Rosa, CA) stent grafts.

The Endurant is Medtronic's next-generation device which, similar to the Aneuryx and Talent devices, is composed of a nitinol polyester fabric and nitinol frame but also incorporates a suprarenal stent with barbs for active fixation. The device is highly flexible, designed to treat challenging neck anatomy, and also reduces the delivery profile to 18–20-F outer diameter. It has been approved in Europe since 2008 and has been recently approved in the USA. The TriVascular Ovation stent graft is a tri-modular, suprarenal device composed of nitinol stents encapsulated in PTFE and maintains the smallest profile of any device (14–15-F outer diameter delivery system). This device also has a novel seal technology which features two inflatable rings in the proximal seal zone that are filled with a polymer to enhance aortic wall apposition. The TriVascular device recently received its CE mark in Europe and is currently in a phase II nonrandomized multicenter trial in the USA.

Advances in EVAR Techniques

As medical device companies forge ahead with significant research and development of next-generation devices, physicians have gained significant experience with EVAR techniques over the past decade. While feasibility of this technology remains limited by some anatomical constraints, certain challenges such as difficult iliac access, hostile proximal aortic neck anatomy, and associated iliac aneurysms can be managed with currently available devices and some appropriate technical maneuvers.

Dealing with Challenging Iliac Artery Access

As previously mentioned, a substantial proportion of potential EVAR candidates has iliac artery anatomy not ideally suited for delivery of large-profile devices. Frequently encountered problems such as excessive vessel calcification, occlusive disease, and tortuosity may be overcome with adjunctive procedures such as iliac artery balloon angioplasty, endoluminal conduit construction (endoconduit), buddy wire techniques, external iliac artery straightening via manual extracorporeal compression or even retroperitoneal dissection and traction, and, occasionally, iliofemoral bypass conduit construction.

For patients with small diameter external iliac arteries (i.e., <7 mm), one should use the lowest possible profile device, and at times, the use of components from different manufacturers may be necessary to achieve aneurysm exclusion with the minimum profile. Several maneuvers may facilitate passage through small, calcified vessels including placement of mineral oil on the outer sheath (though the advent of hydrophilic sheaths makes this less necessary), sequential vessel expansion with gradual dilators, and balloon angioplasty. When performing balloon angioplasty, only the smallest profile necessary to facilitate passage of the main body of the graft is needed (usually an 8 mm balloon), and this vessel segment can often be covered with the stent graft or an adjunctive self-expanding stent following device deployment. Though more commonly needed for thoracic EVAR (TEVAR), an endoconduit may occasionally be the best option for safe delivery of the endograft [57, 58]. In this scenario, a covered stent or a contralateral limb of the device (greater radial force) is deployed in the ipsilateral external and common iliac artery in a primary fashion, and the graft is then balloon dilated to facilitate passage of the device (Fig. 1.2).

Extremely tortuous iliac vessels may be difficult to cross with a stiff wire, even when attempting exchange through a catheter, and in these scenarios, a "buddy wire" technique may be helpful. In this case, leaving a floppy wire and catheter in the proximal thoracic aorta will often provide enough stability to advance a stiff wire through a separate catheter which will straighten the tortuous iliac and facilitate passage of the device into the aorta. One must be mindful of the potential complications caused by the change in anatomical configuration after vessel straightening, including upward (i.e., cephalad) torque and device migration, and iliac limb kinking and occlusion.

Management of the Hostile Aortic Neck

As mentioned previously, the most frequent anatomic features limiting potential EVAR are short and angulated proximal aortic necks, and there is no substitute for length with respect to preventing endoleak and potential device migration [59]. Greater neck length provides increased seal potential, and one of the best ways to maximize seal is optimizing graft positioning. This is facilitated by the use of preoperative 3D imaging for case planning with intraoperative magnification and appropriate adjustment of the fluoroscopy image intensifier to facilitate placement of the device as close to the renal arteries as possible. Future EVAR procedures may be enhanced by the use of novel imaging systems such as the Artis zeego (Siemens, Erlangen, Germany) which is the first robotically controlled multi-axis imaging system that provides simultaneous angiography and large volume 3D DynaCT imaging capacity (Fig. 1.3).

Another technique to maximize the proximal seal zone, termed the "endo-wedge," places wires into the renal artery via a proximal brachial approach and takes advantage of the proximal

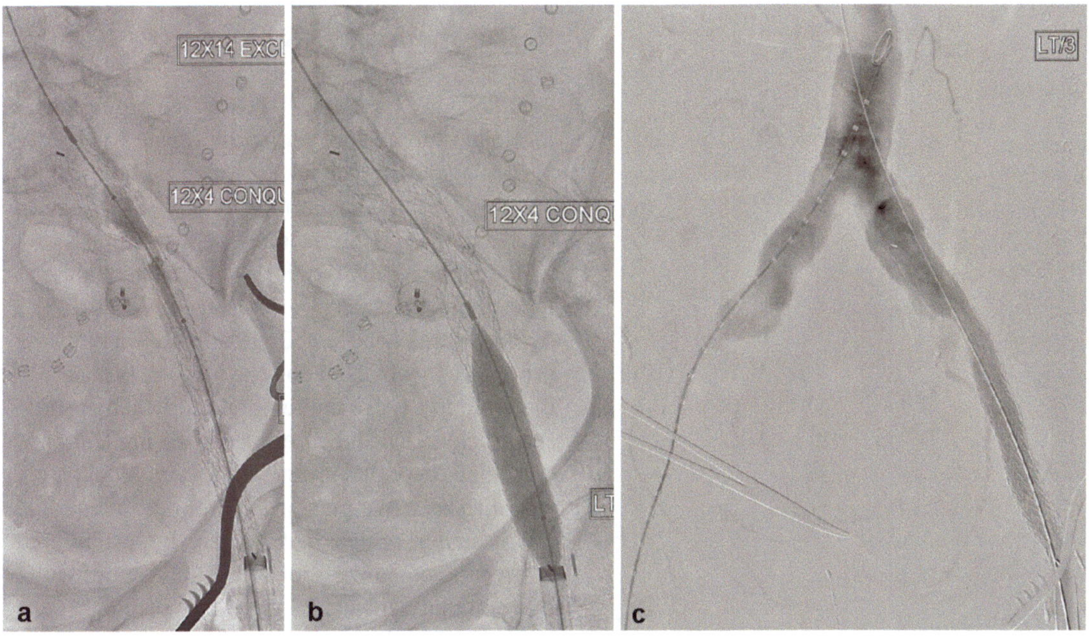

Fig. 1.2 Endoconduit for challenging iliac access. (**a**) Primary stent graft placement followed by balloon angioplasty of a circumferentially calcified stenosis at the iliac artery bifurcation; (**b**) balloon angioplasty of the common and small diameter external iliac arteries; (**c**) completion angiogram demonstrating endoconduit

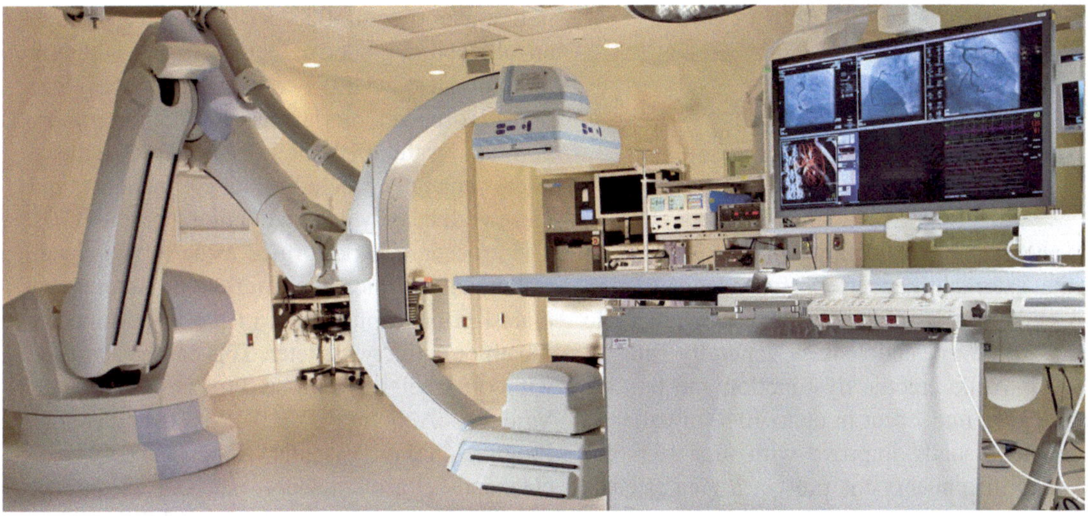

Fig. 1.3 Artis zeego multi-axis imaging system. Artis zeego multi-axis imaging system (Siemens, Erlange, Germany)

scalloped 4 mm of the Excluder device to maximize seal and achieve aneurysm exclusion [60]. For persistant proximal endoleaks, other options include placement of zero-extension aortic cuffs and/or balloon-expandable Palmaz (Cordis Corporation, Miami Lakes, FL) stents.

Iliac Artery Aneurysms

AAA-associated common iliac artery aneurysm occurs in 35 % of patients evaluated for EVAR, and these aneurysms may prevent a suitable seal zone in the distal common iliac artery [61, 62].

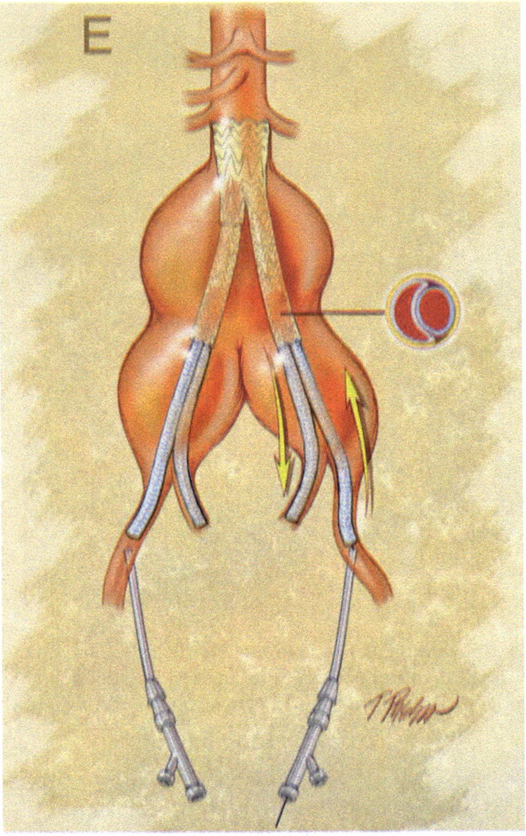

Fig. 1.4 "Snorkel" technique for EVAR. Medical illustration of completed percutaneous repair of aorto-bi-iliac aneurysm using the branched-graft "snorkel" technique

For aneurysms that require unilateral extension to the external iliac artery for adequate seal, coil embolization of the ipsilateral hypogastric artery to prevent endoleak is generally safe [4, 53, 62]. While erectile dysfunction and buttock claudication may occur in up to 40 % of patients, symptoms usually improve with time [63–65]. Bilateral iliac aneurysms present a greater challenge because bilateral coil embolization, even in a staged fashion, is not as well tolerated as unilateral embolization [65, 66]. Options in this setting include internal iliac artery bypass, endovascular repair with an iliac branched device (IBD), or endovascular repair using a "snorkel" technique (Fig. 1.4). This later approach is attractive because it can be performed with the current commercially available devices, but its durability remains unknown.

Percutaneous EVAR

Percutaneous EVAR (PEVAR) is emerging as a feasible approach to endograft repair of AAA, particularly with advancements in both delivery and closure device technology [67]. EVAR device delivery systems range in size from 18 to 24 Fr and generally require external and common iliac artery diameters to be at least 7 mm [68]. Typically this is accessed via a femoral cutdown procedure in which an oblique incision is made in the groin to expose the femoral artery and ensure secure closure of the arteriotomy. Complications contributed to the groin wound, include pain, paresthesias, lymphoceles, wound infection, and scarring, which may greatly impact future interventions via the groin [69]. In keeping with the minimally invasive approach, percutaneous access for EVAR has been used to minimize these postsurgical complications and promote earlier ambulation and shorter procedure time.

The ideal candidate for PEVAR is a nonobese patient with noncalcified femoral arteries >7 mm in diameter. Femoral access is obtained through an ultrasound-guided puncture in the common femoral artery at least 1 cm proximal to the origin of the profunda femoris artery [67]. Some authors note successful PEVAR in suboptimal femoral artery anatomy, including obese patients and those with heavily calcified femoral arteries [70]. The procedure is performed using a "pre-close" technique in which the arteriotomy sutures are placed prior to placement of the large-diameter sheath or delivery catheter. This can be achieved with off-label use of one Prostar XL (Abbott Vascular, Abbott Park, Ill) or two Perclose Proglide (Abbott Vascular, Abbott Park, Ill) percutaneous closure devices, and safe closure of femoral artery defects as large as 24F has been demonstrated [71].

Several moderate-sized single center studies have been published demonstrating acceptable outcomes with PEVAR (Table 1.3). A prospective, randomized controlled pilot study by Torsello et al. compared percutaneous closure with the 10-F Prostar XL to conventional cutdown technique. In one patient (of 30 total), conversion to an open groin incision was necessary due to bleeding

Table 1.3 PEVAR: current literature

	Cases	Sites closed	Complications *N* (%)	Conversions *N* (%)	Technical success *N* (%)
Krajcer and Gregoric [72]	57	112	13 (12)	1 (0.9)	56 (98)
Eisenack et al. [74]	500	903	35 (3.9)	16 (1.8)	868 (96.1)
Jahnke et al. [75]	70	132	2 (1.5)	2 (2.9)	127 (96.2)
Lee et al. [76]	292	432	24 (8.2)	20 (6.8)	408 (94)
Jean-Baptiste et al. [77]	19	38	3 (19)	2 (11)	35 (92)
Starnes et al. [78]	49	79	2 (4.1)	5 (6.3)	74 (94)
Quinn and Kim [79]	63	100	8 (12.7)	0 (0)	96 (96)
Morasch et al. [80]	47	94	6 (12.7)	7 (7.4)	87 (93)
Torsello et al. [69]	15	27	1 (6.7)	1 (3.7)	25 (93)
Rachel et al. [81]	62	100	3 (3.3)	24 (24)	76 (76)
Teh et al. [82]	44	82	2 (4.5)	12 (14)	70 (85)
Howell et al. [83]	144	144	0 (0)	8 (5.6)	136 (94)
Traul et al. [84]	17	29	0 (0)	10 (35)	19 (66)
Haas et al. [67]	12	13	0 (0)	0 (0)	13 (100)

after Prostar device deployment, and three devices initially failed (one due to needle deflection off calcified arterial wall, two due to failure of needles to grasp the arterial wall in obese patients), yet a second device was deployed without complication in all three cases. Postoperative arterial thrombosis occurred in one patient from each study group; however, mean operative time and time to ambulation were significantly shorter in the percutaneous closure group [69].

Aneurysm Surveillance Following EVAR

Postoperative surveillance is required after EVAR to detect and monitor potential complications such as endoleak or endotension, persistent flow inside the aneurysm sac. Endoleak is the most commonly detected complication of EVAR [85, 86]. While the gold standard for post-EVAR surveillance currently relies on contrast-enhanced CT at 1, 6, and 12 months postoperatively with subsequent annual follow-up, other less invasive imaging modalities as well as protocols are emerging [86, 87].

Color duplex US (CDUS) is frequently used for post-EVAR surveillance, but its potential limitations included high false-negative and false-positive results due to reflection from the metallic graft, calcifications, slow-flowing endoleaks, and obesity. Recent prospective studies have shown contrast-enhanced US (CEUS) to be superior to CDUS and a successful alternative to contrast-enhanced CT with the advantage of no additional radiation exposure [86]. CEUS relies on contrast agents composed of microbubbles which resonate upon interrogation with ultrasound and the recent introduction of second-generation agents has greatly improved their diagnostic accuracy. Advantages of CEUS over CT include increased detection capability despite high attenuation caused by extensive calcification and, occasionally, increased sensitivity to slow-flowing leaks [85].

CTA will likely remain a necessary post-EVAR evaluation in order to ensure accurate graft anchoring and integrity, post-repair aneurysm regression, and visceral vessel patency, but CEUS may well serve as an adequate surveillance tool and certainly diminish the number of surveillance CTs required.

Cardiomems Sac Pressure Monitoring

Intra-aneurysm sac pressure is one of the primary determinants of arterial wall stress and subsequent aneurysm expansion or shrinkage. The development of minimally invasive implantable telemetric sensors such as the FDA-approved EndoSure Wireless AAA Pressure Sensor (CardioMems, Atlanta, GA) allows for direct measurement of sac pressure without the added radiation or contrast exposure. The EndoSure sensor responds to changes in surrounding pressure by changing capacitance, and this resonance frequency is detected by an external antenna via radiofrequency impulse [88]. The device is delivered over a super stiff guidewire in the contralateral iliac artery during EVAR and positioned inside the aneurysm sac, held in place by its surrounding wire basket. In the Acute Pressure Measurement to Confirm Aneurysm Sac Exclusion (APEX) trial, the EndoSure sensor demonstrated a sensitivity of 0.939 and specificity of 0.800 for the detection of type I or III endoleaks when compared to intraoperative angiography [89]. The Cardiomems is an exciting new technology and holds the potential to significantly alter our current post-EVAR surveillance protocols, but its exact role in clinical practice remains to be seen.

Medical Management

The current medical management of AAA focuses on pathophysiologic contributors to aneurysmal disease, specifically hemodynamics, inflammation, and proteolytic enzymes. First-line therapy always includes smoking cessation due to its independent association with increased aneurysm growth rate [20]. Unfortunately, beta blockade with propranolol has failed to provide conclusive evidence for attenuated aneurysm growth rate [90, 91]. Statin therapy, despite a lack of association between cholesterol levels and the expansion rate of AAAs, remains a promising and important component of therapy due to a proposed reduction in C-reactive protein levels, matrix metalloproteinase-9 (MMP-9) concentration, and infiltrating inflammatory cells [92–96]. Additionally, tetracycline antibiotics such as doxycycline hold much hope for becoming a mainstay of treatment due to their ability to inhibit MMP activity and attenuate elastin degradation, leading to dose-dependent prevention of aneurysm expansion [97, 98]. In summary, when combined with US surveillance, optimum medical management for patients with small AAA provides a continuum of care prior to definitive repair.

Conclusion

AAAs remain underdiagnosed and a significant killer of the elderly population. Since the introduction of EVAR, the incidence of aneurysm-associated deaths has substantially decreased, correlating with an increase in elective AAA repair and decrease in repair of ruptured AAAs. As device technology and operative experience continue to improve, EVAR-related complications can be expected to decrease. Ultimately, improvements in AAA detection and advances in medical management to retard aneurysm growth remain the greatest potential for the next breakthrough in AAA therapy.

References

1. Best VA, Price JF, Fowkes FG. Persistent increase in the incidence of abdominal aortic aneurysm in Scotland, 1981–2000. Br J Surg. 2003;90(12):1510–5.
2. Nordon IM, Hinchliffe RJ, Holt PJ, Loftus IM, Thompson MM. Review of current theories for abdominal aortic aneurysm pathogenesis. Vascular. 2009; 17(5):253–63.
3. Golledge J, Muller J, Daugherty A, Norman P. Abdominal aortic aneurysm: pathogenesis and implications for management. Arterioscler Thromb Vasc Biol. 2006;26(12):2605–13.
4. Chaikof EL, Brewster DC, Dalman RL, et al. The care of patients with an abdominal aortic aneurysm: the society for vascular surgery practice guidelines. J Vasc Surg. 2009;50(4 Suppl):S2–49.
5. Joels CS, Langan 3rd EM, Daley CA, et al. Changing indications and outcomes for open abdominal aortic aneurysm repair since the advent of endovascular repair. Am Surg. 2009;75(8):665–9; discussion 669–70.
6. De Bruin JL, Baas AF, Buth J, et al. Long-term outcome of open or endovascular repair of abdominal aortic aneurysm. N Engl J Med. 2010;362(20):1881–9.

7. Greenhalgh RM, Brown LC, Kwong GP, Powell JT, Thompson SG. Comparison of endovascular aneurysm repair with open repair in patients with abdominal aortic aneurysm (EVAR trial 1), 30-day operative mortality results: randomised controlled trial. Lancet. 2004;364(9437):843–8.
8. Greenhalgh RM, Brown LC, Powell JT, Thompson SG, Epstein D, Sculpher MJ. Endovascular versus open repair of abdominal aortic aneurysm. N Engl J Med. 2010;362(20):1863–71.
9. Lederle FA, Freischlag JA, Kyriakides TC, et al. Outcomes following endovascular vs open repair of abdominal aortic aneurysm: a randomized trial. JAMA. 2009;302(14):1535–42.
10. Prinssen M, Verhoeven EL, Buth J, et al. A randomized trial comparing conventional and endovascular repair of abdominal aortic aneurysms. N Engl J Med. 2004;351(16):1607–18.
11. Giles KA, Pomposelli F, Hamdan A, Wyers M, Jhaveri A, Schermerhorn ML. Decrease in total aneurysm-related deaths in the era of endovascular aneurysm repair. J Vasc Surg. 2009;49(3):543–50; discussion 550–1.
12. Brewster DC, Cronenwett JL, Hallett Jr JW, Johnston KW, Krupski WC, Matsumura JS. Guidelines for the treatment of abdominal aortic aneurysms. Report of a subcommittee of the Joint Council of the American Association for Vascular Surgery and Society for Vascular Surgery. J Vasc Surg. 2003;37(5):1106–17.
13. Lederle FA, Johnson GR, Wilson SE, et al. Rupture rate of large abdominal aortic aneurysms in patients refusing or unfit for elective repair. JAMA. 2002;287(22):2968–72.
14. Lederle FA, Wilson SE, Johnson GR, et al. Variability in measurement of abdominal aortic aneurysms. Abdominal Aortic Aneurysm Detection and Management Veterans Administration Cooperative Study Group. J Vasc Surg. 1995;21(6):945–52.
15. Wilmink AB, Forshaw M, Quick CR, Hubbard CS, Day NE. Accuracy of serial screening for abdominal aortic aneurysms by ultrasound. J Med Screen. 2002;9(3):125–7.
16. Zhou W. Radiation exposure of vascular surgery patients beyond endovascular procedures. J Vasc Surg. 2011;53:39S–43. Epub 2010 Sept 16.
17. Lederle FA. The natural history of abdominal aortic aneurysm. Acta Chir Belg. 2009;109(1):7–12.
18. Propper BW, Rasmussen TE, Jones WT, Gifford SM, Burkhardt GE, Clouse WD. Temporal changes of aortic neck morphology in abdominal aortic aneurysms. J Vasc Surg. 2010;51(5):1111–5.
19. Schlosser FJ, Tangelder MJ, Verhagen HJ, et al. Growth predictors and prognosis of small abdominal aortic aneurysms. J Vasc Surg. 2008;47(6):1127–33.
20. Baxter BT, Terrin MC, Dalman RL. Medical management of small abdominal aortic aneurysms. Circulation. 2008;117(14):1883–9.
21. Brady AR, Thompson SG, Fowkes FG, Greenhalgh RM, Powell JT. Abdominal aortic aneurysm expansion: risk factors and time intervals for surveillance. Circulation. 2004;110(1):16–21.
22. Eckstein HH, Bockler D, Flessenkamper I, Schmitz-Rixen T, Debus S, Lang W. Ultrasonographic screening for the detection of abdominal aortic aneurysms. Dtsch Arztebl Int. 2009;106(41):657–63.
23. Kim LG, P Scott RA, Ashton HA, Thompson SG. A sustained mortality benefit from screening for abdominal aortic aneurysm. Ann Intern Med. 2007;146(10):699–706.
24. Lee ES, Pickett E, Hedayati N, Dawson DL, Pevec WC. Implementation of an aortic screening program in clinical practice: implications for the Screen for Abdominal Aortic Aneurysms Very Efficiently (SAAAVE) Act. J Vasc Surg. 2009;49(5):1107–11.
25. Lederle FA, Wilson SE, Johnson GR, et al. Immediate repair compared with surveillance of small abdominal aortic aneurysms. N Engl J Med. 2002;346(19):1437–44.
26. Brady AR, Brown LC, Fowkes FG, et al. Long-term outcomes of immediate repair compared with surveillance of small abdominal aortic aneurysms. N Engl J Med. 2002;346(19):1445–52.
27. Powell JT, Brady AR, Brown LC, et al. Mortality results for randomised controlled trial of early elective surgery or ultrasonographic surveillance for small abdominal aortic aneurysms. The UK Small Aneurysm Trial Participants. Lancet. 1998;352(9141):1649–55.
28. Powell JT, Brown LC, Forbes JF, et al. Final 12-year follow-up of surgery versus surveillance in the UK Small Aneurysm Trial. Br J Surg. 2007;94(6):702–8.
29. Welborn 3rd MB, Yau FS, Modrall JG, et al. Endovascular repair of small abdominal aortic aneurysms: a paradigm shift? Vasc Endovascular Surg. 2005;39(5):381–91.
30. Arko FR, Filis KA, Hill BB, Fogarty TJ, Zarins CK. Morphologic changes and outcome following endovascular abdominal aortic aneurysm repair as a function of aneurysm size. Arch Surg. 2003;138(6):651–5; discussion 655–6.
31. Cao P. Comparison of surveillance vs aortic endografting for small aneurysm repair (CAESAR) trial: study design and progress. Eur J Vasc Endovasc Surg. 2005;30(3):245–51.
32. Ouriel K. Randomized clinical trials of endovascular repair versus surveillance for treatment of small abdominal aortic aneurysms. J Endovasc Ther. 2009;16 Suppl 1:I94–105.
33. Ouriel K, Clair DG, Kent KC, Zarins CK. Endovascular repair compared with surveillance for patients with small abdominal aortic aneurysms. J Vasc Surg. 2010;51(5):1081–7.
34. Cao P, De Rango P, Verzini F, Parlani G, Romano L, Cieri E. Comparison of surveillance versus aortic endografting for small aneurysm repair (CAESAR): results from a randomised trial. Eur J Vasc Endovasc Surg. 2011;41:13–25. Epub 2010 Sept 25.
35. Buckley CJ, Rutherford RB, Diethrich EB, Buckley SD. Inherent problems with randomized clinical trials with observational/no treatment arms. J Vasc Surg. 2010;52(1):237–41.
36. Soor GS, Chakrabarti MO, Abraham JR, et al. Aortic stent grafts. J Clin Pathol. 2008;61(7):794–801.

37. Gowda RM, Misra D, Tranbaugh RF, Ohki T, Khan IA. Endovascular stent grafting of descending thoracic aortic aneurysms. Chest. 2003;124(2):714–9.
38. Rutherford RB, Krupski WC. Current status of open versus endovascular stent-graft repair of abdominal aortic aneurysm. J Vasc Surg. 2004;39(5):1129–39.
39. Tan JWC, Yeo KK, Laird JR. Food and drug administration-approved endovascular repair devices for abdominal aortic aneurysms: a review. J Vasc Interv Radiol. 2008;19(6 Suppl 1):S9–17.
40. Jim J, Sanchez LA, Rubin BG, et al. A 5-year evaluation using the talent endovascular graft for endovascular aneurysm repair in short aortic necks. Ann Vasc Surg. 2010;24(7):851–8.
41. Turnbull IC, Criado FJ, Sanchez L, et al. Five-year results for the talent enhanced low profile system abdominal stent graft pivotal trial including early and long-term safety and efficacy. J Vasc Surg. 2010;51(3):537–44, 544 e531–532.
42. Haider SE, Najjar SF, Cho JS, et al. Sac behavior after aneurysm treatment with the gore excluder low-permeability aortic endoprosthesis: 12-month comparison to the original excluder device. J Vasc Surg. 2006;44(4):694–700.
43. Albertini JN, Lahlou Z, Magnan PE, Branchereau A. Endovascular repair of abdominal aortic aneurysms with a unibody stent-graft: 3-year results of the French Powerlink Multicenter Trial. J Endovasc Ther. 2005;12(6):629–37.
44. Carpenter JP. Midterm results of the multicenter trial of the powerlink bifurcated system for endovascular aortic aneurysm repair. J Vasc Surg. 2004;40(5):849–59.
45. Qu L, Raithel D. From clinical trials to clinical practice: 612 cases treated with the Powerlink stent-graft for endovascular repair of AAA. J Cardiovasc Surg (Torino). 2009;50(2):131–7.
46. Ouriel K, Clair DG, Greenberg RK, et al. Endovascular repair of abdominal aortic aneurysms: device-specific outcome. J Vasc Surg. 2003;37(5):991–8.
47. Simons P, van Overhagen H, Nawijn A, Bruijninckx B, Knippenberg B. Endovascular aneurysm repair with a bifurcated endovascular graft at a primary referral center: influence of experience, age, gender, and aneurysm size on suitability. J Vasc Surg. 2003;38(4):758–61.
48. Stella A, Freyrie A, Gargiulo M, Faggioli GL. The advantages of Anaconda endograft for AAA. J Cardiovasc Surg (Torino). 2009;50(2):145–52.
49. Freyrie A, Gargiulo M, Rossi C, et al. Preliminary results of Anaconda aortic endografts: a single center study. Eur J Vasc Endovasc Surg. 2007;34(6):693–8.
50. Saratzis N, Melas N, Saratzis A, et al. Anaconda aortic stent-graft: single-center experience of a new commercially available device for abdominal aortic aneurysms. J Endovasc Ther. 2008;15(1):33–41.
51. Albertini JN, Perdikides T, Soong CV, Hinchliffe RJ, Trojanowska M, Yusuf SW. Endovascular repair of abdominal aortic aneurysms in patients with severe angulation of the proximal neck using a flexible stent-graft: European Multicenter Experience. J Cardiovasc Surg (Torino). 2006;47(3):245–50.
52. Perdikides T, Georgiadis GS, Avgerinos ED, et al. The Aorfix stent-graft to treat infrarenal abdominal aortic aneurysms with angulated necks and/or tortuous iliac arteries: midterm results. J Endovasc Ther. 2009;16(5):567–76.
53. Henretta JP, Karch LA, Hodgson KJ, et al. Special iliac artery considerations during aneurysm endografting. Am J Surg. 1999;178(3):212–8.
54. Cotroneo AR, Iezzi R, Giancristofaro D, et al. Endovascular abdominal aortic aneurysm repair: how many patients are eligible for endovascular repair? Radiol Med. 2006;111(4):597–606.
55. Velazquez OC, Larson RA, Baum RA, et al. Gender-related differences in infrarenal aortic aneurysm morphologic features: issues relevant to Ancure and Talent endografts. J Vasc Surg. 2001;33(2 Suppl):S77–84.
56. Masuda EM, Caps MT, Singh N, et al. Effect of ethnicity on access and device complications during endovascular aneurysm repair. J Vasc Surg. 2004;40(1):24–9.
57. Hinchliffe RJ, Ivancev K, Sonesson B, Malina M. "Paving and cracking": an endovascular technique to facilitate the introduction of aortic stent-grafts through stenosed iliac arteries. J Endovasc Ther. 2007;14(5):630–3.
58. Peterson BG, Matsumura JS. Creative options for large sheath access during aortic endografting. J Vasc Interv Radiol. 2008;19(6 Suppl):S22–6.
59. Leurs LJ, Kievit J, Dagnelie PC, Nelemans PJ, Buth J. Influence of infrarenal neck length on outcome of endovascular abdominal aortic aneurysm repair. J Endovasc Ther. 2006;13(5):640–8.
60. Minion DJ, Yancey A, Patterson DE, Saha S, Endean ED. The endowedge and kilt techniques to achieve additional juxtarenal seal during deployment of the Gore Excluder endoprosthesis. Ann Vasc Surg. 2006;20(4):472–7.
61. Vallabhaneni SR, Harris PL. Lessons learnt from the EUROSTAR registry on endovascular repair of abdominal aortic aneurysm repair. Eur J Radiol. 2001;39(1):34–41.
62. Lee C, Dougherty M, Calligaro K. Concomitant unilateral internal iliac artery embolization and endovascular infrarenal aortic aneurysm repair. J Vasc Surg. 2006;43(5):903–7.
63. Mehta M, Veith FJ, Ohki T, et al. Unilateral and bilateral hypogastric artery interruption during aortoiliac aneurysm repair in 154 patients: a relatively innocuous procedure. J Vasc Surg. 2001;33(2 Suppl): S27–32.
64. Lee WA, O'Dorisio J, Wolf YG, Hill BB, Fogarty TJ, Zarins CK. Outcome after unilateral hypogastric artery occlusion during endovascular aneurysm repair. J Vasc Surg. 2001;33(5):921–6.

65. Rayt HS, Bown MJ, Lambert KV, et al. Buttock claudication and erectile dysfunction after internal iliac artery embolization in patients prior to endovascular aortic aneurysm repair. Cardiovasc Intervent Radiol. 2008;31(4):728–34.
66. Morrissey NJ, Faries PL, Carrocio A, et al. Intentional internal iliac artery occlusion in endovascular repair of abdominal aortic aneurysms. J Invasive Cardiol. 2002;14(12):760–3.
67. Haas PC, Krajcer Z, Diethrich EB. Closure of large percutaneous access sites using the prostar XL percutaneous vascular surgery device. J Endovasc Surg. 1999;6(2):168–70.
68. Berland TL, Cayne NS, Veith FJ. Access complications during endovascular aortic repair. J Cardiovasc Surg (Torino). 2010;51(1):43–52.
69. Torsello GB, Kasprzak B, Klenk E, Tessarek J, Osada N, Torsello G. Endovascular suture versus cutdown for endovascular aneurysm repair: a prospective randomized pilot study. J Vasc Surg. 2003;38(1):78–82.
70. Smith ST, Timaran CH, Valentine RJ, Rosero EB, Clagett GP, Arko FR. Percutaneous access for endovascular abdominal aortic aneurysm repair: can selection criteria be expanded? Ann Vasc Surg. 2009;23(5):621–6.
71. Morasch MD. Percutaneous techniques for aneurysm repair. J Vasc Surg. 2006;43(Suppl a):69A–72.
72. Krajcer Z, Gregoric I. Totally percutaneous aortic aneurysm repair: methods and outcomes using the fully integrated IntuiTrak endovascular system. J Cardiovasc Surg (Torino). 2010;51(4):493–501.
73. Malkawi AH, Hinchliffe RJ, Holt PJ, Loftus IM, Thompson MM. Percutaneous access for endovascular aneurysm repair: a systematic review. Eur J Vasc Endovasc Surg. 2010;39(6):676–82.
74. Eisenack M, Umscheid T, Tessarek J, Torsello GF, Torsello GB. Percutaneous endovascular aortic aneurysm repair: a prospective evaluation of safety, efficiency, and risk factors. J Endovasc Ther. 2009;16(6):708–13.
75. Jahnke T, Schafer JP, Charalambous N, et al. Total percutaneous endovascular aneurysm repair with the dual 6-F Perclose-AT preclosing technique: a case-control study. J Vasc Interv Radiol. 2009;20(10):1292–8.
76. Lee WA, Brown MP, Nelson PR, Huber TS, Seeger JM. Midterm outcomes of femoral arteries after percutaneous endovascular aortic repair using the Preclose technique. J Vasc Surg. 2008;47(5):919–23.
77. Jean-Baptiste E, Hassen-Khodja R, Haudebourg P, Bouillanne PJ, Declemy S, Batt M. Percutaneous closure devices for endovascular repair of infrarenal abdominal aortic aneurysms: a prospective, non-randomized comparative study. Eur J Vasc Endovasc Surg. 2008;35(4):422–8.
78. Starnes BW, Andersen CA, Ronsivalle JA, Stockmaster NR, Mullenix PS, Statler JD. Totally percutaneous aortic aneurysm repair: experience and prudence. J Vasc Surg. 2006;43(2):270–6.
79. Quinn SF, Kim J. Percutaneous femoral closure following stent-graft placement: use of the Perclose device. Cardiovasc Intervent Radiol. 2004;27(3):231–6.
80. Morasch MD, Kibbe MR, Evans ME, et al. Percutaneous repair of abdominal aortic aneurysm. J Vasc Surg. 2004;40(1):12–6.
81. Rachel ES, Bergamini TM, Kinney EV, Jung MT, Kaebnick HW, Mitchell RA. Percutaneous endovascular abdominal aortic aneurysm repair. Ann Vasc Surg. 2002;16(1):43–9.
82. Teh LG, Sieunarine K, van Schie G, et al. Use of the percutaneous vascular surgery device for closure of femoral access sites during endovascular aneurysm repair: lessons from our experience. Eur J Vasc Endovasc Surg. 2001;22(5):418–23.
83. Howell M, Doughtery K, Strickman N, Krajcer Z. Percutaneous repair of abdominal aortic aneurysms using the AneuRx stent graft and the percutaneous vascular surgery device. Catheter Cardiovasc Interv. 2002;55(3):281–7.
84. Traul DK, Clair DG, Gray B, O'Hara PJ, Ouriel K. Percutaneous endovascular repair of infrarenal abdominal aortic aneurysms: a feasibility study. J Vasc Surg. 2000;32(4):770–6.
85. Carrafiello G, Recaldini C, Lagana D, Piffaretti G, Fugazzola C. Endoleak detection and classification after endovascular treatment of abdominal aortic aneurysm: value of CEUS over CTA. Abdom Imaging. 2008;33(3):357–62.
86. Iezzi R, Basilico R, Giancristofaro D, Pascali D, Cotroneo AR, Storto ML. Contrast-enhanced ultrasound versus color duplex ultrasound imaging in the follow-up of patients after endovascular abdominal aortic aneurysm repair. J Vasc Surg. 2009;49(3):552–60.
87. Back MR. Surveillance after endovascular abdominal aortic aneurysm repair. Perspect Vasc Surg Endovasc Ther. 2007;19(4):395–400; discussion 401–2.
88. Springer F, Gunther RW, Schmitz-Rode T. Aneurysm Sac pressure measurement with minimally invasive implantable pressure sensors: an alternative to current surveillance regimes after EVAR? Cardiovasc Intervent Radiol. 2008;31(3):460–7.
89. Ohki T, Ouriel K, Silveira PG, et al. Initial results of wireless pressure sensing for endovascular aneurysm repair: the APEX Trial–Acute Pressure Measurement to Confirm Aneurysm Sac EXclusion. J Vasc Surg. 2007;45(2):236–42.
90. Propanolol Aneurysm Trial Investigators. Propranolol for small abdominal aortic aneurysms: results of a randomized trial. J Vasc Surg. 2002;35(1):72–9.
91. Lindholt JS, Vammen S, Juul S, Henneberg EW, Fasting H. The validity of ultrasonographic scanning as screening method for abdominal aortic aneurysm. Eur J Vasc Endovasc Surg. 1999;17(6):472–5.
92. Gotto Jr AM. Role of C-reactive protein in coronary risk reduction: focus on primary prevention. Am J Cardiol. 2007;99(5):718–25.

93. Evans J, Powell JT, Schwalbe E, Loftus IM, Thompson MM. Simvastatin attenuates the activity of matrix metalloprotease-9 in aneurysmal aortic tissue. Eur J Vasc Endovasc Surg. 2007;34(3):302–3.
94. Nagashima H, Aoka Y, Sakomura Y, et al. A 3-hydroxy-3-methylglutaryl coenzyme A reductase inhibitor, cerivastatin, suppresses production of matrix metalloproteinase-9 in human abdominal aortic aneurysm wall. J Vasc Surg. 2002;36(1):158–63.
95. Schouten O, van Laanen JH, Boersma E, et al. Statins are associated with a reduced infrarenal abdominal aortic aneurysm growth. Eur J Vasc Endovasc Surg. 2006;32(1):21–6.
96. Sukhija R, Aronow WS, Sandhu R, Kakar P, Babu S. Mortality and size of abdominal aortic aneurysm at long-term follow-up of patients not treated surgically and treated with and without statins. Am J Cardiol. 2006;97(2):279–80.
97. Baxter BT, Pearce WH, Waltke EA, et al. Prolonged administration of doxycycline in patients with small asymptomatic abdominal aortic aneurysms: report of a prospective (Phase II) multicenter study. J Vasc Surg. 2002;36(1):1–12.
98. Prall AK, Longo GM, Mayhan WG, et al. Doxycycline in patients with abdominal aortic aneurysms and in mice: comparison of serum levels and effect on aneurysm growth in mice. J Vasc Surg. 2002;35(5):923–9.

2 Treatment of Suprarenal and Juxtarenal AAA with Fenestrated Grafts and Debranching Procedures

Heather P. Park and Mark A. Farber

Abstract

Endovascular aneurysm repair (EVAR) has revolutionized the treatment of infrarenal abdominal aneurysms; however, as many as 45 % of aneurysms are not amenable to standard EVAR due to inadequate sealing zone or involvement of the visceral segment of the aorta. For these patients, advanced endovascular techniques have been developed that allow incorporation of the visceral vessels into the sealing zone while maintaining flow either via stents or with open surgical debranching. Fenestrated techniques are currently available in the USA as part of clinical trial or investigational device protocols or as "surgeon modifications" for urgent or compassionate usage. Successful repair of suprarenal or juxtarenal aneurysms using these techniques requires careful advanced planning based, high-quality intraoperative imaging, and a high level of endovascular expertise.

Keywords

Fenestrated endovascular aortic repair • Complex aortic repair • Aortic debranching • Juxtarenal aneurysm • Suprarenal aneurysm

H.P. Park, M.D.
Department of Surgery,
University of North Carolina Health Care,
Chapel Hill, NC, USA

M.A. Farber, M.D., FACS (✉)
Department of Surgery and Radiology,
UNC Aortic Center,
University of North Carolina Health Care,
3025 Burnett Womack Building, CB# 7212,
Chapel Hill, NC, 27599-7212, USA
e-mail: mark_farber@med.unc.edu

Juxtarenal and pararenal abdominal aortic aneurysms pose complex problems for vascular surgeons involved in their management. Development of endovascular repair of aortic aneurysms has been associated with low perioperative morbidity and mortality, even in high-risk patients. However, as many as 45 % of patients have aneurysms that are not amenable to endovascular techniques based on the instructions for use for each device. Exclusion may be because of short, nonexistent, or angulated necks precluding adequate proximal seal [1]. Good surgical candidates may tolerate the complex open procedure necessary to exclude

J.J. Hoballah, A.B. Lumsden (eds.), *Vascular Surgery*, New Techniques in Surgery Series,
DOI 10.1007/978-1-4471-2912-7_2, © Springer-Verlag London 2012

the aneurysm, but many patients with serious cardiac, pulmonary, or renal comorbidities are unlikely to fully recover from the extensive open procedure. These patients may be best served by a minimally invasive approach to aneurysm exclusion, with the most appropriate treatment determined by an experienced surgeon after consideration of each patient's risk profile.

History

Since the initial reports of endovascular stent grafting for AAA exclusion by Juan Parodi and associates in 1991 [2], there has been significant adoption of endovascular techniques to treat aortic pathology in nearly every subset of patients. However, despite advances in almost all aspects of endovascular technology including preoperative imaging, wires, catheters, balloons, and delivery systems, all available devices are limited by the proximal neck characteristics (length, diameter, angulation, shape, thrombus lining) required to achieve and maintain an effective proximal seal [3]. Of the devices approved by the US Food and Drug Administration (FDA) for treatment of abdominal aortic aneurysms (Cook Zenith [Cook Inc., Indianapolis, IA], Gore Excluder [WL Gore, Flagstaff, AZ], AneurRx [Medtronic Inc., Santa Rosa, CA], Talent [Medtronic Inc.], and Endologix Powerlink [Endologix, Irvine, CA]), all must have a minimal proximal neck length of 1.5 cm for adequate sealing, except the Talent device, which is approved for 1-cm neck lengths. In juxtarenal aneurysms where the neck length is shorter than these approved lengths, the visceral vessels may be incorporated into the proximal sealing zone to lengthen this area, a process known as fenestration. Since the first reports of AAA repair with fenestrated devices in 1996 by Park and associates [4], there have been considerable innovations and improvements in this technology as well. In geographic regions where devices have been less readily available, "hybrid" procedures that combine open debranching procedures with endovascular aneurysm exclusion have been utilized.

Definitions

Aortic aneurysms in the region of the renal arteries are grouped collectively as pararenal aneurysms and further classified into juxtarenal and suprarenal subtypes. There is no universally agreed-upon definition of the term "juxtarenal aneurysm"; however, it is commonly used to describe a complex AAA with either a short infrarenal neck or one which encroaches upon the renal segment of the aorta. Suprarenal aneurysms involve renal arteries and extend up to the splanchnic arteries. Type IV thoracoabdominal aortic aneurysms extend to a variable abdominal length but always involve the visceral aortic segment [5]. Classification systems have been proposed, but none have gained wide acceptance or clinical use [6]. This lends some ambiguity to the terms and makes comparison of clinical studies difficult.

The terms fenestrated and branched endovascular repair describe two similar uses of the same technique. The term fenestrated endovascular repair is used when the sealing region of the stent graft incorporates branched vessels of the aorta itself. In the case of juxtarenal aneurysms where the renal arteries arise from normal aorta, there is no gap between the device and the target vessel. This is contrasted with a branched endovascular repair, in which case the target arteries arise from aneurismal aorta, and there is a gap between the device and the aortic wall at the vessel origin. In this case, the device typically incorporates a cuff, which facilitates the placement of the branch artery stent graft [7].

Indications

Fenestrated stent grafts were originally developed as a minimally invasive alternative to open repair to treat complex aneurysm morphology in patients considered to be unfit or at high risk for open surgery. The criteria for treatment with a fenestrated device are in evolution as the safety and efficacy of available devices and techniques are determined. Generally accepted high-risk characteristics include old age, severe medical comorbidities, prior aortic reconstruction, and the need for suprarenal aortic crossclamping [8]. Currently, there are no FDA-approved fenestrated devices approved for general use in the USA. The use of the internationally available Zenith fenestrated device (Cook Inc.) in the USA is currently limited to a few institutions and patients who are enrolled in a prospective investigational device exemption protocol. Device customization currently requires a 4–8-week waiting period, which has led to advances in techniques for surgeon-customized fenestrated stent grafts. This technique is described primarily for patients who would not be eligible to enroll in one of the prospective trials or who need urgent or emergent repair of their aneurysm and cannot safely undergo standard open repair [9]. While this technique has been reported to be successful, it is not reimbursable currently in the USA.

Techniques

The technique of fenestrated/branched repair has undergone considerable evolution since its inception. This description represents the current standards, but it is subject to change as dictated by a rapidly improving technique.

The most important component of successful fenestrated aneurysm repair is careful and accurate advance planning of the procedure and of the graft construction. Computed tomography (CT) angiography allows measurements of distances using centerline of flow analysis and of the clock position of the target vessel using axial measurements. The criteria for device implantation are essentially unchanged from standard endovascular repairs. The proximal landing zone must consist of at least 2 cm of normal parallel aortic wall, <32 mm in diameter for juxtarenal aneurysms, and <38 mm for thoracoabdominal aneurysms. The centerline measurement from the top of the landing zone to the center of the target vessel origin is recorded, as are the clock position, orientation, and diameter of each target vessel origin. The device configuration can consist of single or multiple fenestrations, depending on patient characteristics. Small fenestrations (6 mm × 8 mm) are preferentially designed for branched stent grafts or vessels arising from aneurismal aorta. Large fenestrations (8 mm × 10 mm) are used preferentially for fenestrated stent grafts, or vessels arising in the proximal seal zone of normal aorta.

Regardless of the presence of a gap between the graft and the aortic wall, all fenestrations are bridged with a balloon-expandable stent or stent graft to reduce any misalignment between the fenestration and the vessel origin. The device design for internationally available Cook Zenith or TX2 platform fenestrated devices is based on these measurements, and customized devices based on individual patient specifications are available from the manufacturer in 4–8 weeks outside the USA.

For patients in the USA unable to be enrolled in a clinical trial with a manufactured fenestrated graft, techniques are available that allow surgeons to customize available stent grafts. These techniques are generally offered selectively to patients in whom open repair poses prohibitive risk and who are unable to travel to a center where a manufactured device is available through a clinical trial. These techniques are also being offered on a compassionate basis to patients who have impending or contained rupture and therefore cannot wait the required weeks for manufacturer customization [7]. Efforts are ongoing to provide an "off-the-shelf" fenestrated or branched device which would obviate the need for individual customization in time-sensitive situations in a majority of patients [10].

Surgeon customization of stent grafts is performed in the operating room under sterile conditions. The process generally ranges from 30 to 120 min. In general, most device modifications have used the Cook Zenith or TX2 platform (Cook Medical Inc., Bloomington, IN), but modifications have also been performed using Talent stent grafts and W.L. Gore Excluder stent grafts. Knowledge of the grafts, their material components, and their deployment and design is critical in determining what can be accomplished with each device.

The planned fenestrations and scallops are marked on the stent graft based on previously documented measurements from the centerline of flow analysis. The fenestrations are created with an ophthalmologic cautery device to prevent unraveling of the graft material. Ideally, the fenestrations should be round, but occasionally, the position of stent struts dictates a more oval shape. Radiopaque markers are used to note the location of the fenestrations, and in some cases, longitudinal and transverse markers can be used to assist with orientation during deployment.

A constraining wire or tie may be used to allow rotational and axial movement of the Zenith graft during deployment. Some authors have described use of the same wire provided to secure the uncovered stent into the top cap. This wire can be carefully retrieved from inside the device and rerouted posteriorly. A series of silk ties are then used to collapse each of the Z stents, and the device is re-sheathed [7].

Prior to commencing any fenestrated endovascular aneurysm repair, it is imperative that the surgeon has access to excellent imaging equipment and a complete endovascular inventory. A wide range of catheters, wires, sheaths, stents, and stent grafts may be required to safely and effectively complete this procedure. Preoperatively, the patient is medically optimized. Consideration for preoperative hydration with or without bicarbonate infusion and oral acetylcysteine is appropriate in the patient with baseline renal insufficiency. Intraoperatively, contrast is routinely diluted to 50 % strength with normal saline. Attempts are made to minimize contrast administration by using hand injections for selective arteriographies. A spinal drain should be considered in patients in whom extensive aortic coverage will be required or in those patients with other risk factors for paraplegia including those with prior aortic grafting or hypogastric artery occlusion.

Graft implantation generally requires bilateral femoral and left brachial arterial access. The larger femoral artery is generally used for main body device implantation, and the contralateral femoral artery is used for the target vessels. A large sheath is introduced via the contralateral femoral artery, and the sheath valve is accessed with multiple 5-F sheaths. These sheaths are used for selective catheterization of the renal and superior mesenteric arteries. The target vessels are then catheterized using selective contrast injections. Once all target branches are accessed, the main stent graft is oriented and introduced via the femoral artery. Via a sheath, a balloon-expandable stent graft is introduced into each target vessel after it has been selectively catheterized through the stent graft fenestration. Once all bridging stent grafts are in place, the main body stent graft is fully deployed. The balloon-expandable stent grafts are then deployed to profile and flared proximally with a balloon.

A high level of endovascular surgical expertise is required to safely perform fenestrated procedures. It is imperative that the surgeon be facile with salvage or "bail out" maneuvers that may be required for device design or deployment errors. Access to the target vessel cannot always be regained when significant misalignment occurs. Some authors describe the use of a flush catheter left between the main aortic stent graft and the aortic wall during the entire procedure. In the case of device misalignment, this catheter may be exchanged for a balloon, allowing enough space for wire and catheter manipulation to make catheterization of the target vessel possible [9]. Use of microcatheters, microwires, and a variety of catheter shapes may be necessary.

In selected patients, it may be helpful to perform a debranching procedure prior to fenestrated endovascular aneurysm repair. In patients with anatomy that precludes a separate fenestration for each visceral vessel, standard techniques do not permit fenestrated/branched repair. This is seen most commonly in patients with paired renal arteries, which supply comparable fractions of the kidney, but can also be seen when separate target vessels lie in close proximity to one another. In these circumstances, an open bypass, such as a hepatorenal or splenorenal bypass, may be performed. This allows endovascular coverage of the bypassed artery and thereby makes the patient's anatomy amenable to endovascular repair. There are no large series reporting outcomes with this "hybrid" method, but in case reports, the technique has been well tolerated by patients otherwise at high risk for extensive aortic surgery.

Outcomes

No randomized controlled trial has compared fenestrated/branched endovascular aneurysm repair with conventional open repair. However, multiple case series and cohort studies have documented the safety and efficacy of the technique. In a recent review, Nordon and associates analyzed 8 studies with a total of 368 cases of FEVAR and compared them with 12 studies representing 1,164 open repairs of juxtarenal aneurysms. Cumulative mortality was similar in the two groups. There was statistically significant increase in transient renal failure in the open group compared with the FEVAR group; however, there was no difference in the rate of dialysis requirement in the two groups (1.4 % in both) [11]. Multiple case series from different institutions, both internationally and in the USA, have been published. These series routinely document target vessel patency rates in excess of 96 %. No patients experienced aneurysm rupture or increase in aneurysm size during documented follow-up [12–15].

Future Directions

Endovascular repair of aneurysms involving the visceral aorta has become a reality. More than 1,000 cases have been performed worldwide with midterm results that demonstrate safety and success. Continued success with fenestrated and branched endografting will require continued appropriate patient selection, high-resolution imaging, proper device design, and technical expertise on the part of the endovascular surgeon. However, as technology and techniques evolve, the endovascular treatment of juxtarenal aneurysms is certain to become more widespread. The continued efforts to provide safe, prefabricated devices available to more patients will certainly allow greater ease of treating patients. Finally, surgeon customization of devices should only be performed in certain urgent or emergent settings for patients with unusual anatomy when standard open surgical repair is of prohibitive risk. These customized repairs should not be attempted unless significant training and experience have been obtained. These customized repairs currently cannot be reimbursed.

References

1. EVAR trial participants. Endovascular aneurysm repair versus open repair in patients with abdominal aortic aneurysm (EVAR trial 1): randomized controlled trial. Lancet. 2005;365(9478):2179–86.
2. Parodi JC, Palmaz JC, Barone HD. Transfemoral intraluminal graft implantation for abdominal aortic aneurysms. Ann Vasc Surg. 1991;5:491–9.
3. Chisci E, Kristmundsson T, de Donato G, Resch T, Setacci F, Sonesson B, Setacci C, Malina M. The AAA with a challenging neck: outcome of open versus endovascular repair with standard and fenestrated stent-grafts. J Endovasc Ther. 2009;16(2):137–46.
4. Park JH, Chung JW, Choo IW, Kim SJ, Lee JY, Han MC. Fenestrated stent-grafts for preserving the visceral arterial branches in the treatment of abdominal aortic aneurysms: preliminary experience. J Vasc Interv Radiol. 1996;7:819–23.
5. Chaikof EL, Blankensteijn JD, Harris PL, White GH, Zarins CK, Bernhard VM, et al. Reporting standards for endovascular aortic aneurysm repair. J Vasc Surg. 2002;35(5):1048–60.
6. Johnston KW, Rutherford RB, Tilson MD, Shah DM, Hollier L, Stanley JC. Suggested standards for reporting on arterial aneurysms. Subcommittee on Reporting Standards for Arterial Aneurysms, Ad Hoc Committee on Reporting Standards, Society for Vascular Surgery and North American Chapter, International Society for Cardiovascular Surgery. J Vasc Surg. 1991;13(3):452–8.
7. Ricotta JJ, Oderich GS. Fenestrated and branched stent grafts. Perspect Vasc Surg Endovasc Ther. 2008;20(2):174–87.
8. Dias NV, Ivancev K, Malina M, Resch T, Lindblad B, Sonesson B. Does the wide application of endovascular AAA repair affect the results of open surgery? Eur J Vasc Endovasc Surg. 2003;26:188–94.
9. Oderich GS, Ricotta JJ. Modified fenestrated stent grafts: device dedisgn, modifications, implantation, and current applications. Perspect Vasc Surg Endovasc Ther. 2009;21(3):157–67.
10. Nordon IM, Hinchliffe RJ, Manning B, Ivancev K, Holt PJ, Loftus IM, Thompson MM. Toward an "off-the-shelf" fenestrated endograft for management of short-necked abdominal aortic aneurysms: an analysis

of current graft morphological diversity. J Endovasc Ther. 2010;17(1):78–85.
11. Nordon IM, Hinchliffe RJ, Holt PJ, Loftus IM, Thompson MM. Modern treatment of juxtarenal abdominal aortic aneurysms with fenestrated endografting and open repair- a systematic review. Eur J Vasc Endovasc Surg. 2009;38:35–41.
12. Greenberg RK, Sternbergh WC, Makaroun M, Ohki T, Chuter T, Bharadwaj P, Saunders A. Intermediate results of a United States Multicenter trial of fenestrated endograft repair for juxtarenal abdominal aortic aneurysms. J Vasc Surg. 2009;50(4):730–7.
13. Amiot S, Haulon S, Becquemin JP, Magnan PE, Lermusiaux P, Goueffic Y, Jean-Baptiste E, Cochennec F, Favre JP. Association Universitaire de Recherche en Chirurgie Vascularie. Fenestrated Endovascular Grafting: the French Multicentre Experience. Eur J Vasc Endovasc Surg. 2010;39:537–44.
14. Scurr JRH, Brennan JA, Gilling-Smith GL, Harris PL, Vallabhaneni SR, McWilliams RG. Fenestrated endovascular repair for juxtarenal aortic aneurysm. Br J Surg. 2008;95:326–32. Verhoeven ELG, Vourliotakis G, Bos WTGJ, Tielliu IFJ, Zeebregts CJ, Prins TR, Bracale UM, van den Dungen JJAM. Fenestrated stent grafting for short-necked and juxtarenal abdominal aortic aneurysm: an 8-year single-centre experience. Eur J Vasc Endovasc Surg. 2010;39:529–36.
15. Kristmundsson T, Sonesson B, Malina M, Bjorses K, Dias N, Resch T. Fenestrated endovascular repair for juxtarenal aortic pathology. J Vasc Surg. 2009;49: 568–75.

Surgeon-Modified Fenestrated and Branched Stent Grafts

3

Nikolaos Tsilimparis and Joseph J. Ricotta II

Abstract

Endovascular repair of aneurysms involving the visceral and thoracoabdominal aorta and iliac arteries has become a reality with over 1,000 cases performed worldwide. Sm-FBSG for pararenal, thoracoabdominal, and aortoiliac aneurysms have emerged as a viable endovascular alternative for patients unfit for open repair in circumstances not allowing the use of customized stent grafts or suitable off-the-shelf devices. The major limitation for widespread of this technique is the fact that a time window of 1–2 h is needed to construct the graft and the fact that it is rather complex to complete when not performed routinely.

Until standardized off-the-shelf devices become widely available, sm-FBSG represent the best option for patients requiring urgent and emergent repair, especially because outcome and durability of these repairs appears to be similar to that of commercially available devices.

Keywords

Aortic aneurysm • Surgeon-modified fenestrated-branched stent grafts Thoracoabdominal aneurysm • Complex aneurysm • Stent

Introduction: Background

Infrarenal abdominal aortic aneurysms (AAA) represent the simplest form of aortic aneurysmal disease. Techniques of open repair of infrarenal AAAs have been mastered with excellent results, good functional results, and reduced perioperative morbidity and mortality. However, involvement of the renal and visceral arteries requires higher exposure of the aorta proximal to the renal arteries and temporary suprarenal or supramesenteric aortic cross-clamping, which increases the

N. Tsilimparis, M.D. • J.J. Ricotta II, M.D., M.S., FACS (✉)
Department of Vascular and Endovascular Surgery, Heart and Vascular Institute, Northside Hospital Health System, 1000 Johnson Ferry Road NE, Atlanta, GA 30322, USA
e-mail: joseph.ricotta@northside.com

J.J. Hoballah, A.B. Lumsden (eds.), *Vascular Surgery*, New Techniques in Surgery Series, DOI 10.1007/978-1-4471-2912-7_3, © Springer-Verlag London 2012 complexity of the operation and carries higher risk of complications. These aneurysms together with the thoracoabdominal aortic aneurysms (TAAA) are generally classified with the term complex aortic aneurysms (CAA).

Despite advancement in preoperative evaluation and perioperative care of patients with CAA, open surgical repair remains a formidable challenge for the vascular surgeon. In a recent meta-analysis from our group of 7,833 patients who underwent open surgical repair of TAAA between the years 2000 and 2010, the overall risk of death within 30 days was 7 %, while in-hospital mortality was 10 % [1]. The 30-day mortality was 5 % for elective cases, with significant associated morbidity ranging from a 7.5 % incidence of spinal cord ischemia, to 19 % rate of renal failure and 36 % rate of pulmonary dysfunction. The 30-day mortality for open repair of ruptured TAAA has been reported as high as 40 %, with an average of 19 % in this meta-analysis. These data clearly demonstrate the high morbidity and mortality of the open procedure, particularly in the urgent or emergent setting, even in patients considered to be at low or moderate risk for open surgery. As a consequence, many high-risk patients with significant comorbidities will be denied elective open surgery.

Open repair of juxta- and pararenal aneurysms has produced much better results in centers of excellence with outcome comparable to those of standard infrarenal aortic aneurysm repairs according to a publication from the American College of Surgeons National Quality Improvement Program database [2]. Several published reviews of pararenal aneurysms report that suprarenal clamping was associated with a mortality of 3–6 % for elective cases as well as a new onset of dialysis of another 3–4.5 %, with 18 % of the patients experiencing postoperative renal dysfunction [3]. In the urgent setting, early mortality after repair of a ruptured pararenal aneurysm has been described between 40 and 80 % [4]. Again, it must be emphasized that these results come from centers of excellence and reflect a population of low or moderate perioperative risk.

Endovascular aneurysm repair (EVAR) has been shown to be safe and effective in treating uncomplicated infrarenal and thoracic aneurysms in both the elective [5–9] and urgent setting [10, 11], yet there is limited experience with this technology in complex conditions. It is estimated that the rate of ineligibility for infrarenal endovascular repair using standard devices is 25–40 % among patients with aneurysms whose maximum diameter has met operative threshold [12, 13]. Anatomic characteristics of the proximal neck is the most likely cause for ineligibility along with access issues [12]. Between 1999 and 2008, only 69 % of treated AAA in the USA met the most liberal definition of device instructions for use in the treatment of abdominal aortic aneurysms resulting in 41 % of the patients having sac enlargement at 5-year follow-up [14].

These patients would obviously profit from an open repair when suitable for it or from the implantation of a stent graft with fenestrations or branches to the visceral arteries to facilitate adequate seal zone.

Indications for Fenestrated-Branched Stent Grafts

The indication for fenestrated-branched stent grafts is not clearly defined beyond the typical characterization of patients as "unfit for open surgery." The criteria, however, that are used to characterize a patient as "unfit" or "high risk" for open surgery even for AAA differ significantly among studies [15–17]. Generally, major limitations that would preclude patients from open repair are mainly cardiac or pulmonary. Chronic obstructive pulmonary disease (COPD) is typically encountered in 20–60 % of patients with complex AAA or TAAA, while 20–50 % had a previous PTCA or coronary artery bypass graft [1, 18]. Medical conditions that most surgeons would consider discouraging for open surgery include the following:

1. American Society of Anesthesiologists score ≥ 3
2. Society of Vascular Surgery score ≥ 8

3. Patients requiring oxygen supplementation
4. Pulmonary dysfunction with an FEV1 < 1 l
5. Recent myocardial infarction (<6 months)
6. Congestive heart failure (CHF) with an ejection fraction <35 %
7. Symptomatic CHF, age > 79
8. Myocardial infarction within 6 months
9. Coronary revascularization with bypass in past 6 months
10. Coronary revascularization with angioplasty/stent in past 6 weeks
11. Unstable angina, valvular heart disease
12. Cancer with <50 % 5-year survival

Size Threshold for Repair

In contrary to infrarenal aortic repair, where the threshold for open repair has been defined well at 5–5.5 cm for intact aneurysms, the threshold for repair of thoracoabdominal or any complex aortic aneurysms is not well defined. Elefteriades et al. [19] were able to demonstrate that by the time the descending aorta reaches a size of 7.0 cm, 43 % of the patients have suffered rupture or dissection. Davies et al. [20] found that patients with a 6.0-cm TAAA have a 5-year survival of 54 %, yielding a risk for rupture of 3.7 % per year, and risk of death of 12 % per year. Cambria et al. [21] on the other hand found a significantly higher aneurysm-related mortality for untreated patients with TAAA with a 2- and 4-year risk of rupture of 12 and 32 %, respectively, and a median expansion rate of 0.2 cm/year. Most of the studies evaluating the diameter threshold for operating a TAAA considered a diameter between 5 and 6 cm as the right point to operate on an intact TAAA [20–23]. Other critical confounders that affect the decision to treat or not a patient with a TAAA include the extent and morphology of the aneurysm and patient-specific characteristics such as age, glomerular filtration rate, and comorbidities [23, 24]. The aneurysm size threshold for repair should not be different for elective endovascular repair, although more severe comorbidities can be tolerated.

Alternative Options for Management of CAA and Concept for Use of Surgeon-Modified Fenestrated-Branched Stent Grafts

Fenestrated and branched endografts have been developed as a minimally invasive, total endovascular alternative for the treatment of complex aortic aneurysms in high-risk patients [25–27]. However, construction of these devices requires that they are custom-made to fit the specific anatomical requirements of each patient. As a result, it can take as much as 6–12 weeks to manufacture these devices. Restricted access to investigational devices and delays in device customization limit treatment with these endografts to a group of patients with relatively stable aneurysms. Patients who present emergently with ruptured or symptomatic complex aortic aneurysms cannot be treated with the current commercially available fenestrated-branched endograft technology because of the degree of customization required to treat each individual patient.

The question then arises of how to treat patients unfit for open repair who present with symptomatic or ruptured complex aortic aneurysms and cannot wait for a custom fenestrated/branched endograft to be created.

Emergency Treatment Options for High-Risk Patients with Complex Aortic Aneurysms

Patients at high risk for open surgery who present with complex aortic aneurysms requiring urgent or emergent treatment could be considered candidates for the following treatment options:

Conventional EVAR for Short-Neck AAA

Short-neck AAA and juxtarenal aneurysms represent the simplest form of complex aortic aneurysms. The feasibility of EVAR in these cases has been described along with a worse long-term outcome in terms of endoleaks and reintervention rates, when compared with normal neck AAA [28].

On the other hand, Verhoeven et al. [29] reviewed their series of 100 fenestrated grafts for short-necked and juxtarenal aneurysms and were able to demonstrate good long-term outcome. The role of standard EVAR in patients with short-neck or juxtarenal aneurysms should be approached with great caution in an era with good results of open repair for low- to medium-risk patients [30] and excellent results of total endovascular repair with fenestrated grafts [29].

Abdominal Aortic Debranching Combined with Endografting ("Hybrid Approach")

This treatment approach for high-risk patients combines conventional visceral artery bypass with stent-graft implantation, the so-called debranching or hybrid technique [31–34]. The potential advantages of this technique are that it substitutes a laparotomy for thoracoabdominal exposure, eliminates aortic mobilization and cross-clamping, and reduces the duration of visceral ischemia compared to conventional open repair. However, despite these theoretical advantages, it is still an extensive intra-abdominal operation with high complication rates, especially in high-risk patients who would not tolerate conventional open repair. A recent meta-analysis on the outcomes of the hybrid approach demonstrated a 30-day mortality of 12.8 %, renal failure of 9 %, spinal cord ischemia of 7.5 %, and an endoleak rate of 23 % at a mean follow-up of 34.5 months [35]. While the hybrid approach of visceral debranching and overstenting of the aneurysmal segments represents a viable alternative to open surgery for patients with TAAA, other less invasive alternatives may be more beneficial in this fragile patient cohort.

Parallel Graft Endovascular Repair (Snorkel/Chimney/Periscope/Sandwich)

As endovascular techniques have become a routine in the daily practice of vascular surgeons and interventionalists, many feel confident using the technique of parallel grafts (snorkel/chimney/periscope/sandwich techniques) as a quick "bail-out" procedure. Over the last years, several reports have been published describing repair mostly of juxtarenal but also thoracoabdominal aneurysms in patients with acute pathologies [36, 37]. Most of the authors concluded that this treatment option is technically feasible and useful in settings requiring emergent repair, but any mid- or long-term results were poorly described in most cases. However, the authors did emphasize the importance of distinguishing in complexity of repair between juxtarenal aneurysms and TAAA and acknowledge the lack of mid- and long-term follow-up and the issue of unknown durability in these repairs. In a review of 93 patients who were treated with chimney stent grafts, a total of 134 branch stents were implanted in 72 pararenal, 5 thoracoabdominal, and 8 anastomotic aneurysms, as well as in six patients for sealing of a proximal endoleak or other indications [38]. The incidence of intraoperative and early postoperative type I endoleak was 14 and 11 %, respectively.

Customized Fenestrated Endografts

While the Zenith custom-made fenestrated stent graft (Cook Medical, Bloomington, IN) still awaits FDA approval in the USA as this chapter is written, a substantial experience with treatment of elective cases in high-risk patients has been acquired worldwide [39–42]. Custom-made fenestrated-branched grafts are patient tailored, and an interval of 6–12 weeks is required between measurement and delivery of the graft from the producing company. This is acceptable in high-risk patients who do not have the alternative of open surgery but cannot be implemented in patients requiring urgent repair.

Standardized (Off-the-Shelf) Fenestrated-Branched Stent Grafts

Stent grafts that have been constructed to fit a population with typical visceral anatomy and thus are not patient tailored (custom-made) are referred to as standardized grafts. A standardized stent graft would not only prevent ruptures from occurring during the waiting period of graft manufacture but would also allow treatment of patients presenting with ruptures and/or symptoms that currently can only be treated with surgeon-modified fenestrated-branched stent grafts (sm-FBSG) [43, 44]. In 2009, Sweet et al. [42] demonstrated that 88 % of the patients treated with stent grafts customized to patient's anatomy could also have been treated with standardized endografts. Ever since the group continued to report its experience on the transition from customized to standardized stent grafts without any perioperative events [45, 46]. However, Azzaoui et al. [47] in their retrospective analysis of 289 patients with juxtarenal aneurysms that would require two renal branches and a scallop for the SMA concluded that only 20–50 % of the patients could be treated with a standard fenestrated module, depending on the size of the fenestrations. Sobocinski et al. [48] evaluated the applicability of two different "off-the-shelf" standardized fenestrated endografts with two fenestrations for the renal arteries, one for the superior mesenteric artery (SMA), and a scallop for the celiac trunk to conclude that one or both "off-the-shelf" endografts could possibly treat >70 % of the patients. The devices currently in the pipeline or under investigation are designed to treat juxtarenal, pararenal, but also thoracoabdominal aneurysms using different approaches and designs [49–52].

Although the concept of a standardized, off-the-shelf, multibranched stent graft is exciting, its use could compromise the principle of perfect alignment of the graft to the target vessels with unknown results on long-term branch patency. The routine use of plugs to occlude unused branches could potentially lead to higher risk of endoleak. Furthermore, the efficacy of these grafts in the emergent setting is unknown.

Surgeon-Modified Fenestrated-Branched Stent Grafts

The value of fenestrated-branched stent grafts in the management of high-risk patients with TAAA unfit for open surgery is indisputable. Lower perioperative morbidity and mortality with good mid- and long-term results have been demonstrated [39, 40, 53, 54].

Since the first report by Park and associates in 1996 of two patients with infrarenal aortic aneurysms treated with fenestrated devices, the group from Perth, Australia, developed a fenestrated stent graft based on the Cook Zenith® lineage [55]. The addition of a constraining wire allowed more accurate deployment of the main stent graft across the renal and mesenteric arteries [56]. Subsequently, Anderson and associates [57] reported the first clinical experience using this device in 13 patients with juxtarenal and pararenal aortic aneurysms.

Sm-FBSG were introduced because of the need to provide acute care in symptomatic or ruptured complex aortic aneurysms of patients who were unfit for surgery. Surgeons modify commercially available stent grafts to create scallops and fenestrations utilizing techniques similar to those used by industry for the manufacture of a fenestrated-branched stent graft and apply them in a way that fits the resources and materials available in every institution performing endovascular surgery. Key elements in the modification of stent grafts through surgeons are:

1. The accurate construction of the fenestrations without rupture of destruction of the fabric
2. The construction of mechanism for partial constraining that would allow easier orientation and reposition of the stent graft when more than two fenestrations are constructed to achieve optimal alignment of the fenestrations with the branches
3. A proper technique for resheathing the stent graft to prevent damage of the device and ensure accurate and safe deployment in the human aorta

Indication for Sm-FBSG

The indications for sm-FBSG are similar to those for commercially available fenestrated endografts and were earlier described. However, given the fact that modified stent grafts are an off-label use of the devices, certain restrictions apply [58, 59]:

1. The patient is considered at excessive risk of morbidity and mortality with other alternative methods of treatment (e.g., open surgical repair, aortic debranching) [43].

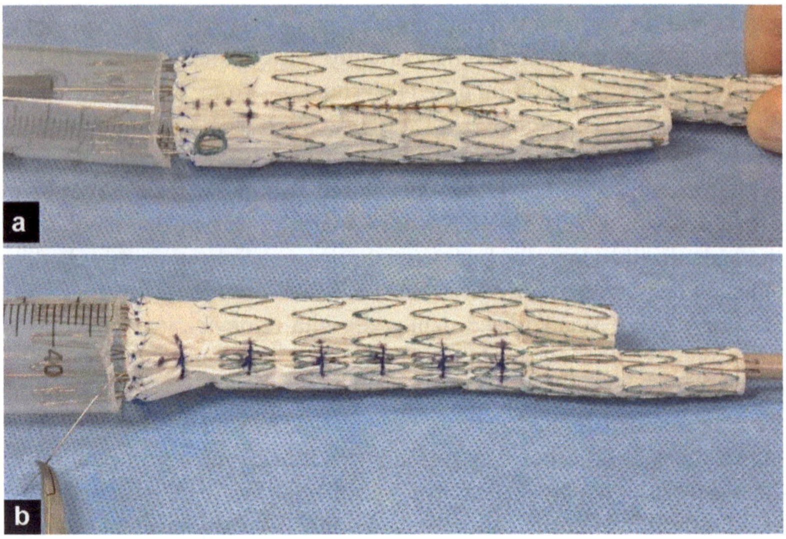

Fig. 3.1 Surgeon-modified fenestrated-branched stent graft (bifurcated Zenith Cook device) from anterior (**a**) and posterior (**b**) view

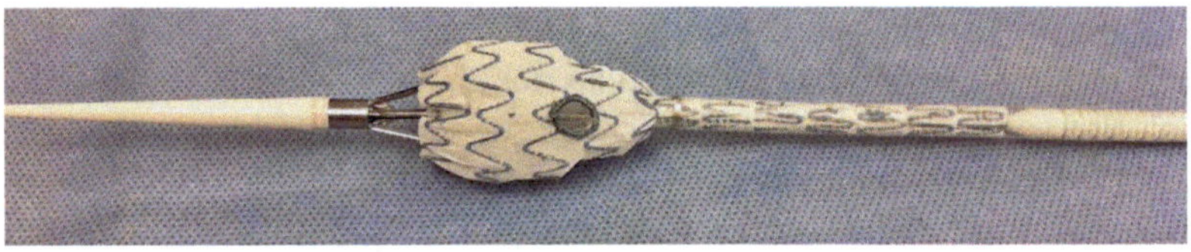

Fig. 3.2 Surgeon-modified Endurant Medtronic stent graft with a single renal fenestration

2. The patient has a symptomatic or contained-ruptured complex aneurysm, yet treatment may be delayed by an additional 1–2 h to allow device design, modification, and implantation.
3. Endovascular repair cannot be accomplished using commercially available stent grafts.
4. The patient cannot be transferred to a regional center of excellence for care using a manufactured device.
5. The patient is treated within a study protocol of an investigational device exemption.
6. Procedural consent from the patient after extensive informative discussion for the off-label use of the device and the associated risks is mandatory.

Choice of Stent Graft for Modification

The technique of fenestrated-branched repair is currently mostly performed using the Cook Zenith® stent graft lineage. The characteristics of the thoracic Zenith TX2 and the abdominal AAA Zenith device (Cook Medical) are optimal for modification due to the morphology of the Z-stents and the availability of multiple wires that can be used as a constraining wire to achieve partial constraining of the sm-FBSG (Fig. 3.1a, b). This facilitates better orientation and alignment of the visceral branches to the fenestrations.
The Medtronic Endurant device has also been frequently used in our experience for patients requiring 1–3 fenestrations to the visceral arteries (Fig. 3.2). Limitation of the Endurant stent graft is the lack of additional wires in the native graft that could be used as a constraining wire. Lack of a constraining wire would limit the ability to rotate the device and therefore jeopardize alignment of all branches.

The following flowchart (Fig. 3.3) illustrates the decision tree in our practice, which determines the stent graft to be used in each case. In general, patients requiring more than three fenestrations, those with severe aortic angulation or when difficult branch alignment is anticipated, the Zenith device is used.

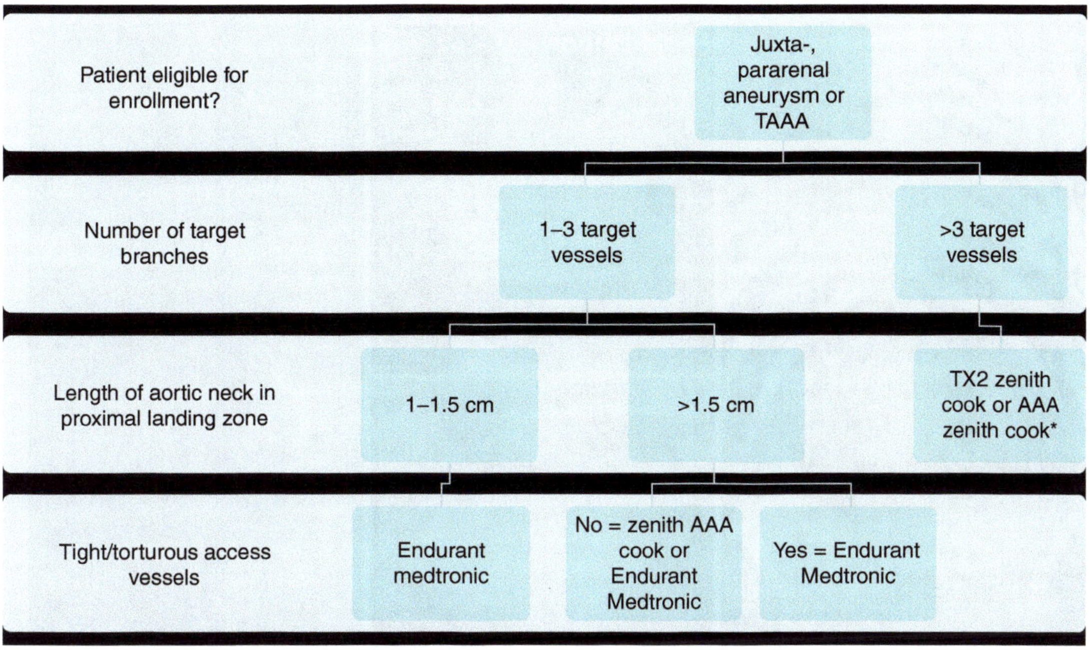

Fig. 3.3 Algorithm for choice of device type for modification

The thoracic TX2 Zenith device is preferred when a stent graft of diameter >36 mm is necessary or when the extent of the coverage is such that a bifurcated graft cannot facilitate. Prior repair of the infrarenal aorta also typically requires the use of the TX2 thoracic stent graft. The Endurant device (Medtronic) is reserved for cases where the aortic neck in the proximal landing zone is <10 mm or the iliac vessels are very torturous and/or tight.

Adjunctive Materials Required

The introduction of long, flexible hydrophilic sheaths to facilitate cannulation of the fenestrations and target vessels and the delivery and implantation of branch stents, along with the introduction of dedicated catheters, wires, and peripheral stents for the aortic branches, have substantially contributed to simplifying the complicated steps of fenestrated and branched graft repair.

With regard to branch stents, currently only the ICAST stent graft (Atrium Medical Corp., Hudson, New Hampshire) is commercially available in the USA as a balloon-expandable covered stent, and the only available covered self-expanding stent grafts are the Viabahn (Gore Medical, Flagstaff, AZ) and the Fluency stent (Bard Peripheral Vascular, Tempe, AZ). However, use of these covered stents during FEVAR is an off-label use of these devices. As a result, Cook Medical was obliged to manufacture a dedicated self-expanding stent called ConnectSX for the aortic branches to use in its clinical trials for the fenestrated-branched endografts. This stent is currently part of the Preserve Iliac Branch IDE trial in the USA.

Preoperative Planning and Measurements

The most important component of the technique is adequate planning and design of the stent graft. Computed tomography angiography allows accurate measurements of lengths using centerline of flow analysis, and the clock position of vessel origin is assessed using axial imaging. While obtaining measurements for sm-FBSG, we also tend to measure arc lengths of the branches from

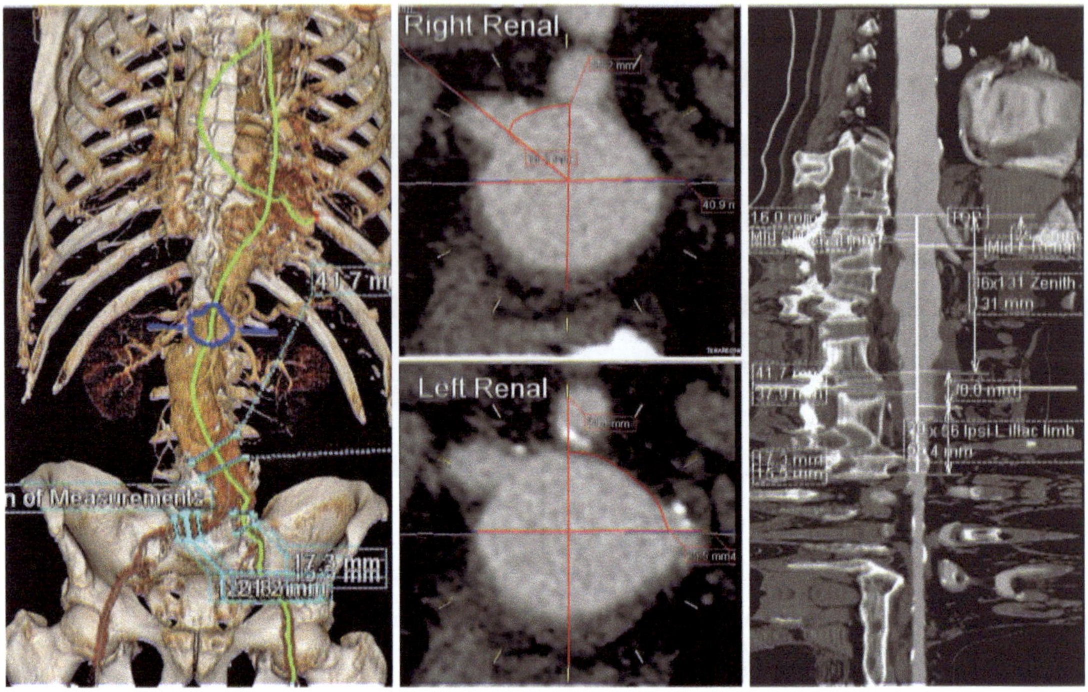

Fig. 3.4 3-D reconstruction and centerline of flow analysis of a CT scan to facilitate accurate preoperative arc and length measurements for proper device modification

the 12 o'clock position instead of clock position alone because we found them to be more accurate in identifying the optimal fenestration position at grafts of different sizes.

Several software programs are currently available to create a centerline of flow, but the TeraRecon Aquarius Workstation (TeraRecon, San Mateo, CA) is currently dominating the field (Fig. 3.4) [60]. The reason for that is the straightened view reconstruction which significantly simplifies calculation of length and arc length measurements and which is to our knowledge not available in other software programs.

Technical Aspects of Sm-FBSG

The main stent graft is designed with a minimum proximal landing zone length of 2 cm. The landing zone should be located within normal aorta in an area of parallel aortic wall diameter and free of thrombus, angulation, or ectasia. Each fenestration is created using the length from the start of the landing zone (fabric) to the middle of the target vessel and the clock position of the target vessel based on centerline of flow reconstructions. Fenestrations are reinforced and marked with a radiopaque ring to allow visualization under fluoroscopy. Additional markers are placed in the anterior aspect of the stent graft to allow orientation prior to deployment (Fig. 3.5).

While creating the fenestrations in a stent graft is a relatively straightforward procedure in patients requiring 1–2 branches fenestration, it is not adequate for cases where more than two branches need to be addressed. The use of a mechanism that would allow partial deployment of the graft facilitating cannulation of the branches through the fenestrations while still preserving the ability to rotate the graft is essential to achieve perfect alignment and optimal outcome. From the currently commercially available devices, only the Zenith devices are suitable for modification with a constraining wire.

Modification of a stent graft to produce 1–4 fenestrations, constrain the device, and resheath it

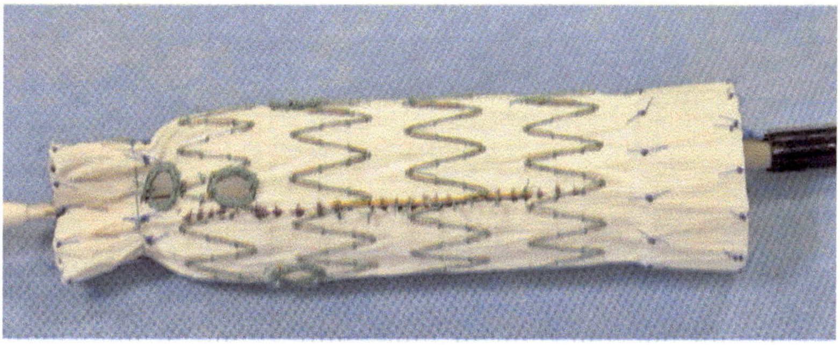

Fig. 3.5 Surgeon-modified fenestrated-branched stent graft (TX2 Zenith Cook device) with four fenestrations and the longitudinal radiopaque marker anteriorly

varies in our experience from 32 to 140 min with an average of 90 min. This represents the major drawback of this technique in the management of aortic emergencies in hemodynamically unstable patients. A window of 1–2 h has to be available to enable safe management of the patients. Nevertheless, modification of the graft can begin independently of the procedure as soon as the CT scan is available and measurements are made. This time interval often coincides with the preparation of the patient from the anesthesiology team and the time needed for bilateral femoral artery exposure and branch access. In cases of high-risk contained ruptures, an aortic occlusion balloon is ready for deployment while waiting for completion of the modified graft.

The use of sm-FBSG is an alternative, which is more complicated than use of the parallel graft technique but is validated through better long-term results. The experience required to modify these grafts will likely be an obstacle in achieving widespread application of this technique in vascular practice, but this is currently the option that best serves the short-term goal of rescuing the patient, as well as the long-term goal of providing a durable exclusion of the aneurysm.

Anatomical Challenges for Sm-FBSG

The anatomic limitations of sm-FBSG are grossly similar to those of commercially available devices. Post dissection aneurysmal degeneration is exceptionally difficult to treat in the setting of a narrow true lumen that cannot accommodate the size of a fenestrated endograft. Angulation at the level of the visceral aorta also represents a formidable challenge both for measurement and alignment of the branches to the fenestrations.

Especially in the case of four-vessel fenestrated-branched procedures, adequate access from both iliac arteries as well as from one brachial artery is essential. In case any of these sites cannot be accessed with or without use of conduit, the procedure is almost impossible to complete.

Patients with prior renal stents protruding in the aortic lumen, as well as patients with significant renal artery stenosis, require management of these conditions, either with balloon dilatation or removal of the stents [61].

Another issue that is especially relevant for patients with thoracoabdominal aortic aneurysms is the distance between the stent graft and the branches of the aorta. In aneurysms with larger maximal diameter, the gap that the branch stents need to cover is longer, and they are therefore more susceptible to cranial and caudal forces that occur during the cardiac circle. This could potentially result in higher rates of kinking, components separation, and branch occlusion, in cases where the branches do not appose the aortic wall. The use of surgeon-manufacted cuffed branches has been suggested to provide better seal between the main stent graft and each bridging branch artery stent to help dealing with this issue.

The primary advantage is that the cuff provides at least 2 cm of overlapping seal zone between the branch artery stent and the main stent graft, as compared to the use of a nitinol ring and a flared stent in which there is no zone of overlap. There are several potential advantages of this technique over fenestrated-branched stent grafts, however only in selected cases. In our experience with both techniques, the advantage

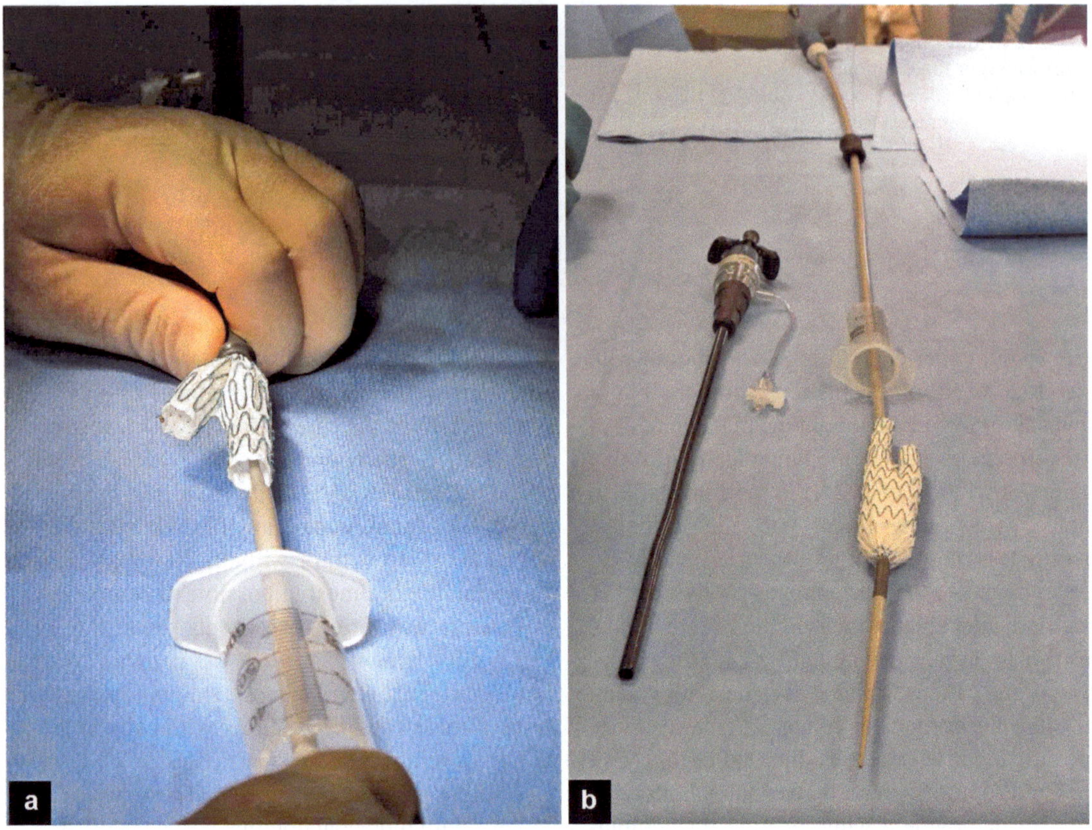

Fig. 3.6 The Zenith stent graft during (**a**) and after (**b**) back-table deployment from the back of the delivery sheath

of cuffs was not that obvious when all necessary steps were taken to ensure perfect alignment of fenestrations with branches including flaring of branch stents to secure attachment to the main graft and appropriate length of branch stents protrusion in the aneurysm.

Another option to further reinforce a branch stent bridging a longer gap and add stability is to add another covered balloon-expandable stent (Icast, Atrium) or a self-expandable bare metal stent to prevent kinking at the distal landing point in the renal artery.

Technique of Graft Modification

The technique of sm-FBSG has been previously published [59, 62]. Here, we describe the process of modifying a bifurcated Zenith AAA prosthesis.

The sm-FBSG is constructed under strict sterile conditions in the operating room on the back table using basic surgical instruments and preoperative measurements obtained from reconstructed CT scans using centerline of flow analysis software. The Cook Zenith bifurcated device is deployed on the back table by pulling it out of the back of the delivery sheath (Fig. 3.6). A 60-cc syringe is cut in half and used to capture the uncovered stent of the device so that the endograft can be modified while temporary constraining the sharp barbs. The site of the fenestrations and of the 12 o'clock longitudinal marking wire is drawn on the stent graft based on the preoperative CT scan measurements. Six by 8-mm fenestrations are created at the pre-marked positions using ophthalmic cautery. The fenestrations are reinforced using the radiopaque wire from an Amplatz GooseNeck® Snare Kit, which is sewn in place with a locking 5.0 Ethibond suture to

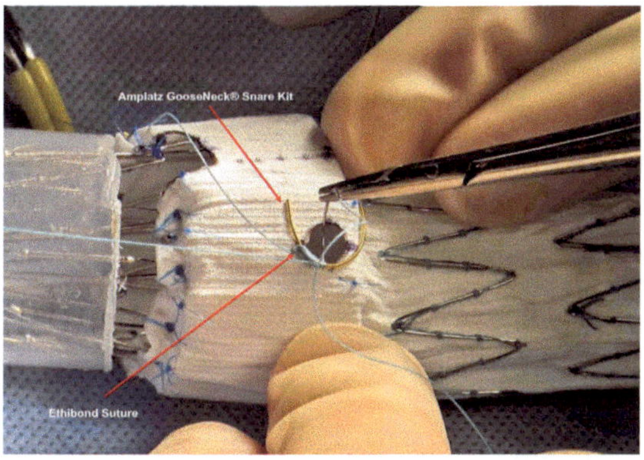

Fig. 3.7 Reinforcement of a fenestration with a radiopaque wire

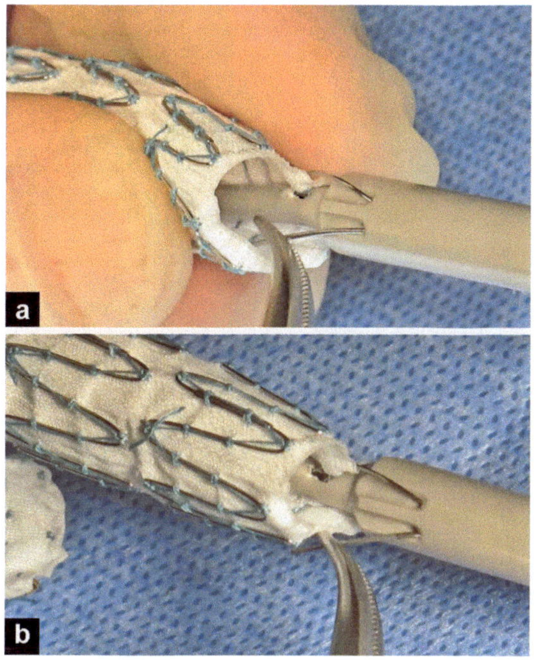

Fig. 3.8 The wire of the top stent trigger-wire release mechanism is retracted to its exit point from the gray positioner (**a**), captured and rerouted to use as a constraining wire (**b**)

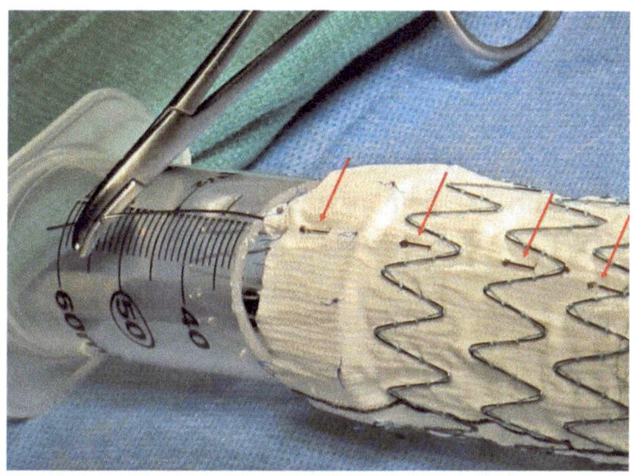

Fig. 3.9 *Red arrows* show the rerouted wire that will be used for constraining of the stent graft, running in and out of the stent graft fabric

completely cover the radiopaque wire and preventing wires from catching at that site during the procedure (Fig. 3.7). A longitudinal radiopaque marking wire is sewn at the anterior 12 o'clock portion of the graft to facilitate accurate orientation of the graft during the procedure. At the posterior portion of the graft, at the 6 o' clock position, the course of the constraining wire is marked on the graft. By pulling the top stent trigger-wire release mechanism, the wire is carefully retracted all the way down to its exit point from the gray positioner, captured and advanced outside of the stent graft to use as a constraining wire (Fig. 3.8). Using a 20-gauge spinal needle, the fabric of the graft is perforated in and out at each stent segment along the pre-marked 6 o'clock line. The extracted wire is inserted in the spinal needle and rerouted through it as a running wire in and out of the graft (Fig. 3.9).

To constrain the graft, a 3.0 polypropylene suture is sewn 2 stent peaks away from the constraining wire and then looped around the constraining wire using the back end of the needle to assure that no fabric is captured during this maneuver. The first loop is tied down to constrain the left two parts of the stent. To create the second loop, another 3.0 polypropylene suture is sewn 2 stent peaks away from the constraining wire on the other side. This second loop is rerouted below the first loop and not around the wire to make sure that no fabric or the other suture is caught during this maneuver that would prevent the graft from total deployment. The second loop is then tied down to achieve partial constraining of the graft diameter. The same procedure is applied for the rest of the stents in a similar fashion (Fig. 3.10a–c).

At this point, the modification of the stent graft is complete, and the maximal diameter of

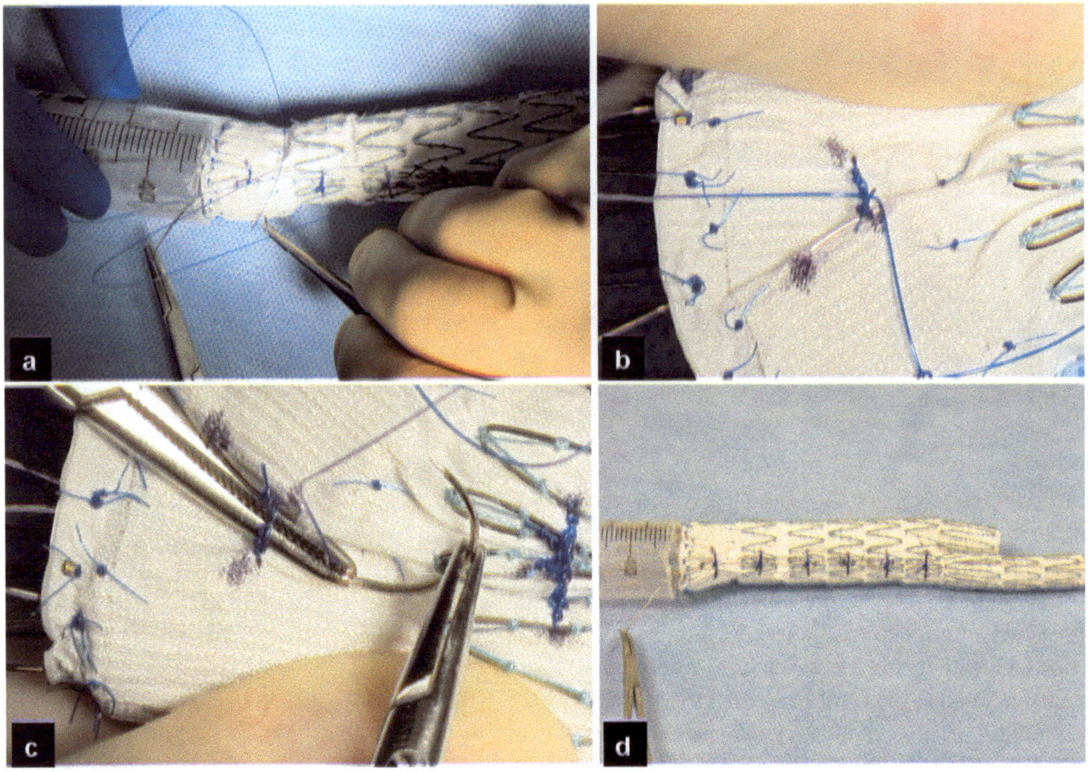

Fig. 3.10 (**a–d**) To constrain the graft, a suture is sewn two stent peaks away from the constraining wire (**a**) and then looped around the constraining wire (**b**) using the back end of the needle (**c**) to assure that no fabric is captured during this maneuver

the graft has been reduced by approximately 30 % with the help of the constraining wire (Fig. 3.10d). This allows the graft to be partially deployed within the aorta and permits repositioning of the graft if needed. The top uncovered stent of the graft is then recaptured in the top cap, and the tip of the constraining wire is relocated in its original position within the top cap.

Using umbilical tape, the stents of the graft are sequentially constrained and resheathed through the back of the peel-away sheath, thereby completing the device modification and returning the graft to its original packaged form (Fig. 3.11a–d).

Procedure

Bilateral femoral and left brachial approach is required in most cases. The right femoral access is usually used for the branches and the left femoral approach for introduction of the main stent graft. A large (20–24-Fr) Check-Flo sheath (Cook Medical, Inc., Bloomington, IN) is introduced via the right femoral artery (Fig. 3.12). A conduit to the iliac artery over a retroperitoneal access is used; when an endoconduit is not feasible, the native vessels cannot facilitate safe advance of the stent graft. The sheath valve is accessed with multiple (two or three) short 5 Fr sheaths, which are used for selective catheterization of the renal and superior mesenteric arteries. The celiac axis is typically accessed using the left brachial artery approach with a 7–8 Fr Raabe sheath and a 5 Fr MPA catheter (Cook Medical, Inc., Bloomington, IN). Contrast injection is used diligently during this part of the procedure. Selective renal and mesenteric angiography using 5 ml of diluted contrast avoids unnecessary use of 30 ml boluses of contrast per injection. Once all the target

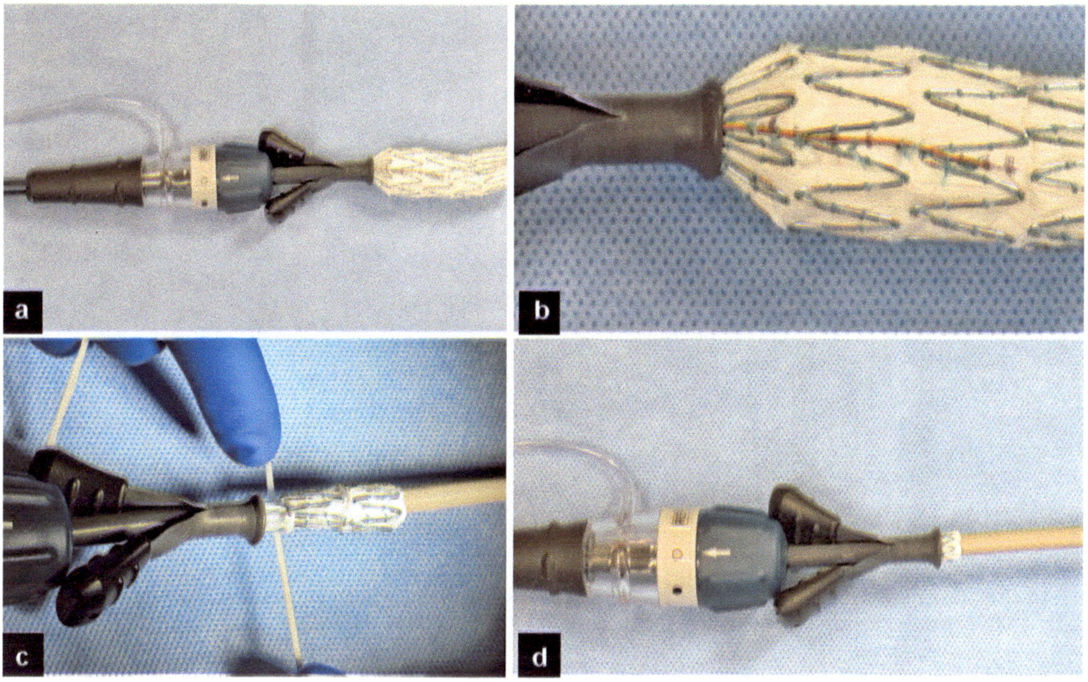

Fig. 3.11 (**a–d**) The stents of the graft are sequentially constrained and resheathed through the back of the peel-away sheath

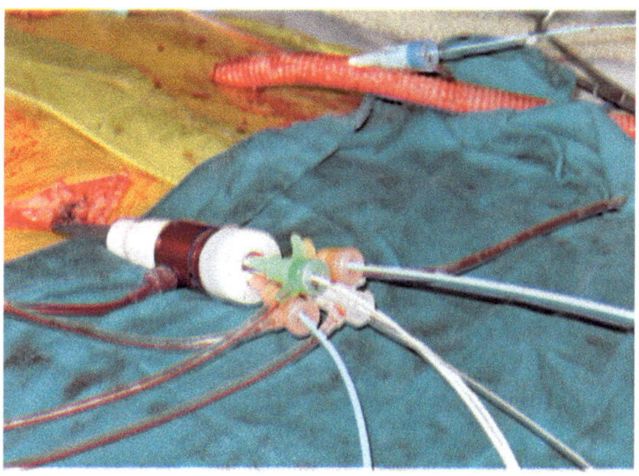

Fig. 3.12 The valve of a 25-cm 22-Fr Check-Flo sheath is punctured in all four quadrants and smaller sheaths, and wires and catheters are placed to gain access to the visceral branches. A conduit is placed on demand

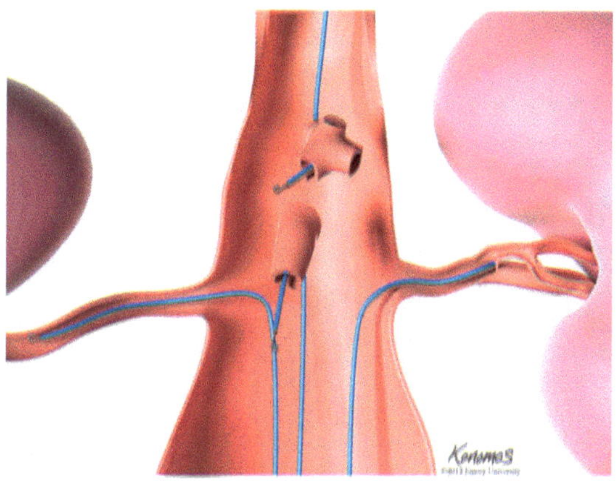

Fig. 3.13 Graphic showing catheterization and marking of all visceral branches with sheaths before stent-graft implantation

branches are catheterized (Fig. 3.13), the main stent graft is oriented extracorporeally and subsequently introduced via the left femoral approach. The fenestrations of the stent graft are then aligned to the visceral branches that are marked with wires and sheaths and deployed (Fig. 3.14). The device remains constrained by a wire, which allows rotational and cranial-caudal movement of the main stent graft to optimize alignment. Each selective catheter is serially removed from the respective vessel and used to regain access into the main stent graft, fenestration, and

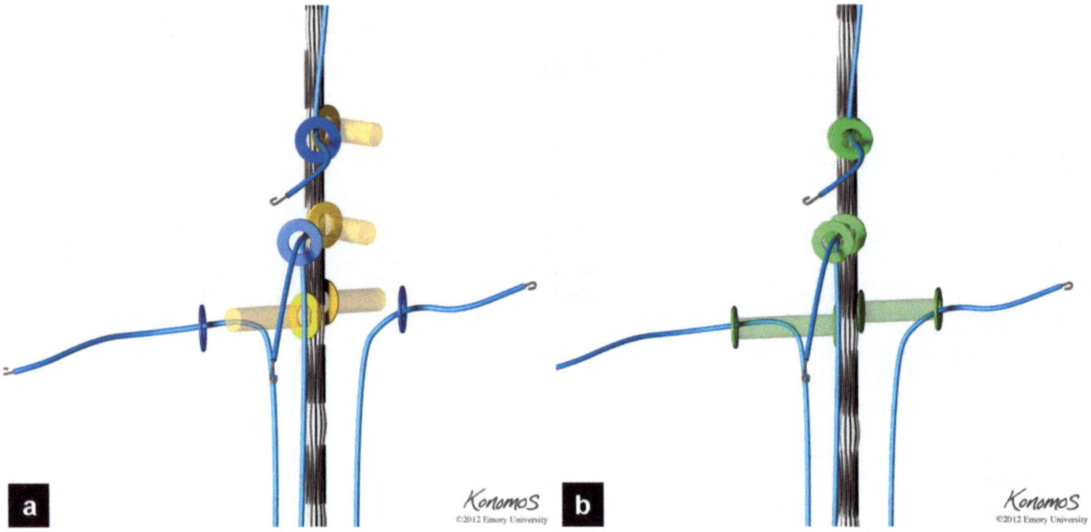

Fig. 3.14 Before deployment of the graft, the catheterized branches (**a**) allow perfect alignment of the fenestrations of the stent graft with the targeted visceral branches (**b**)

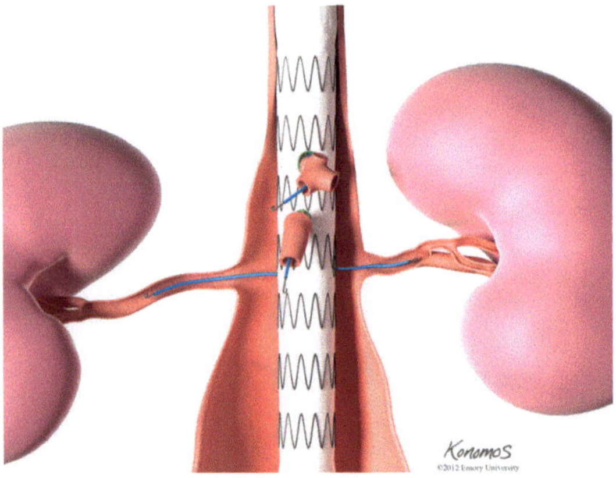

Fig. 3.15 The wires and sheaths are removed, and the visceral branches are recannulated, this time through the fenestrations of the stent graft

target vessel (Fig. 3.15). A 7 Fr Ansel or Raabe sheath (Cook Medical, Inc., Bloomington, IN) is advanced through the femoral sheath to renal and superior mesenteric arteries, followed by a balloon-expandable stent graft. The celiac fenestration and artery are accessed using the 7–8 Fr Raabe sheath from the left brachial artery. Once all the target vessels are accessed and the bridging stent grafts are ready for deployment, the main stent graft is fully unconstrained. Each branched stent graft is deployed and flared proximally with a 10 mm × 2-cm balloon, starting with the renal arteries (Fig. 3.16), followed by the superior mesenteric and celiac axis (Fig. 3.17). If the repair needs to be extended distally to achieve an adequate seal, this is accomplished by placement of a commercially available bifurcated modular device into both iliac arteries (Fig. 3.18). Extension into the proximal thoracic aorta may be necessary for more extensive thoracoabdominal aneurysms.

Surgeon-Modified Iliac Branch Stent Graft

Endovascular approach is not feasible in many aortic cases because of an adequate landing zone in the area of the iliac arteries. Aneurysmal degeneration of the common or/and internal iliac arteries often necessitates exclusion of the ipsilateral hypogastric artery. This could however have potentially detrimental results in the setting of atherosclerotic disease or occlusion of the contralateral hypogastric artery including symptoms of buttock claudication and pelvic ischemia.

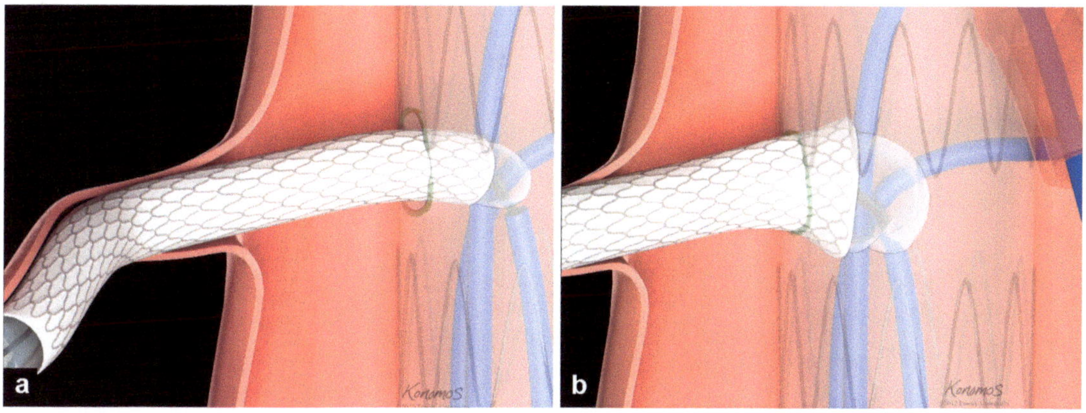

Fig. 3.16 Stent grafts are deployed in the renal and mesenteric branches (**a**) and flared proximally to achieve better seal and stability (**b**)

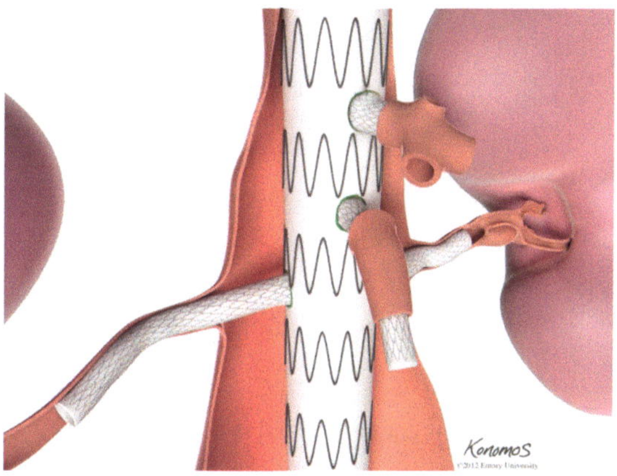

Fig. 3.17 Fenestrated-branched stent graft with all stents to the visceral branches in place

Buttock claudication occurs in 30–40 % of patients with unilateral hypogastric embolization and >50 % of patients with bilateral hypogastric artery exclusion.

While numerous options exist for open surgical revascularization of the hypogastric artery, open repair is associated with higher perioperative mortality and morbidity [63]. Endovascular options include use of chimney stent techniques, bell-bottom stent grafts, and back-table reversed limb technique [64–66]. The endovascular approach with iliac branch devices (IBD) has significantly extended the spectrum of endovascular aortoiliac surgery with excellent short- and long-term results [67]. Different designs of IBD are available including the straight sidearm IBD, the helical branch IBD, and the bifurcated-bifurcated IBD. Currently, the straight sidearm IBD is the one commercially widely available.

However, the same problems that arise for fenestrated-branched stent grafts for complex aortic aneurysms arise also for aortoiliac aneurysms with extension to the iliac arteries. The lack of availability of these grafts outside study protocols in many countries including the USA, as well as the fact that these devices are not always available off-the-shelf, creates a shortage of endovascular alternatives that can be filled by the technique of surgeon-modified hypogastric branched stent grafts.

We have previously described the technique for modification of a Zenith iliac limb stent graft (Cook, Bloomington, IN) [68].

In our experience, the iliac limb of the Endurant Medtronic device can also be modified in a similar fashion to accommodate a side branch for the hypogastric artery.

In brief, the procedure of modifying a Medtronic iliac branch is described below.

Device Modification for Surgeon-Modified Iliac Branch Stent Graft

The iliac limb device (16F sheath) is introduced together with a 4F Kumpe catheter (Cook) into a 20F Performer Check-Flo sheath (Cook Medical).

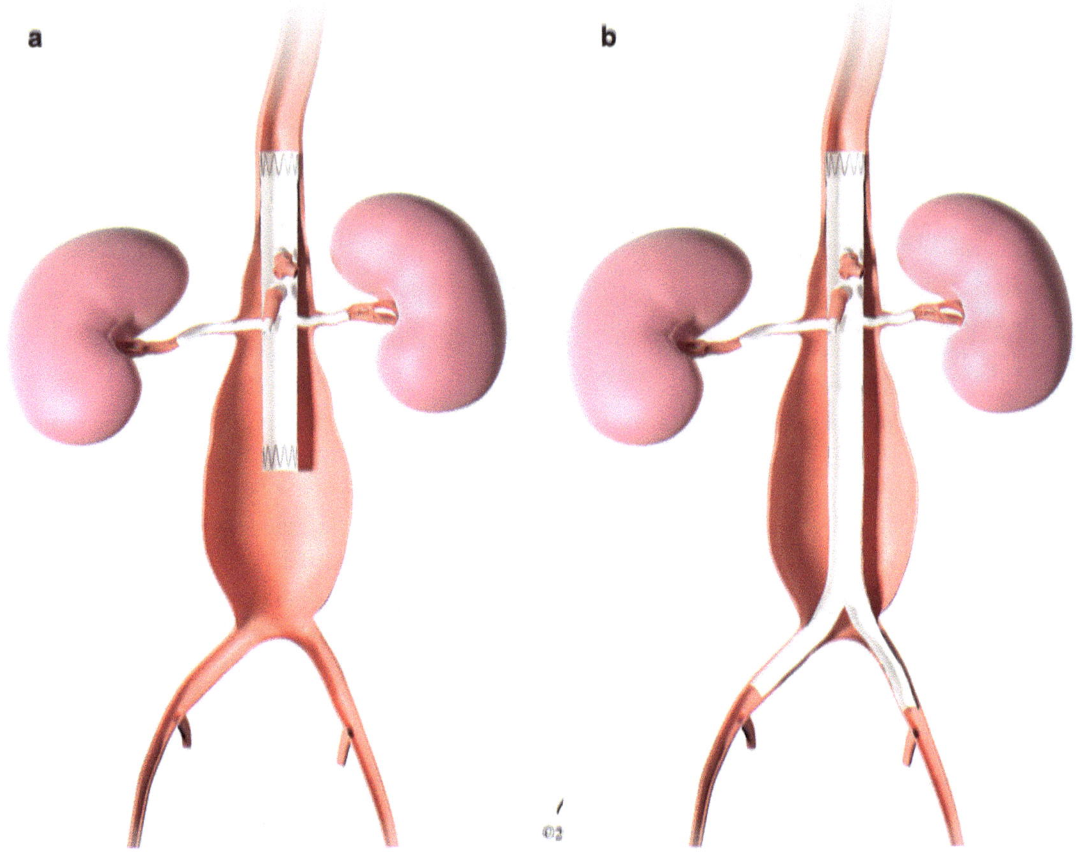

Fig. 3.18 Once the proximal part of the repair with a modified TX2 Zenith stent graft is finished (**a**), the repair can be extended distally with a bifurcated modular device if needed (**b**)

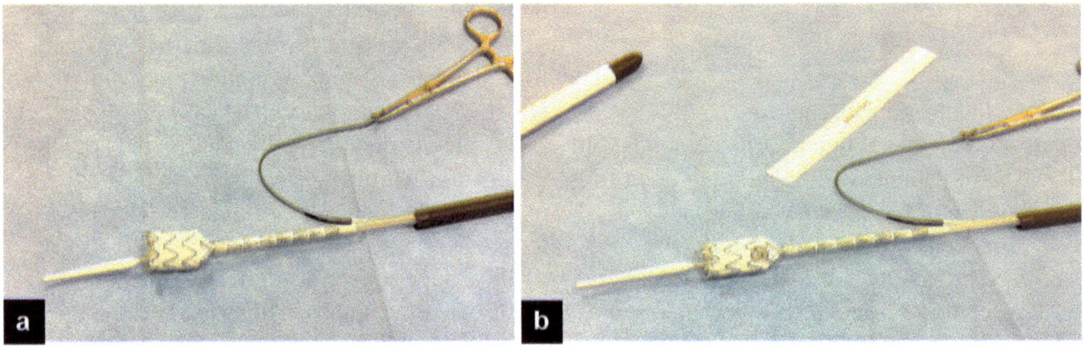

Fig. 3.19 The iliac limb device is introduced with a 4F Kumpe catheter in a 20F Performer Check-Flo sheath (**a**), and a fenestration is created (**b**)

The 4F catheter is placed through the valve in the sheath, and the iliac limb is placed through the center hole. The proximal 3 stents of the iliac stent graft are then deployed so that an adequate proximal sealing zone is exposed (Fig. 3.19a). Below that area and at a "valley" of the struts, a hole is constructed in the fabric of the graft to facilitate the beveled anastomosis of a 6–8-mm

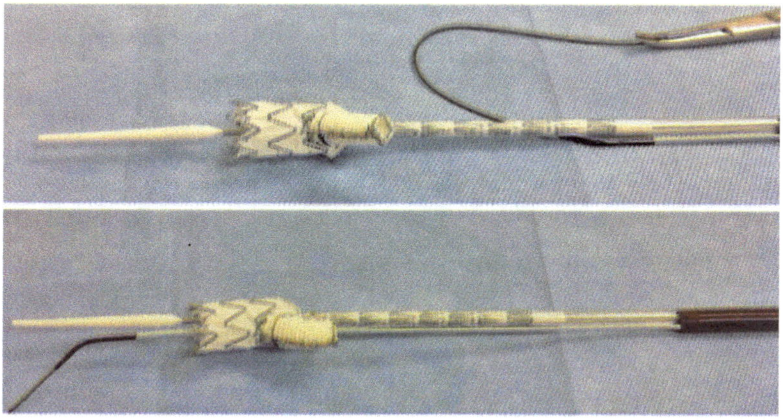

Fig. 3.20 A directional sidearm branch using a Dacron conduit is sewn at the fenestration (**a**), and the 4 Fr Kumpe catheter is loaded through the sidearm branch (**b**)

downward-oriented Dacron conduit (Fig. 3.19b). The Dacron graft is shortened to 10–30 mm and reinforced with a circumferentially running radiopaque wire at the distal part of the Dacron conduit as well as at the junction with the iliac limb. A longitudinal marker is placed anteriorly to facilitate better orientation intraoperatively (Fig. 3.20a). The 4F Kumpe catheter is loaded via the sidearm graft into the iliac stent graft (Fig. 3.20b), thereby "preloading" the sidearm branch and iliac limb. The modified device is resheathed into the 20F sheath using interrupted silk sutures or umbilical tape to collapse each one of the three self-expandable Z-stents which are removed prior to resheathing. The tip of the 4F Kumpe catheter is positioned slightly over the top of the 20F sheath.

Procedure for Surgeon-Modified Hypogastric Branched Stent Graft

Following bilateral femoral artery cut-down, sheaths are placed in both common femoral arteries. The iliac branch endograft is placed through the ipsilateral groin with the branch directed to the hypogastric branch and positioned above the iliac bifurcation. The wire that is preloaded through the hypogastric branch is advanced to the abdominal aorta and snared from the contralateral femoral artery and brought out the right femoral artery for through-and-through access (we prefer to use a 480-cm Tracer® Metro Wire Guide, Cook Medical). Over this femoral-femoral access wire, a 12-French Ansel-1 sheath is advanced up and over the aortic bifurcation and into the hypogastric branch. A wire and a catheter are then placed through this sheath, and the left hypogastric artery is selectively catheterized, and the wire and catheter are advanced into the tertiary branches of the left internal iliac artery. Selective internal iliac artery angiogram is obtained, demonstrating its patency of the main trunk and all of its branches and the distance between the iliac bifurcation and the branches of the internal iliac artery. A stiff Amplatz wire is then advanced into the tertiary branches of the hypogastric artery, and over this wire, a balloon- or a self-expandable stent graft is placed into the left internal iliac artery, through the hypogastric branched graft (Fig. 3.21). Balloon angioplasty of the stent in the internal iliac artery is performed. The branch stent is typically reinforced by placement of another self-expanding stent that extends into the distal internal iliac artery beyond the covered stent. The remainder of the iliac limb is then deployed into the ipsilateral external iliac artery, and the limb is then balloon angioplastied simultaneously with balloon angioplasty of the hypogastric branched stent in a "kissing balloon fashion." Implantation of the abdominal component of the stent graft completes the procedure (Fig. 3.22).

Results of Sm-FBSG

Data on sm-FBSG are limited to reports from few institutions with larger experience on sm-FBSG.

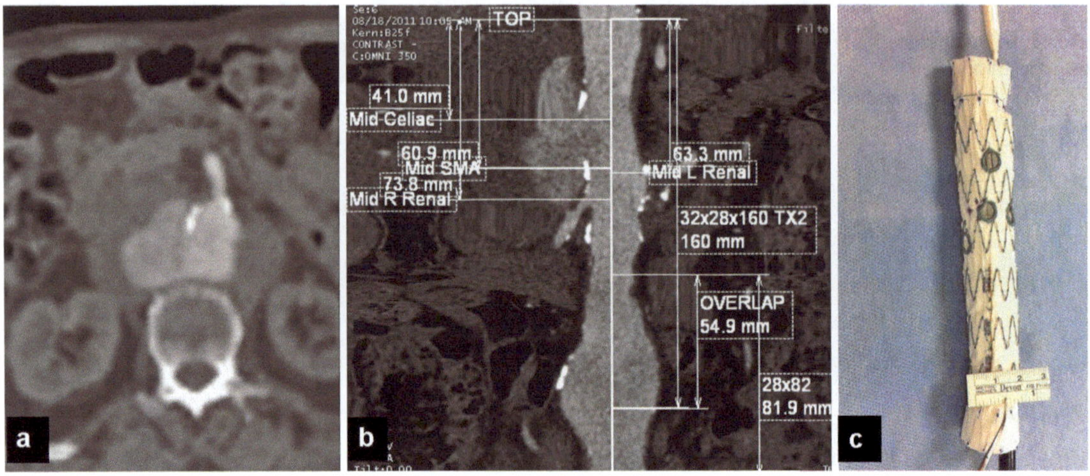

Fig. 3.21 After CT scan of a contained-ruptured type IV thoracoabdominal aneurysm (**a**), centerline of flow analysis reconstruction was performed and measurements were made (**b**) to modify a Zenith TX2 stent graft with four fenestrations for the visceral branches (**c**)

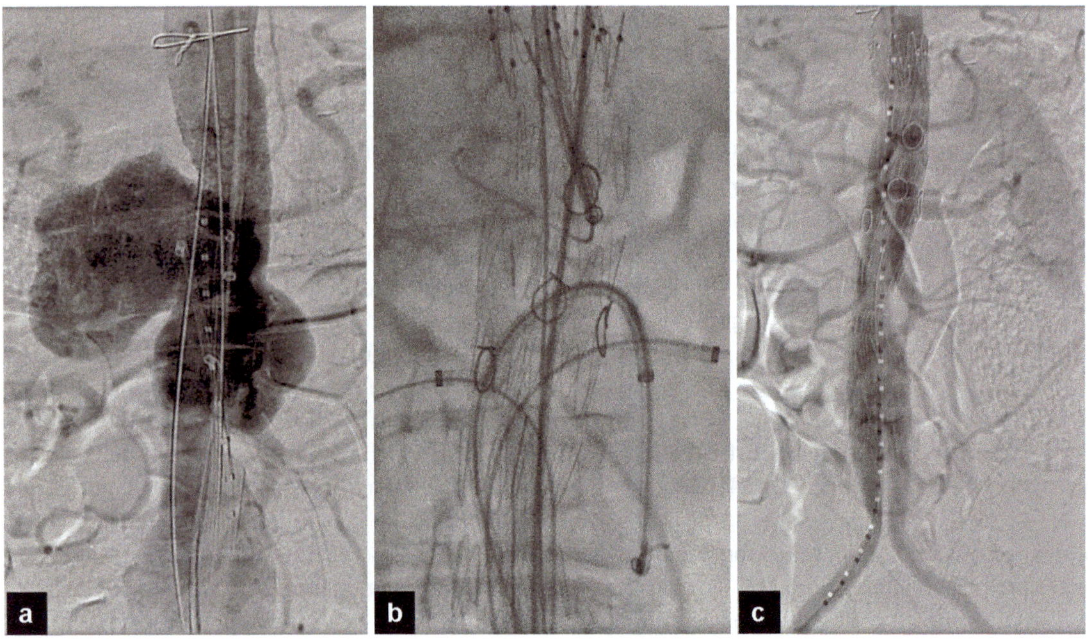

Fig. 3.22 Intraoperative angiograms demonstrating rupture of the aorta at the visceral segment (**a**), successful catheterization of all four fenestrations and target visceral branches with wires and sheaths before release of diameter-reducing ties and complete deployment of the graft (**b**), and successful repair of the ruptured type IV TAAA with patent branches and no evidence of endoleak (**c**)

Recently the group from University of Washington [69] presented a series of 47 consecutive patients who were treated with sm-FBSG over a 3-year period for juxtarenal aortic aneurysms. Eighty-two fenestrations were created for 58 renal arteries, 16 SMAs, 3 celiacs, and 5 for accessory vessels. Early complications included three access site-related and three procedure-related complications including a

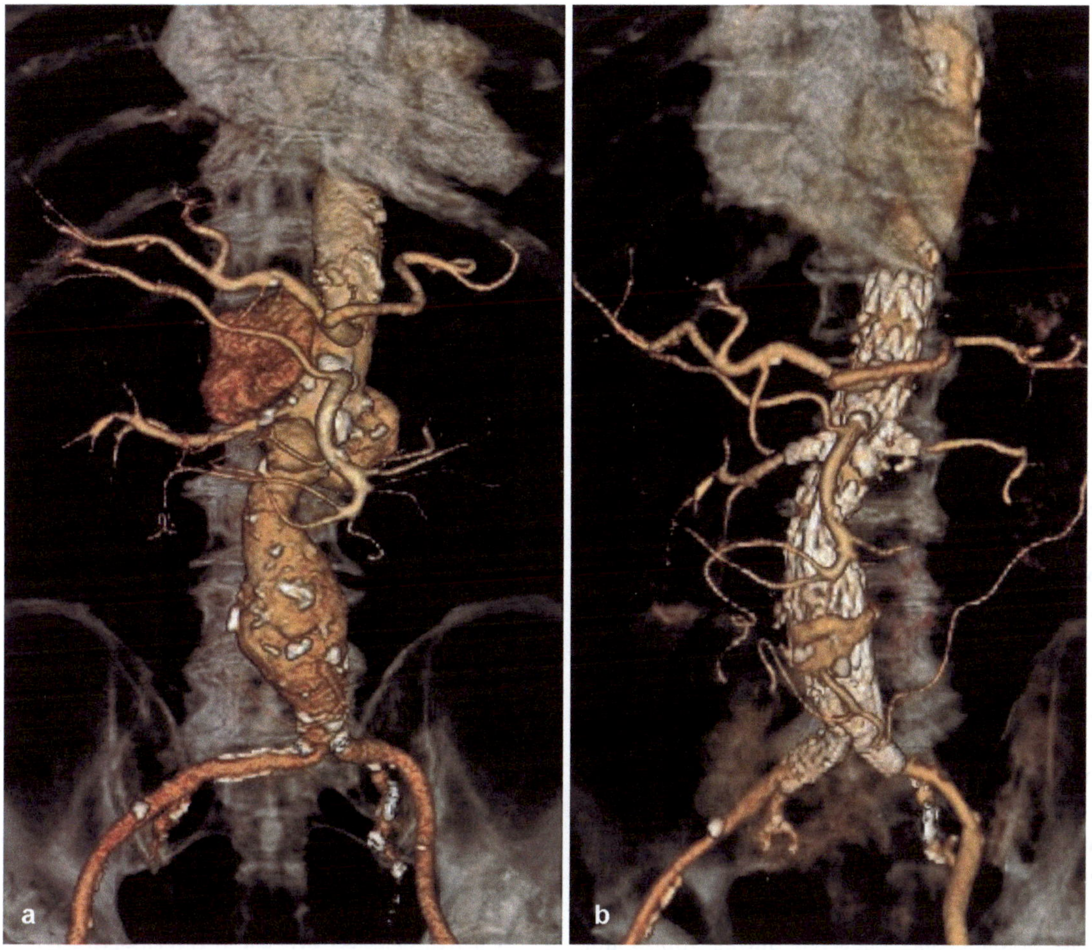

Fig. 3.23 (**a**) Preoperative 3-D CTA in a patient with ruptured visceral aorta. (**b**) CTA at 6 months postoperatively demonstrating no endoleak and patent branch stents to the visceral vessels

stroke, one branch artery dissection, and one renal failure. There was one in-hospital death (2 %) due to aspiration. The authors reported one procedure-related death on follow-up due to distal migration of the graft and SMA occlusion. 12.8 % of the patients had endoleak on follow-up with one patient requiring reintervention.

In 2009, Oderich et al. [70] reviewed their experience of 20 high-risk patients with juxtarenal aneurysm or TAAA, who had 1- to 4-vessel sm-FBSG with branch artery stenting of 52 vessels (32 renal, 18 mesenteric, 2 hypogastric) with reduced mortality (1 %), any morbidity (40 %), and paraplegia rate (5 %).

Sm-FBSG are particularly well suited for the treatment of patients with complex AAA who present urgently or emergently with ruptured or symptomatic aneurysms [43]. We have reported the first series of patients who underwent sm-FBSG repair in the emergency setting [44]. Twelve high-risk patients (7 ASA IV and 5 ASA III) (9 male) presented with symptomatic ($n=7$) or ruptured ($n=5$) aortic aneurysms (Fig. 3.22, and 3.23). Mean age was 71 years (range 52–86 years) and mean maximal aneurysm size 8.1 cm (range 5–12 cm). Six patients (50 %) had prior aortic surgery or a hostile abdomen. Relevant comorbidities included coronary disease in all 12 patients and 7 patients (58 %) with an ejection fraction ≤35 %. Nine patients (75 %) had severe pulmonary dysfunction. Four aneurysms were pararenal and 8 thoracoabdominal

(2 type II, 3 type III, and 3 type IV). The average number of visceral vessels treated per patient was 3 (range 2–4) with 35 total branches revascularized. One renal artery could not be accessed and was sacrificed. Endografts were successfully implanted in all patients. There were no cases of paraplegia, no intraoperative deaths, and one death occurred within 30 days (8.3 %) due to subarachnoid hemorrhage. Reintervention was necessary in two patients, for a type 3 endoleak and for evacuation of retroperitoneal hematoma. Morbidity included one myocardial infarction, two patients with transient respiratory failure, and two with transient renal insufficiency not requiring dialysis. Mean postoperative stay in ICU was 4 days and in-hospital 8 days. At a mean follow-up of 9 months (range 3–18), two patients died of non-aneurysm-related causes.

There were no late reinterventions and all branches, patent at the conclusion of the procedure, remained patent on follow-up (100 %). No type I or III endoleaks occurred, and one type II endoleak is under observation.

So far, none of the groups performing surgeon-modified hypogastric branched stent grafts have published their results. However, in our experience with more than 15 cases, no branch occlusions or endoleaks occurred during follow-up, and all procedures were completed successfully (unpublished data).

Ethical/Legal Implications of Sm-BSG

If one is to perform these procedures, it is imperative to consult their institutional legal department and institutional review board (IRB). In addition, customized operative consent forms must be created detailing that the procedure is performed under "compassionate use" because the patient has no other surgical or endovascular options and their aneurysm is at increased risk of rupture. Ideally, one should obtain a physician-sponsored investigational device exemption (IDE) from the Food and Drug Administration (FDA) as we have done. It should be clearly documented that patients are at an excessive risk for open surgery, have no endovascular alternatives, and are at increased risk of aneurysm rupture. All patients in our practice who were candidates to undergo fenestrated repair of their complex aneurysm with the compassionate use of a sm-FBSG were informed that the use of the grafts were not according to IFU and had an extensive discussion with the primary surgeon with respect to the risks of graft modification, durability of the repair, safety, and efficacy of the procedure. The procedures resulting in this chapter were performed under an IRB protocol and subsequently led to approval of a physician-sponsored IDE by the FDA for pararenal aneurysms and TAAA (MO-dified STE-nt GRA-ft Trial – MOSTEGRA Trial, IDE: G120071).

References

1. Piazza M, Ricotta 2nd JJ. Open surgical repair of thoracoabdominal aortic aneurysms. Ann Vasc Surg. 2011;26:600–5.
2. Patel VI, Lancaster RT, Conrad MF, et al. Comparable mortality with open repair of complex and infrarenal aortic aneurysm. J Vasc Surg. 2011;54:952–9.
3. Jongkind V, Akkersdijk GJ, Yeung KK, Wisselink W. A systematic review of endovascular treatment of extensive aortoiliac occlusive disease. J Vasc Surg. 2010;52:1376–83.
4. Yeung KK, Tangelder GJ, Fung WY, et al. Open surgical repair of ruptured juxtarenal aortic aneurysms with and without renal cooling: observations regarding morbidity and mortality. J Vasc Surg. 2010;51:551–8.
5. Giles KA, Schermerhorn ML, O'Malley AJ, et al. Risk prediction for perioperative mortality of endovascular vs open repair of abdominal aortic aneurysms using the Medicare population. J Vasc Surg. 2009;50:256–62.
6. Brown LC, Thompson SG, Greenhalgh RM, Powell JT. Incidence of cardiovascular events and death after open or endovascular repair of abdominal aortic aneurysm in the randomized EVAR trial 1. Br J Surg. 2011;98: 935–42.
7. De Bruin JL, Baas AF, Buth J, et al. Long-term outcome of open or endovascular repair of abdominal aortic aneurysm. N Engl J Med. 2010;362:1881–9.
8. Greenhalgh RM, Brown LC, Kwong GP, Powell JT, Thompson SG. Comparison of endovascular aneurysm repair with open repair in patients with abdominal aortic aneurysm (EVAR trial 1), 30-day operative mortality results: randomised controlled trial. Lancet. 2004;364:843–8.
9. Lee WA, Daniels MJ, Beaver TM, Klodell CT, Raghinaru DE, Hess Jr PJ. Late outcomes of a single-center experience of 400 consecutive thoracic endovascular aortic repairs. Circulation. 2011;123:2938–45.

10. Veith FJ, Lachat M, Mayer D, et al. Collected world and single center experience with endovascular treatment of ruptured abdominal aortic aneurysms. Ann Surg. 2009;250:818–24.
11. Jonker FH, Verhagen HJ, Lin PH, et al. Outcomes of endovascular repair of ruptured descending thoracic aortic aneurysms. Circulation. 2010;121:2718–23.
12. Arko FR, Filis KA, Seidel SA, et al. How many patients with infrarenal aneurysms are candidates for endovascular repair? The Northern California experience. J Endovasc Ther. 2004;11:33–40.
13. Cotroneo AR, Iezzi R, Giancristofaro D, et al. Endovascular abdominal aortic aneurysm repair: how many patients are eligible for endovascular repair? Radiol Med. 2006;111:597–606.
14. Schanzer A, Greenberg RK, Hevelone N, et al. Predictors of abdominal aortic aneurysm sac enlargement after endovascular repair. Circulation. 2011;123: 2848–55.
15. Kertai MD, Steyerberg EW, Boersma E, et al. Validation of two risk models for perioperative mortality in patients undergoing elective abdominal aortic aneurysm surgery. Vasc Endovascular Surg. 2003;37:13–21.
16. Brown LC, Greenhalgh RM, Howell S, Powell JT, Thompson SG. Patient fitness and survival after abdominal aortic aneurysm repair in patients from the UK EVAR trials. Br J Surg. 2007;94:709–16.
17. Greenberg RK, Chuter TA, Cambria RP, Sternbergh 3rd WC, Fearnot NE. Zenith abdominal aortic aneurysm endovascular graft. J Vasc Surg. 2008;48:1–9.
18. Ehsan O, Murray D, Farquharson F, Serracino-Inglott F. Endovascular repair of complex aortic aneurysms. Ann Vasc Surg. 2011;25:716–25.
19. Elefteriades JA. Natural history of thoracic aortic aneurysms: indications for surgery, and surgical versus nonsurgical risks. Ann Thorac Surg. 2002;74: S1877–80; discussion S92–8.
20. Davies RR, Goldstein LJ, Coady MA, et al. Yearly rupture or dissection rates for thoracic aortic aneurysms: simple prediction based on size. Ann Thorac Surg. 2002;73:17–27; discussion 27–8.
21. Cambria RA, Gloviczki P, Stanson AW, et al. Outcome and expansion rate of 57 thoracoabdominal aortic aneurysms managed nonoperatively. Am J Surg. 1995;170:213–7.
22. Ricco JB, Cau J, Marchand C, et al. Stent-graft repair for thoracic aortic disease: results of an independent nationwide study in France from 1999 to 2001. J Thorac Cardiovasc Surg. 2006;131:131–7.
23. Escobar GA, Upchurch Jr GR. Management of thoracoabdominal aortic aneurysms. Curr Probl Surg. 2011;48:70–133.
24. Huynh TT, van Eps RG, Miller 3rd CC, et al. Glomerular filtration rate is superior to serum creatinine for prediction of mortality after thoracoabdominal aortic surgery. J Vasc Surg. 2005;42:206–12.
25. Chuter TA. Branched and fenestrated stent grafts for endovascular repair of thoracic aortic aneurysms. J Vasc Surg. 2006;43(Suppl A):111A–5A.
26. Chuter TA, Reilly LM. Endovascular treatment of thoracoabdominal aortic aneurysms. J Cardiovasc Surg (Torino). 2006;47:619–28.
27. Verhoeven EL, Tielliu IF, Muhs BE, et al. Fenestrated and branched stent-grafting: a 5-years experience. Acta Chir Belg. 2006;106:317–22.
28. AbuRahma AF, Campbell J, Stone PA, et al. The correlation of aortic neck length to early and late outcomes in endovascular aneurysm repair patients. J Vasc Surg. 2009;50:738–48.
29. Verhoeven EL, Vourliotakis G, Bos WT, et al. Fenestrated stent grafting for short-necked and juxtarenal abdominal aortic aneurysm: an 8-year single-centre experience. Eur J Vasc Endovasc Surg. 2010;39: 529–36.
30. Ricotta II JJ, Duncan AA, Harbuzariu C, et al. SS37. Open surgical repair of pararenal abdominal aortic aneurysms: long-term outcomes of renal function. J Vasc Surg. 2009;49:S13.
31. Bockler D, Kotelis D, Geisbusch P, et al. Hybrid procedures for thoracoabdominal aortic aneurysms and chronic aortic dissections - a single center experience in 28 patients. J Vasc Surg. 2008;47:724–32.
32. Drinkwater SL, Bockler D, Eckstein H, et al. The visceral hybrid repair of thoraco-abdominal aortic aneurysms–a collaborative approach. Eur J Vasc Endovasc Surg. 2009;38:578–85.
33. Patel R, Conrad MF, Paruchuri V, Kwolek CJ, Chung TK, Cambria RP. Thoracoabdominal aneurysm repair: hybrid versus open repair. J Vasc Surg. 2009;50:15–22.
34. Chiesa R, Tshomba Y, Marone EM, et al. Hybrid procedures for the treatment of thoracoabdominal aortic aneurysms and dissections. J Cardiovasc Surg (Torino). 2010;51:821–32.
35. Moulakakis KG, Mylonas SN, Avgerinos ED, Kakisis JD, Brunkwall J, Liapis CD. Hybrid open endovascular technique for aortic thoracoabdominal pathologies. Circulation. 2011;124:2670–80.
36. Bruen KJ, Feezor RJ, Daniels MJ, Beck AW, Lee WA. Endovascular chimney technique versus open repair of juxtarenal and suprarenal aneurysms. J Vasc Surg. 2011;53:895–904; discussion904–5.
37. Brechtel K, Ketelsen D, Endisch A, et al. Endovascular repair of acute symptomatic pararenal aortic aneurysm with three chimney and one periscope graft for complete visceral artery revascularization. Cardiovasc Intervent Radiol. 2011;35:413–7.
38. Moulakakis KG, Mylonas SN, Avgerinos E, et al. The chimney graft technique for preserving visceral vessels during endovascular treatment of aortic pathologies. J Vasc Surg. 2012;55:1497–503.
39. Verhoeven E, Tielliu IF, Zeebregts CJ, et al. Results of endovascular repair of TAAA in the first 50 patients. Zentralbl Chir. 2011;136:451–7.
40. Greenberg R, Eagleton M, Mastracci T. Branched endografts for thoracoabdominal aneurysms. J Thorac Cardiovasc Surg. 2010;140:S171–8.
41. Greenberg RK, Sternbergh 3rd WC, Makaroun M, et al. Intermediate results of a United States multicenter trial of fenestrated endograft repair for juxtarenal

abdominal aortic aneurysms. J Vasc Surg. 2009;50: 730–7.e1.
42. Sweet MP, Hiramoto JS, Park KH, Reilly LM, Chuter TA. A standardized multi-branched thoracoabdominal stent-graft for endovascular aneurysm repair. J Endovasc Ther. 2009;16:359–64.
43. Ricotta JJ, Tsilimparis N. Surgeon-modified fenestrated and branched stent grafts – an alternative method for treating complex aortic emergencies in patients who are unfit for surgery. J Endovasc Today. 2011;11:55–60.
44. Ricotta II JJ, Tsilimparis N. Outcomes of surgeon-modified fenestrated-branched stent-grafts to emergently treat ruptured and symptomatic complex aortic aneurysms in high risk-patients. J Vasc Surg. 2012;in press.
45. Chuter TA, Hiramoto JS, Park KH, Reilly LM. The transition from custom-made to standardized multi-branched thoracoabdominal aortic stent grafts. J Vasc Surg. 2011;54:660–8.
46. Chuter T, Greenberg RK. Standardized off-the-shelf components for multibranched endovascular repair of thoracoabdominal aortic aneurysms. Perspect Vasc Surg Endovasc Ther. 2011;23:195–201.
47. Azzaoui R, Sobocinski J, Maurel B, et al. Anatomic study of juxta renal aneurysms: impact on fenestrated stent-grafts. Ann Vasc Surg. 2011;25:315–21.
48. Sobocinski J, d'Utra G, O'Brien N, et al. Off-the-shelf fenestrated endografts: a realistic option for more than 70 % of patients with juxtarenal aneurysms. J Endovasc Ther. 2012;19:165–72.
49. Resch TA, Dias NV, Sobocinski J, Sonesson B, Roeder B, Haulon S. Development of off-the-shelf stent grafts for juxtarenal abdominal aortic aneurysms. Eur J Vasc Endovasc Surg. 2012;43:655–60.
50. Clair D, Holden A, Hill A, Mertens R, Marine L. Initial pilot study outcomes of the Ventana fenestrated stent graft system for endovascular repair of juxtarenal and pararenal aortic aneurysms. In: SCVS, Las Vegas, 2012.
51. Greenberg RK, Qureshi M. Fenestrated and branched devices in the pipeline. J Vasc Surg. 2010;52:15S–21S.
52. Bungay PM, Burfitt N, Sritharan K, et al. Initial experience with a new fenestrated stent graft. J Vasc Surg. 2011;54:1832–8.
53. Chuter TA. Fenestrated and branched stent-grafts for thoracoabdominal, pararenal and juxtarenal aortic aneurysm repair. Semin Vasc Surg. 2007;20:90–6.
54. Haulon S, Amiot S, Magnan PE, et al. An analysis of the French multicentre experience of fenestrated aortic endografts: medium-term outcomes. Ann Surg. 2010;251:357–62.
55. Park JH, Chung JW, Choo IW, Kim SJ, Lee JY, Han MC. Fenestrated stent-grafts for preserving visceral arterial branches in the treatment of abdominal aortic aneurysms: preliminary experience. J Vasc Interv Radiol. 1996;7:819–23.
56. Browne TF, Hartley D, Purchas S, Rosenberg M, Van Schie G, Lawrence-Brown M. A fenestrated covered suprarenal aortic stent. Eur J Vasc Endovasc Surg. 1999;18:445–9.
57. Anderson JL, Berce M, Hartley DE. Endoluminal aortic grafting with renal and superior mesenteric artery incorporation by graft fenestration. J Endovasc Ther. 2001;8:3–15.
58. Ricotta 2nd JJ, Oderich GS. Fenestrated and branched stent grafts. Perspect Vasc Surg Endovasc Ther. 2008;20:174–87; discussion 88–9.
59. Oderich GS, Ricotta 2nd JJ. Modified fenestrated stent grafts: device design, modifications, implantation, and current applications. Perspect Vasc Surg Endovasc Ther. 2009;21:157–67.
60. Lee WA. Endovascular abdominal aortic aneurysm sizing and case planning using the TeraRecon Aquarius workstation. Vasc Endovascular Surg. 2007; 41:61–7.
61. Morgan-Rowe L, Simring D, Raja J, Agu O, Ivancev K, Hague J. Techniques for removing bilateral renal artery stents prior to fenestrated endovascular aneurysm repair. J Endovasc Ther. 2012;19:96–9.
62. Ricotta 2nd JJ. Commentary: fenestrated and branched stent-grafts for the treatment of thoracoabdominal aortic aneurysms: the future is now. J Endovasc Ther. 2010;17:212–5.
63. Donas KP, Torsello G, Pitoulias GA, Austermann M, Papadimitriou DK. Surgical versus endovascular repair by iliac branch device of aneurysms involving the iliac bifurcation. J Vasc Surg. 2011;53: 1223–9.
64. Torsello G, Schonefeld E, Osada N, Austermann M, Pennekamp C, Donas KP. Endovascular treatment of common iliac artery aneurysms using the bell-bottom technique: long-term results. J Endovasc Ther. 2010; 17:504–9.
65. Hiramoto JS, Reilly LM, Schneider DB, Rapp JH, Chuter TAM. The upside-down zenith stent graft limb. Vascular. 2009;17:93–5.
66. Arochena NJM, Feijoo GR, Fernandez CC, et al. Use of modified sandwich-graft technique to preserve hypogastric artery in EVAR treatment of complex aortic aneurysm anatomy. J Cardiovasc Surg. 2011;52: 643–9.
67. Verzini F, Parlani G, Romano L, De Rango P, Panuccio G, Cao P. Endovascular treatment of iliac aneurysm: concurrent comparison of side branch endograft versus hypogastric exclusion. J Vasc Surg. 2009;49: 1154–61.
68. Oderich GS, Ricotta 2nd JJ. Novel surgeon-modified hypogastric branch stent graft to preserve pelvic perfusion. Ann Vasc Surg. 2010;24:278–86.
69. Starnes BW. Physician-modified endovascular grafts for the treatment of elective, symptomatic, or ruptured juxtarenal aortic aneurysms. J Vasc Surg. 2012;56:601–7. Epub 2012 May 2.
70. Oderich GS, Ricotta II JJ, Hofer J, et al. RR11. Surgeon-modified fenestrated and branched stent grafts for high risk patients with juxtarenal, paravisceral and thoracoabdominal aortic aneurysms: comparison with open abdominal debranching in a single center. J Vasc Surg. 2009;49:S48–S9.

Pelvic Revascularization During Endovascular Aortic Aneurysm Repair

4

Javairiah Fatima and Gustavo S. Oderich

Abstract

Endovascular repair of aortic aneurysms (EVAR) has gained widespread acceptance in the treatment of abdominal aortic aneurysms (AAAs). Prospective randomized studies have shown several short-term advantages compared to open surgical repair, including less blood loss, operating time, length of stay, morbidity, and mortality. The long-term efficacy of EVAR is dependent upon careful selection of patients with respect to anatomical factors such as excessive angulation, vessel tortuosity, or involvement of visceral or iliac arteries. Although many of these anatomical constraints were previously considered to be relative contraindications to EVAR, technological advances have expanded the indications to include patients with more challenging anatomy. This chapter summarizes the evolution of methods used for preservation of pelvic flow in patients with aortoiliac aneurysms involving one or both common iliac arteries.

Keywords

Iliac artery • Stent graft • Bypass • EVAR • Artery

Background

Endovascular repair of aortic aneurysms (EVAR) has gained widespread acceptance in the treatment of abdominal aortic aneurysms (AAAs). Prospective randomized studies have shown several short-term advantages compared to open surgical repair, including less blood loss, operating time, length of stay, morbidity, and mortality. The long-term efficacy of EVAR is dependent upon careful selection of patients with respect to anatomical factors such as excessive angulation, vessel tortuosity, or involvement of visceral or iliac arteries. Although many of these anatomical constraints were previously considered to be relative contraindications to EVAR, technological advances have expanded the indications to include patients with more challenging anatomy. This chapter summarizes the evolution of methods used for preservation of pelvic flow in patients with aortoiliac aneurysms involving one or both common iliac arteries.

J. Fatima
Department of Surgery, Mayo Clinic,
Rochester, MN, USA

G.S. Oderich, M.D., FACS (✉)
Department of Vascular and Endovascular Surgery,
Gonda Vascular Center, Mayo Clinic Medical College,
200 First Street SW, Rochester, MN 55905, USA
e-mail: oderich.gustavo@mayo.edu

J.J. Hoballah, A.B. Lumsden (eds.), *Vascular Surgery*, New Techniques in Surgery Series,
DOI 10.1007/978-1-4471-2912-7_4, © Springer-Verlag London 2012

Scope of the Problem

Approximately 30 % of patients treated by EVAR have ectatic or aneurysmal common iliac arteries not suitable for distal sealing zone [1, 2]. Common iliac artery aneurysms affect one iliac artery in 43 % of patients and both iliac arteries in 11 % [1, 3]. One of the most frequently utilized options in these patients is exclusion of the internal iliac artery by placement of coils or endovascular plugs, allowing placement of iliac limbs into the external iliac artery without retrograde type II endoleak. While unilateral and bilateral internal iliac artery exclusions can be safely done in most patients, decreased pelvic perfusion carries risk of ischemic complications. A frequently underreported event is buttock claudication, which occurs in 16–50 % of patients treated by unilateral and up to 80 % of those undergoing bilateral embolization [4–7]. Sexual dysfunction is noted in 10–17 % [4, 5, 8, 9]. In addition, although uncommon, devastating complications include spinal cord injury, ischemic colitis, and gluteal muscle necrosis [10]. Among patients requiring extensive aortic coverage of the thoracic or thoracoabdominal aorta, preservation of pelvic flow via the internal iliac arteries has been shown to be an important collateral network, reducing rates of spinal cord injury [11–13].

"Bell-Bottom" or Flared Iliac Stent Graft Limbs

Flared iliac stent graft limbs are typically utilized in patients with small common iliac artery aneurysms up to 21 mm in diameter (Fig. 4.1). The technique can also be done with off-label use of aortic extension cuffs, allowing treatment of larger common iliac aneurysms. Ideally, the common iliac artery should not be affected by thrombus or excessive calcification. In these patients, a shorter bifurcated device may be selected and introduced via the contralateral side, allowing a longer working length for precise deployment of the intended flared iliac limb close to the iliac bifurcation. Table 4.1 summarizes the sizes and indications of commercially available iliac stent graft limbs. Although the use of "bell-bottom" grafts simplifies the repair, the durability of this procedure remains questionable and few clinical reports have shown long-term data.

Lawrence-Brown and colleagues from Western Australia reported that iliac arteries between 16

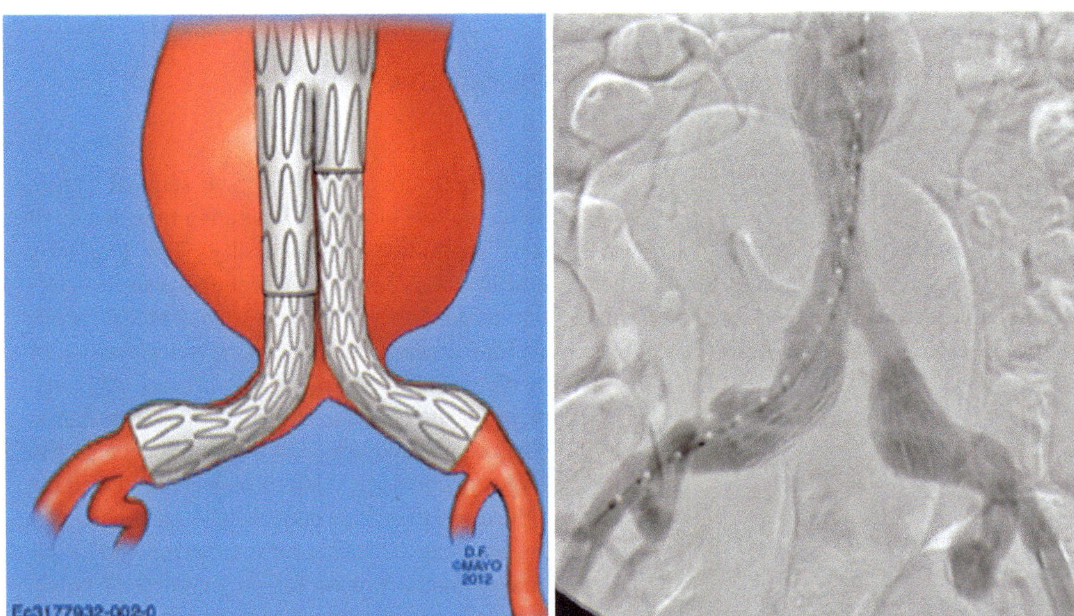

Fig. 4.1 "Bell-bottom" technique using flared iliac stent graft limbs for treatment of bilateral common iliac aneurysms

and 22 mm in diameter can be treated with 90 % efficacy using "bell-bottom" grafts [14]. However, after a mean follow-up of 30 months, endoleaks were noted in 40 % of patients, including type Ib endoleaks in 7 %. Secondary re-interventions for iliac artery-related problems were needed in 10 % of the patients. Woo and associates reviewed the prospective cohort of patients treated by Cook Zenith stent grafts (Cook Medical Inc, Bloomington, IN) in the Cook Zenith US multicenter trial of 671 patients. In that study, 220 patients required flared iliac limbs in common iliac arteries with landing zone >20 mm. They did not find a higher rate of increase in iliac artery diameter, endoleaks, or re-interventions compared to patients with "normal" iliac diameter. A type Ib endoleak occurred in only 2.2 % of patients [15]. However, a recent report by the Mayo Clinic group showed that use of "bell-bottom" outside the recommendations for use is potentially associated with higher rates of complications. In that report, 71 patients treated by 93 limbs with mean iliac artery diameter of 23 mm were followed for mean follow-up of 29 months. Continued iliac artery enlargement >5 mm was noted in 86 % of the patients, and 17 % had iliac limb events, which included sac growth >5 mm, type Ib endoleak, and re-intervention. Freedom from iliac limb events and iliac limb re-interventions at 2 years were 87 ± 6 % and 96 ± 6 %, respectively (unpublished data).

Table 4.1 Commercially available iliac stent graft limbs

Device	Iliac limb diameters (mm)	Minimal iliac landing zone length (mm)	Distal iliac diameters (mm)
Cook Zenith	8–24	10	7–20
Gore Excluder	10–20	10	8–18
Medtronic AneuRx	12–24	15	8–20
Medtronic Talent	8–24	15	7–20
Endologix Powerlink	16–25	15	10–22

Internal Iliac Artery Bypass or Transposition

Open surgical revascularization of the internal iliac artery can be performed using retroperitoneal approach with a small curvilinear flank incision (Fig. 4.2). Since its first description in 1999

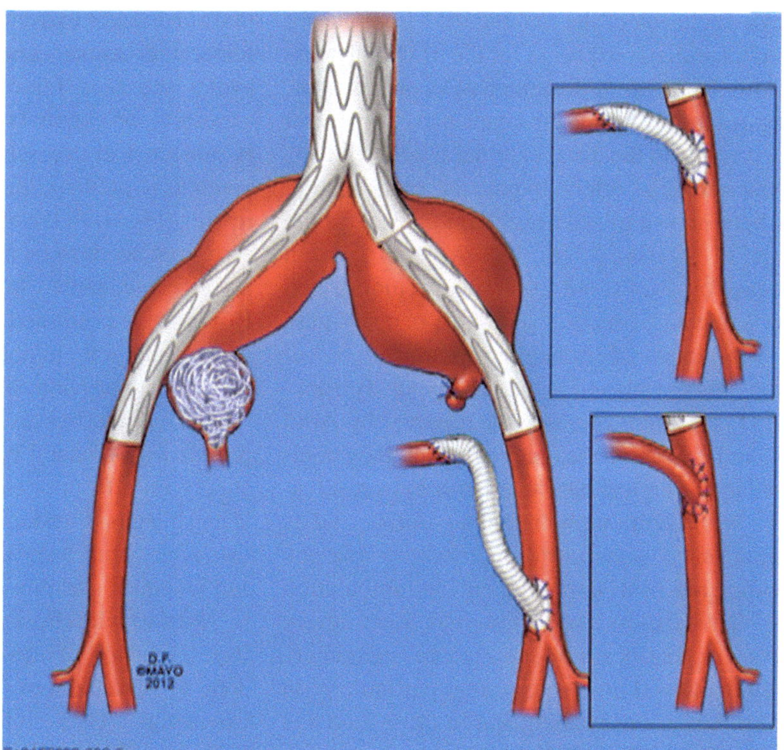

Fig. 4.2 Techniques of open surgical internal iliac artery revascularization using bypass or translocation

by Juan Parodi and Marcelo Ferreira, hybrid revascularization of the internal iliac artery has been widely adopted as an alternative to coil embolization [16]. The technique is also useful in patients with small iliac artery diameter who require iliac artery conduit.

The iliac arteries are exposed using retroperitoneal approach. The ureter should be identified and protected, avoiding excessive manipulation or devascularization of soft tissue. After exposure and dissection of the common, internal, and iliac arteries, the patient is systemically heparinized. The proximal internal iliac artery is ligated with 1-0 Ethibond suture, clamped distally, and transected. The proximal stump should be oversewn with running 4-0 Prolene suture. A 6- or 7-mm polyester graft is anastomosed end to end to the internal iliac arteries using 4- or 5-0 Prolene and "parachute technique." After the anastomosis is tested, the graft is clamped and attention is directed to the proximal anastomosis. A useful technique is to proceed with EVAR using femoral approach and to perform the proximal anastomosis of the internal iliac graft in the location of the femoral puncture at the end of the procedure. This avoids occlusion of the internal iliac graft during EVAR, facilitates exposure for the proximal anastomosis, and allows documentation of graft patency. Alternatively, the proximal anastomosis can also be done to the distal external iliac artery.

Internal iliac artery bypass or transposition has been shown to offer excellent patency in the range of 80–100 % [6, 16]. A report of ten patients by Faries and associates demonstrated 100 % technical success and graft patency with no symptoms of ischemic complications of colon, gluteal claudication, or sexual dysfunction [17]. Similar results were reported by Arko [18] and Lee and colleagues [6] when they compared open surgical internal iliac artery preservation with coil embolization. Both studies demonstrated significant decrease in buttock claudication and improvement in ambulation [19]. Nonetheless, open internal iliac artery bypass or transposition can also be technically challenging and time consuming, particularly in the morbidly obese patient and in those who had prior pelvic operations or radiation.

Endovascular Pelvic Revascularization

One of the basic tenets of vascular reconstruction is to preserve normal anatomy and end-organ flow whenever possible. A variety of creative methods have been described to preserve pelvic flow in patients with aortoiliac aneurysms using total endovascular techniques. Iliac branch devices designed to preserve flow into the internal iliac artery have been shown to be clinically effective and safe. However, access to these devices is still limited, and long-term follow-up is needed to determine branch patency and rates of iliac-related secondary interventions. Total endovascular techniques utilized to preserve iliac flow are described below.

External to Internal Iliac Artery Stenting with Femoral Crossover Grafts

The technique of external to internal iliac artery stenting was described by Bergamini and associates [20] and used successfully by Woo and colleagues [21]. The original description included aneurysm exclusion with aorto-uni-iliac stent graft and lower extremity revascularization with femoral crossover graft. While this technique avoids the need for retroperitoneal iliac artery exposure, the external to internal iliac artery stent is subjected to excessive tortuosity and kinking, potentially predisposing to late occlusion or narrowing (Fig. 4.3). It is not infrequent that the covered stent needs to be reinforced by placement of a self-expandable stent to prevent kinking. However, it is limited in being a viable option when only one hypogastric artery patency is sufficient to provide adequate pelvic perfusion.

The author has used this technique in one patient with bilateral common iliac artery stump aneurysms after prior aortofemoral graft (Fig. 4.4). Using bilateral transfemoral approach, the internal iliac artery branches were selectively catheterized and an Ansel sheath was advanced over a 0.035-in. Amplatz wire (Boston Scientific, Bloomington, IN). Exclusion of the common iliac artery was done by placement of Fluency stent grafts (Bard, Covington, GA) with reinforcement using Wallstents (Boston Scientific, Bloomington, IN).

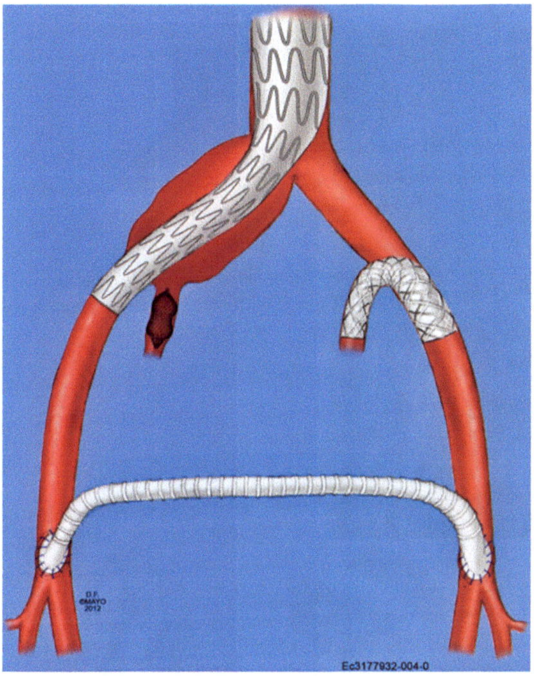

Fig. 4.3 External to internal iliac artery stent graft with femoral crossover bypass

A modification of the technique was described by Delle and associates. The authors described placement of an internal iliac artery stent using transbrachial approach, originated from one of the iliac docking limbs of the bifurcated graft to the internal iliac artery. A femoral crossover graft was used to revascularize the lower extremity (Fig. 4.5). While these techniques allow pelvic revascularization by endovascular techniques, limitations include need for extra-anatomic open surgical reconstruction of the femoral arteries, which is potentially associated with decreased patency and risk of graft infection.

Iliac Sandwich or Parallel Stent Grafts

The "sandwich" technique applies the principle of chimney or parallel stent grafts to preserve flow into one or both internal iliac arteries. The technique was introduced by Armando Lobato, allowing endovascular repair with commercially available iliac limb extensions and stent grafts (Fig. 4.6) [22].

The "sandwich" technique requires transbrachial approach for placement of a covered stent from one or both docking limbs of the bifurcated aortic stent graft into the internal iliac artery, while a parallel stent graft maintains flow into the external iliac artery. Ipsilateral femoral artery approach is used to introduce the main stent graft body with iliac limb positioned 1 cm above the IIA takeoff. The IIA is then cannulated via brachial access, and a covered self-expanding stent is introduced over an extra-stiff guidewire with floppy tip. Iliac limb extension is positioned 1 cm below the IIA stent and deployed, followed by deployment and angioplasty of the IIA covered stent. Lobato advocates an overlap of at least 5 cm between the internal iliac and the external iliac stents to minimize risk of endoleak within the gutters of both stents [22]. Limitations of the technique include the need to use longer internal iliac stents as compared to branched devices, the potential for compression of one of the parallel grafts, and lack of long-term controlled data on limb occlusion and endoleaks. Despite these considerations, the technique has been endorsed by several centers with low rates of limb occlusion and endoleaks in early follow-up [23–25].

Double Bifurcated Aortic Stent Graft

The use of two aortic bifurcated stent grafts has been described to preserve internal iliac artery flow. The technique has been described using two Gore Excluder stent grafts (WL Gore, Flagstaff, AZ). The first aortic stent graft is deployed, followed by a short 20-mm iliac limb extension. A second 23-mm Gore Excluder aortic stent graft is deployed into the 20-mm iliac limb (Fig. 4.7). Using the brachial approach, the shorter docking limb of the second bifurcated device is bridged into the internal iliac artery using Excluder iliac limb extension or Viabahn stent grafts (WL Gore, Flagstaff, AZ). A limitation of the technique is the added cost and need for longer lengths between the renal arteries and the aortic and iliac bifurcations.

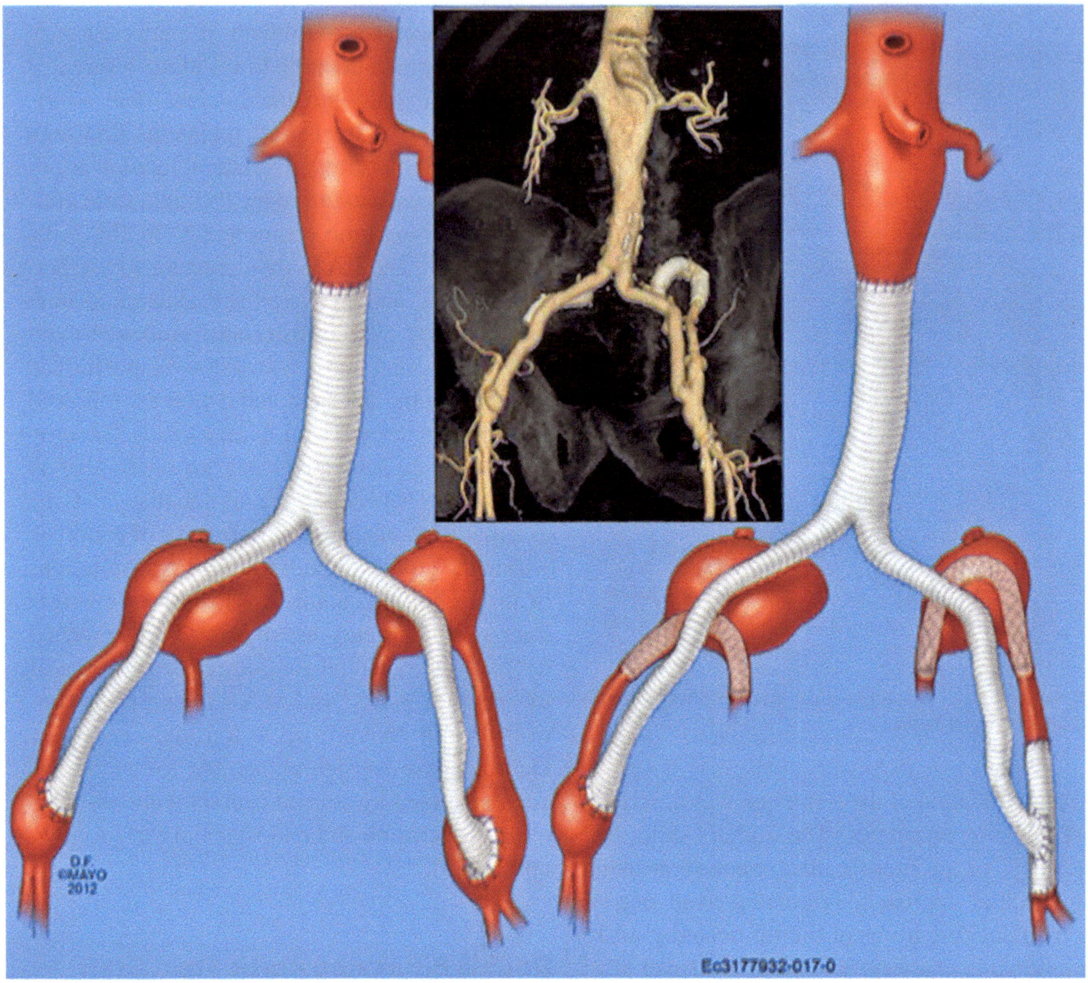

Fig. 4.4 Treatment of bilateral common iliac artery stump aneurysms with external to internal iliac artery stent grafts. Note follow-up CTA revealing no endoleak and occlusion of the right side stent

Iliac Bifurcation Devices (IBDs)

IBDs allow total endovascular repair of aortoiliac aneurysms using specifically designed stent graft configuration to provide optimal seal and flow dynamics into the internal and external iliac arteries. IBDs are designed for patients with inadequate distal landing zone at the common iliac artery, allowing incorporation of the internal iliac artery by preserving pelvic flow via the iliac side branch. The IBD is mated to the internal iliac artery using a balloon-expandable or self-expandable stent graft. Current clinical experience is limited to designs by Cook Medical Inc. The pipeline has evolved to three main types of IBDs (Fig. 4.8) [26]. The designs are the Zenith bifurcated iliac side (ZBIS) branch device, also known as straight side-arm (S-IBD) IBD, the helical branch (H-IBD), and the bifurcated-bifurcated IBD (BB-IBD). The straight side-arm has a relatively short overlapping zone and is intended for use with a balloon-expandable stent graft. A modification of the S-IBD using a flexible longer straight arm akin to a non-wrapped H-IBD has also been applied clinically using a self-expandable stent graft. The H-IBD design is intended for use with a self-expandable stent graft by providing a longer overlapping zone. Both devices maintain the modular concept and are joined to a conventional Zenith

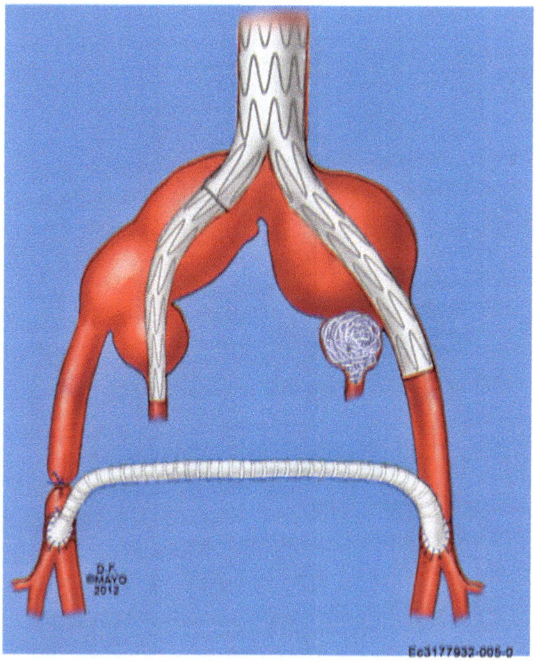

Fig. 4.5 Aortic stent graft to internal iliac artery stent graft with femoral crossover graft

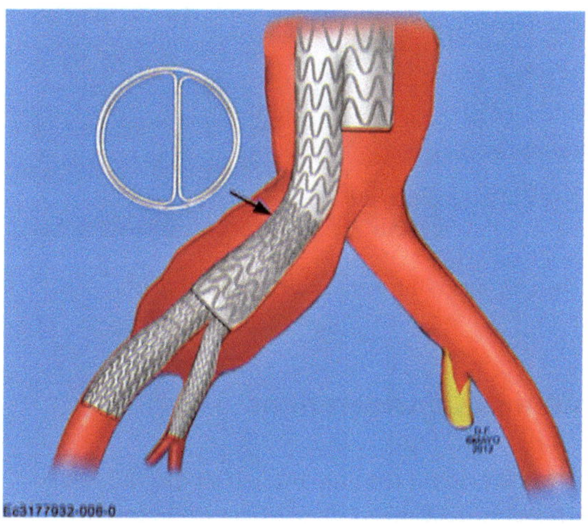

Fig. 4.6 "Sandwich" technique using parallel stent grafts. Note in the inset the gutters and partial compression of the stent graft

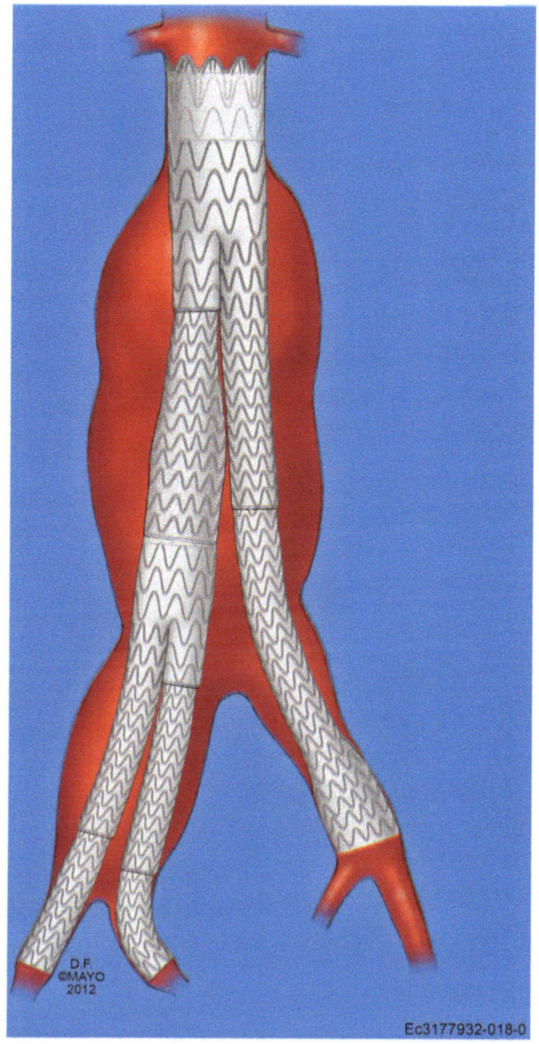

Fig. 4.7 Double bifurcated stent graft technique using Gore Excluder stent grafts (WL Gore, Flagstaff, AZ)

bifurcated stent graft (Cook Medical, Bloomington, IN) by an extension limb component. The S- and H-IBD utilize the same 20 Fr delivery system that includes a preloaded catheter through the branch and out of the proximal aspect of the device. The preloaded catheter allows introduction of a wire, which is snared from an alternative site (usually the contralateral groin but also the brachial approach) and provides ready access through the branch with a sheath.

The third and latest development is the bifurcated-bifurcated IBD or BB-IBD (Fig. 4.8). This device involves a combination of the H-IBD with the distal bifurcated component of a fenestrated device. The addition of the helical sidearm to the ipsilateral (long) limb of a bifurcated aortic device makes conceptual sense, as it

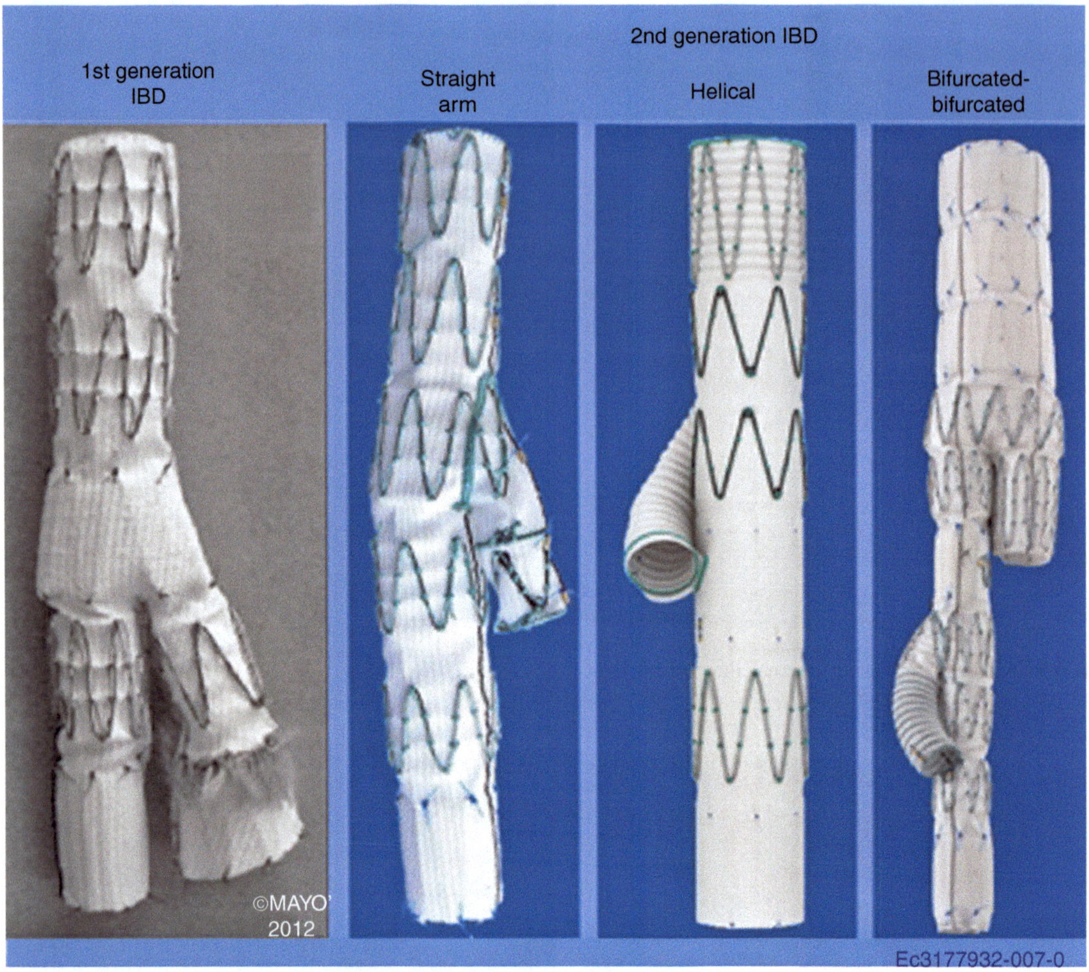

Fig. 4.8 Iliac branch devices (*IBD*) designs include the straight, helical, and bifurcated-bifurcated stent grafts

eliminates two modular joints from an IBD repair but relegates access into the internal iliac branch to the brachial/axillary circulation. The limitation is overcome by the development of a self-sealing fenestration immediately cranially to the ostium of the helical branch origin on the medial wall of the iliac limb. The self-sealing fenestration is used in conjunction with a preloaded wire, which is snared in a manner identical to that with standard IBD devices. Matting of the helical limb is completed as above, and when the preloaded wire is removed, the sealing segment (a covered Z-stent) then resides over the fenestration, functionally excluding the aneurysm.

Anatomic Considerations

Anatomic criteria for iliac branch stent grafts have not been standardized or validated. Factors to be considered include the presence of excessive iliac tortuosity, calcifications, or stenosis, and characteristics of the distal internal iliac artery, including aneurysmal involvement with inadequate distal landing zone for the IBD or poor runoff because of distal branch vessel disease. In most reports, IBDs are indicated in patients with common iliac aneurysms greater than 20–24 mm. In general, the distal fixation in the external iliac artery requires a minimum length of 20 mm and a "normal diameter" of 8–12 mm – and this is rarely a problem. For the H-IBD and S-IBD, the common iliac artery should have a minimum length of 50 mm, or else the IBD device will extend high up into the abdominal aorta, potentially destabilizing the more proximal repair. The presence of internal iliac artery stenosis is not a contraindication but may increase technical difficulty. The internal iliac artery should have a non-aneurysmal segment (fixation site) of >10 mm length and inner-wall diameter of 6–10 mm. However, the latter can be overcome with use of smaller-diameter matting stent grafts. It is important to note that there is considerable tortuosity in many internal and external iliac arteries particularly in the setting of a large common iliac artery aneurysm; as such, aneurysms grow in length as well as diameter. As they do so, they distort the origin of the internal iliac artery, creating tortuosity of the main internal iliac artery trunk and also creating potentially extreme tortuosity in the external iliac system.

Technique

Assuming that the repair involves an aortic component as well as an IBD, the femoral arteries are exposed and the patient is systemically anticoagulated with intravenous heparin. The ipsilateral femoral artery is accessed using two femoral punctures (Fig. 4.9). The main aortic device is usually introduced via the side opposite to the IBD, which can be done prior or after placement of the proximal aortic component. The target internal iliac artery should be imaged prior to deploying an IBD above the vessel. This can be done prior to introduction of the IBD device or afterward, following snaring of the preloaded wire. Following insertion of the IBD over a stiff wire, it is oriented such that the three markers immediately distal to the distal branch ostium align with the internal iliac ostium clock position on an axial image (usually 5:00 for a right internal iliac orifice and 7:00 for the left). This should result in the preloaded catheter oriented at the 3:00 position for right-sided devices and 9:00 for left-sided devices. This facilitates snaring of the preloaded wire. BB-IBD devices are oriented such that the preloaded fenestrations are above the aortic bifurcation. Care must be taken with a BB-IBD in the setting of very short common iliac artery that the three markers distal to the branch exit are above the origin of the target internal iliac artery. Contralateral femoral access is established, and a 12 Fr modified Ansel sheath (Cook Inc., Bloomington, Indiana) is inserted and placed at the origin of the common iliac artery. A second puncture is made in the sheath valve, and a 5F sheath placed in that location through which an over-the-wire snare will be used (Indy Snare, Cook Inc.). The preloaded wire within the IBD is exchanged for a long glidewire, and the wire is snared and withdrawn through the contralateral groin. The H-IBD or S-IBD is advanced to the desired location with the branch terminus immediately above the target internal iliac artery, and the sheath is withdrawn to expose the branch. The 12 Fr sheath is then advanced from the contralateral side up and over the aortic bifurcation into the target branch using the preloaded wire. The preloaded catheter and wire can be withdrawn as a unit as the 12F sheath is advanced into the branch. A second puncture is then made in the valve of the 12F sheath, and a 5F sheath is placed, through which a steerable guidewire-catheter combination (Kumpe catheter, Cook Medical, Bloomington, Indiana) is advanced alongside the through-and-through wire within the 12F sheath. The "buddy" catheter and wire are used to cannulate internal iliac artery and preferably advanced into the posterior (Gluteal) branch of the target vessel. A stiff wire (Rosen or Amplatz, Cook Medical, Bloomington, Indiana) is then placed through the catheter and the catheter removed. The internal iliac artery is imaged in a manner that will demonstrate the branch terminus as well as the target sealing zone. An appropriate length matting self-expandable stent graft (Fluency stent graft, Bard Peripheral Vascular Inc., Tempe, Arizona) for H-IBDs or balloon-expandable stent graft (iCAST, Atrium Medical, Hudson, NH; or Jomed, Abbott Labs, Red Oaks, CA) for S-IBDs is inserted over the stiff wire. Caution must be taken when advancing balloon-expandable stent grafts beyond the protecting sheath, and sometimes an 8 or 9F sheath will be needed to gain purchase to the desired level of sealing within the internal iliac circulation. During this process,

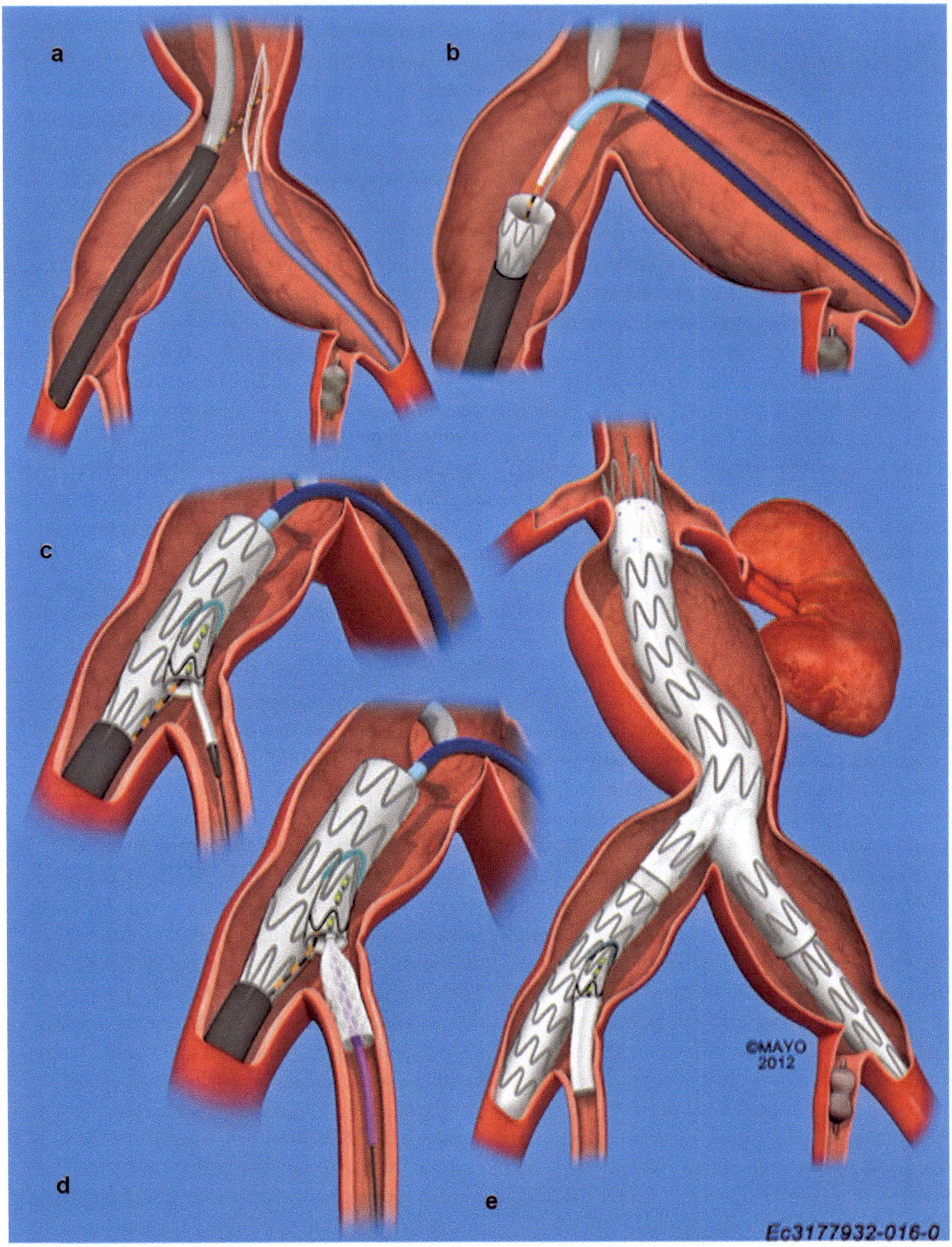

Fig. 4.9 Illustration of the technique of placement of straight arm iliac branch device (S-IBD). A guidewire is advanced into the preloaded catheter and snared via the contralateral femoral approach (**a**), allowing advancement of a 12 Fr modified Ansel sheath (**b**, Cook Medical Inc., Bloomington, IN). Once access is established into the internal iliac artery, a self-expandable stent graft is positioned for deployment (**c**). Following deployment of the matting stent graft (**d**) and completion iliac angiography, the repair is completed using a bifurcated aortic stent graft via the contralateral side (**e**)

traction on the through-and-through wire stabilizes the 12F sheath, such that the delivery of mating devices is not treacherous. Prior to deployment, the through-and-through wire is removed. For helical branches, the self-expandable stent graft is deployed with at least 2 cm overlap with the helical branch and 2-cm seal within the internal iliac artery. Additional radial force may be required in some cases where there is marked tortuosity or minimal luminal size within the common iliac artery. In these cases, the matting stent graft is reinforced with a second self-expanding stent or a balloon-expandable stent, but removal of the through-and-through wire should precede this step. Once the IBD and matting stent graft are fully deployed, the remainder of the branch is deployed by sheath withdrawal and the trigger wires are then deployed, leaving the internal iliac wire over which the mating stent graft was deployed in place, with an 8-mm balloon transcending the internal iliac and external iliac junctions. The 8-mm balloon is then inflated, protecting the branch, and the delivery system is removed. A 12-mm balloon can then be inflated at the junction of the two iliac arteries in a kissing balloon fashion to ensure patency of the internal and external iliac arteries. The repair is then imaged by injecting through the 12F sheath. The remainder of the repair is carried using a standard bifurcated modular component, which is introduced via the contralateral. The IBD is mated to the remainder of the Zenith stent graft (Cook Medical Inc., Bloomington, Indiana) with a short iliac extension.

Deployment of the BB-IBD differs in some ways from the H-IBD and S-IBD deployments. Once the BB-IBD is inserted and oriented such that the contralateral limb and self-sealing fenestration are positioned properly, the sheath is withdrawn while tension is being applied to the through-and-through preloaded wire. This will prevent the preloaded wire from getting caught on any Z-stents as the device is deployed. A 12F sheath is advanced over the preloaded wire, but it is not brought through the valve (although it can be, if it goes in easily). An 8 or 9F sheath is used to cross the valve and transcend the branch. The valve hub is double punctured, and a catheter and wire are brought to the branch terminus and used to cannulate the posterior branch of the target vessel. The 8 or 9F sheath is then removed entirely, and the mating self-expanding stent graft is then advanced through the 12F sheath, self-sealing fenestration, and branch to its target location. The remainder of the repair is akin to that with the H-IBD or S-IBD.

The ideal type of mating stent graft for the internal iliac artery is controversial. While balloon-expandable stent grafts have greater radial force that is sometimes necessary to dilate tight internal iliac artery origins (and are intended for use with S-IBD), they are not ideal for confronting tortuosity within the internal iliac bed or diameter discrepancies that may exist. Joint strength in the overlapping segments becomes an issue, as there is inadequate length to achieve a durable modular interface between the standard S-IBD and a self-expanding stent graft. Thus, an S-IBD coupled with a balloon-expandable stent graft may require non-tortuous anatomy or may be coupled with a self-expanding stent graft in addition to the balloon-expandable stent graft. The reverse situation may occur with the H-IBD.

Results

Although over 1,000 IBDs have been implanted worldwide, published literature is scarce with only a few clinical series [7, 27–32]. However, results of iliac branch stent grafts have been encouraging with technical success rates of greater than 95 % in most reports [29, 31]. The first reported series by Greenberg and associates in 2006 included 21 patients with three technical failures (14 %), all caused by inability to visualize the origin of the internal iliac artery due to significant stenosis [27]. Since its initial conception, results of IBD have improved with newer generation devices. Ziegler and associates analyzed 46 patients treated with S-IBDs, but the first 26 patients were treated using an early generation uni-body configuration, and only the last 20 utilized the S-IBD system [33]. Technical success improved from 58 % with the early generation device to 85 % with the current S-IBD. There were no perioperative deaths, and of the 35 IBDs successfully implanted, none developed endoleak, component separations, or migration. There were four branch occlusions after a mean follow-up of 26 months. Other groups have reported excellent results with the newer generation S-IBD, with technical success rates of 91–100 % and primary patency rates of 74–100 % from 6 to 20 months follow-up [4, 29–31].

The anatomical challenges frequently imposed by the tortuous anatomy of the iliac arteries, particularly in the setting of large aneurysms, have led to the development of the helical design by Roy Greenberg and the group at the Cleveland Clinic [27, 34]. The helical branch provides a longer overlapping zone (>20 mm) between the common iliac device and the mating self-expandable stent graft. In addition, by using a self-expandable stent instead of the balloon-expandable stent, the mating stent graft adapts better to the iliac tortuosity and to the acute angle at the internal iliac artery origin, which potentially reduce kinks and late stent graft occlusion. The results of a multicenter prospective study in 52 patients treated with 53 helical branched stent grafts included a technical success rate of 94 %, with no endoleaks or component separations [34]. There were six branch occlusions, all within the first month. Importantly, whereas none of the patients with patent branches developed claudication, all of those who occluded their branches could pinpoint the date of thrombosis based upon the development of claudication.

Verzini and associates from Perugia, Italy, reported the only comparative analysis of IBDs versus hypogastric exclusion in 74 patients [4]. In this study, there were no differences in procedure time, contrast use, and technical success and no early deaths. However, there was a trend toward more endoleaks (19 % vs. 4 %) and pelvic ischemic symptoms (22 % vs. 4 %) among patients treated with coil embolization compared to IBDs.

Karthikesalingam and associates reported a systematic analysis of nine studies including 196 patients treated with IBDs [35]. The anatomical suitability for IBD was not detailed in most studies, but Tielliu et al. described that only 27 (52 %) of their 52 potential candidates for IBD met all the following anatomical criteria: common iliac diameter >18 mm, absence of excessive iliac tortuosity or internal iliac aneurysm, or severe stenosis [34]. The median operative time ranged from 101 to 290 min and the contrast load 58–208 ml. Technical success ranged from 85 to 100 %. There were no aneurysm-related deaths. Only one patient with patent IBD complained of buttock claudication. However, late thrombosis of the IBD occurred in 24 patients (12 %) and resulted in buttock claudication in 12 (50 %). Endoleak rates were exceedingly low, with only one type I (0.5 %) and two type III endoleaks (1 %). Type II endoleaks were treated conservatively and were not associated with sac expansion. Re-interventions were required in 12 patients (6 %), including 5 with occlusion stent graft limbs to the external iliac artery.

Modified Internal Iliac Artery Branched Stent Graft

In the absence of commercially available IBDs, the technique of modification of Cook Zenith (Cook Medical, Bloomington, IN) iliac extension limb was described by Oderich in 2010 (Fig. 4.7) [36]. The procedure may be used selectively in high-risk patients with bilateral internal iliac artery aneurysms who do not have access to a manufactured IBD. The technique of device modification is reported elsewhere, and device implantation is nearly identical to that already described for manufactured IBDs.

Conclusion

Endovascular treatment of aortoiliac aneurysms can be challenging, particularly in patients who are felt not to be ideally suited for any open surgical procedure. The option of unilateral or bilateral internal iliac artery embolization has a predictable risk of complication, most notably buttock claudication and erectile dysfunction but also rarely serious complications such as ischemic colitis, gluteal muscle necrosis, and spinal cord injury. IBDs represent a significant improvement in the treatment of aortoiliac aneurysms by allowing preservation of pelvic flow with a totally endovascular technique. Furthermore, they ameliorate the need for techniques whereby aneurysmal tissue is left pressurized and prone to rupture (such as the bell-bottom technique) and avoid the need for retroperitoneal incisions. The procedure can be performed with high technical success rates and similar morbidity and mortality compared to standard EVAR. However, widespread utilization of IBD still faces several challenges including regulatory approval, physician training, and an evaluation of the late results of IBDs including device integrity, re-interventions, and occlusion rates.

References

1. Armon MP, et al. Common iliac artery aneurysms in patients with abdominal aortic aneurysms. Eur J Vasc Endovasc Surg. 1998;15(3):255–7.
2. Wyers MC, et al. Internal iliac occlusion without coil embolization during endovascular abdominal aortic aneurysm repair. J Vasc Surg. 2002;36(6):1138–45.
3. Hobo R, et al. Endovascular repair of abdominal aortic aneurysms with concomitant common iliac artery aneurysm: outcome analysis of the EUROSTAR Experience. J Endovasc Ther. 2008;15(1):12–22.
4. Verzini F, et al. Endovascular treatment of iliac aneurysm: concurrent comparison of side branch endograft versus hypogastric exclusion. J Vasc Surg. 2009;49(5):1154–61.
5. Mehta M, et al. Effects of bilateral hypogastric artery interruption during endovascular and open aortoiliac aneurysm repair. J Vasc Surg. 2004;40(4):698–702.
6. Lee WA, et al. Outcome after hypogastric artery bypass and embolization during endovascular aneurysm repair. J Vasc Surg. 2006;44(6):1162–8; discussion 1168–9.
7. Ghosh J, et al. Contemporary management of aorto-iliac aneurysms in the endovascular era. Eur J Vasc Endovasc Surg. 2009;37(2):182–8.
8. Lee WA, et al. Outcome after unilateral hypogastric artery occlusion during endovascular aneurysm repair. J Vasc Surg. 2001;33(5):921–6.
9. Rayt HS, et al. Buttock claudication and erectile dysfunction after internal iliac artery embolization in patients prior to endovascular aortic aneurysm repair. Cardiovasc Intervent Radiol. 2008;31(4):728–34.
10. Maldonado TS, et al. Ischemic complications after endovascular abdominal aortic aneurysm repair. J Vasc Surg. 2004;40(4):703–9; discussion 709–10.
11. Bischoff MS, et al. Spinal cord preservation in thoracoabdominal aneurysm repair. Perspect Vasc Surg Endovasc Ther. 2011;23(3):214–22.
12. Bischoff MS, et al. Staged approach prevents spinal cord injury in hybrid surgical-endovascular thoracoabdominal aortic aneurysm repair: an experimental model. Ann Thorac Surg. 2011;92(1):138–46; discussion 146.
13. Griepp RB, Griepp EB. Spinal cord perfusion and protection during descending thoracic and thoracoabdominal aortic surgery: the collateral network concept. Ann Thorac Surg. 2007;83(2):S865–9; discussion S890–2.
14. McDonnell CO, et al. Large iliac arteries: a high-risk group for endovascular aortic aneurysm repair. J Endovasc Ther. 2007;14(5):625–9.
15. Kirkwood ML, et al. Aneurysmal iliac arteries do not portend future iliac aneurysmal enlargement after endovascular aneurysm repair for abdominal aortic aneurysm. J Vasc Surg. 2011;53(2):269–73.
16. Parodi JC, Ferreira M. Relocation of the iliac artery bifurcation to facilitate endoluminal treatment of abdominal aortic aneurysms. J Endovasc Surg. 1999;6(4):342–7.
17. Faries PL, et al. Internal iliac artery revascularization as an adjunct to endovascular repair of aortoiliac aneurysms. J Vasc Surg. 2001;34(5):892–9.
18. Arko FR, et al. Hypogastric artery bypass to preserve pelvic circulation: improved outcome after endovascular abdominal aortic aneurysm repair. J Vasc Surg. 2004;39(2):404–8.
19. Lee WA, et al. A technique for combined hypogastric artery bypass and endovascular repair of complex aortoiliac aneurysms. J Vasc Surg. 2002;35(6):1289–91.
20. Bergamini TM, et al. External iliac artery-to-internal iliac artery endograft: a novel approach to preserve pelvic inflow in aortoiliac stent grafting. J Vasc Surg. 2002;35(1):120–4.
21. Woo EY, Lombardi JV, Carpenter JP. Endovascular external-to-internal iliac bypass as an adjunct to endovascular aneurysm repair for patients with extensive common iliac artery aneurysmal disease. J Vasc Surg. 2004;39(2):470.
22. Lobato AC. Sandwich technique for aortoiliac aneurysms extending to the internal iliac artery or isolated common/internal iliac artery aneurysms: a new endovascular approach to preserve pelvic circulation. J Endovasc Ther. 2011;18(1):106–11.
23. Parodi JC, Parodi FE. Commentary: the sandwich technique to preserve the hypogastric artery during EVAR. J Endovasc Ther. 2011;18(1):112–3.
24. Yoshida RD, et al. Modified "stent-graft sandwich" technique for treatment of isolated common iliac artery aneurysm in patient with marfan syndrome. Ann Vasc Surg. 2012;26:419.e7–9. Epub 2012 Feb 8.
25. Mosquera Arochena N, et al. Use of modified sandwich-graft technique to preserve hypogastric artery in EVAR treatment of complex aortic aneurysm anatomy. J Cardiovasc Surg. 2011;52(5):643–9.
26. Greenberg RK, Qureshi M. Fenestrated and branched devices in the pipeline. J Vasc Surg. 2010;52(4 Suppl):15S–21.
27. Greenberg RK, et al. Beyond the aortic bifurcation: branched endovascular grafts for thoracoabdominal

and aortoiliac aneurysms. J Vasc Surg. 2006;43(5): 879–86; discussion 886–7.
28. Malina M, et al. Feasibility of a branched stent-graft in common iliac artery aneurysms. J Endovasc Ther. 2006;13(4):496–500.
29. Ferreira M, Monteiro M, Lanziotti L. Technical aspects and midterm patency of iliac branched devices. J Vasc Surg. 2010;51(3):545–50; discussion 550.
30. Tielliu IF, et al. The role of branched endografts in preserving internal iliac arteries. J Cardiovasc Surg. 2009;50(2):213–8.
31. Serracino-Inglott F, Bray AE, Myers P. Endovascular abdominal aortic aneurysm repair in patients with common iliac artery aneurysms–initial experience with the Zenith bifurcated iliac side branch device. J Vasc Surg. 2007;46(2):211–7.
32. Huilgol RL, Denton MJ, Cohen T. The iliac bifurcation device for endovascular iliac aneurysm repair: indications, deployment options and results at 1-year follow-up of 25 cases. ANZ J Surg. 2009;79(11):844–9.
33. Ziegler P, et al. Branched iliac bifurcation: 6 years experience with endovascular preservation of internal iliac artery flow. J Vasc Surg. 2007;46(2): 204–10.
34. Haulon S, et al. Branched grafting for aortoiliac aneurysms. Eur J Vasc Endovasc Surg. 2007;33(5): 567–74.
35. Karthikesalingam A, et al. Endovascular aneurysm repair with preservation of the internal iliac artery using the iliac branch graft device. Eur J Vasc Endovasc Surg. 2010;39(3):285–94.
36. Oderich GS, Ricotta 2nd JJ. Novel surgeon-modified hypogastric branch stent graft to preserve pelvic perfusion. Ann Vasc Surg. 2010;24(2):278–86.

Management of Endoleak Following Endovascular Aneurysm Repair

5

Andrew Misselt and Jafar Golzarian

Abstract

In 1991, Parodi et al. described their initial venture into stent-graft placement for the treatment of aortic aneurysms. The purpose of aneurysm treatment is to prolong life by preventing aneurysm rupture. Given the less invasive approach of the endograft procedure compared to open surgical repair, it is not surprising that endovascular treatment has gained momentum in recent years. However, endograft treatment is not without complication. The most common complication following endograft placement is endoleak. This chapter will focus on the detection and management of endoleak following endovascular treatment of abdominal aortic aneurysms.

Keywords

Endovascular repair • Vascular • Endoleak • Endograft • Catheter

Introduction

In 1991, Parodi et al. described their initial venture into stent-graft placement for the treatment of aortic aneurysms [1]. The purpose of aneurysm treatment is to prolong life by preventing aneurysm rupture. Given the less invasive approach of the endograft procedure compared to open surgical repair, it is not surprising that endovascular treatment has gained momentum in recent years. The rapid advancement of endografts for the treatment of aortic aneurysms has been well documented, and, to date, thousands of individuals in the United States alone have been treated with this method [2].

The placement of an endograft for aneurysm treatment has been shown to be a durable procedure with less mortality and morbidity than open surgical repair [3]. However, endograft placement is not without complication. The most common complication following endograft placement is endoleak. Endoleak, a term described by White et al., refers to blood flow within the aneurysm sac despite placement of an endograft [4]. Endoleaks have been further subdivided into a five-type schema. Briefly, type I endoleaks refer to improper sealing of either the proximal or distal endograft components leading to persistent filling of the aneurysm sac. Type II endoleaks are

A. Misselt, M.D. (✉) • J. Golzarian, M.D.
Department of Radiology, University of Minnesota,
420 Delaware Street SE, MMC 292, Minneapolis,
MN 55435, USA
e-mail: misse001@umn.edu

J.J. Hoballah, A.B. Lumsden (eds.), *Vascular Surgery*, New Techniques in Surgery Series,
DOI 10.1007/978-1-4471-2912-7_5, © Springer-Verlag London 2012

described as filling of the aneurysm sac due to retrograde flow within a collateral vessel [5]. Type III endoleaks are caused by either a tear in the graft material or separation of the graft components. Type IV endoleaks refer to intrinsic porosity of the graft material [6]. Finally, type V endoleaks are described as "endotension," a state of persistent pressure within the aneurysm sac without a discernable source of blood flow [7].

The presence of an endoleak is a relatively common phenomenon occurring in approximately 20 % of patients with endograft repair of abdominal aortic aneurysm [8]. However, as will be described shortly, not all endoleaks are alike, and only a small portion of endoleaks will require intervention. In the subsequent sections, we will discuss various aspects of endoleaks including their classification, surveillance and detection, and treatment.

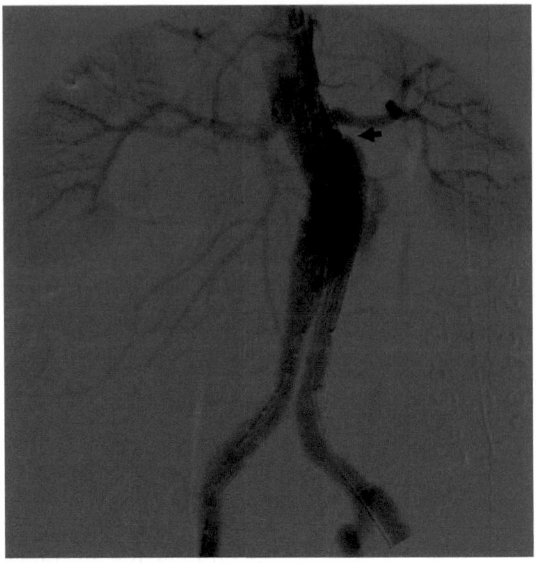

Fig. 5.1 Endograft with suprarenal fixation and type IA endoleak arising from the proximal aspect of the covered portion of the endograft (*black arrow*)

Classification of Endoleak

Endoleak refers to the persistent flow of blood within the aneurysm sac despite placement of an endograft. Originally described and expanded upon by White et al. in the mid to late 1990s, the current endoleak classification system characterizes endoleaks by etiology. In addition to classifying endoleaks etiology, one can also describe these leaks in terms of their chronology of onset. For example, an endoleak which appears immediately after endograft placement is referred to as an immediate endoleak. While an endoleak that becomes apparent later during follow-up imaging is described as a delayed or late endoleak.

Type I Endoleak

Type I endoleak occurs when there is persistent blood flow within the aneurysm sac originating from the site of graft attachment. The point of leak can occur either proximally at the superior margin of the graft in the abdominal aorta or distally where the graft limbs attach to the iliac arteries. These two manifestations have been subdivided into proximal type 1A (Fig. 5.1) or distal type IB. The separation of the graft body from the aneurysm wall in a type I endoleak allows blood to flow alongside the graft, thus perfusing the aneurysm. There is a third, more exotic form of type 1 endoleak, the type IC, which occurs in the setting of an aorta-uniiliac graft. In this scenario, a type 1C endoleak results in back filling of the aneurysm sac from the contralateral (non-stent-grafted) iliac artery. Typically, the contralateral iliac artery is either thrombosed or has been embolized. For a type IC endoleak to occur, blood must flow through the endograft conduit to the ipsilateral femoral artery, across a femoral-to-femoral artery bypass, then retrograde through the contralateral iliac artery and past the point of embolization to fill the residual aneurysm sac.

Whether due to a proximal type IA, distal type IB, or contralateral type IC, type I endoleak is a serious finding because the residual aneurysm sac continues to be perfused with systemic level blood pressure. Consequently, the pressurized residual aneurysm sac remains unprotected and at risk for rupture.

Type II Endoleak

Overall, type II endoleaks are the most common, occurring in approximately 10–25 % of

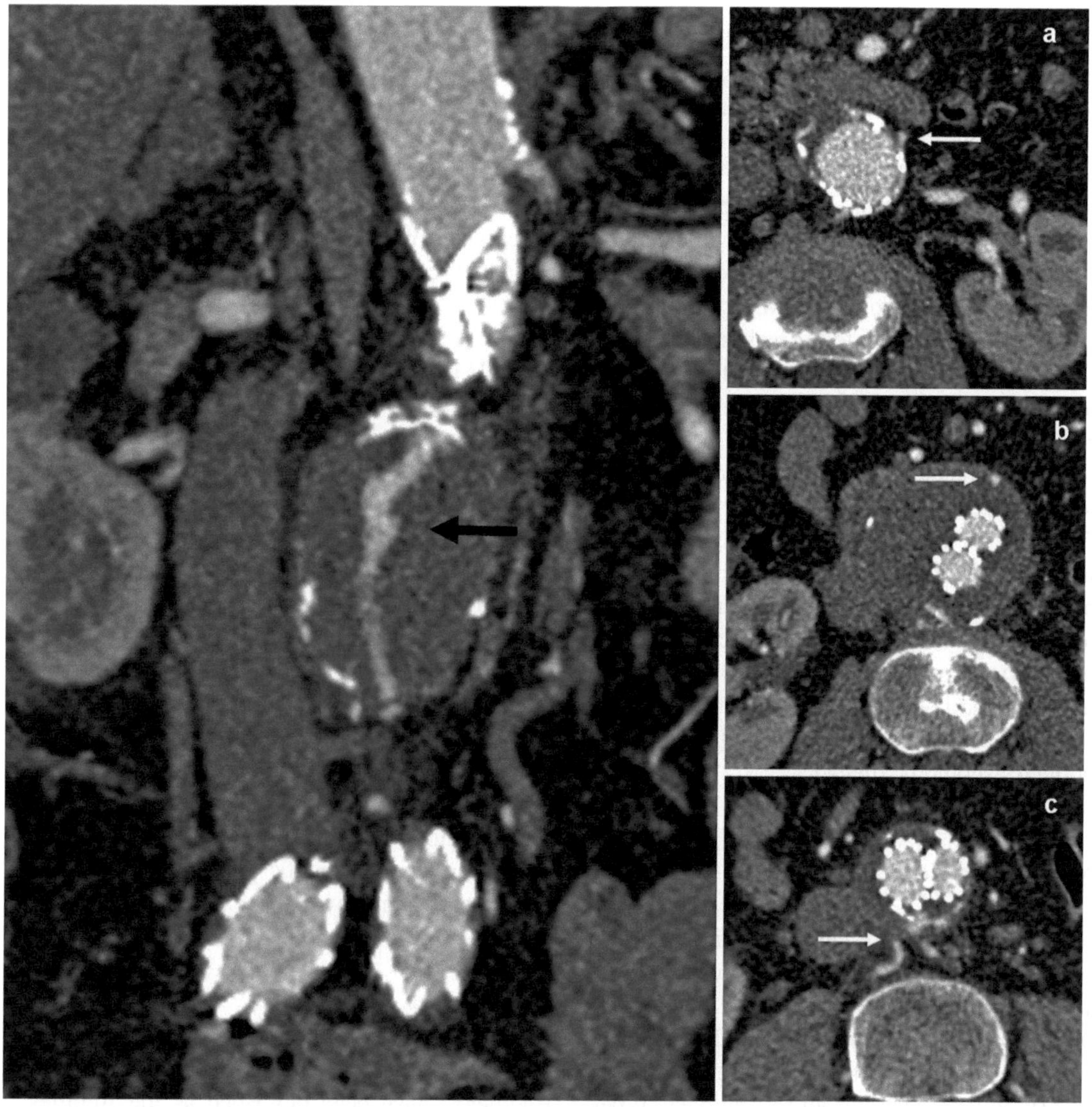

Fig. 5.2 Type IIB endoleak. Note the channel of flow within the residual aneurysm sac (*black arrow*). Contributing vessels include an accessory renal artery (image **a**, *white arrow*), inferior mesenteric artery (image **b**, *white arrow*), and lumbar arteries (image **c**, *white arrow*)

abdominal endograft cases [9]. Type II endoleaks are due to collateral flow. They occur from retrograde perfusion of the residual aneurysm sac via aortic branch arteries that arise from the covered portion of the aorta. In the typical abdominal aortic aneurysm treated by endografting, the aneurysm arises distal to the renal arteries and extends to the aortic bifurcation or perhaps into the iliac arteries. As such, successful treatment of the aneurysm may require covering multiple branch vessels arising from the aorta including the internal iliac arteries, the inferior mesenteric artery, the multiple lumbar and iliolumbar arteries, and the median sacral artery. These aortic branch vessels are the culprits in type II endoleak. Type II endoleaks occur in two varieties: simple (type IIA) and complex (type IIB) (Fig. 5.2). Simple type IIA endoleaks occur when a single vessel supplies both the inflow and outflow of the leak. These leaks tend to be relatively slow flow with the inflow occurring during systole and outflow during diastole. Complex type IIB endoleaks have one or more arteries providing inflow into the aneurysm sac with additional arteries providing the outflow. In this way, the type IIB endoleak looks and behaves much like an arteriovenous malformation. An example might be retrograde filling of the inferior mesenteric arteries via collaterals from the superior mesenteric artery. The blood then flows from the inferior mesenteric artery into the residual aneurysm sac, through vascular channels within the sac, and finally out via antegrade flow through a vessel such as a lumbar artery.

The significance of a type II endoleak is subject to considerable debate. Type II endoleaks are often transient and elusive. They may be seen on one follow-up study, only to resolve on the next, and then return months or even years later [10]. However, type II endoleaks are associated with at least diastolic pressure loads within the residual aneurysm sac [11], and when persistent [12] or accompanied by sac enlargement [13], type II endoleaks should be treated.

Type III Endoleak

Type III endoleaks are caused by failure of the structural integrity of the endograft device. Such failures include modular separation of the graft components (type IIIA) and leaks through tears in the graft fabric or through suture lines of the graft (type IIIB) [10]. Of all the endoleak types, type III leaks are considered to be among the most dangerous in terms of rupture risk. This is due to the acute repressurization of the aneurysm sac that often accompanies the development of this type of device failure [14]. Accordingly, diagnosis and prompt management is essential.

Type IV Endoleak

Type IV endoleaks refer to the passage of blood through the pores of the graft and into the residual aneurysm sac. This is notably different than the larger type III endoleak that accompanies a tear in the graft fabric. Historically, type IV endoleaks were commonly observed during the immediate postplacement angiogram of a systemically heparinized patient. Currently, however, with advancements in graft construction, type IV endoleaks have practically ceased to exist. Consequently, any endoleak with the appearance of a type IV should be thoroughly evaluated for a more sinister etiology.

Type V Endoleak

In some regard, the term type V endoleak is a misnomer. A type V endoleak refers to the phenomenon of residual aneurysm sac expansion despite visualization of an endoleak using all available imaging means. This state of unexplained aneurysm expansion is also known as endotension. Several theories have been developed to explain this occurrence including the following: the presence of a radiographically occult endoleak (types I–IV), transmission of the arterial pulse wave through perigraft space to the residual aneurysm sac, or the development of an ultrafiltration of seroma through the graft porosity perhaps due to oncotic pressure from degradation of thrombus in the excluded aneurysm [10, 15, 16].

Endoleak Diagnosis and Surveillance

Endoleaks have been described as the Achilles heel of endoluminal aneurysm repair [9]. Thus, it is critically important for the vascular interventionalist to know how to effectively diagnose and manage the various types of endoleaks.

In our practice, we begin considering possible sources of endoleak during the pre-procedure planning stage with a thorough review of the sizing computed tomography angiogram (CTA). Close attention should be paid to landing zone measurements and to short, highly angulated, or conical necks as these may herald fixation difficulties which may lead to type I endoleaks. Attention needs also to be paid to the patency of the internal iliac arteries and their relationship to the proposed landing zone. The internal iliac arteries should be preemptively embolized when needed to avoid a type II endoleak through this vessel. Some have also suggested that preemptive embolization of other aortic branch vessels such as the inferior mesenteric artery, lumbar artery, and median sacral artery may be warranted [17, 18], though this practice has not been widely adopted as its efficacy is not conclusively supported [18]. Other authors have described injection of thrombin or glue within the residual aneurysm sac at the time of endograft placement to decrease the incidence of endoleak [19–21]. While these techniques may prove beneficial, their use is not yet widespread.

The first opportunity to identify an endoleak is during the post-endograft placement angiogram. The initial injection should be performed with the catheter above the superior margin of the graft. Any contrast opacification seen outside the endograft lumen and within the residual aneurysm sac is by definition an endoleak. To discern which type of endoleak is present, careful attention should be paid to the location from which the sac fills as well as the timing of the opacification. If for instance, the aneurysm sac fills concomitantly with the passage of the main contrast bolus and the point of filling is near the proximal or distal seal zones, then a type I endoleak should be invoked. Alternatively, if one clearly observes the filling of the residual aneurysm sac in a delayed fashion relative to the main contrast bolus, one should look closely for retrograde flow in aortic branch vessels as the cause of a probable type II endoleak.

Following the initial injection, subsequent injections may be needed to perform a conclusive investigation, particularly with an indeterminate type of endoleak. The catheter is next withdrawn within the graft main body and modular attachment sites to search for type III endoleak. If the type of leak is still unknown, selective injections may be performed to search for type III endoleaks.

If no endoleak is identified at the time of endograft placement, it is important to maintain vigilance during follow-up imaging. At our institution, we obtain a follow-up CTA at 1 month, 6 months, and then annually. CTA is performed in three phases including noncontrast, arterial, and delayed phase. The noncontrast phase is useful for assessing changes in size of the residual aneurysm sac and to evaluate for calcification that may simulate the appearance of a leak. The contrast phases are used in conjunction with the noncontrast images for the diagnosis of endoleak [22, 23].

CTA provides a static, rather than dynamic, appraisal of the anatomy. Thus, CTA can identify the presence of endoleak but may not be able to establish the primary type. Further, noninvasive imaging methods often underrepresent the size and complexity of endoleak; thus, angiography, which is the gold standard imaging test for endoleak, may be needed to conclusively classify the source [24, 25].

If poor renal function precludes the use of intravenous iodinated contrast, we rely on the measurements of the noncontrast CT scan to determine changes in sac diameter, and we also use duplex ultrasonography to look for flow within the residual aneurysm sac [26, 27].

Magnetic resonance imaging (MRI) has also been used as a surveillance method following endograft placement. MRI has the obvious benefit of being a robust technique that uses nonionizing radiation. Other drawbacks include longer imaging time and the potential for image artifact from the metallic components of grafts. Time-resolved MRA is a relatively new technique in which the contrast bolus is imaged in dynamic fashion as it flows through the body. This method has a clear advantage over the static display of a CTA as it provides temporal data similar to a catheter angiogram. As such, one can see the direction of flow within aortic branch vessels as location of leak origin. Undoubtedly MRI will play a larger role in the imaging of post-endograft patients in the future.

Implanted pressure monitoring devices have also been utilized as a means of post-endograft placement surveillance. A wireless pressure monitor implanted inside the residual aneurysm sac at the time of endograft placement provides a nonimaging method of monitoring the residual sac pressure. A residual aneurysm sac with low or no pressure is indicative of a graft with no endoleak. While an implanted monitoring device that reports a pressure near the level of the measured blood pressure indicates an endoleak [28, 29].

Endoleak Treatment

Type I endoleaks require immediate attention to prevent aneurysm rupture. Occasionally a type I leak is observed during the initial angiogram following endograft deployment. The first step in this situation is balloon angioplasty at the level of the leak to oppose the graft to the wall of the aneurysm. If this is unsuccessful, it may be necessary to use an extension cuff to achieve the requisite seal. When a type I endoleak is appreciated during follow-up surveillance imaging, one should carefully scrutinize the available comparison images to see if there has been any migration of the graft or expansion of the aneurysm because these will likely require cuff extension to re-oppose the graft to the aortic wall. If there has been no change in graft position, a trial of balloon angioplasty alone is warranted before progressing to cuff placement. The placement of a cuff extender is similar to the placement of the initial graft in that it typically requires a surgical cut-down and large introducer sheaths. Occasionally, a Palmaz bare metal stent is used to augment the graft seal at the site of a type I endoleak. This step can be used alone or in conjunction with a cuff extender if necessary. To safely deliver the Palmaz stent, it should be carefully crimped upon a large compliant balloon. The balloon and stent combination should then be delivered to the proximal seal zone via a long introducer sheath, typically 12 Fr. It is vital to bring the stent all the way to the deployment site within the sheath, before withdrawing the sheath and inflating the balloon. Failure to observe this technique may result in premature dislodgement of the stent from the balloon.

If a type I endoleak persists despite the use of repeat balloon angioplasty, placement of cuff extendors, or use of large bare metal stents, the next step is to attempt to seal the leak entry and exit sites with catheter-based delivery of an embolic agent such as coils. Typically, blood enters a type IA endoleak site alongside a portion of graft which has not adhered to the aortic wall. The blood then continues to flow into the residual aneurysm sac before exiting through one or more aortic branch outflow vessels such as the inferior mesenteric artery or the lumbar arteries. To successfully treat a type I endoleak with the transcatheter embolization technique, one must first fully understand the anatomy. Based on the angle of the aorta and the position of the proximal leak site, it may be better to access the leak using a reverse curve catheter from the femoral approach or a simple curved catheter from a brachial approach. After angiographically confirming the endoleak origin, the leak site is gently probed with a catheter and wire combination. Once wire access has been gained within the residual aneurysm sac, the catheter is advanced as deep into the sac as possible. Imaging with the catheter placed within the sac will demonstrate the full complexity of the aneurysm sac. Next, a catheter is advanced through the residual aneurysm sac and into the origins of the outflow aortic branch vessels. A microcatheter is frequently needed to accomplish the outflow vessel cannulation. Once in place, the outflow vessels are embolized at their origin from the aorta. This is typically accomplished using coils. The catheter is then returned to the aneurysm sac, and repeat angiography is performed. This step is essential as additional outflow vessels may become apparent as the primary egress of flow is eliminated. After the outflow is eliminated or disrupted, the catheter is withdrawn to the level of the inflow leak. At this point, a dense coil pack is created to buttress the graft material to the aortic wall and eliminate the space through which the type 1 endoleak occurred. This type of endoleak treatment, while technically challenging, is often successful [30, 31]. In summary, the key to successful embolization is to alter or occlude the communication between the inflow and the outflow.

If endovascular treatment attempts have all failed, open conversion is the next and final step in the treatment of type I endoleak.

Type II endoleaks, when present for longer than 6 months and associated with an expanding residual aneurysm sac, should be treated. In general, there are two different strategies for

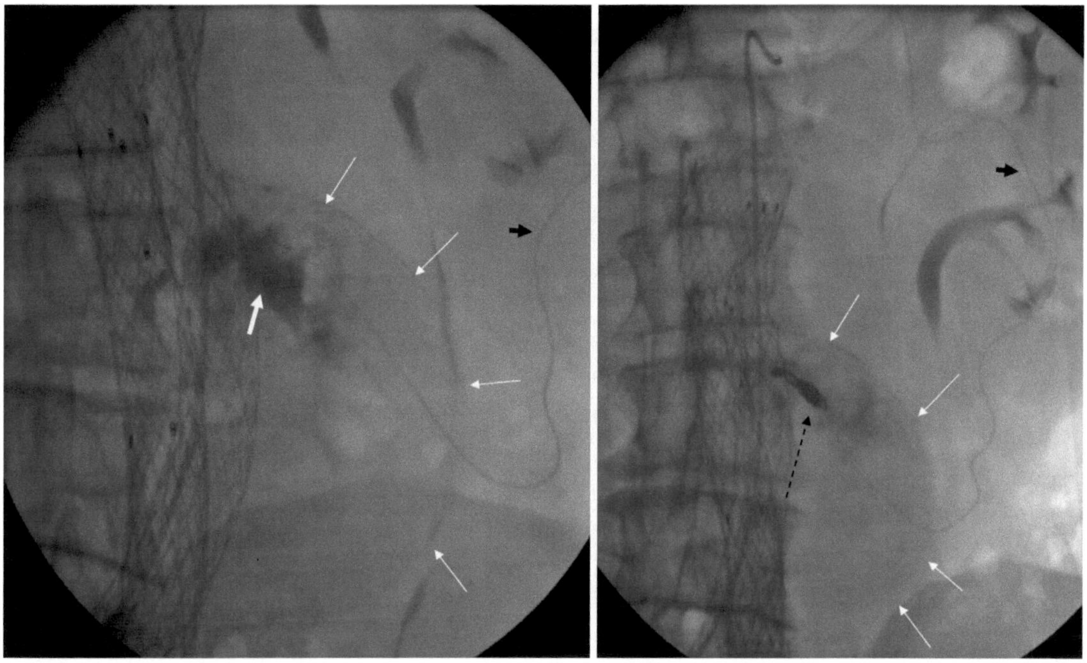

Fig. 5.3 Repair of type IIB endoleak. Note microcatheter course from superior mesenteric artery to inferior mesenteric artery (*small black arrows*), outline of aneurysm sac (*thin white arrows*), embolic glue disrupting the endoleak channel (*thick white arrow*), and coil embolization of the inferior mesenteric origin (*dashed black arrow*)

treatment: transarterial [32] and translumbar [10, 33]. In our practice, we attempt transarterial treatment first.

Suspicion of type II endoleak should be confirmed at angiography. If the precise pathway of the endoleak is not obvious, angiographic confirmation will often require multiple injections. Typically, the first injection is an aortogram with the catheter above the superior margin of the graft, usually near the level of the superior mesenteric artery. If a type II leak is not seen, injections within the graft, both at the proximal margin and at the level of the modular component junction, should be performed to exclude type III endoleak. Next, selective and subselective injections of the superior mesenteric artery should be performed. If these injections fail to demonstrate the leak, the angiographer should proceed to injections of the internal iliac arteries to look for iliolumbar arteries refilling the aneurysm sac.

If an inferior mesenteric artery leak is visible via a superior mesenteric artery, injection of microcatheter is advanced through the mesenteric collaterals to the origin of the inferior mesenteric artery. Then the microcatheter is advanced past the inferior mesenteric artery origin and into the residual aneurysm sac where an injection of the sac itself is performed. If the injection reveals only a single source of leak, then the inferior mesenteric artery origin can be embolized and the leak will resolve (Fig. 5.3). However, it has been our experience that type IIA (simple) endoleaks will thrombose spontaneously and do not typically need treatment.

Oftentimes, however, the injection of the sac will demonstrate a complex channel of flow with multiple inflow and outflow vessels. This is a type IIB (complex) endoleak. In the case of complexity, the channel must be disrupted. This can be accomplished with coils, cyanoacrylate, particles, thrombin, and onyx or any combination of these materials. Next, the microcatheter is withdrawn to the level of the IMA origin, and the vessel is coil occluded at this level. Care must be taken to ensure that only the origin of the IMA is occluded as distal embolization of the IMA is related to risk of ischemic colitis [34]. A repeat injection is performed within the IMA to confirm

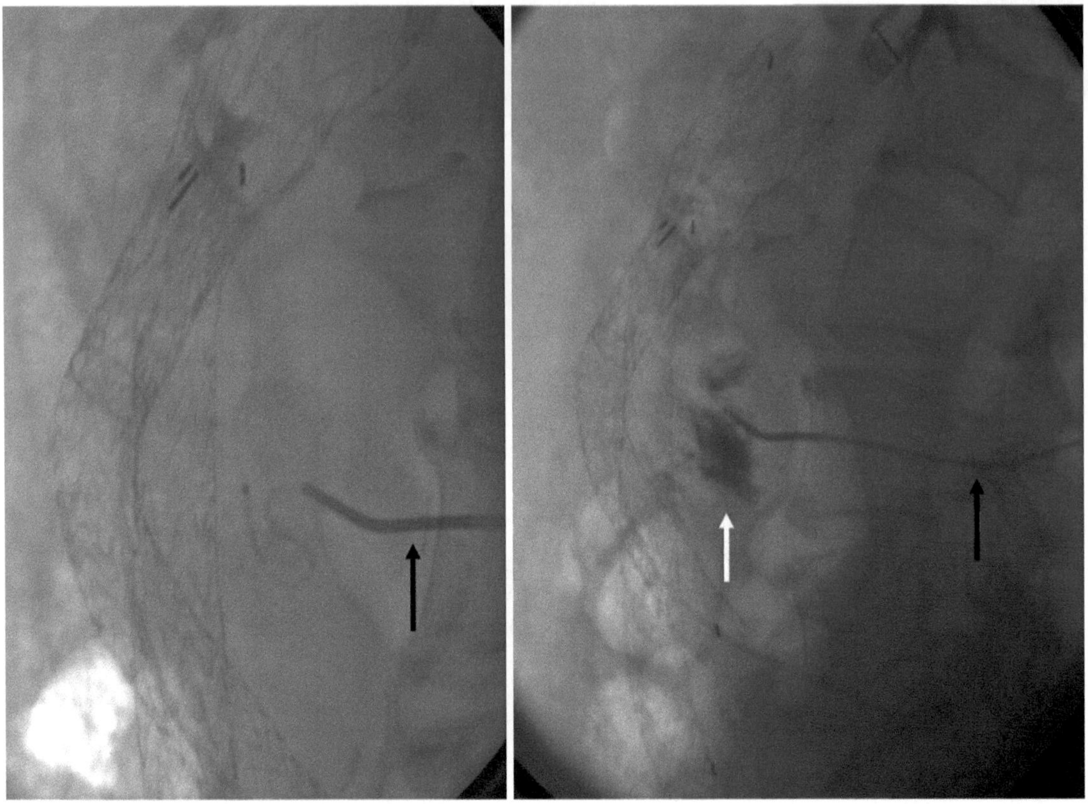

Fig. 5.4 Translumbar repair of type II endoleak. Note translumbar access (*black arrows*) for the administration of embolic glue (*white arrow*)

occlusion of the inflow before the catheter is withdrawn to the aorta to once again evaluate for endoleak. If additional type II endoleak is demonstrated or access from the superior mesenteric artery is not possible, then treatment should proceed via iliolumbar artery catheterization. The process is then repeated with the intent of closing this new leak source.

If the type II endoleak does not abate despite transcatheter therapy, the translumbar approach is attempted next. In this method, the residual aneurysm sac is accessed directly via a percutaneous puncture (Fig. 5.4). Depending on where the bulk of the endoleak is seen on pre-procedural CT, either a left or right translumbar approach will be required. In general, the left translumbar approach is preferred as there is direct access through the psoas muscle into the sac. If, however, a right translumbar approach is required, the pathway of the needle may traverse the inferior vena cava. While somewhat disconcerting, this approach has been shown to be safe and effective [35]. Regardless of whether a left or right translumbar approach has been chosen, the idea is to place a 21-gauge needle into the residual aneurysm sac itself. This is accomplished using fluoroscopic or CT guidance. Once in place, blood is aspirated from the needle and fluoroscopy is used to perform an aortogram. If needed, needle access could be exchanged for catheter access for more selective imaging and embolization. Typically, however, we carry out our embolization directly through the access needle using coils and cyanoacrylate or onyx. The goal of the embolization is to disrupt the channel of flow within the sac and possibly occlude the origins of the inflow and outflow vessels. Care should be taken not to extrude the embolization material distally within the aortic branch vessels to avoid ischemic complications. If the translumbar route does not provide suitable access to the leak, one may also consider a direct anterior transabdominal puncture into the residual aneurysm sac, followed by standard embolization through the needle [10].

A third innovative approach at residual aneurysm sac embolization has emerged in which the aorta is approached using a catheter-based transvenous puncture into the aorta [36, 37]. In this technique, catheter access in the femoral vein is used to introduce a puncture needle which is then directed through the IVC to the residual aneurysm sac. Once access is gained, embolization is carried out in standard fashion.

Laparoscopic clipping of the offending aortic branch vessels has also been described as a treatment method of type II endoleak [38].

Type III endoleaks, when present, are treated by relining the graft with additional endograft components. A successful repair of a type III leak depends on finding the leak site. Because the leak site is only rarely apparent on CT imaging, aortography is often needed to confidently identify the problem. Injections should be performed at the top of the graft and adjacent to modular component interfaces. Once the leak site is identified, treatment is straightforward.

Type IV endoleaks have all but disappeared with newer generations of endografts. Type V endoleaks are a rare occurrence that seldom require treatment. If one feels compelled to intervene upon a type V endoleak, treatment options include draining the aneurysm sac, relining the endograft with a new endograft, or open conversion.

Conclusion

Endograft repair of aneurysm has continued to mature and has become the preferred means of aneurysm treatment. More endograft procedures have led to more endoleaks, which remain an ongoing complication of endovascular repair. An established imaging and surveillance protocol is needed to safely monitor patients with endograft. When an endoleak is present, correct classification is critical to triage the treatment approach. A full complement of endovascular treatment options is available, and when appropriately applied, open conversion will be rare.

References

1. Parodi JC, Palmaz JC, Barone HD. Transfemoral intraluminal graft implantation for abdominal aortic aneurysms. Ann Vasc Surg. 1991;5(6):491–9.
2. Baum RA, Stavropoulos SW, Fairman RM, Carpenter JP. Endoleaks after endovascular repair of abdominal aortic aneurysms. J Vasc Interv Radiol. 2003; 14(9, Part 1):1111–7.
3. Lovegrove RE, Javid M, Magee TR, Galland RB. A meta-analysis of 21,178 patients undergoing open or endovascular repair of abdominal aortic aneurysm. Br J Surg. 2008;95(6):677–84.
4. White GH, Yu W, May J. Endoleak – a proposed new terminology to describe incomplete aneurysm exclusion by an endoluminal graft. J Endovasc Surg. 1996; 3(1):124–5.
5. White GH, May J, Waugh RC, Yu W. Type I and type II endoleaks: a more useful classification for reporting results of endoluminal AAA repair. J Endovasc Surg. 1998;5(2):189–91.
6. White GH, May J, Waugh RC, Chaufour X, Yu W. Type III and type IV endoleak: toward a complete definition of blood flow in the sac after endoluminal AAA repair. J Endovasc Surg. 1998;5(4): 305–9.
7. Gilling-Smith G, Brennan J, Harris P, Bakran A, Gould D, McWilliams R. Endotension after endovascular aneurysm repair: definition, classification, and strategies for surveillance and intervention. J Endovasc Surg. 1999;6(4):305–7.
8. van Marrewijk C, Buth J, Harris P, Norgren L, Nevelsteen A, Wyatt M. Significance of endoleaks after endovascular repair of abdominal aortic aneurysms: the EUROSTAR experience. J Vasc Surg. 2002;35(3):461–73.
9. Veith FJ, Baum RA, Ohki T, et al. Nature and significance of endoleaks and endotension: summary of opinions expressed at an international conference. J Vasc Surg. 2002;35(5):1029–35.
10. Rosen RJ, Green RM. Endoleak management following endovascular aneurysm repair. J Vasc Interv Radiol. 2008;19(6, Suppl 1):S37–43.
11. Schurink GW, Aarts NJ, Wilde J, et al. Endoleakage after stent-graft treatment of abdominal aneurysm: implications on pressure and imaging – an in vitro study. J Vasc Surg. 1998;28(2):234–41.
12. Jones J, Atkins M, Brewster D, et al. Persistent type 2 endoleak after endovascular repair of abdominal aortic aneurysm is associated with adverse late outcomes. J Vasc Surg. 2007;46(1):1–8.
13. Bernhard V, Mitchell RS, Matsumura J, et al. Ruptured abdominal aortic aneurysm after endovascular repair. J Vasc Surg. 2002;35(6):1155–62.
14. Golzarian J, Maes EB, Sun S. Endoleak: treatment options. Tech Vasc Interv Radiol. 2005;8(1):41–9.
15. Heikkinen MA, Arko FR, Zarins CK. What is the significance of endoleaks and endotension. Surg Clin North Am. 2004;84(5):1337–52.

16. Toya N, Fujita T, Kanaoka Y, Ohki T. Endotension following endovascular aneurysm repair. Vasc Med. 2008;13(4):305–11.
17. Axelrod D, Lookstein R, Guller J, et al. Inferior mesenteric artery embolization before endovascular aneurysm repair: technique and initial results. J Vasc Interv Radiol. 2004;15(11):1263–7.
18. Gould DA, McWilliams R, Edwards RD, et al. Aortic side branch embolization before endovascular aneurysm repair: incidence of type II endoleak. J Vasc Interv Radiol. 2001;12(3):337–41.
19. Hill C, Hill CA. Strategies to reduce the rate of type II endoleaks: routine intraoperative embolization of the inferior mesenteric artery and thrombin injection into the aneurysm sac. J Endovasc Ther. 2007;14(5):661–8.
20. Zanchetta M, Faresin F, Pedon L, Ronsivalle S. Intraoperative intrasac thrombin injection to prevent type II endoleak after endovascular abdominal aortic aneurysm repair. J Endovasc Ther. 2007;14(2):176–83.
21. Zanchetta M, Faresin F, Pedon L, Riggi M, Ronsivalle S. Fibrin glue aneurysm sac embolization at the time of endografting. J Endovasc Ther. 2005;12(5):579–82.
22. Golzarian J, Dussaussois L, Abada HT, et al. Helical CT of aorta after endoluminal stent-graft therapy: value of biphasic acquisition. AJR Am J Roentgenol. 1998;171(2):329–31.
23. Abada H, Golzarian J. Multidetector CT in abdominal aortic aneurysm following endovascular repair: How to consider the value of a delayed phase. Radiology. 2007;245(2):610–1.
24. Golzarian J, Struyven J, Abada HT, et al. Endovascular aortic stent-grafts: transcatheter embolization of persistent perigraft leaks. Radiology. 1997;202(3):731–4.
25. Grich J, Rilinger N, Krmer S, et al. Angiography of leaks after endovascular repair of infrarenal aortic aneurysms. AJR Am J Roentgenol. 2000;174(3):811–4.
26. McLafferty RB, McCrary BS, Mattos MA, et al. The use of color-flow duplex scan for the detection of endoleaks. J Vasc Surg. 2002;36(1):100–4.
27. Mirza TA, Karthikesalingam A, Jackson D, et al. Duplex ultrasound and contrast-enhanced ultrasound versus computed tomography for the detection of endoleak after EVAR: systematic review and bivariate meta-analysis. Eur J Vasc Endovasc Surg. 2010;39(4): 418–28.
28. Ellozy S, Carroccio A, Lookstein R, et al. First experience in human beings with a permanently implantable intrasac pressure transducer for monitoring endovascular repair of abdominal aortic aneurysms. J Vasc Surg. 2004;40(3):405–12. doi:10.1016/j.jvs.2004.06.027.
29. Ohki T, Ouriel K, Silveira P, et al. Initial results of wireless pressure sensing for endovascular aneurysm repair: the APEX trial – acute pressure measurement to confirm aneurysm sac EXclusion. J Vasc Surg. 2007;45(2):236–42. doi:10.1016/j.jvs.2006.09.060.
30. Golzarian J, Valenti D. Endoleakage after endovascular treatment of abdominal aortic aneurysms: diagnosis, significance and treatment. Eur Radiol. 2006; 16(12):2849–57.
31. Gorich J, Rilinger N, Sokiranski R, et al. Treatment of leaks after endovascular repair of aortic aneurysms. Radiology. 2000;215(2):414–20.
32. LaBerge JM, Sawhney R, Wall SD, et al. Retrograde catheterization of the inferior mesenteric artery to treat endoleaks: anatomic and technical considerations. J Vasc Interv Radiol. 2000;11(1):55–9.
33. Baum RA, Carpenter JP, Golden MA, et al. Treatment of type 2 endoleaks after endovascular repair of abdominal aortic aneurysms: comparison of transarterial and translumbar techniques. J Vasc Surg. 2002; 35(1):23–9.
34. Gambaro E, Abou-Zamzam Jr AM, Teruya TH, Bianchi C, Hopewell J, Ballard JL. Ischemic colitis following translumbar thrombin injection for treatment of endoleak. Ann Vasc Surg. 2004;18(1):74–8.
35. Stavropoulos SW, Carpenter JP, Fairman RM, Golden MA, Baum RA. Inferior vena cava traversal for translumbar endoleak embolization after endovascular abdominal aortic aneurysm repair. J Vasc Interv Radiol. 2003;14(9 Pt 1):1191–4.
36. Mansueto G, Cenzi D, D'Onofrio M, Petrella E, Gumbs AA, Mucelli RP. Treatment of type II endoleaks after endovascular repair of abdominal aortic aneurysms: transcaval approach. Cardiovasc Intervent Radiol. 2005;28(5):641–5.
37. Mansueto G, Cenzi D, Scuro A, et al. Treatment of type II endoleak with a transcatheter transcaval approach: results at 1-year follow-up. J Vasc Surg. 2007;45(6):1120–7.
38. Ho P, Law WL, Tung PH, Poon JT, Ting AC, Cheng SW. Laparoscopic transperitoneal clipping of the inferior mesenteric artery for the management of type II endoleak after endovascular repair of an aneurysm. Surg Endosc. 2004;18(5):870.

Thoracic Endovascular Aortic Repair (TEVAR): New Horizons

6

Jonathan Bath and Jae-Sung Cho

Abstract

Thoracic aortic aneurysm repair utilizing endovascular approaches has been in clinical existence for close to two decades and has quickly become the preferred treatment for anatomically suitable candidates. The modern vascular surgeon must, therefore, be familiar with new and changing treatment modalities for this formidable disease.

This chapter describes the advances in endovascular treatments for DTAA, TAAA, as well as aortic arch aneurysms, with a special emphasis on novel endovascular techniques that are emerging to treat the complex array of aortic disease encountered in current practice. Hybrid open and endovascular operations, branched and fenestrated endograft techniques, chimney graft and sandwich approaches, and application in thoracic aortic trauma are included in this comprehensive overview of new horizons for thoracic endovascular repair.

Keywords

Chimney and sandwich technique • TEVAR • Hybrid repair Thoracoabdominal and thoracic aneurysm • Branched and fenestrated endograft

Etiology, Classification, and Pathophysiology of Aortic Aneurysms

Aortic disease, manifest in the form of aneurysmal degeneration, has been estimated to be responsible for approximately 15,000–30,000 deaths per year in the USA [1]. Population studies of mortality in the USA rank death from aortic aneurysm as the 12th leading cause, mirroring the rate seen in other Western countries. Aortic aneurysms are typically classified anatomically, which also provides the most important clinical distinction when

J. Bath, MBBS (✉) • J.-S. Cho, M.D.
Division of Vascular Surgery
and Endovascular Therapy,
Loyola University Chicago-Stritch
School of Medicine, 2160 S First Ave., EMS Bldg
110-Rm 3215, Maywood, Ilinois 60153,
USA
e-mail: bathj@upmc.edu; jaecho@lumc.edu

J.J. Hoballah, A.B. Lumsden (eds.), *Vascular Surgery*, New Techniques in Surgery Series,
DOI 10.1007/978-1-4471-2912-7_6, © Springer-Verlag London 2012

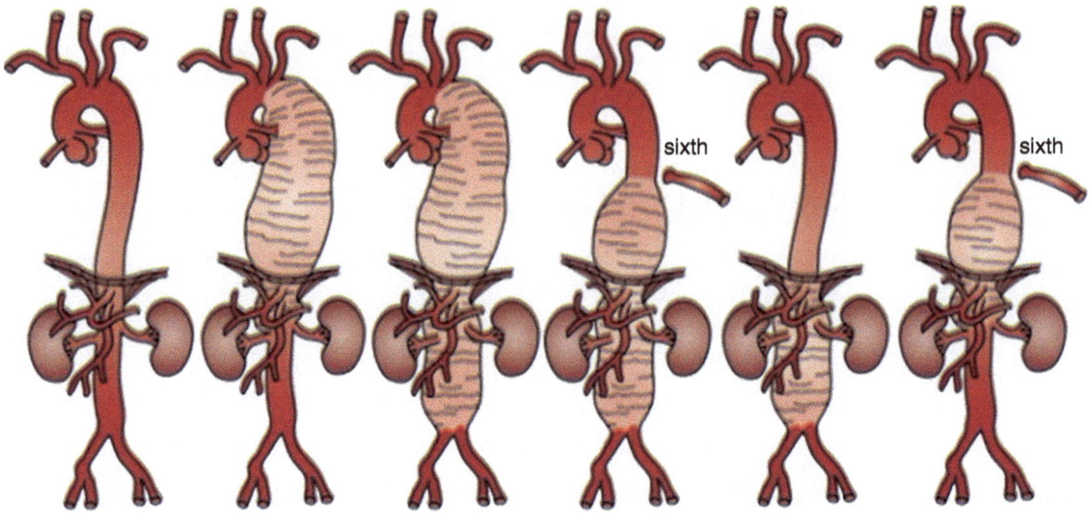

Fig. 6.1 Crawford classification scheme for thoracic and thoracoabdominal aortic aneurysms (This figure was published in Upchurch and Patel [5])

approaching aneurysmal disease from a treatment perspective. Ascending, descending thoracic (DTAA), and thoracoabdominal aortic aneurysms (TAAA) are less commonly encountered than abdominal aortic aneurysms (AAA). For the vascular surgeon, DTAA, TAAA, and AAA are the most common clinically relevant entity and will be the focus of this chapter. DTAA and TAAA have been estimated to occur with an incidence of 4.5–5.9 per 100,000 person-years [2, 3]. Interestingly, abdominal aortic aneurysms are more frequently seen in clinical practice with a reported prevalence of approximately 2.5 % in individuals over 65 years of age, although this likely represents an underestimation of the true prevalence [4].

The Crawford classification scheme for DTAA and TAAA is the most widely used system (Fig. 6.1). The scheme has proven useful clinically for standardized reporting of aneurysm outcomes by aneurysm type and extent and allows comparison of neurological deficit and aneurysm-related mortality, and additionally influences the type of treatment offered with respect to surgical approach, endovascular feasibility, and need for adjunctive procedures based upon proximity to branch vessels.

The relative rarity of DTAA and TAAA compared to AAA has been subject to scrutiny for many years, and many differing theories regarding the pathophysiologic difference in aortic segments leading to predilection for aneurysmal degeneration of the infrarenal aorta have been postulated. Differential matrix metalloproteinase (MMP) activities in the thoracic versus infrarenal aortic segments have been cited in rat experiments as a putative etiologic factor [6], although authors of previous reports of aortic composition argue that a change in the elastin to collagen ratio from proximal to distal aorta is the cause of the greater prevalence of infrarenal aortic aneurysms [7]. In addition, there are proponents of a theory of reduced vasa vasorum observed in the infrarenal segment leading to a predisposition to degeneration and a model of aneurysmal degeneration based upon pulse-flow dynamics specific to the aortic bifurcation [8, 9].

Thoracic aortic aneurysm repair utilizing endovascular approaches has been in clinical existence for close to two decades. Custom-designed patient-specific devices have been used on a trial basis since 1994 shortly after work by Parodi and colleagues demonstrating the feasibility of an endovascular treatment modality for infrarenal abdominal aortic aneurysms (EVAR) was described [10]. Dake and colleagues extended the concept to the thoracic aorta using similar self-expanding stents with a woven Dacron graft exoskeleton [11]. Since the introduction of a commercially available thoracic endograft in 2005, the range of devices and delivery systems has increased rapidly. In a similar fashion to infrarenal endografts, TEVAR has quickly become the preferred treatment for anatomically suitable candidates, in part by reports of a reduction in perioperative mortality, paraplegia rate, and cardiovascular complications [12–17]. In contrast to EVAR, however, the challenges faced by endovascular repair of the thoracic aorta are far greater. Anatomic limitations imposed by the great vessels with respect to adequate proximal landing zones and similarly, consideration of the distal end point in relation to the visceral segment of the thoracic aorta provide unique challenges when assessing the feasibility of TEVAR.

Indications for Endovascular Repair

The indications for TEVAR have also grown as experience with more complex endovascular techniques has proven to be durable in patients who might not tolerate the physiological insult of a traditional open DTAA or TAAA repair. The lack of large multicenter randomized prospective trials and rarity of the disease had, up until the last 5 years, limited expansion of usage of commercial devices. This was partly due to the paucity of device sizes, long-term results, and experience with difficult or hostile aneurysm anatomy. Recent advances in device technology, range of device diameters, and greater comfort with TEVAR have allowed expansion of its application to aneurysms involving the supra-aortic trunk (also referred to as the great vessels) and renovisceral vessels, either entirely or with adjunctive covered stents using chimney (also known as snorkel) techniques, and other pathologies such as intramural hematoma, penetrating ulcers, complicated type B aortic dissection, Kommerell's diverticulum, and traumatic aortic injury. The application of endovascular repair to paravisceral aneurysm repair ushered in an era of innovation leading to introduction of branched and fenestrated endografts in 2001 [18].

Table 6.1 Indications for repair of thoracic and thoracoabdominal aortic aneurysms

Absolute minor axis diameter > 6 cm
Rate of growth > 0.5 cm over 6 months
Thromboembolic aneurysm
Pain related to the presence of aneurysm
Connective tissue disorder-related aneurysms, e.g., Marfan's syndrome, Ehlers-Danlos syndrome >5.5 cm on the minor axis
Penetrating aortic ulceration
Saccular aneurysm
Acute traumatic false aneurysm
Post-dissection aneurysm

General Considerations for TEVAR

Patient selection for TEVAR is in part constrained by the same limitations encountered in EVAR. Anatomic feasibility is derived from accurate imaging, usually involving contrast-enhanced computed tomography angiography (CTA). The rate of growth, minimum diameter of an aneurysm, location, and proximity to important visceral and cerebral branches dictate the need and ability to undergo successful endograft repair. Accepted criteria for repair include rapid expansion greater than 5 mm over 6 months or absolute diameter greater than 6 cm in the absence of symptoms. Symptomatic aneurysms may require repair at sizes less than 6 cm. Ulceration, saccular conformation, or thromboembolic aneurysms are all considerations in the decision to intervene upon a thoracic aneurysm (Table 6.1). Open repair in adequate-risk patients may prove preferable to endovascular approaches where need for complex branch revascularization or concern for adequacy of endograft fixation is a possibility, despite the greater operative risk faced by the patient. The range of devices now commercially available has expanded indications for previously difficult or hostile aortic necks, small aortic neck size, and severe tortuosity. In addition, the better trackability of newer devices appears to make TEVAR more widely applicable for those with anatomically difficult aneurysm configuration.

In the preoperative assessment of patients considered for endovascular repair should be a discussion of patient comorbidities that might complicate or even obviate the benefit of elective repair. Chronic renal failure not yet requiring dialysis in a patient who is not prepared to risk postoperative hemodialysis might dissuade one from endovascular repair. Contrast-induced nephropathy (CIN) is recognized as a significant entity in vascular patients with a recent systematic review of preoperative angiography in a vascular population citing a frequency of CIN of 9.2 % [19]. Identified risk factors for CIN include age greater than 70 years, high contrast volume, preexisting renal disease, and the use of antihypertensive agents. Similar studies in a coronary population have identified a contrast volume to calculated creatinine clearance ratio of greater than 3 as highly predictive of CIN [20].

Technical Considerations for TEVAR

The length of coverage of thoracic aortic segment should also be taken into consideration with respect to the potential for spinal cord ischemia (SCI) and paraplegia. Data regarding paraplegia rates between TEVAR and open thoracic aneurysm repair is controversial but suggests a lower incidence in TEVAR [21, 22]; however, the rate is not insignificant with estimates around 3–6.6 % of all thoracic endograft repairs reported [23, 24]. In a similar manner to open thoracic aneurysm repair, cerebrospinal fluid (CSF) drainage may confer protection against SCI in certain selected cases, such as extensive coverage of the thoracic aorta (>20 cm coverage) [25] and bilateral hypogastric artery occlusion, in the setting of previous infrarenal abdominal aortic repair. It also has been demonstrated to reverse postoperative paraplegia after TEVAR [26]. Anatomical considerations for endograft repair, although expanded and altering with the advent of newer commercial device, can essentially be broken down into three main areas: endovascular access, proximal and distal landing zone, and endograft sizing.

Access to the thoracic aorta is most commonly favored via the femoral arteries, and thus size of the iliofemoral segment, tortuosity, calcification, and absence of occlusion or severe stenosis should be taken into account when planning TEVAR. Traditionally, an adequate size of iliofemoral artery would be around 8 mm, minimizing the risk of iliac artery tear and allowing device sheath placement safely without complete occlusion to flow during the procedure. Smaller device profiles and thus smaller delivery sheaths will likely make placement of TEVAR through smaller caliber arteries feasible; however, present recommendations place this size as the lower limit of acceptable conduit. Options for delivery conduit in the presence of contraindications as pointed above include delivery of TEVAR via open iliac access or even distal aortic access, when the iliofemoral segment is not available [27]. Retroperitoneal access to the iliac artery with anastomosis of a 10-mm Dacron graft to the distal common iliac artery is a well-recognized means of establishing an endovascular conduit for TEVAR (Fig. 6.2).

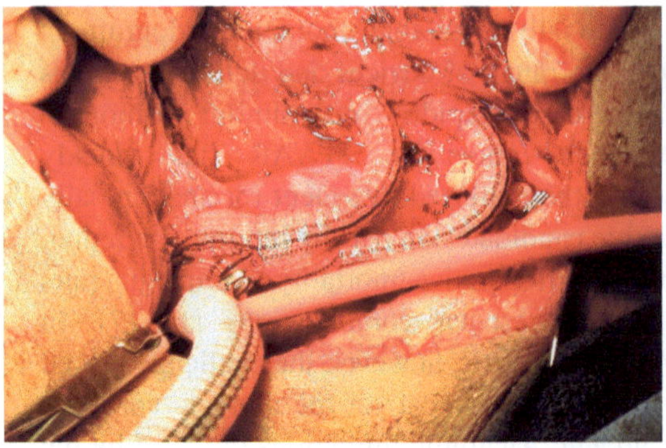

Fig. 6.2 Dacron conduit anastomosed to a bifurcated graft to accommodate TEVAR sheath access (Courtesy of Dr. Robert Rhee, M.D.)

The proximal landing zone for TEVAR is classified according to coverage of the arch vessels and can be represented by five discrete zones. The Ishimaru classification of thoracic landing zones is represented in the Fig. 6.3 [29]. Zone 0 requires coverage of all three arch vessels with proximal fixation in the ascending aorta. Zone 1 abuts the innominate artery and covers both the left common carotid artery (LCCA) and the left subclavian artery (LSA). Zone 2 abuts the LCCA and covers the LSA. Zone 3 abuts the LSA but does not cover any branch vessels. Zone 4 represents a proximal landing zone in the descending thoracic aorta.

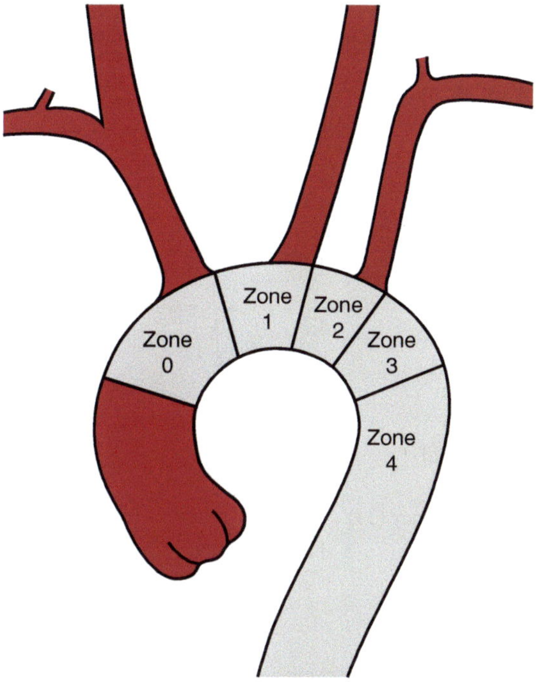

Fig. 6.3 Ishimaru classification of thoracic aortic proximal landing zones (This figure was published in Cho and Makaroun [28])

The classification of proximal landing zone represents more than just an anatomic delineation in that the decision to repair thoracic aneurysms requiring adjunctive procedures to revascularize arch vessels may influence the assessment of operative risk and therefore approach to management. An adequate seal zone proximally is generally respected at 2–3 cm; however, arch angulation, device type, and other anatomic features of an aneurysm may make achieving a proximal seal more complex. Proximal coverage increases the complexity of TEVAR with carotid to carotid and carotid to subclavian bypasses bringing additional morbidity to the operation. Hybrid approaches to arch revascularization with debranching of the great vessels followed by TEVAR have been well described, although the magnitude of operation in this high-risk population is often comparable to a more traditional repair, leading to mixed enthusiasm for this approach [27, 30, 31]. Table 6.2 provides an overview of recent published studies of left subclavian coverage during TEVAR without revascularization with respect to neurological outcomes of stroke and spinal cord injury.

Distal landing zones are determined by the distal extent of the thoracic aneurysm and may present a similar challenge if the thoracic aorta is aneurysmal at the level of the visceral segment. Collateralization of the celiac axis and superior mesenteric artery (SMA) via the gastroduodenal artery and others may allow coverage of the celiac with minimal adverse effects to the midgut organs. More distal coverage of the visceral segment involves a similar attitude to that regarding the arch vessels. The greater coverage that is required, the greater the endovascular complexity of TEVAR becomes. Newer techniques such as chimney or snorkel grafts in addition to TEVAR may assist in a completely endovascular solution in high-risk patients; however, the durability of these approaches is still being evaluated. Hybrid debranching procedures for the visceral segment have been described with rerouting of visceral flow from distal targets such as the infrarenal aorta, iliac arteries, and prior infrarenal aortic bypass grafts [30, 40] (Fig. 6.4).

Endograft sizing has altered dramatically over the decade of clinical use, and currently available devices range from 22 to 46 mm in diameter providing the ability to repair aortic inner diameters of 16–42 mm. The original Gore (W.L. Gore & Associates, Flagstaff, AZ) TAG, Medtronic (Medtronic, Santa Rosa, CA) Talent/Valiant, and Cook (Cook Medical, Indianapolis, IN) Zenith TX2 devices were configured for larger aortic sizes designed to be used in patients with thoracic aneurysms. The recent advent of smaller endograft diameters has been driven by the continued interest in the treatment of thoracic aortic trauma, where smaller aortic diameters are encountered. TEVAR sizing typically involves an element of oversizing, 10–20 % greater than the intended aortic landing zone diameter. This approximation, however, varies slightly by device type and intended placement within the aorta. Curved or angulated aortic landing zones often require careful sizing to avoid infolding, bird's beak, or high shear or stress forces. Consideration of the expected conformation of the endograft within a particular aneurysm requires experience and

Table 6.2 Summary of results from selected recent published reports of left subclavian coverage without revascularization during TEVAR and neurologic outcomes

Author	No. patients	Device	Urgency	% stroke	% SCI
Schoder et al. [32]	58	Talent, TAG, Endofit	Elective (39) Urgent (19)	3.1	9.4
Marcheix et al. [33]	45	Talent, TAG	Elective (37) Urgent (8)	16.7	0
Feezor et al. [34]	196	TAG	Elective (138) Urgent (30)	4	12.1
Buth et al. [35]	606	Various devices	Various	4.2	5
Rodriguez et al. [36]	324	TAG	Elective (224) Urgent (100)	8.3	8.3
Woo et al. [37]	70	TAG, Talent, TX2	Elective (47) Emergency (23)	11	0
Kotelis et al. [38]	88	TAG, Talent, Zenith, Endofit	Elective (54) Urgent/emergency (34)	3	1.5
Holt et al. [39]	78	Talent, TAG, TX2	Elective (50) Emergency (28)	11.6	6.9

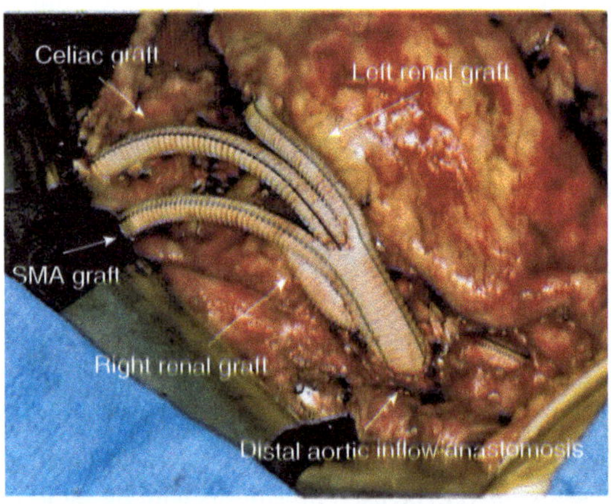

Fig. 6.4 Hybrid debranching of visceral segment with inflow from distal aorta. *SMA* superior mesenteric artery

judgment in order to select the correct device type and size and is aided by accurate three-dimensional reconstructions.

Operative Techniques in TEVAR

Based upon the criteria outlined above, the intended access vessel is chosen for delivery. In most cases, the common femoral artery on the right side provides the most direct route to the aorta and is favored. Although open access to the common femoral artery may be considered, percutaneous approaches utilizing predelivered closure devices are commonly employed. Given the large sheath diameters that are required depending on endograft size, Perclose (Abbott Vascular, Abbott Park, IL) suture technique or similar closure techniques are reliable percutaneous options [41]. Contralateral access is obtained for placement of a marker pigtail catheter. Stiff wires (Lunderquist [Cook Medical, Bloomington, IN] or Amplatz [Boston Scientific, Natick, MS]) are placed in the ascending aorta to allow tracking of device sheaths through areas of tortuosity and calcification. Fluoroscopic visualization of wire placement is recommended to avoid inadvertent arch vessel cannulation or intracardiac placement. Marking of the distal end of the wire on the angiography drapes allows the angiography team to ensure relatively constant positioning of the proximal tip without need for repeated fluoroscopy. Imaging of the thoracic aorta at the level of interest is performed . Accurate imaging at the level of the arch may be facilitated by left anterior oblique projection, while at the visceral segment, lateral or oblique views may demonstrate celiac or SMA orifices more clearly, and cranial-caudal views may provide better identification of the aorta at the renal orifices.

Intravenous heparin is given prior to introduction of large delivery sheaths and under fluoroscopic visualization directed to the proximal area of interest in the thoracic aorta. The selected thoracic endograft is introduced through the sheath and placed fluoroscopically just beyond (proximal to) the proximal neck to be withdrawn to the desired level prior to deployment. This maneuver is critical in allowing any proximal stored energy to be dissipated with withdrawing of the device. Inadvertent forward movement of the endograft can occur if proximal advancement followed by distal realignment is not attended to prior to device deployment. Accurate placement is essential when deploying the endograft near or over branch vessels, and it is often helpful to have wire access in the branch vessel from a femoral or brachial route.

TEVAR may involve the use of more than a single device component. In these cases, overlap between segments as per device manufacturer's recommendation should be adhered to prevent type III endoleaks. If devices are of the same size and in tortuous area, a longer overlap is necessary to avoid type III endoleaks. The order of deployment of devices with respect to distal or proximal landing zones is dependent on the particular anatomy and device used. When more than two devices are used, it is recommended to treat the proximal and the distal landing zones first, followed by the third larger device connecting the two. When treating a large proximal aneurysm, the distal endograft may be deployed first followed by proximal deployment so as to stabilize the proximal endograft and facilitate accurate placement. In case of treatment for acute aortic dissection, deployment should occur from proximal to distal direction as retrograde dissection leading to fatal pericardial tamponade and aortic root disruption have been reported when the distal endograft was deployed first [40, 42, 43]. Molding of the seal zones proximally and distally and additionally at component zones is often performed with compliant balloons depending on the technical result after endograft deployment.

The different commercial devices have idiosyncrasies to deployment that are beyond the scope of this chapter, however, generally adhere to similar general principles after following the steps outlined above. The Gore TAG endoprosthesis is an expanded polytetrafluoroethylene (ePTFE) graft with an external nickel-titanium (nitinol) self-expanding stent component attached to the graft. The Medtronic Valiant Thoracic Stent Graft is a modular device composed of a woven polyester fabric within a nitinol stent frame and incorporated bare-metal struts at the proximal and distal extent that are designed to maintain perfusion to major branch vessels while extending landing zones. The Cook Zenith TX2 device is a modular device composed of Dacron graft sewn to a set of stainless steel Z-stents. The device has active fixation barbs at both proximal and distal ends to reduce the risk of migration; the proximal barbs are oriented caudally and the distal proximally. The steel skeleton is exoskeleton except at the proximal end where the stents are inside in an effort to optimize graft apposition to the aortic wall. The Bolton Relay thoracic graft (Bolton Medical, Sunrise, FL) is made of self-expanding nitinol exoskeleton covered with Dacron. The proximal portion of the device has an exposed bare-metal stent. There is a double "S" configuration of the support bar along the length of the device that is designed to follow the natural curve of the aorta while providing columnar strength.

After successful deployment of the endograft, completion angiography is performed to assess the proximal, distal, and component seal zones. This may be undertaken before or after balloon apposition but should be focused on the presence or absence of endoleaks, adequate fixation in proximity to branch vessels without occlusion of the branch, and acceptable configuration within the aorta, i.e., no evidence of critical narrowing, crimping or folding, or poor apposition along the lesser curvature of the aortic arch (bird's beak). The presence of endoleaks can be difficult to appreciate when subtle, and incorporating a delay into the subtracted imaging may assist in detecting this occurrence. Lateral or oblique projections may be required to image visceral orifices to ensure patency. Extension cuffs or balloon apposition of inadequate seal zones for endoleaks will usually suffice in the absence of a gross technical

Table 6.3 Outcomes from recent thoracic endograft trials

Series	No. patients	Device	30-day mortality (%)	SCI (%)	MAE (%)	Late endoleak (%)	Aneurysm growth (%)	1 year aneurysm-related survival (%)
Thompson et al. [46]	46	Excluder	4	0	23	NR	0	100
Riesenman et al. [47]	50	Various	8	0	NR	21.8	0	NR
Rodriguez et al. [36]	406	TAG	5.5	1.9	22.7	4	NR	94.4
Gore TAG [16]	140	TAG	1.5	2.8	28	3.9	9	97
TX2 investigators [17]	160	TX2	1.9	5.6	41.9	3.9	7.1	94.2
VALOR trial [13]	195	Talent	2.1	8.7	30	12.2	8.5	96.9
Murphy et al. [48]	58	Talent, TAG, TX2	3.4	3.4	24.1	13.8	8.6	96.6

SCI spinal cord injury, *MAE* major adverse event as defined per Sacks criteria [49], *NR* not reported (includes studies where standardization of outcome between studies is not suitable to be included as a comparison)

misadventure and correct graft placement. Type I to III endoleaks have been described in reports of TEVAR outcomes, similar to that experienced in EVAR, with a frequency of 19–40 % [44, 45]. Table 6.3 details recent thoracic endograft trials with respect to neurological and aneurysm-related outcomes and mortality.

New Horizons for TEVAR Application

Branched and Fenestrated Endograft Repair

Following along the continuum of endovascular solutions for complex TAAA repair, a clinical focus had been established in a completely endovascular solution that attempted to reproduce normal thoracoabdominal aortic morphology with durable renovisceral branch preservation. Branched endografts represent an important step in the evolution of TEVAR toward an aneurysm-specific endovascular repair. The interest in these specific devices has grown from physician-championed trials at selected institutions under investigational device exemption (IDE) protocols to industry-sponsored multicenter trials such as the Ventana™ (Endologix, Irvine, CA) fenestrated stent graft trial with the intent of bringing branched and fenestrated thoracoabdominal grafts to commercial viability.

The ability to perform a completely endovascular repair of a TAAA was first demonstrated in 2001 with visceral perfusion to both renal arteries, celiac, and SMA maintained by branched grafts from the endograft (Fig. 6.5) [18]. The clinical realization of this pioneering concept has since led to the application of branched and fenestrated endografts to selected patients who were precluded from standard endovascular repair based on anatomical constraints and who also were not favorable candidates for open repair [50–57]. Contraindications to complete endovascular repair vary within trial exclusion criteria and physician selection, however, generally include patients with significant stenosis or visceral branch angulation relative to the aortic centerline, patients who present as an emergency or urgently, primarily due to the complex technical nature and duration of the procedure, and patients who are not able to tolerate the greater amounts of contrast dye administered due to severe underlying renal failure.

Technique

Technical considerations regarding the use of endovascular stent grafts with branch perfusion include the decision to use a custom-made fenestrated or

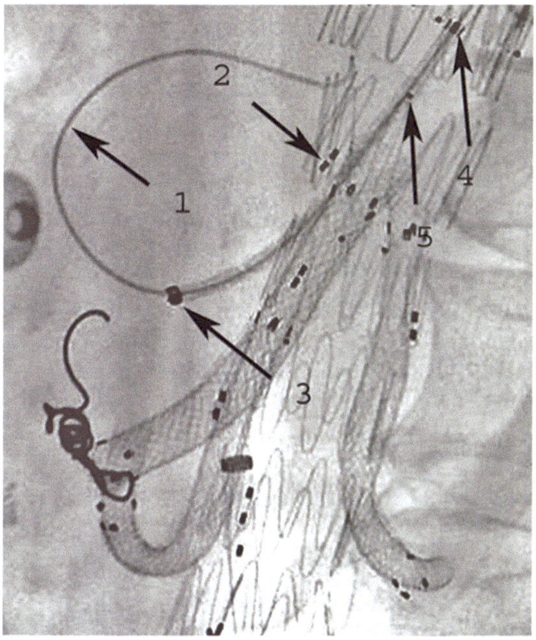

Fig. 6.5 Quadruple-branched endograft repair of thoracoabdominal aneurysm. *1* – Guidewire access to right renal artery. *2* – Radiopaque marker at outer edge of branch cuff. *3* – Distal end of the undeployed Fluency™ graft. *4* – Proximal end of the undeployed Fluency™ graft. *5* – Inner end of the branch cuff (Courtesy of Dr. Timothy A.M. Chuter, DM)

branched device or a combination branched and fenestrated device. The use of fenestrations is more relevant in discussion regarding para- or juxtarenal aneurysms that have a significant infrarenal component and a short or unfavorable proximal neck that requires fixation at or above some of the visceral branches. Fenestrations at the level of the renal artery might allow adequate sealing for a short proximal neck, however, more likely would be the use of a branched graft to one or more renal arteries with scallop or fenestration of the endograft to celiac and SMA segments, respectively [58–60]. Access from the femoral route is required for delivery of the larger diameter branched thoracic endograft, and contralateral placement of a large sheath (20 Fr or similar) facilitates placement of branch wire access and delivery systems (Fig. 6.6).

Axillary or brachial access is required for placement of a branch stent if oriented caudally and is best facilitated by a coaxial technique using two wires via upper extremity access with one of the wires traversing from brachial to femoral artery. The choice of balloon-expandable or self-expandable stents and whether to use covered or uncovered stents is highly dependent on aneurysm configuration, although the use of covered

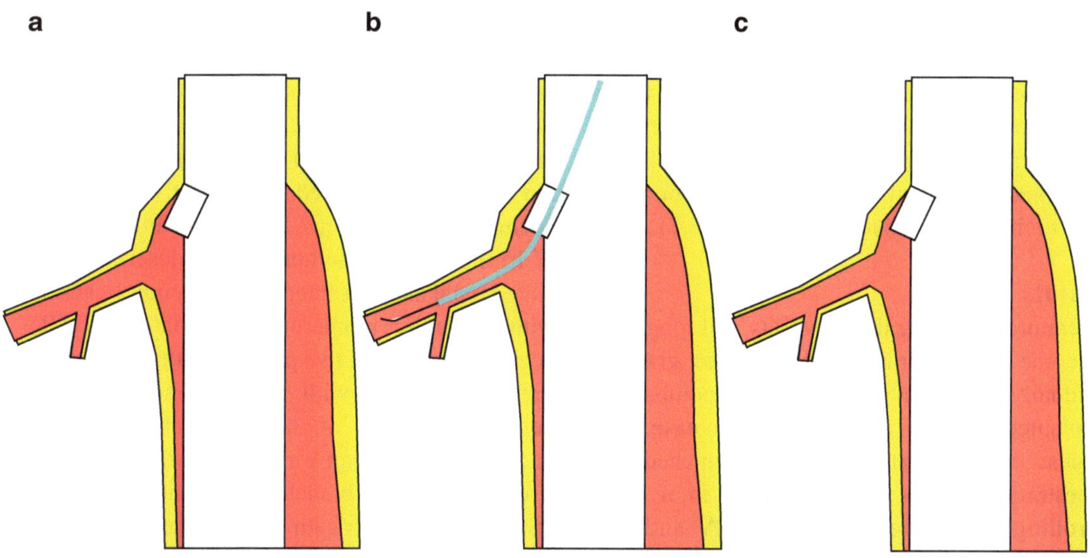

Fig. 6.6 Cannulation of branched endograft cuff with placement of branch graft within visceral vessel. (**a**) Branched endograft positioned with cuff directed toward visceral vessel takeoff. (**b**) Wire access and stabilizing sheath placed within visceral vessel. (**c**) Branched graft deployed within visceral vessel with proximal portion within branched endograft cuff (Courtesy of Dr. Timothy A.M. Chuter, DM)

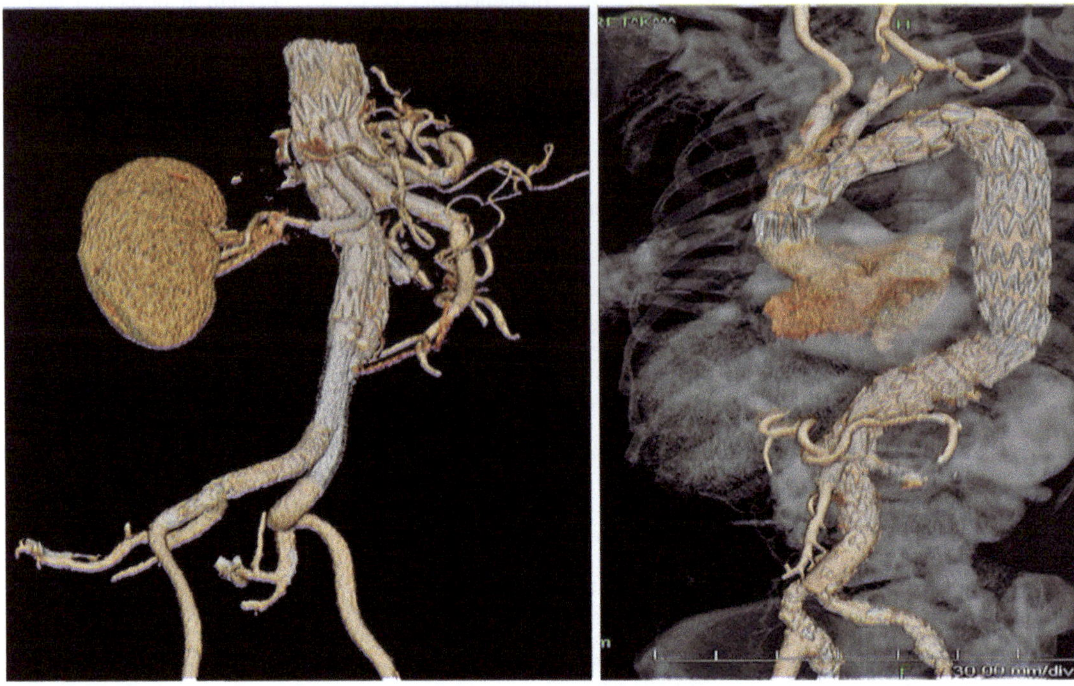

Fig. 6.7 CT reconstruction following complete endovascular thoracoabdominal branch graft repair with four vessel branch preservation (*left*) and innominate and left common carotid branch preservation with left carotid to subclavian bypass (*right*) (Courtesy of Dr. Timothy A.M. Chuter, DM)

stents is appropriate for branch revascularization in situations where the branch lies within aneurysmal aorta so as to exclude branch flow from the aneurysm sac [56]. Balloon-expandable stents, when used, are placed with enough length inside the aortic graft to allow overdilation and flaring of the internal segment. This functions to provide additional stability of the stent by functioning as a rivet to the main aortic graft [54] (Fig. 6.7).

Results

Literature regarding the durability and long-term outcome of fenestrated and branched grafts is gradually accumulating as the number of implanted devices continues to increase. The largest contemporary series of branched and fenestrated devices was described in a study enrolling 406 patients with TAAA and 227 patients with juxtarenal aneurysms over a 9-year period. The total 30-day mortality for all variants of juxtarenal and TAAA was 3.2 % with the highest mortality seen in the group of patients undergoing type I TAAA endovascular repair (12.5 %), although only 16 patients underwent repair of this type. The lowest 30-day mortality was seen in juxtarenal aneurysm repair (1.8 %). Late aneurysm rupture after endovascular repairs was very rare (0.8 %) and was due to component separation in two of the six patients. A combination of branched celiac and SMA with reinforced renal fenestrations was placed with a renal fenestration occlusion incidence of 2.2 % at a mean follow-up of 15 months. The authors further describe associated renal and mesenteric branch complications with worsening glomerular filtration rate (GFR) occurring in four of five patients with renal fenestration occlusion with two patients requiring hemodialysis, one of these permanently. Only one branch occlusion was noted in this series, as a result of sidearm branch compression; however, this led to patient death [61]. Regarding SCI, a 4.3 % rate was reported which is not significantly different when examined against a matched surgical cohort (7.5 %) [62].

The Fenestrated Investigators trial reported the intermediate outcomes (24 months) of a prospective, multicenter trial designed to assess the Zenith Fenestrated AAA Endovascular Graft (Cook Medical, Bloomington, IN) in 2009. The trial was specifically aimed at juxtarenal aneurysms with short proximal necks with image-guided patient-customized endografts. The most common configuration of the device incorporated two renal arteries and a fenestration for the SMA. The investigators report no aneurysm-related death, aneurysm rupture, or open conversion in the 24-month follow-up period. Type II endoleaks were noted in 26.1 % of patients; however, no patients sustained an increase in aneurysm size during this period. Renal events occurred in 26.7 % of patients: specifically four renal artery stenosis, two renal artery occlusions, and two renal infarcts. There were no incidences of dialysis-dependent renal failure during the 24-month follow-up period [59].

A systematic review of the current literature from 2000 to 2009 regarding fenestrated or branched endograft repair of TAAA highlighted the outcomes published regarding endovascular repair. The authors reviewed a total of 155 patients described in seven studies with a mean follow-up of 11.8 months. In 94.2 % of patients, technical success was achieved, in line with previous reports. There was a 7.1 % 30-day mortality overall, and 82.6 % of patients survived at 1 year. Interestingly, the authors describe a low incidence of permanent paraplegia of 1.9 % with 1.3 % incidence of paraparesis. The overall follow-up mortality in the reviewed period was 16.1 %. The authors conclude that endovascular repair is encouraging for patients who are unfit for traditional open surgical repair [51].

A recent small review of a single-institution experience describes a series of 50 patients treated using a custom-made Zenith device with fixed branches. The authors point to primary and primary-assisted technical successes of 88 and 92 %, respectively. There was a single intraoperative death due to aneurysm rupture. The authors highlighted the challenges of total endovascular repair with loss of two renal arteries during the initial procedure, loss of one celiac axis due to cannulation failure, and inability to cannulate the renal arteries in two patients who subsequently required laparotomy and retrograde renal bypass in one patient and splenorenal bypass in the other. The authors pointed to a moderate 30-day mortality of 8 and a 73.7 % freedom from further intervention at 2 years as evidence of feasibility of this approach [63].

While complete endovascular repair of TAAA shows feasibility and satisfactory early outcomes, the technology is not readily available for general use. The technology involved is complex and difficult. The device requires about 6 weeks of manufacturing time and thus is not applicable for emergent or urgent situations, although safety and efficacy of standardized "off-the-shelf" devices are being evaluated at the present time [60]. For patients who may not tolerate an open thoracoabdominal or thoracic operation but whose anatomy and extent of aneurysm mandate coverage of visceral or supra-aortic trunk and do not have access to complete endovascular repair, alternative approaches have been developed.

Hybrid Repair

The term hybrid repair describes the performance of an open surgical debranching or rerouting of branch vessel inflow to allow placement of a thoracic endograft either during the same operation or as a second stage once recovery from the open operation has occurred. For visceral vessel debranching, the inflow sources are commonly from the common iliac artery, infrarenal aorta, or previous aortic graft. For great vessel debranching, the inflow sources may be the common carotid or the ascending aorta. This effectively extends the potential landing zone for TEVAR either proximally or distally while preserving blood flow to the critical branch vessels.

Debranching for Lesions Involving the Renovisceral Vessels

Technique

Visceral debranching takes place via a standard abdominal exposure of the paravisceral aorta. If a complete thoracic endograft repair of the paravisceral segment is anticipated with coverage of all four visceral vessels, then exposure of SMA, celiac, and both renal arteries is obtained. A bifurcated, trifurcated, or hand-fashioned configuration of Dacron or ePTFE graft is anastomosed to the distal inflow source, and sequential bypasses to the visceral vessels are performed to minimize individual vessel ischemic time. Bypass can be performed end-to-end or side-to-end with ligation of the proximal segment of the vessel to prevent a type II endoleak. Similar to mesenteric revascularization procedures, the celiac axis bypass graft is usually routed retropancreatic with the celiac trunk or common hepatic artery as targets. Bypass to the infrapancreatic portion of the SMA is the usual configuration (Fig. 6.8). Access for TEVAR is then performed after completion of the debranching or most usually within the same hospitalization via the contralateral iliofemoral artery. In the event that the iliac arteries are not of sufficient size to accommodate the larger sheath required for the thoracic endograft, a conduit can be added to the branched Dacron graft that can be placed in a subcutaneous pocket for simple exposure and endograft delivery at the second stage.

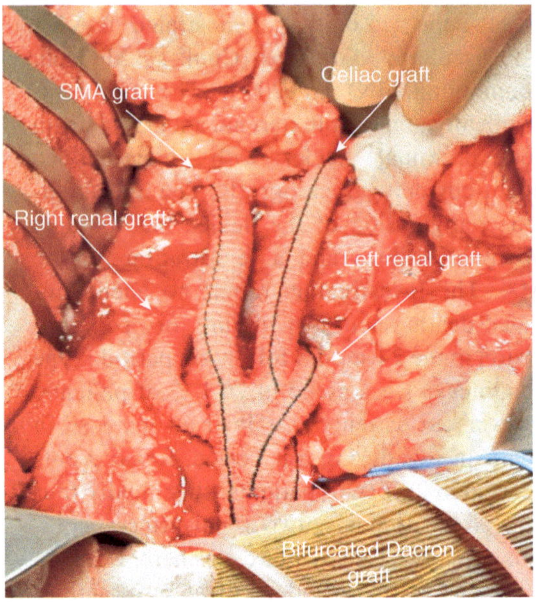

Fig. 6.8 Intraoperative photograph illustrating visceral debranching with retrograde bypass grafting to all four visceral vessels from the distal aorta. *SMA* superior mesenteric artery

Results

The timing of thoracic endografting was addressed in a small series by Lin et al. where 27 patients who underwent staged hybrid repair were compared with 31 patients undergoing a concomitant combined repair [64]. The results demonstrated a clear benefit to a staged rather than combined approach, in terms of perioperative morbidity, mostly due to the incidence of renal complications. The authors concluded that combined hybrid treatment strategies should be approached with caution for this reason. Interestingly, the staged approach was associated with a not insignificant incidence of aneurysm rupture of 6 % when the duration between stages was prolonged and, thus the authors suggest same-admission two-stage repair as the preferred approach.

A meta-analysis of recent reports of hybrid approaches to thoracoabdominal aortic pathologies attempted to assess outcomes across the spectrum of published experience. Moulakakis et al. reported on 19 publications with a total of 507 patients and demonstrated excellent pooled estimates of primary technical success and visceral graft patency of 96.2 and 96.5 %, respectively [65]. The pooled outcome estimates for irreversible paraplegia of 4.5 % and renal failure of 8.8 % are similar to previously reported outcomes with hybrid and open repair of TAAA; however, the authors reported a pooled 30-day/inhospital mortality rate of 12.8 %, concluding that the hybrid approach is still associated with significant mortality rates, and cited this uncertainty of its potential benefits as the cause of hesitation for wide application. Salient features of the hybrid repair have been reported in publications mainly from single institutional experiences and focus on the benefit of a less morbid abdominal procedure and endografting over the more invasive thoracoabdominal incision.

Quinones-Baldrich et al. reported their 10-year outcomes and experience with a combined endovascular and surgical approach at a single institution in 20 patients. The authors pointed to a 2-year all-cause mortality of 76.5 %, paraplegia incidence of 6.6 %, and absence of graft thrombosis at a mean follow-up of 16.6 months as comparable to that of contemporary series of open thoracoabdominal repair [40]. Perioperative complications were described by the authors to comprise acute renal failure not requiring dialysis in one patient, reoperation for enterotomy with prolonged respiratory failure, and chylous ascites managed conservatively in another patient. Three patients were readmitted within 30 days of the operation; one for a type IB endoleak that was managed with endovascular extension of the thoracic endograft and two patients for partial small-bowel obstruction requiring laparotomy and lysis of adhesions. The authors performed 13 single-stage repairs, where both abdominal debranching and thoracic endografting occurred during the same operation, and six two-stage repairs, with thoracic endografting occurring during the same admission after a short period of recovery from the abdominal stage. The authors concluded that the hybrid approach is a durable solution for patients with significant comorbidities; however, in younger, better-surgical-risk patients, the conventional open approach should be the preferred treatment.

Debranching for Lesions Involving the Aortic Arch

The presence of great vessels, arch angulation, and high blood flow in the arch all render the management of diseases involving or near the arch a great challenge for both the surgeon and the patient. Traditional open reconstruction requires cardiopulmonary bypass and often deep hypothermic circulatory arrest with their attendant morbidities and mortality. Aortic cross-clamping in the arch is associated with neurologic complications including stroke, paraplegia, and retrograde aortic dissection. Thus, high-risk patients who are not candidates for conventional open repair may be treated by hybrid approach.

A variety of ways exists for debranching the great vessels depending on involvement of the aortic arch with the disease process and the number of the vessels requiring revascularization. The management of the LSA, however, remains a controversial issue. Management has swung pendulously from initial revascularization of all LSA undergoing planned proximal landing zone in Zone 2 through selective revascularization. Coverage of the LSA is generally well tolerated by most patients; however, attendant risks in selective or non-revascularization strategies have recently been demonstrated to be associated with increased stroke and SCI. A higher overall stroke rate of 12–13 % was noted with coverage of the LSA compared with 0–2 % with LSA revascularization [34, 39, 66]. The combined stroke and SCI rate was noted to be significantly higher (8.4 % without versus 0 % with LSA revascularization) in a review of the European Collaborators on Stent-Graft Techniques for Aortic Aneurysm Repair (EUROSTAR) registry data [35]. The rationale for revascularization is that occlusion of the LSA may lead to vertebrobasilar ischemia with resultant posterior circulation strokes as well as anterior circulation strokes by compromising perfusion pressure to the Circle of Willis. Due to the added complexity and cost with potential complications, selective LSA revascularization has been advocated [41–44]. The Society for Vascular Surgery, however, has issued the following guidelines [67]: routine LSA revascularization is suggested when coverage is planned in an elective setting. LSA revascularization is recommended in the following circumstances: patent LIMA to coronary graft, left upper extremity hemodialysis fistula, diminutive or absent right vertebral arteries, left hand ischemia, extensive coverage (>20 cm) of the descending thoracic aorta, hypogastric artery occlusion, and termination of the left vertebral artery into the posterior inferior cerebellar artery. In emergency situations, individualized and expectant management is recommended.

Technique

The LSA can be revascularized by either LCCA to LSA interposition grafting using a 7- or 8-mm prosthetic bypass graft or LSA transposition to the LCCA [68]. The latter cannot be done when the vertebral artery (VA) originates from a very proximal segment of the LSA or in the presence of a patent internal mammary artery to coronary artery bypass graft. The first segment of the LSA is exposed for transposition through a transverse cervical incision above the clavicle. Dissection is carried between the two heads of the sternocleidomastoid muscle [45]. Alternatively, the sternal head can be detached to facilitate the exposure [69]. The omohyoid muscle is divided and the internal jugular vein retracted laterally. On the left side, care is taken to identify, divide, and ligate the thoracic duct and other small lymphatics. The small multiple lymphatics should be similarly handled on the right. The phrenic nerve, located on the anterior surface of the scalenus anticus muscle as it runs from a lateral to medial direction toward the mediastinum, must be preserved. The common carotid artery is mobilized for a sufficient length. The vertebral vein is ligated as it crosses the LSA anterior to the VA. The LSA and its branches are isolated and dissected free. The medial aspect of the scalenus anticus muscle may be divided or retracted when more distal segment of the LSA is necessary. Following systemic heparinization, the LSA proximal to the vertebral origin is ligated and divided. The vessel is then brought into approximation with the common carotid artery and anastomosed to the posterolateral aspect using the standard technique.

When a bypass is planned, the LSA is exposed in its second or third portion. Exposure of the artery is achieved by dividing the clavicular head of the sternocleidomastoid muscle, the omohyoid, and detaching the scalenus anticus muscle. Other precautionary measures with respect to the lymphatics and nerves are applied. A prosthetic interposition graft of appropriate size, usually 7 mm, is then anastomosed in the standard fashion.

As the disease involves more proximal arch such that proximal landing in zone 1 or 0 becomes necessary, more extensive revascularization should be performed. When landing in zone 1, preservation of blood flow to the LCCA and the LSA can be accomplished by extra-anatomic bypass grafting: right common carotid artery (RCCA) to LCCA bypass grafting with either sequential bypass to the LSA or transposition of the LSA to the LCCA (Fig. 6.9).

These extrathoracic procedures are less invasive and better tolerated than intrathoracic debranching procedures performed through a median sternotomy. Carotid to carotid bypass can be tunneled either anterior or posterior to the pharynx.

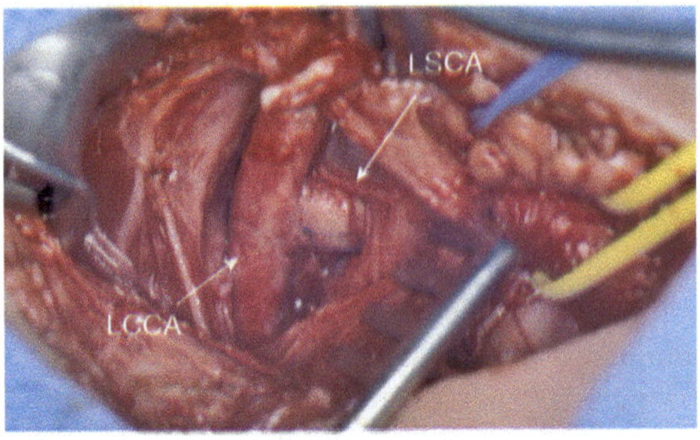

Fig. 6.9 Left subclavian to left carotid transposition in preparation for thoracic endograft delivery with proximal landing in arch zone 2

While it is technically a bit easier to place the graft anteriorly, it carries the risk of being exposed in subsequent median sternotomy or neck dissections. For this reason, the authors prefer to place it in a retropharyngeal fashion.

To assure adequate landing in zone 0, inflow is originated from the ascending aorta through a sternotomy. The ascending aorta should be evaluated with a preoperative CTA to assure that it is free of embolic burden such as atheroma or calcification so as to minimize the risk of cerebral embolic complication. A mini-sternotomy with extension to the fourth intercostal space may be utilized with adequate exposure. The pericardium is opened, and the ascending aorta is exposed and inspected (Fig. 6.10). Intraoperative transesophageal echocardiography can also be very helpful to evaluate the quality of the ascending aorta if there remains a clinical suspicion.

When TEVAR is planned at the same setting as a debranching procedure, as is required in complicated type B aortic dissection or in the setting of severe iliac stenosis, an 8-mm conduit for a stent graft should be pre-sewn to the hood of the aorto-innominate graft. The systolic blood pressure is then lowered to about 100 mmHg before a side-biting clamp is applied as far laterally over the ascending aorta as possible. The latter maneuver is important to avoid compression of the aorto-innominate graft by the sternum once it is reapproximated. A flanged Dacron graft of 10–12 mm in diameter is anastomosed in the usual fashion. Once hemostasis is assured, the patient is systemically heparinized

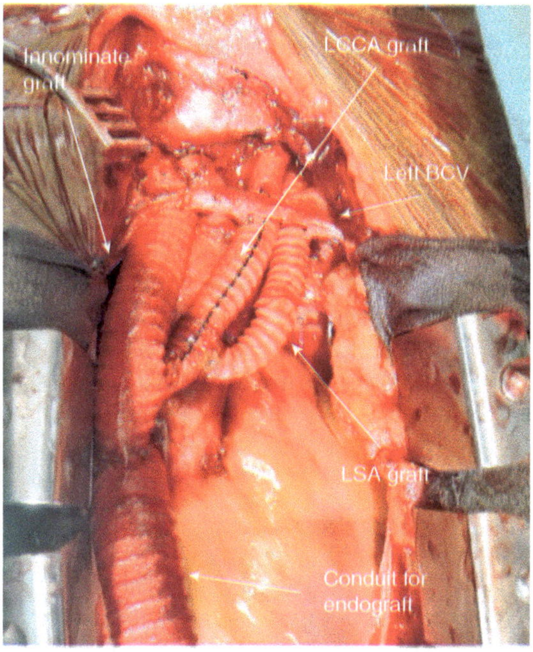

Fig. 6.10 Ascending aorta as inflow for complete arch debranching prior to thoracic endograft delivery with proximal landing in zone 0. Conduit can be seen attached to the ascending graft for antegrade endograft deployment. *LSA* left subclavian artery, *CCA* common carotid artery, *BCV* brachiocephalic vein

[70]. The graft is placed posterior to the innominate vein and anastomosed to the innominate artery in the usual fashion. Physiologic monitoring of the brain function is helpful to detect and treat cerebral ischemia. If the LCCA or the LSA needs to be revascularized, then a 7- or 8-mm sidearm graft(s) can be originated from the aorto-innominate graft. This reduces the risk of kinking of one of the limbs in the event a bifurcated graft is sewn to the aorta as well as bulk effect posterior to the sternum and consequent compression of the grafts by the reapproximated sternum.

TEVAR is then performed through a conduit using the standard technique in the same setting. Alternatively, it can be performed in a staged fashion through femoral access.

Results

Bergeron et al. reported their experience with 102 patients with TAAA with emphasis on a subgroup of 25 patients who required open adjunctive procedures to create a suitable proximal landing zone for thoracic endografting [71]. The authors performed partial arch debranching in ten patients and a complete arch debranching in 15 patients. Thoracic endografting was undertaken within 1–2 weeks from the open operation. Interestingly, the authors did not perform left subclavian bypass, instead selectively coiling the left subclavian only when a type II endoleak was apparent. In their reported series, there was one minor stroke at the time of partial arch debranching and one proximal aortic dissection as a result of clamp injury that resolved spontaneously. Postoperatively from the initial open operation, a minor stroke was observed in one patient due to occlusion of the LCCA bypass, which was treated with carotid to carotid bypass. The overall stroke rate was 8 % in this series. The 30-day mortality was 8 %; one patient died from wire perforation of the left ventricle and the other from multi-organ failure due to iliac artery rupture during thoracic endograft deployment. The endoleak rate in this series was 17 %, which the authors describe as three minor type I endoleaks, of which one was managed with graft extension, and one type II endoleak from the left subclavian artery, which was coiled at 1 week.

Melissano et al. reported their outcomes with 64 patients with TAAA involving part of all of the aortic arch [72]. The authors categorized the proximal landing zones of the proposed thoracic endograft using the Ishimaru classification; 14 cases required deployment in zone 0, 12 cases zone 1, and 38 cases in zone 2. The authors report 30-day mortality, stroke, and spinal cord ischemia rates of 6.3, 3.1, and 3.1 %, respectively. A policy of selective revascularization of the left subclavian artery was instituted for patients who had previously undergone left internal mammary coronary bypass, when the contralateral vertebral artery was inadequate, in young patients, in left-handed professionals, and in cases of previous abdominal aortic surgery to prevent paraplegia. The incidence of type I endoleak in this series was 12.5 % and aneurysm-related death rate was 16.5 % [49]. It is of note that the shortest landing zone was associated with the highest incidence rate of type IA endoleak at 33.3 %. The authors discuss their concern over the durability of extrathoracic bypass for the left carotid artery when compared to intrathoracic bypass. Carotid to carotid bypasses have patency rates of 88 % at 3 years and 84 at 5 years; [49, 73] however, experience with atherosclerotic bypass of the supra-aortic vessels does imply a better patency rate with intrathoracic bypass [74].

In a pooled analysis of selected studies of aortic arch debranching procedures (excluding case reports, series with less than five patients, mixed studies, studies in which cardiopulmonary bypass was used), a mean mortality rate of 15 %, stroke rate of 8 %, and paraplegia rate of 2 % were noted [75, 76]. Occlusion or hemodynamically significant stenosis of a bypass graft in this location can have devastating consequences. The long-term patency rate was estimated at 96 %. It should be noted, however, that the literature is sparse on the long-term data of debranching grafts. Notwithstanding, the patency rates following debranching are similar to patency rates of bypass grafts performed for occlusive disease and offer promise for excellent long-term durability.

Chimney/Snorkel Technique

The chimney graft was first conceptualized by Greenberg et al. in 2003 [77]. The concept was the use of self-expanding stents running parallel to the aortic wall to preserve blood flow to the renal artery while extending proximal landing zone for aortic stent graft. Hiramoto et al. then reported salvage of the inadvertently covered left common carotid artery during TEVAR using a stent [78]. Subsequently, Larzon et al. described "the top fenestrating technique" which reopened the renal, left common carotid, or the left subclavian arteries by preplaced stents [79]. Uncovered stents were predominantly used until Ohrlander et al. introduced the term "chimney graft" using a covered stent [80].

The chimney (also known as snorkel) strategy consists of placing parallel stents or stent grafts adjacent to the main body endograft to preserve blood flow to renal, visceral, and great vessels after exclusion of the aortic lesion. This approach can be used in patients who cannot tolerate open abdominal or thoracic operation in a planned fashion or as a bailout from inadvertent coverage of critical branch vessels during endovascular repair.

An extended application of the chimney technique is a "telescoping" chimney grafts in which multiple chimney grafts are used to provide the length needed to provide antegrade flow to the visceral vessels [81]. To extend the distal landing zone, a variant of the chimney technique, the "periscope" technique, in which the graft is reversed and the direction of blood flow to the target vessel is retrograde can be applied [82]. Another variant of this concept is the "sandwich "technique described first by Lobato et al. in 2010 [83]. The concept of this technique is to have the chimney grafts sandwiched between two aortic endografts. First, the main aortic stent graft is deployed with the distal end above the origins of the visceral/renal vessels of interest. Next, the target vessels are chimney grafted followed by deployment of another main aortic graft distal to the target vessels. The area between the proximal aspect of the chimney grafts and the gap between the two aortic grafts are then bridged by deployment of another aortic stent graft.

The successful chimney EVAR is predicated on thrombosis/closure of the "gutters," the space created by the presence of chimney stent/graft between the main aortic endograft and the aortic wall, or closure of the gutters around the chimney, a phenomenon that is affected by a variety of factors such as aortic wall rigidity, the number of chimneys, the length of the gutters, morphology of the neck, and size of the aorta.

Interactions between the aortic wall, chimney graft(s), and aortic endograft lead to conformation of these structures around each other, thereby closing/thrombosing the gutters. Local deformation of the aortic wall around the chimney graft is one example. If the aortic wall is calcified and rigid, it may not accommodate the chimney graft(s) and may contribute to an inadequate seal. The endograft also accommodates the chimney graft(s) by infolding and wrapping around it (them). To account for the additional fabric infolding to accommodate the chimney graft(s), the main body endograft is oversized by 20–30 % [84, 85]. Although the minimum length of the gutters to assure closure/thrombosis has not been evaluated, the longer the gutters, the higher the chances are for spontaneous thrombosis as resistance to flow is proportional to the length of flow channel. At least 10–15 mm of sealing zone is thought to be necessary [84, 86], although some authors recommend 20 mm [87].

The maximal number of chimney grafts that can be safely used has not been evaluated. Most studies report the use of two or less chimney grafts per patient. The use of three or more chimney grafts has been reported rarely and is associated with higher technical failure and endoleak rates [80, 81, 84, 85, 87]. Some investigators have limited their chimney grafts to two and intentionally covered the lower renal artery or coil embolized it if it originated from the aneurysm in order to prevent a type II endoleak. Other investigators, however, have reported successful use of three or more stent grafts [88–90]. It should be noted, however, as the number of chimney/periscope grafts used in a given patient increases, there is a progressive reduction in the cross-sectional area of the aortic lumen. This can be a problem with a small (<16 mm) aortic diameter in terms of crowding of the lumen [86].

Aortic neck morphology may play an important role. It is important to recognize that proximal fixation length is not necessarily the same as sealing zone when employing the chimney technique. The fixation length will be the sealing zone only when the gutters thrombose or close around the chimney graft(s), which may not occur in the setting of a reverse-tapered aortic neck. The presence of a sealing "ring" or segment below the chimney graft (or proximal to the chimney in the setting of periscope graft) would be helpful to achieve a seal, although not mandatory. In such settings, use of covered stents would be recommended over bare stents to maximize the chance of seal around the gutters.

The ideal choice of stent type has not been clarified. The areas of controversy include the use of balloon-expandable versus self-expanding stents, covered versus bare stents, and the order of deployment. Balloon-expandable stent provides superior radial strength and allows more precise deployment compared with self-expanding stents. It also allows deployment and balloon apposition at the same time, whereas self-expanding stents require one more step in order to balloon the stent to profile. The benefit of self-expanding stents includes a lower risk of compression on the main aortic endograft. Both types of devices have been used successfully as chimney grafts [91, 92].

With respect to the issue of bare stents versus covered stents (stent graft), theoretically, a covered stent would reduce the risk of a type IA endoleak; however, some investigators have reported no type IA endoleak associated with bare stent [85, 93]. Some investigators promote the use of bare stents as covered stents require larger introducers and are more likely to interrupt the cerebral blood flow in the setting of chimney grafting of the left common carotid or innominate artery [94, 95]. Proponents of stent grafts raise the concern for embolic complication into the target vessels from thrombus that is formed in the "gutters" or "cul-de-sac" [91]. Routine use of clopidogrel is advocated for this reason. At our institution, the current preference is to use covered stents. If self-expanding stents are used, placement of an additional bare-metal balloon expandable stent may be needed to increase radial force [81, 84].

Malperfusion to the target vessels may occur due to compression of the chimney graft by the main aortic graft. Conversely, lower extremity perfusion may be compromised due to narrowing of the main graft by multiple chimney grafts. Thus, selective pressure measurement may be necessary to rule out malperfusion of the vessel in concern. If a significant pressure gradient is noted, additional stenting or stent grafting should be performed to increase the radial force. In the setting of significant aortic graft stenosis and distal malperfusion, axillobifemoral bypass grafting may be considered [82].

Technique

The procedure proceeds in a similar fashion to standard TEVAR. Under general anesthesia, bilateral groins and the left upper extremity are prepared and draped in the sterile field. Antegrade access to the branch vessels is gained usually through the left brachial, axillary, or subclavian artery. Although percutaneous approaches may be used for the brachial artery, the authors prefer open exposure to minimize postoperative complications such as hematoma or thrombosis. If more than one branch vessel is to undergo chimney grafting, then the placement of two separate sheaths is usually required. Exposure of more than one vessel or a long segment of an access vessel may be necessary in such settings. Percutaneous access of femoral arteries is preferred over open exposure.

Careful attention is paid to assure placement of the chimney graft 1–2 cm proximal to the proximal leading edge of the main body endograft. Short chimney grafts may migrate over time, and longer grafts may become kinked or folded with aortic motion both leading to a risk of catastrophic branch occlusion. Ensuring wire access at all times until the completion of the TEVAR is critical in case a technical misadventure occurs, requiring further grafts to be placed in the branch vessels. Loss of wire access may result in stent graft deployment failure. Particular caution should be made when choosing the length of branch graft to account for significant foreshortening of the graft during deployment of the thoracic endograft occurs. The thoracic endograft tends to draw the branch graft into the aneurysm sac, and thus, length is often lost at the proximal leading edge of the main body endograft. When access via the axillary or brachial artery is impossible, access of the visceral vessels can be gained via the femoral artery with the branch graft deployed in a downward direction, thus, maintaining retrograde flow into the vessel.

Chimney Technique for Lesions Involving the Visceral Vessels

While open repair of pararenal/juxtarenal AAA and TAAA has been proven to be an effective and durable in centers of excellence [96–98], not all patients can undergo this physiologically challenging operation. For patients who are not fit to undergo any open abdominal procedure chimney technique, periscope technique or combination of the two may be an alternate strategy until fenestrated or branched grafts become available.

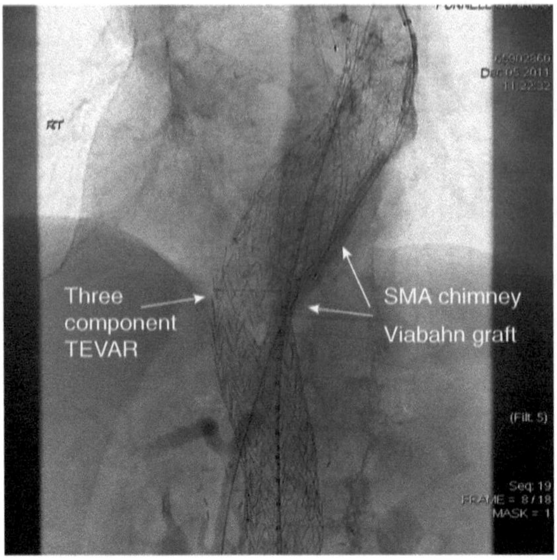

Fig. 6.11 Long superior mesenteric artery (*SMA*) chimney graft during TEVAR for thoracoabdominal aneurysm. Bilateral retrograde renal bypass grafts from the distal aorta were already performed prior to TEVAR

The chimney graft technique, however, is in general not applicable in TAAA due to the number of and the length of the chimney grafts needed. Thus, depending on the extent of the TAAA and preoperative patency of the visceral/renal vessels, the management strategy can be tailored to meet the individual patient's need. For instance, an extent 1 TAAA, in which the celiac axis and the SMA need to be revascularized, can be managed by periscope technique so as to avoid long length of chimney grafts that would have been required. For extent 5 TAAA, either chimney or periscope technique may be utilized. In selected cases, the renal arteries may be surgically revascularized followed by TEVAR with chimney grafting to the celiac axis and/or SMA (Fig. 6.11).

For cases in which more than three vessels need to be revascularized by chimney grafts, the "sandwich" technique can be applied. Kolvenbach et al. reported a series of five patients treated for symptomatic TAAA using that technique [88]. The sandwich technique holds unique advantages

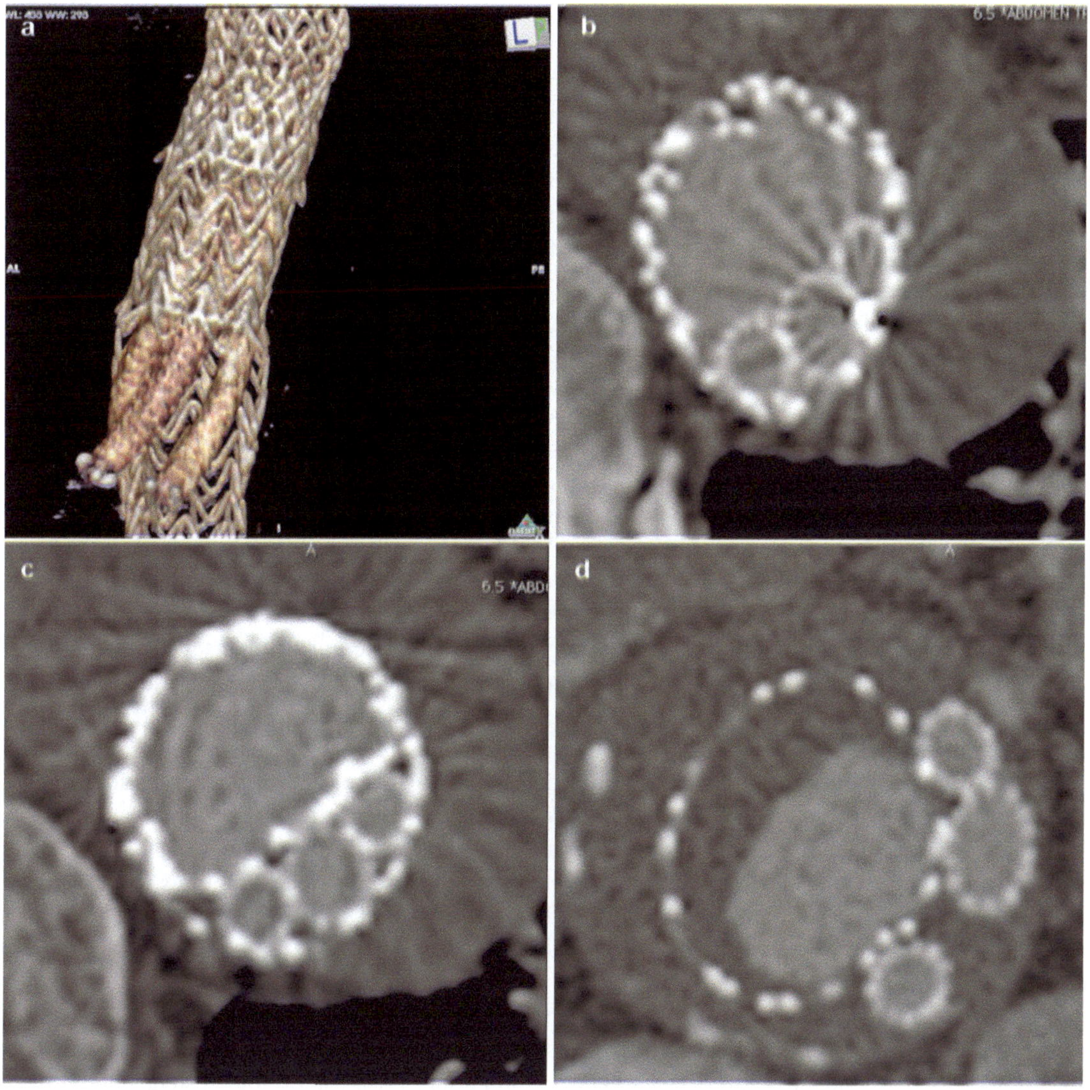

Fig. 6.12 (**a**) Sandwich technique using three Viabahn stent grafts 'sandwiched' between three thoracic endograft components. (**b**) At the superior aspect of the repair the Viabahn stent grafts lie within the cranial-most endograft. (**c**) At the middle of the repair the Viabahn stent grafts lie within the cranial-most endograft and outside of the middle endograft. (**d**) At the inferior aspect of the repair the Viabahn stent grafts lie outside of the caudal-most endograft (Courtesy of Dr. Armando C. Lobato, M.D., Ph.D.)

over fenestrated or branched repairs in that the components are cheap and readily available in large well-stocked endovascular centers and the devices are familiar to the procedural surgeon (Fig. 6.12). The technique does remain experimental at present, however, and requires longer-term follow-up, and larger patient cohorts before recommendations can be made regarding the durability of this approach.

Results

Despite the initial concern for proximal endoleak (type IA) due to an inadequate seal from the chimney stent, the so-called gutters, chimney grafts have shown to be safe and effective without a significant risk of type IA endoleaks. Another concern is that juxtaposition of two endografts (the main body endograft and the chimney graft) may result in material fatigue from the two endografts interacting with each other manifested by stent fracture or vessel injury that in turn will cause catastrophic events such as hemorrhage, stroke, or pseudoaneurysm formation [99, 100].

A recent publication examining the role of open and endovascular modalities for treatment of juxtarenal aortic aneurysms highlights the technical challenges and outcomes associated with totally endovascular repair of these aneurysms. For chimney graft placement, 30 patients were evaluated with 97.4 % technical success for target vessel preservation. Subsequent computed tomography scanning revealed two type II endoleaks in the chimney graft group. The 30-day mortality comparison between open and endovascular was 6.4 % in the open group versus 0 % in the endovascular group with significantly less transfusion and length of hospital stay in the endovascular group. One occluded renal chimney graft was detected at 45 days postoperatively with the development of left flank pain, and the patient underwent open thrombectomy of the left renal artery with subsequent iliorenal bypass. The authors discussed the issue of gutter leak and the significance with respect to long-term outcomes. In their reported series, balloon-mounted covered stents were used with a high radial force and excellent seal achieved in all cases. The authors hypothesized that longer gutter lengths may in fact reduce the rate of type I endoleaks by virtue of increased resistance within the gutter that promotes thrombosis of the gutter flow channel, thus, obliterating the endoleak over time [101]. Table 6.4 below examines the recent literature and outcomes regarding chimney/periscope grafting of the visceral aorta.

Chimney Technique for Lesions Involving the Aortic Arch

The aortic arch remains a challenging arena whether one approaches with a traditional open technique, endovascular means, or a combination thereof. A complete endovascular solution is not currently available and open reconstruction may present with significant risks especially with respect to cerebral ischemic complication. The hybrid approach to aortic arch lesions offers reduced morbidity and mortality by avoiding hypothermic circulatory arrest and aortic cross-clamping. However, it has its own attendant risks related to sternotomy, especially when redo-sternotomy is required and access to the ascending aorta is limited from prior coronary bypass grafting. For patients with prohibitively high surgical risks for hybrid or traditional repair, chimney grafts into the arch vessels can be utilized at the time of TEVAR. In the presence of a significant amount of thrombus in the arch, shaggy arch, or severe branch vessel stenosis, however, one should lean against the use of the chimney technique because of a significant risk of stroke.

When the proximal landing zone needs to be in zone 3, only the LSA needs to be revascularized. Access to the LSA can be gained via either percutaneous puncture or open exposure of the left brachial artery. A 6-French introducer sheath is then inserted so as to allow retrograde hand injection of contrast to delineate the anatomy and determine the site of chimney graft deployment. When the brachial artery is too small, the left axillary artery may be used.

When the disease process requires coverage of the arch proximal to the LSA, double-chimney technique may be used; even complete coverage of the aortic arch can be achieved without a sternotomy [91]. First described as a "bailout" procedure after inadvertent coverage of the left common carotid artery [78], use of branch stent/stent graft to preserve great vessel patency has gained popularity since open arch debranching may be accompanied by increased complexity and morbidity, mitigating the benefits of TEVAR. This can be performed with concomitant cervical bypass grafting and/or vessel transposition. Access to either common carotid artery is gained by open exposure of the vessel, and retrograde chimney stenting can be performed in this manner. Similarly, via a transbrachial approach the left subclavian artery can be chimney stented at the same time as thoracic endograft placement [102].

When the left common or innominate artery needs to be chimney grafted, controlled hypotension can be achieved with inflation and downward

Table 6.4 Outcomes from recent chimney/periscope grafting in the setting of visceral aortic aneurysm repair

Author	No. patients	Technical success rate	No. of covered arteries	Endoleak rate (type)	Stent type	30-day mortality rate	Primary patency rate	Complications
Donas et al. [101]	30	97.4 %	35 renal 3 SMA	6.7 % (all type II)	BES	0 %	97.4 % at 24 months	1 renal chimney occlusion
Ohrlander et al. [80]	6	NR	7 renal 2 SMA	0 %	BES SES	0 %	100 % at 30 days	2 SMA graft accidental coverage with aortic graft 1 death at 4 months
Coscas et al. [86]	16	94 %	20 renal 6 SMA	12.5 % (all type IA)	BES SES	12.5 %	96 % at 10.5 months	2 retroperitoneal hematoma 2 iliac dissection 1 seizure 3 renal infarctions 1 stroke 2 deaths
Lee et al. [84]	28	98.2 %	22 renal 6 SMA/CA/renal comb.	25 % (2 type I, 3 type II, 2 type III)	BES SES	7.1 %	98.2 % at 10.7 months	2 perinephric hematoma 3 deaths 1 permanent hemodialysis 1 iliac artery injury 1 brachial plexus nerve injury 1 myocardial infarction 1 stroke
Bruen et al. [87]	21	97.3 %	20 renal 9 SMA	19 % (1 type IA, 3 type II)	BES	4.8 %	84 % at 12 months	6 acute kidney injuries 2 strokes 2 deaths 1 asymptomatic SMA stent occlusion 3 access site PSA 3 ileus 1 renal artery occlusion 1 myocardial infarction 3 arterial thrombosis
Donas et al. [100]	72	99.2 %	107 renal 14 SMA 6 CA	16.7 % (6 type I, 6 type II)	BES SES	0 %	99.2 % at 15.9 months	1 renal stent occlusion 1 myocardial infarction 1 renal hematoma

BES balloon-expandable stent, *SES* self-expanding stent, *SMA* superior mesenteric artery, *CA* celiac artery, *PSA* pseudoaneurysm, *NR* not reported

traction of an occlusion balloon at the right atrial-caval junction via femoral vein access [103]. Alternatively, adenosine-induced temporary cardiac arrest can be utilized.

In the setting of complete arch coverage, the sequence of device deployment may be an important consideration. In order to minimize ischemic time to the brain, some authors recommend deploying the chimney graft into the left common carotid or innominate artery before implantation of the thoracic endograft to avoid complete interruption of the blood flow to the brain [94].

Results

Gehringhoff and colleagues described a small contemporary series of nine patients undergoing TEVAR for symptomatic aortic arch pathologies. The authors reported the application of TEVAR in five urgent aortic arch aneurysms, a mobile aortic thrombus with peripheral embolism, symptomatic type B dissection, penetrating aortic ulceration, and a persistent type I endoleak following TEVAR. The LSA underwent chimney grafting in eight cases with the LCCA undergoing chimney grafts in five patients. The immediate technical success, as measured by the patency of the target branch vessel after TEVAR and absence of large type I endoleak, was 88.9 %. The authors reported a 30-day mortality of 11 % from one patient suffering cardiac insufficiency. In this small series, there were two access site complications: a brachial artery pseudoaneurysm requiring repair and repair of a heavily calcified femoral artery puncture. In addition, one patient sustained a persistent type I endoleak that required surgical conversion via an open approach. The early follow-up results demonstrated a 15-month patency of 78 % for arch chimney stents in the remaining seven patients [104].

Shu et al. recently reported their outcomes from a similar small series of TEVAR and chimney grafts for acute arch dissections [105]. A total of eight patients were treated with TEVAR and LCCA chimney grafting with intentional coverage of the LSA after cerebrovascular assessment. Particularly noteworthy is the absence of major complication in this series; the authors reported no stroke, paralysis, death, or access site complications, albeit in a limited number of patients. Patency was 100 % for the LCCA stents at a mean follow-up interval of 11.4 months. Accordingly, the assessment of true- and false-lumen flow demonstrated enlargement of the true lumen and compression of the false lumen in this follow-up period with two conservatively managed type II endoleaks eventually resolving by the end of 11 months. The authors tentatively suggested that chimney grafting in the setting of TEVAR for acute dissections appears promising as a therapy for patients without adequate proximal landing zones.

These above results are in line with other literature reports of high early technical success and branch patency rates for acute aortic arch pathologies with relatively low incidence of endoleak and pave the way for the growing experience with the chimney technique and wider applicability to more elective settings [95, 106].

Multilayer Stent

Multilayer stent is the latest technology that is being evaluated in the treatment of vascular pathologies including aneurysms and dissections. The Cardiatis Multilayer Stent (Cardiatis, Isnes, Belgium) is a cobalt self-expandable bare stent that consists of a three-dimensional braided tube made of two interconnected layers. It is a type of flow-diverter stent in which optimal flow modulation through the layers was reached with a 65 % mean porosity, which allows the exclusion of aneurysm by promoting laminar flow in the main artery and the branch vessels while reducing flow velocity and vortex into the sac [107–112] (Fig. 6.13). The laminar flow in the main sac decreases shear stress on the wall, results in around a 90 % reduction in flow velocity outside the stent and decreased risk of rupture. In an aneurysm sac with branches, the flow is redirected to the collaterals due to the Venturi effects, with regression of the sac at a rate that is dependent on the diameter of the branch vessels and the compliance of the sac. The device is currently available in 22–44 mm in diameter for treatment of aortic aneurysms.

There are several reports of these stents being used to treat aortic [108, 110, 113] and peripheral aneurysms [107, 109, 111, 112, 114]. In France, application of this device for the treatment of TAAA is under investigation (Agence Française de Sécurité Sanitaire des Produits de Santé [AFSSAPS], protocol# 2008-A01396-49/A) [110]. Most of these reports are case reports with very short-term follow-up. Ruffino et al. reported on 19 patients with visceral aneurysms treated at 12 different centers. Initial technical success was 100 %; however, two stent thromboses occurred within 1 month, resulting in 6-month stent patency and sac thrombosis rate of 87.5 % [114]. Other stent-related complications such as migration, component separation, and fracture rates have not been reported. One of the major limitations of this technology is that the branch vessel orifices cannot be accessed during follow-up should that become necessary to treat subsequent stenosis of the overstented vessels.

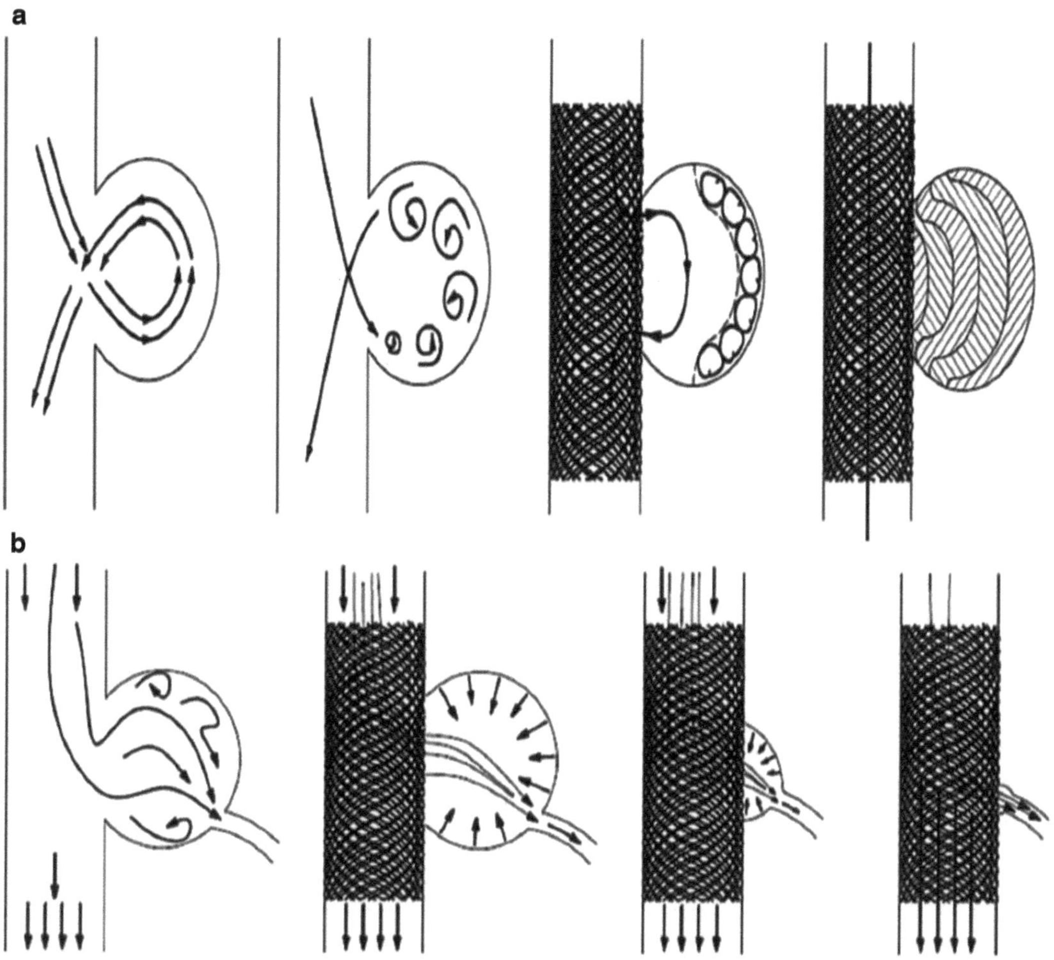

Fig. 6.13 (**a**) Representation of the effect on vortex velocity within an aneurysm sac once the multilayer stent is placed. A reduction of 90 % vortex velocity allows organized thrombus to form in layers thus excluding pressurization of the aneurysm sac. (**b**) Similar effect occurs in aneurysm sac with a branched vessel. Flow is redirected into the branch allowing branch patency with surrounding aneurysm sac shrinkage (Reproduced with permission from Allen Press. Benjelloun et al. [108])

While these case reports show promising early results, due to its extremely small numbers, no definitive conclusion can be made about early results, let alone long-term performance data.

Thoracic Endograft Application in Traumatic Thoracic Aortic Injury (TTAI)

In patients with blunt trauma, head injury is the prime cause of mortality. Second to this is TTAI. Estimates of the mortality due to TTAI in a trauma population range from 75 to 85 % during the initial phases of injury or subsequent resuscitation [114–117]. Compounding the fatality of such injuries is the observation that major head, abdominal, and pelvic injuries, each of which may be life threatening, often coexist with thoracic aortic trauma [115]. The clear benefit of TEVAR over open aneurysm repair in the elective and emergency setting provided the impetus for application of TEVAR to TTAI. The trauma population provided an ideal opportunity to utilize an endovascular mode of therapy given the relative underlying health of the patients, other additive traumatic issues, and the need for a procedure that would allow repair to be undertaken with minimal physiological insult and without disturbance of the delicate tissues surrounding a contained traumatic rupture.

A small series of 11 patients treated with stent grafts for acute thoracic aortic rupture demonstrated the feasibility of this approach to traumatic thoracic aortic injury. In this series, only three patients suffered aortic rupture due to trauma that underwent TEVAR, and there were no significant perioperative complications noted [118]. Since this early report, the use of TEVAR for blunt traumatic thoracic aortic injuries has increased exponentially [119]. Reflecting this trend, a recent American Association for the Surgery of Trauma (AAST) multicenter trial was completed, in which open versus endovascular repair of TTAI were prospectively compared and found to favor endovascular repair with respect to mortality and paraplegia rate [120]. Now, TEVAR has supplanted open repair for the treatment of TTAI at the authors' institution, a trend that is observed across the country [121].

However, due to the lack of commercially available device specifically engineered for TTAI to accommodate typically small (average of 19 mm diameter) and acutely angulated aortic arch, stent grafts implanted for treatment of TTAI often suffered from poor apposition to the aortic arch ("bird's beak" appearance). Thus, in addition to the usual plethora of endograft-related complications (endoleaks, migration, material fatigue), physiologic aortic coarctation with distal organ malperfusion, reperfusion of the pseudoaneurysm, and endograft collapse have been reported to occur [122–124].

The underlying mechanism of collapse is multifactorial and includes a small aortic diameter, a tight arch angulation, excessive oversizing (even up to 90 %) [125], a bird's beak phenomenon, low radial force devices, and material fatigue. It usually occurs within 30 days of implantation with reported incidence ranging from 0.4 to 19 % and most are asymptomatic, (Fig. 6.14), although delayed collapse at 38 months has been reported [126–128]. When diagnosed it should be corrected whether symptomatic or not. Reintervention can be undertaken by either open conversion with stent graft explantation in case of compression or by endovascular means in case of invagination [127]. Open conversion can be performed safely once the patient has recovered from the initial traumatic injuries [123]. In a large series of 139 TAG collapses, an 80 % successful reintervention rate was observed [127].

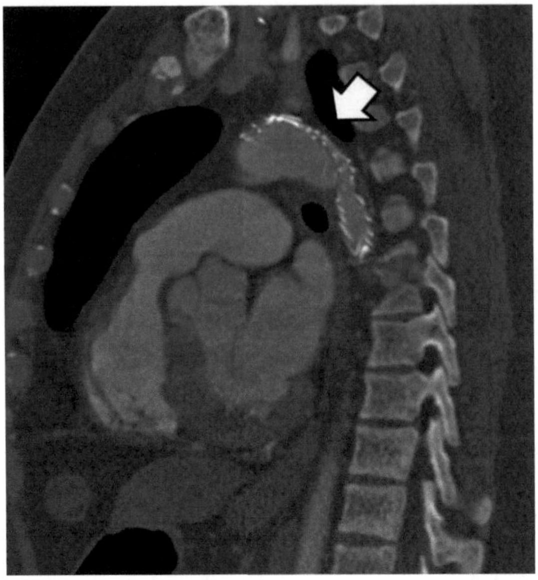

Fig. 6.14 CT angiogram of thoracic aortic stent graft collapse 38 months after TEVAR for traumatic aortic transection. Collapse (*arrow*) was associated with spinal-cord injury that recovered with re-expansion of endograft (Reproduced with permission from Elsevier. Shukla et al. [126])

Recently, newer generation devices designed to accommodate tight aortic angulation have become available. Cook TX2 Pro-Form device and Gore Conformable TAG devices allow greater flexibility at the aortic arch and wider range of oversizing as well as aortic diameter changes with tapered grafts to better accommodate challenging aortic morphology.

Conclusions

Thoracic endograft techniques are evolving and their use rapidly increasing. As EVAR has supplanted open infrarenal aortic aneurysm repair, so has the trend toward anatomically favorable candidates being primarily offered an endovascular solution. The recent innovations and techniques highlighted in this chapter serve to describe the advances in endovascular capability for those patients who are not well suited to open repair but who are not traditional candidates for TEVAR. The use of chimney techniques has increased and adequate short-term results have been demonstrated; however, the expansion of this technique to the repertoire of thoracic aortic surgeons may be curtailed in the future with the advent and introduction of branched and fenestrated endografts into the clinical arena.

Broadening the indications for TEVAR to include acute traumatic injuries to the thoracic aorta has led to the realization that older generation devices were not ideally suited for placement in relatively normal aorta, and therefore, clinical application has driven innovation and newer devices that are able to successfully treat a wider range of pathologies.

Although endovascular repair is fast becoming the preferred modality for treatment of thoracic aortic diseases, the physician should apply sound judgment when counseling individual patients and select the approach, device, and timing of surgery most suited to a particular individual. This will remain one of the most challenging aspects of thoracic aortic surgery in the modern era of endovascular surgery.

References

1. Kent KC, Zwolak RM, Jaff MR, Hollenbeck ST, Thompson RW, Schermerhorn ML, et al. Screening for abdominal aortic aneurysm: a consensus statement. J Vasc Surg. 2004;39(1):267–9.
2. Coady MA, Rizzo JA, Goldstein LJ, Elefteriades JA. Natural history, pathogenesis, and etiology of thoracic aortic aneurysms and dissections. Cardiol Clin. 1999;17(4):615–35.
3. Bickerstaff LK, Pairolero PC, Hollier LH, Melton LJ, Van Peenen HJ, Cherry KJ, et al. Thoracic aortic aneurysms: a population-based study. Surgery. 1982; 92(6):1103–8.
4. Lederle FA, Johnson GR, Wilson SE, Chute EP, Littooy FN, Bandyk D, et al. Prevalence and associations of abdominal aortic aneurysm detected through screening. Aneurysm Detection and Management (ADAM) Veterans Affairs Cooperative Study Group. Ann Intern Med. 1997;126(6):441–9.
5. Upchurch Jr GR, Patel HJ. Thoracic and thoracoabdominal aortic aneurysms: evaluation and decision making. In: Rutherford's vascular surgery. 7th ed. Philadelphia: Copyright Saunders Elsevier; 2010. p. 2021.
6. Ailawadi G, Knipp BS, Lu G, Roelofs KJ, Ford JW, Hannawa KK, et al. A nonintrinsic regional basis for increased infrarenal aortic MMP-9 expression and activity. J Vasc Surg. 2003;37(5):1059–66.
7. Halloran BG, Davis VA, McManus BM, Lynch TG, Baxter BT. Localization of aortic disease is associated with intrinsic differences in aortic structure. J Surg Res. 1995;59(1):17–22.
8. Moore Jr JE, Ku DN, Zarins CK, Glagov S. Pulsatile flow visualization in the abdominal aorta under differing physiologic conditions: implications for increased susceptibility to atherosclerosis. J Biomech Eng. 1992;114(3):391–7.
9. Pedersen EM, Sung HW, Yoganathan AP. Influence of abdominal aortic curvature and resting versus exercise conditions on velocity fields in the normal abdominal aortic bifurcation. J Biomech Eng. 1994;116(3): 347–54.
10. Parodi JC, Palmaz JC, Barone HD. Transfemoral intraluminal graft implantation for abdominal aortic aneurysms. AVS. 1991;5(6):491–9.
11. Dake MD, Miller DC, Semba CP, Mitchell RS, Walker PJ, Liddell RP. Transluminal placement of endovascular stent-grafts for the treatment of descending thoracic aortic aneurysms. N Engl J Med. 1994;331:1729–34.
12. Cho JS, Haider S, Makaroun MS. US multi-center trials of endoprostheses for the endovascular treatment of descending thoracic aneurysms. JVS. 2006;43(Suppl A):12A–9.
13. Fairman RM, Criado F, Farber M, Kwolek C, Mehta M, White R, et al. Pivotal results of the Medtronic Vascular Talent Thoracic Stent Graft System: the VALOR trial. JVS. 2008;48(3):546–54.
14. Leurs LJ, Bell R, Degrieck Y, Thomas S, Hobo R, Lundbom J. Endovascular treatment of thoracic aortic diseases: combined experience from the EUROSTAR and United Kingdom Thoracic Endograft registries. JVS. 2004;40(4):670–9.
15. Makaroun MS, Dillavou ED, Kee ST, Sicard G, Chaikof E, Bavaria J, et al. Endovascular treatment of thoracic aortic aneurysms: results of the phase II multicenter trial of the GORE TAG thoracic endoprosthesis. JVS. 2005;41(1):1–9.
16. Makaroun MS, Dillavou ED, Wheatley GH, Cambria RP. Five-year results of endovascular treatment with the Gore TAG device compared with open repair of thoracic aortic aneurysms. JVS. 2008;47(5):912–8.
17. Matsumura JS, Cambria RP, Dake MD, Moore RD, Svensson LG, Snyder S. International controlled clinical trial of thoracic endovascular aneurysm repair with the Zenith TX2 endovascular graft: 1-year results. JVS. 2008;47(2):247–57.
18. Chuter TAM, Gordon RL, Reilly LM, Goodman JD, Messina LM. An endovascular system for thoracoabdominal aortic aneurysm repair. J Endovasc Ther. 2001;8:25–33.
19. Zaraca F, Wiedermann CJ, Ebner H. Contrast media-induced nephropathy in patients undergoing

angiography prior to or during vascular surgery: a systematic review. Minerva Chir. 2011;66(6):553–60.
20. Gurm HS, Dixon SR, Smith DE, Share D, Lalonde T, Greenbaum A, et al. Renal function-based contrast dosing to define safe limits of radiographic contrast media in patients undergoing percutaneous coronary interventions. J Am Coll Cardiol. 2011;58(9):907–14.
21. Cheng D, Martin J, Shennib H, Dunning J, Muneretto C, Schueler S, et al. Endovascular aortic repair versus open surgical repair for descending thoracic aortic disease a systematic review and meta-analysis of comparative studies. J Am Coll Cardiol. 2010;55(10):986–1001.
22. Walsh SR, Tang TY, Sadat U, Naik J, Gaunt ME, Boyle JR, et al. Endovascular stenting versus open surgery for thoracic aortic disease: systematic review and meta-analysis of perioperative results. J Vasc Surg. 2008;47(5):1094–8.
23. Cheung AT, Pochettino A, McGarvey ML, Appoo JJ, Fairman RM, Carpenter JP, et al. Strategies to manage paraplegia risk after endovascular stent repair of descending thoracic aortic aneurysms. Ann Thorac Surg. 2005;80(4):1280–8.
24. Ullery BW, Cheung AT, Fairman RM, Jackson BM, Woo EY, Bavaria J, et al. Risk factors, outcomes, and clinical manifestations of spinal cord ischemia following thoracic endovascular aortic repair. J Vasc Surg. 2011;54(3):677–84.
25. Lam CH, Vatakencherry G. Spinal cord protection with a cerebrospinal fluid drain in a patient undergoing thoracic endovascular aortic repair. J Vasc Interv Radiol. 2010;21(9):1343–6.
26. Chiesa R, Melissano G, Marrocco-Trischitta MM, Civilini E, Setacci F. Spinal cord ischemia after elective stent-graft repair of the thoracic aorta. J Vasc Surg. 2005;42(1):11–7.
27. Chiesa R, Tshomba Y, Melissano G, Marone EM, Bertoglio L, Setacci F, et al. Hybrid approach to thoracoabdominal aortic aneurysms in patients with prior aortic surgery. JVS. 2007;45(6):1128–35.
28. Cho JS, Makaroun MS. Thoracic and thoracoabdominal aortic aneurysms: endovascular treatment. In: Rutherford's vascular surgery. 7th ed. Philadelphia: Copyright Saunders Elsevier; 2010. p. 2057.
29. Mitchell RS, Ishimaru S, Ehrlich MP, Iwase T, Lauterjung L, Shimono T, et al. First international summit on thoracic aortic endografting: roundtable on thoracic aortic dissection as an indication for endografting. J Endovasc Ther. 2002;9 Suppl 2:II98–105.
30. Hughes GC, Nienaber JJ, Bush EL, Daneshmand MA, McCann RL. Use of custom Dacron branch grafts for "hybrid" aortic debranching during endovascular repair of thoracic and thoracoabdominal aortic aneurysms. J Thorac Cardiovasc Surg. 2008;136(1):21–8, 28.
31. Vallejo N, Rodriguez-Lopez JA, Heidari P, Wheatley G, Caparrelli D, Ramaiah V, et al. Hybrid repair of thoracic aortic lesions for zone 0 and 1 in high-risk patients. J Vasc Surg. 2012;55(2):318–25.
32. Schoder M, Grabenwoger M, Holzenbein T, Cejna M, Ehrlich MP, Rand T, et al. Endovascular repair of the thoracic aorta necessitating anchoring of the stent graft across the arch vessels. J Thorac Cardiovasc Surg. 2006;131(2):380–7.
33. Marcheix B, Dambrin C, Bolduc JP, Arnaud C, Cron C, Hollington L, et al. Midterm results of endovascular treatment of atherosclerotic aneurysms of the descending thoracic aorta. J Thorac Cardiovasc Surg. 2006;132(5):1030–6.
34. Feezor RJ, Martin TD, Hess PJ, Klodell CT, Beaver TM, Huber TS, et al. Risk factors for perioperative stroke during thoracic endovascular aortic repairs (TEVAR). J Endovasc Ther. 2007;14(4):568–73.
35. Buth J, Harris PL, Hobo R, van Eps R, Cuypers P, Duijm L, et al. Neurologic complications associated with endovascular repair of thoracic aortic pathology: incidence and risk factors. A study from the European Collaborators on Stent/Graft Techniques for Aortic Aneurysm Repair (EUROSTAR) registry. JVS. 2007;46(6):1103–10.
36. Rodriguez JA, Olsen DM, Shtutman A, Lucas LA, Wheatley G, Alpern J, et al. Application of endograft to treat thoracic aortic pathologies: a single center experience. JVS. 2007;46(3):413–20.
37. Woo EY, Carpenter JP, Jackson BM, Pochettino A, Bavaria JE, Szeto WY, et al. Left subclavian artery coverage during thoracic endovascular aortic repair: a single-center experience. J Vasc Surg. 2008;48(3):555–60.
38. Kotelis D, Geisbusch P, Hinz U, Hyhlik-Durr A, von Tengg-Kobligk H, Allenberg JR, et al. Short and midterm results after left subclavian artery coverage during endovascular repair of the thoracic aorta. J Vasc Surg. 2009;50(6):1285–92.
39. Holt PJ, Johnson C, Hinchliffe RJ, Morgan R, Jahingiri M, Loftus IM, et al. Outcomes of the endovascular management of aortic arch aneurysm: implications for management of the left subclavian artery. JVS. 2010;51(6):1329–38.
40. Quinones-Baldrich W, Jimenez JC, DeRubertis B, Moore WS. Combined endovascular and surgical approach (CESA) to thoracoabdominal aortic pathology: a 10-year experience. J Vasc Surg. 2009;49(5):1125–34.
41. Perdikides TP, Georgiadis GS, Avgerinos ED, Paraskevas KI, Siafakas KX, Katsargyris A, et al. Percutaneous endovascular treatment of aortic aneurysms: clinical evaluation and literature results. Minim Invasive Ther Allied Technol. 2011 Nov 29 [ePub ahead of print].
42. Bellos JK, Petrosyan A, Abdulamit T, Trastour JC, Bergeron P. Retrograde type A aortic dissections after endovascular stent-graft placement for type B dissection. J Cardiovasc Surg (Torino). 2010;51(1):85–93.
43. Eggebrecht H, Thompson M, Rousseau H, Czerny M, Lonn L, Mehta RH, et al. Retrograde ascending aortic dissection during or after thoracic aortic stent graft placement: insight from the European registry on endovascular aortic repair complications. Circulation. 2009;120(11 Suppl):S276–81.

44. Alsac JM, Khantalin I, Julia P, Achouh P, Farahmand P, Capdevila C, et al. The significance of endoleaks in thoracic endovascular aneurysm repair. Ann Vasc Surg. 2011;25(3):345–51.
45. Ueda T, Fleischmann D, Dake MD, Rubin GD, Sze DY. Incomplete endograft apposition to the aortic arch: bird-beak configuration increases risk of endoleak formation after thoracic endovascular aortic repair. Radiology. 2010;255(2):645–52.
46. Thompson CS, Rodriguez JA, Ramaiah VG, DiMugno L, Shafique S, Olsen D, et al. Acute traumatic rupture of the thoracic aorta treated with endoluminal stent grafts. J Trauma. 2002;52(6):1173–7.
47. Riesenman PJ, Farber MA, Mendes RR, Marston WA, Fulton JJ, Mauro M, et al. Endovascular repair of lesions involving the descending thoracic aorta. JVS. 2005;42(6):1063–74.
48. Murphy EH, Stanley GA, Ilves M, Knowles M, Dimaio JM, Jessen ME, et al. Thoracic endovascular repair (TEVAR) in the management of aortic arch pathology. AVS. 2012;26(1):55–66.
49. Ozsvath KJ, Roddy SP, Darling III RC, Byrne J, Kreienberg PB, Choi D, et al. Carotid-carotid crossover bypass: is it a durable procedure? JVS. 2003; 37(3):582–5.
50. Anderson JL, Adam DJ, Berce M, Hartley DE. Repair of thoracoabdominal aortic aneurysms with fenestrated and branched endovascular stent grafts. J Vasc Surg. 2005;42(4):600–7.
51. Bakoyiannis CN, Economopoulos KP, Georgopoulos S, Klonaris C, Shialarou M, Kafeza M, et al. Fenestrated and branched endografts for the treatment of thoracoabdominal aortic aneurysms: a systematic review. J Endovasc Ther. 2010;17(2):201–9.
52. Black SA, Wolfe JH, Clark M, Hamady M, Cheshire NJ, Jenkins MP. Complex thoracoabdominal aortic aneurysms: endovascular exclusion with visceral revascularization. J Vasc Surg. 2006;43(6):1081–9.
53. Chuter TA, Rapp JH, Hiramoto JS, Schneider DB, Howell B, Reilly LM. Endovascular treatment of thoracoabdominal aortic aneurysms. J Vasc Surg. 2008;47(1):6–16.
54. Haddad F, Greenberg RK, Walker E, Nally J, O'Neill S, Kolin G, et al. Fenestrated endovascular grafting: the renal side of the story. J Vasc Surg. 2005;41(2):181–90.
55. Linsen MA, Vos AW, Diks J, Rauwerda JA, Wisselink W. Fenestrated and branched endografts: assessment of proximal aortic neck fixation. J Endovasc Ther. 2005;12(6):647–53.
56. Muhs BE, Verhoeven EL, Zeebregts CJ, Tielliu IF, Prins TR, Verhagen HJ, et al. Mid-term results of endovascular aneurysm repair with branched and fenestrated endografts. J Vasc Surg. 2006;44(1):9–15.
57. Vourliotakis G, Bos WT, Beck AW, van den Dungen JJ, Prins TR, Verhoeven EL. Fenestrated stent-grafting after previous endovascular abdominal aortic aneurysm repair. J Cardiovasc Surg (Torino). 2010;51(3):383–9.
58. Beck AW, Bos WT, Vourliotakis G, Zeebregts CJ, Tielliu IF, Verhoeven EL. Fenestrated and branched endograft repair of juxtarenal aneurysms after previous open aortic reconstruction. J Vasc Surg. 2009;49(6):1387–94.
59. Greenberg RK, Sternbergh III WC, Makaroun M, Ohki T, Chuter T, Bharadwaj P, et al. Intermediate results of a United States multicenter trial of fenestrated endograft repair for juxtarenal abdominal aortic aneurysms. J Vasc Surg. 2009;50(4):730–7.
60. Chuter TA, Hiramoto JS, Park KH, Reilly LM. The transition from custom-made to standardized multibranched thoracoabdominal aortic stent grafts. JVS. 2011;54(3):660–7.
61. Greenberg R, Eagleton M, Mastracci T. Branched endografts for thoracoabdominal aneurysms. J Thorac Cardiovasc Surg. 2010;140(6 Suppl):S171–8.
62. Greenberg RK, Lu Q, Roselli EE, Svensson LG, Moon MC, Hernandez AV, et al. Contemporary analysis of descending thoracic and thoracoabdominal aneurysm repair: a comparison of endovascular and open techniques. Circulation. 2008;118(8):808–17.
63. Verhoeven E, Tielliu IF, Zeebregts CJ, Bekkema F, Vourliotakis G, Ritter W, et al. Results of endovascular repair of TAAA in the first 50 patients. Zentralbl Chir. 2011;136(5):451–7.
64. Lin PH, Kougias P, Bechara CF, Weakley SM, Bakaeen FG, LeMaire SA, et al. Clinical outcome of staged versus combined treatment approach of hybrid repair of thoracoabdominal aortic aneurysm with visceral vessel debranching and aortic endograft exclusion. Perspect Vasc Surg Endovasc Ther. 2012;24: 5–13.
65. Moulakakis KG, Mylonas SN, Avgerinos ED, Kakisis JD, Brunkwall J, Liapis CD. Hybrid open endovascular technique for aortic thoracoabdominal pathologies. Circulation. 2011;124(24):2670–80.
66. Peterson BG, Eskandari MK, Gleason TG, Morasch MD. Utility of left subclavian artery revascularization in association with endoluminal repair of acute and chronic thoracic aortic pathology. JVS. 2006;43(3): 433–9.
67. Matsumura JS, Rizvi AZ. Left subclavian artery revascularization: society for vascular surgery practice guidelines. JVS. 2010;52(4 Suppl):65S–70.
68. Morasch MD. Technique for subclavian to carotid transposition, tips, and tricks. J Vasc Surg. 2009;49(1):251–4.
69. Berguer R, Kline RA. Methods for reconstruction of proximal subclavian artery lesions: transposition and bypass. Semin Vasc Surg. 1996;9(2):98–104.
70. Whitley D, Cherry Jr KJ. Innominate artery reconstruction for occlusive disease. Semin Vasc Surg. 1996;9(2):84–92.
71. Bergeron P, Mangialardi N, Costa P, Coulon P, Douillez V, Serreo E, et al. Great vessel management for endovascular exclusion of aortic arch aneurysms and dissections. Eur J Vasc Endovasc Surg. 2006;32(1):38–45.

72. Melissano G, Tshomba Y, Bertoglio L, Rinaldi E, Chiesa R. Analysis of stroke after TEVAR involving the aortic arch. Eur J Vasc Endovasc Surg. 2012;43(3):269–75.
73. Czerny M, Zimpfer D, Fleck T, Hofmann W, Schoder M, Cejna M, et al. Initial results after combined repair of aortic arch aneurysms by sequential transposition of the supra-aortic branches and consecutive endovascular stent-graft placement. Ann Thorac Surg. 2004;78(4):1256–60.
74. Takach TJ, Reul GJ, Cooley DA, Duncan JM, Livesay JJ, Gregoric ID, et al. Brachiocephalic reconstruction I: operative and long-term results for complex disease. JVS. 2005;42(1):47–54.
75. Antoniou GA, El SK, Hamady M, Wolfe JH. Hybrid treatment of complex aortic arch disease with supra-aortic debranching and endovascular stent graft repair. Eur J Vasc Endovasc Surg. 2010;39(6):683–90.
76. Lotfi S, Clough RE, Ali T, Salter R, Young CP, Bell R, et al. Hybrid repair of complex thoracic aortic arch pathology: long-term outcomes of extra-anatomic bypass grafting of the supra-aortic trunk. Cardiovasc Intervent Radiol. 2012. Apr 21 [ePub ahead of print].
77. Greenberg RK, Clair D, Srivastava S, Bhandari G, Turc A, Hampton J, et al. Should patients with challenging anatomy be offered endovascular aneurysm repair? J Vasc Surg. 2003;38(5):990–6.
78. Hiramoto JS, Schneider DB, Reilly LM, Chuter TA. A double-barrel stent-graft for endovascular repair of the aortic arch. J Endovasc Ther. 2006;13(1):72–6.
79. Larzon T, Eliasson K, Gruber G. Top-fenestrating technique in stentgrafting of aortic diseases with mid-term follow-up. J Cardiovasc Surg (Torino). 2008;49(3):317–22.
80. Ohrlander T, Sonesson B, Ivancev K, Resch T, Dias N, Malina M. The chimney graft: a technique for preserving or rescuing aortic branch vessels in stent-graft sealing zones. J Endovasc Ther. 2008;15(4): 427–32.
81. Richardson S, Popori RK, Pichel AC, Farquharson F, Serracino-Inglott F. A ruptured thoracoabdominal aortic aneurysm managed endovascularly using the telescoping chimney technique. Ann Vasc Surg. 2011;25(3):384.
82. Rancic Z, Pfammatter T, Lachat M, Hechelhammer L, Frauenfelder T, Veith FJ, et al. Periscope graft to extend distal landing zone in ruptured thoracoabdominal aneurysms with short distal necks. J Vasc Surg. 2010;51(5):1293–6.
83. Lobato AC. Sandwich technique for aortoiliac aneurysms extending to the internal iliac artery or isolated common/internal iliac artery aneurysms: a new endovascular approach to preserve pelvic circulation. J Endovasc Ther. 2011;18(1):106–11.
84. Lee JT, Greenberg JI, Dalman RL. Early experience with the snorkel technique for juxtarenal aneurysms. J Vasc Surg. 2012;55(4):935–46.
85. Moulakakis KG, Mylonas SN, Avgerinos E, Papapetrou A, Kakisis JD, Brountzos EN, et al. The chimney graft technique for preserving visceral vessels during endovascular treatment of aortic pathologies. JVS. 2012;55(5):1497–503.
86. Coscas R, Kobeiter H, Desgranges P, Becquemin JP. Technical aspects, current indications, and results of chimney grafts for juxtarenal aortic aneurysms. JVS. 2011;53(6):1520–7.
87. Bruen KJ, Feezor RJ, Daniels MJ, Beck AW, Lee WA. Endovascular chimney technique versus open repair of juxtarenal and suprarenal aneurysms. JVS. 2011;53(4):895–904.
88. Kolvenbach RR, Yoshida R, Pinter L, Zhu Y, Lin F. Urgent endovascular treatment of thoraco-abdominal aneurysms using a sandwich technique and chimney grafts–a technical description. Eur J Vasc Endovasc Surg. 2011;41(1):54–60.
89. Pecoraro F, Pfammatter T, Mayer D, Frauenfelder T, Papadimitriou D, Hechelhammer L, et al. Multiple periscope and chimney grafts to treat ruptured thoracoabdominal and pararenal aortic aneurysms. J Endovasc Ther. 2011;18(5):642–9.
90. Lachat M, Frauenfelder T, Mayer D, Pfiffner R, Veith FJ, Rancic Z, et al. Complete endovascular renal and visceral artery revascularization and exclusion of a ruptured type IV thoracoabdominal aortic aneurysm. J Endovasc Ther. 2010;17(2): 216–20.
91. Baldwin ZK, Chuter TA, Hiramoto JS, Reilly LM, Schneider DB. Double-barrel technique for preservation of aortic arch branches during thoracic endovascular aortic repair. Ann Vasc Surg. 2008;22(6): 703–9.
92. Criado FJ, Barnatan MF, Rizk Y, Clark NS, Wang CF. Technical strategies to expand stent-graft applicability in the aortic arch and proximal descending thoracic aorta. J Endovasc Ther. 2002;9 Suppl 2:II32–8.
93. Tolenaar JL, van Keulen JW, Trimarchi S, Muhs BE, Moll FL, van Herwaarden JA. The chimney graft, a systematic review. AVS. 2012. Apr 10 [ePub ahead of print].
94. Feng R, Zhao Z, Bao J, Wei X, Wang L, Jing Z. Double-chimney technology for treating secondary type I endoleak after endovascular repair for complicated thoracic aortic dissection. J Vasc Surg. 2011;54(1):212–5.
95. Criado FJ. A percutaneous technique for preservation of arch branch patency during thoracic endovascular aortic repair (TEVAR): retrograde catheterization and stenting. J Endovasc Ther. 2007; 14(1):54–8.
96. Estrera AL, Miller III CC, Chen EP, Meada R, Torres RH, Porat EE, et al. Descending thoracic aortic aneurysm repair: 12-year experience using distal aortic perfusion and cerebrospinal fluid drainage. Ann Thorac Surg. 2005;80(4):1290–6.
97. Jeyabalan G, Park T, Rhee RY, Makaroun MS, Cho JS. Comparison of modern open infrarenal and pararenal abdominal aortic aneurysm repair on early

outcomes and renal dysfunction at one year. JVS. 2011;54(3):654–9.
98. Tsai S, Conrad MF, Patel VI, Kwolek CJ, Lamuraglia GM, Brewster DC, et al. Long-term durability of open repair of juxtarenal abdominal aortic aneurysms. JVS 2012;56(1):2–7.
99. Coscas R, Kobeiter H, Desgranges P, Becquemin JP. Technical aspects, current indications, and results of chimney grafts for juxtarenal aortic aneurysms. J Vasc Surg. 2011;53(6):1520–7.
100. Donas KP, Pecoraro F, Torsello G, Lachat M, Austermann M, Mayer D, et al. Use of covered chimney stents for pararenal aortic pathologies is safe and feasible with excellent patency and low incidence of endoleaks. JVS. 2012;55(3):659–65.
101. Donas KP, Eisenack M, Panuccio G, Austermann M, Osada N, Torsello G. The role of open and endovascular treatment with fenestrated and chimney endografts for patients with juxtarenal aortic aneurysms. JVS. 2012;56(2):285–90.
102. Longo GM, Pipinos II. Endovascular techniques for arch vessel reconstruction. JVS. 2010;52(4 Suppl): 77S–81.
103. Lee WA, Martin TD, Gravenstein N. Partial right atrial inflow occlusion for controlled systemic hypotension during thoracic endovascular aortic repair. J Vasc Surg. 2008;48(2):494–8.
104. Gehringhoff B, Torsello G, Pitoulias GA, Austermann M, Donas KP. Use of chimney grafts in aortic arch pathologies involving the supra-aortic branches. J Endovasc Ther. 2011;18(5):650–5.
105. Shu C, Luo MY, Li QM, Li M, Wang T, He H. Early results of left carotid chimney technique in endovascular repair of acute non-a-non-B aortic dissections. J Endovasc Ther. 2011;18(4): 477–84.
106. Sugiura K, Sonesson B, Akesson M, Bjorses K, Holst J, Malina M. The applicability of chimney grafts in the aortic arch. J Cardiovasc Surg (Torino). 2009;50(4):475–81.
107. Balderi A, Antonietti A, Pedrazzini F, Ferro L, Leotta L, Peano E, et al. Treatment of a hepatic artery aneurysm by endovascular exclusion using the multilayer cardiatis stent. Cardiovasc Intervent Radiol. 2010;33(6):1282–6.
108. Benjelloun A, Henry M, Ghannam A, Vaislic C, Azzouzi A, Maazouzi W, et al. Endovascular treatment of a tuberculous thoracoabdominal aneurysm with the Multilayer stent. J Endovasc Ther. 2012;19(1):115–20.
109. Carrafiello G, Rivolta N, Annoni M, Fontana F, Piffaretti G. Endovascular repair of a celiac trunk aneurysm with a new multilayer stent. J Vasc Surg. 2011;54(4):1148–50.
110. Chocron S, Vaislic C, Kaili D, Bonneville JF. Multilayer stents in the treatment of thoraco-abdominal residual type B dissection. Interact Cardiovasc Thorac Surg. 2011;12(6):1057–9.
111. Henry M, Polydorou A, Frid N, Gruffaz P, Cavet A, Henry I, et al. Treatment of renal artery aneurysm with the multilayer stent. J Endovasc Ther. 2008; 15(2):231–6.
112. Meyer C, Verrel F, Weyer G, Wilhelm K. Endovascular management of complex renal artery aneurysms using the multilayer stent. Cardiovasc Intervent Radiol. 2011;34(3):637–41.
113. Natrella M, Castagnola M, Navarretta F, Cristoferi M, Fanelli G, Meloni T, et al. Treatment of juxtarenal aortic aneurysm with the Multilayer stent. J Endovasc Ther. 2012;19(1):121–4.
114. Ruffino M, Rabbia C. Endovascular treatment of visceral artery aneurysms with Cardiatis multilayer flow modulator: preliminary results at six-month follow-up. J Cardiovasc Surg (Torino). 2011;52(3): 311–21.
115. Arthurs ZM, Starnes BW, Sohn VY, Singh N, Martin MJ, Andersen CA. Functional and survival outcomes in traumatic blunt thoracic aortic injuries: an analysis of the National Trauma Databank. J Vasc Surg. 2009;49(4):988–94.
116. Fabian TC, Richardson JD, Croce MA, Smith Jr JS, Rodman Jr G, Kearney PA, et al. Prospective study of blunt aortic injury: Multicenter Trial of the American Association for the Surgery of Trauma. J Trauma. 1997;42(3):374–80.
117. Neschis DG, Scalea TM, Flinn WR, Griffith BP. Blunt aortic injury. N Engl J Med. 2008;359(16): 1708–16.
118. Semba CP, Kato N, Kee ST, Lee GK, Mitchell RS, Miller DC, et al. Acute rupture of the descending thoracic aorta: repair with use of endovascular stent-grafts. J Vasc Interv Radiol. 1997;8(3):337–42.
119. Go MR, Barbato JE, Dillavou ED, Gupta N, Rhee RY, Makaroun MS, et al. Thoracic endovascular aortic repair for traumatic aortic transection. JVS. 2007;46(5):928–33.
120. Demetriades D, Velmahos GC, Scalea TM, Jurkovich GJ, Karmy-Jones R, Teixeira PG, et al. Operative repair or endovascular stent graft in blunt traumatic thoracic aortic injuries: results of an American Association for the Surgery of Trauma Multicenter Study. J Trauma. 2008;64(3):561–70.
121. Celis R, Park SC, Zenati MS, Chaer RA, Rhee RY, Makaroun MS, et al. Evolution of treatment for traumatic thoracic aortic injuries in a single institution. JVS. 2012;56:74–80.
122. Go MR, Siegenthaler MP, Rhee RY, Gupta N, Makaroun MS, Cho JS. Physiologic coarctation of the aorta resulting from proximal protrusion of thoracic aortic stent grafts into the arch. JVS. 2008;48(4):1007–11.
123. Tadros RO, Lipsitz EC, Chaer RA, Faries PL, Marin ML, Cho JS. A multicenter experience of the management of collapsed thoracic endografts. JVS. 2011;53(5):1217–22.
124. Neschis DG, Moainie S, Flinn WR, Scalea TM, Bartlett ST, Griffith BP. Endograft repair of traumatic aortic injury-a technique in evolution: a single institution's experience. Ann Surg. 2009;250(3):377–82.

125. Muhs BE, Balm R, White GH, Verhagen HJ. Anatomic factors associated with acute endograft collapse after Gore TAG treatment of thoracic aortic dissection or traumatic rupture. JVS. 2007;45(4):655–61.
126. Shukla AJ, Jeyabalan G, Cho JS. Late collapse of a thoracic endoprosthesis. JVS. 2011;53(3):798–801.
127. Kasirajan K, Dake MD, Lumsden A, Bavaria J, Makaroun MS. Incidence and outcomes after infolding or collapse of thoracic stent grafts. JVS. 2012;55(3):652–8.
128. Jonker FH, Schlosser FJ, Geirsson A, Sumpio BE, Moll FL, Muhs BE. Endograft collapse after thoracic endovascular aortic repair. J Endovasc Ther. 2010; 17(6):725–34.

7 Thoracic Aneurysms: Endovascular Procedures for Debranching of Ascending and Isolated Arch Aneurysms

Basel Ramlawi, Michael J. Reardon, and Alan B. Lumsden

Abstract

Open surgical repair of thoracic aortic arch aneurysm is a well-established technique for aneurysms involving the aorta arch or the aortic arch and ascending aorta. Open repair generally requires sternotomy, cardiopulmonary bypass, cardiac arrest, profound hypothermia, and circulatory arrest to complete the repair. Hybrid procedures using arch debranching techniques and thoracic endografting have been developed that can eliminate the need for cardiopulmonary bypass, cardiac arrest, profound hypothermia, and circulatory arrest and occasionally sternotomy also. We will describe the approach used at the Methodist DeBakey Heart & Vascular Center for hybrid repair of thoracic aortic arch aneurysm with and without ascending aortic involvement.

Keywords

Thoracic aneurysm • Arch aneurysm • Hybrid procedure • Thoracic endografting • Minimally invasive • Debranching

Introduction

Thoracic aortic aneurysm is a progressive, life-threatening disease that occurs with an incidence of about 10/100,000 [1]. Progressive expansion and subsequent rupture will lead to death in 45–85 % of untreated patients by 5 years [2]. This dismal prognosis has led our surgical department to an early interest in the repair of thoracic aortic aneurysm that persists today [3]. The earliest repairs of aortic arch aneurysm required extra anatomic bypass to maintain cerebral blood flow, cardiopulmonary bypass with resection and reconstruction of the aortic arch aneurysm, and

B. Ramlawi, M.D. • A.B. Lumsden, M.D.
Department of Cardiovascular Surgery,
The Methodist Hospital,
Houston, TX, USA

M.J. Reardon, M.D., FACC, FACS (✉)
The Methodist Hospital,
The Methodist DeBakey Heart and Vascular Center,
Weill Medical College of Cornell University,
6550 Fannin Street, Smith Tower Suite 1401,
Houston, TX 77030, USA

Department of Cardiovascular Surgery,
The Methodist Hospital,
Houston, TX, USA
e-mail: mreardon@tmhs.org

J.J. Hoballah, A.B. Lumsden (eds.), *Vascular Surgery*, New Techniques in Surgery Series,
DOI 10.1007/978-1-4471-2912-7_7, © Springer-Verlag London 2012

subsequent take down of the previously created extra anatomic bypass. This was simplified by Griepp with the introduction of profound hypothermia and circulatory arrest to allow cerebral protection during aortic arch resection [4]. Despite continued improvement of surgical techniques, open aortic arch repair remains a challenge to the surgeon and the patient. Current results from the Mayo Group in a series of 95 open aortic arch repairs revealed a mortality of 16.8 % and a stroke rate of 9.5 % [5]. The introduction of axillary cannulation and antegrade cerebral perfusion did allow a decrease in mortality to 6 % and stroke rate to 6 % but still highlights the complexity of this disease. For our increasingly elderly and often frail patient population, open aortic arch repair continues to be associated with an in-hospital mortality of up to 20 % and stroke rate of up to 12 % [6, 7]. For patients with significant comorbidities such as severe chronic obstructive lung disease, dialysis-dependent renal failure, heart failure, diabetes, or previous stroke, open surgical repair may not be a viable option due to prohibitive estimated mortality and permanent morbidity. Hybrid repair of aortic arch aneurysm has been developed by our group and others to address this high-risk patient cohort without the use of circulatory arrest and often cardiopulmonary bypass which can be poorly tolerated [8–11].

Rational for Hybrid Approach

It is clear from the previous discussion that traditional open repair of aortic arch aneurysms is possible but comes at a significant cost to the patient [12–17]. This cost is not only dependent on the magnitude of the incision and dissection needed for open repair but heavily influenced by the need for cardiopulmonary bypass, cardiac arrest, and profound hypothermia with circulatory arrest. Hybrid procedures were developed to help minimize or eliminate these whenever possible in hopes of decreasing mortality and morbidity and allowing us to extend therapy to a group previously believed to have a prohibitive risk using standard repair techniques [18–25]. The endovascular repair of infrarenal abdominal aortic aneurysm and descending thoracic aortic aneurysm with adequate landing zones has become commonplace and well accepted as an alternative to traditional open repair in appropriate cases [26–28]. Thoracic aneurysms that would require coverage of the innominate artery or the left common carotid artery for proper graft fixation are not amenable to standard, isolated endovascular techniques. Aortic arch aneurysm can be isolated or involve the ascending and/or descending thoracic aorta. When isolated or involving the descending thoracic aorta, these aneurysms can be repaired by extra anatomic bypass of the cerebral vessels and the left subclavian when desired and antegrade or retrograde endograft deployment without cardiopulmonary bypass, cardiac arrest, or circulatory arrest, removing many of the technical risks factors. For arch aneurysm that also involves the ascending thoracic aorta, cardiopulmonary bypass and cardiac arrest is necessary for ascending aortic replacement, but debranching and endograft repair will eliminate the need for profound hypothermia and circulatory arrest and can shorten the overall procedure (Fig. 7.1).

Technical Issues with Arch Aneurysms

Endograft repair of aneurysms requires anatomically appropriate necks or landing zones for the proper fixation and sealing of the aneurysm at its proximal and distal extent. It also requires that critically important arteries not be covered unless revascularized by some method as well as access to deliver the graft for deployment. Aortic arch aneurysms can provide challenges in each of these areas. The thoracic aorta has been divided into four zones. Zone 0 includes the ascending aorta to just beyond the takeoff of the innominate artery. Zone 1 begins at the end of zone 0 and extends to just beyond the takeoff of the left carotid artery. Zone 2 begins at the end of zone 1 and extends to just beyond the takeoff of the left subclavian artery. Zone 3 represents the proximal descending thoracic aorta from just beyond the left subclavian to the mid-descending thoracic aorta, and finally, zone 4

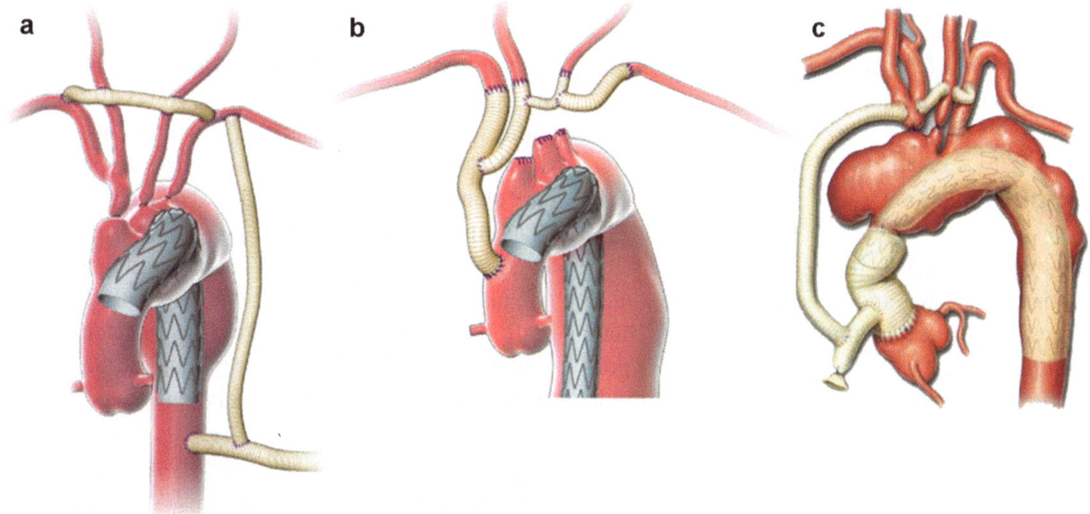

Fig. 7.1 (**a**) Arch vessels debranching using 14-mm inflow conduit from ascending aorta followed by 10-mm bypass graft to the innominate, left common carotid, and left subclavian arteries; (**b**) Arch vessels debranching using 10-mm Dacron graft with retrograde inflow through 10-mm graft. Endograft was delivered using 14-mm conduit; (**c**) Arch vessels showing a 10-mm lib being sutured to a 14-mm trunk. The 10-mm limb is tunneled superiorly to revascularize the supra-aortic trunks, whereas the 14-mm trunk is used as the conduit for antegrade stent-graft placement. The 14-mm stump is oversewn after completion of the stent-graft deployment [9, 10]

comprises the rest of the descending thoracic aorta (Fig. 7.2). Endograft coverage of zones 0 or 1 will of necessity cover vital cerebral blood flow from the innominate and/or left carotid arteries and cannot be done without establishing an extra anatomic route of blood flow that will not be covered. Endografts that cover zone 2 will cover the left subclavian artery. Although the left subclavian artery can be covered without untoward effect in some patients, there is a growing belief that revascularization of the left subclavian in these circumstances may improve outcomes [29]. Even when appropriately revascularized, landing an endograft in the aortic arch may pose a technical challenge due to the curvature of the arch and potential "bird beaking" of the graft [30]. Each of the techniques used to allow endograft coverage of the aortic arch is in effect extending the proximal "branchless" section of the descending thoracic aorta to allow an appropriate proximal landing zone. The final technical consideration is delivering the stent graft to the site of deployment. This can be done in an antegrade or a retrograde fashion. In some tall patients, the current endograft delivery

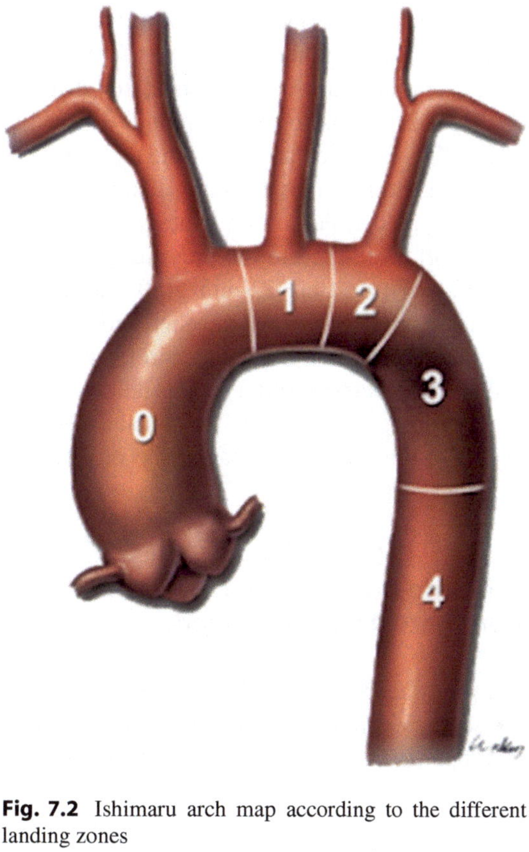

Fig. 7.2 Ishimaru arch map according to the different landing zones

systems may not be long enough to land in the ascending aorta from a retrograde approach and must be considered during the planning phase.

Techniques Used

Available approaches depend if the ascending aorta is aneurysmal and must be replaced and if the innominate artery must be covered. These techniques have also been applied to various presentations of aortic dissections. The following is our management strategy at the MDHVC as it applies to the anatomy of the patient:

Ascending Aortic Involvement

Evaluation of the quality of the ascending aorta is critical. Is it calcified? Is it aneurismal? Is there luminal thrombus? If the ascending aorta is involved and must be replaced, we use a standard median sternotomy or (mini-sternotomy) for surgical access. Cardiopulmonary bypass with cardioplegic cardiac arrest and standard distal ascending aortic cross-clamp technique is used for ascending aortic replacement. The arch aneurysm is left in place thus avoiding the need for profound hypothermia and circulatory arrest. A 12-mm graft is attached to the proximal ascending graft, and from this 12-mm graft, separate side arms are constructed and attached end to end to the innominate artery, the left carotid artery, and the left subclavian artery. This allows the proximal stent graft to land in the distal ascending graft to provide a safe seal of the proximal component of the repair (Fig. 7.3a).

Ascending Aorta Not Involved but Innominate Artery Involved

When the ascending aorta does not need to be replaced, the entire procedure can be done without stopping the heart at any point. Surgical access may be via a standard median sternotomy, or mini-sternotomy or via mini right anterior thoracotomy and cervical incisions [43]. Median sternotomy allows attachment of a 12-mm graft to the proximal ascending aorta using a side-biting clamp. Care must be taken to lower the systemic blood pressure prior to applying the side-biting clamp to avoid dissection or premature clamp release. Care must also be taken to attach this graft far enough proximally to allow an adequate landing zone in the ascending aorta. Because this graft is used for antegrade stent-graft deployment, we bolster the anastomosis with a pledgeted suture at the toe and at the heel of the ascending aortic attachment to prevent disruption.

Sidearm grafts are individually constructed and attached to the innominate, left carotid, and left subclavian arteries. Technically, it is easiest to attach a graft end to end to the left subclavian prior to constructing the end-to-end anastomoses to the innominate and left carotid arteries since these will obscure the left subclavian. After the innominate and left carotid grafts are complete, it is an easy matter to attach the left subclavian graft previously sewn to the left subclavian in an end-to-side manner to the existing left carotid graft. Once the arch has been completely reconstructed in this extra anatomic fashion, the stent graft is deployed in an antegrade fashion through the 12-mm graft attached to the ascending aorta. The distal extent of the stent graft is dependent on the distal extent of the aneurysm and achieving an adequate distal landing zone. We have used this approach to debranch the entire aortic arch and the celiac and superior mesenteric arteries, allowing a distal graft landing at just above the renal arteries (Figs. 7.3b and 7.4).

Innominate Not Involved

If the endograft has a proximal landing zone that must cover the left carotid and left subclavian arteries, then cervical incisions only for right carotid to left carotid bypass as well as left carotid-subclavian bypass can be carried out with retrograde endograft deployment. We routinely use transcranial Doppler and cerebral oximetry to monitor cerebral blood flow during these procedures.

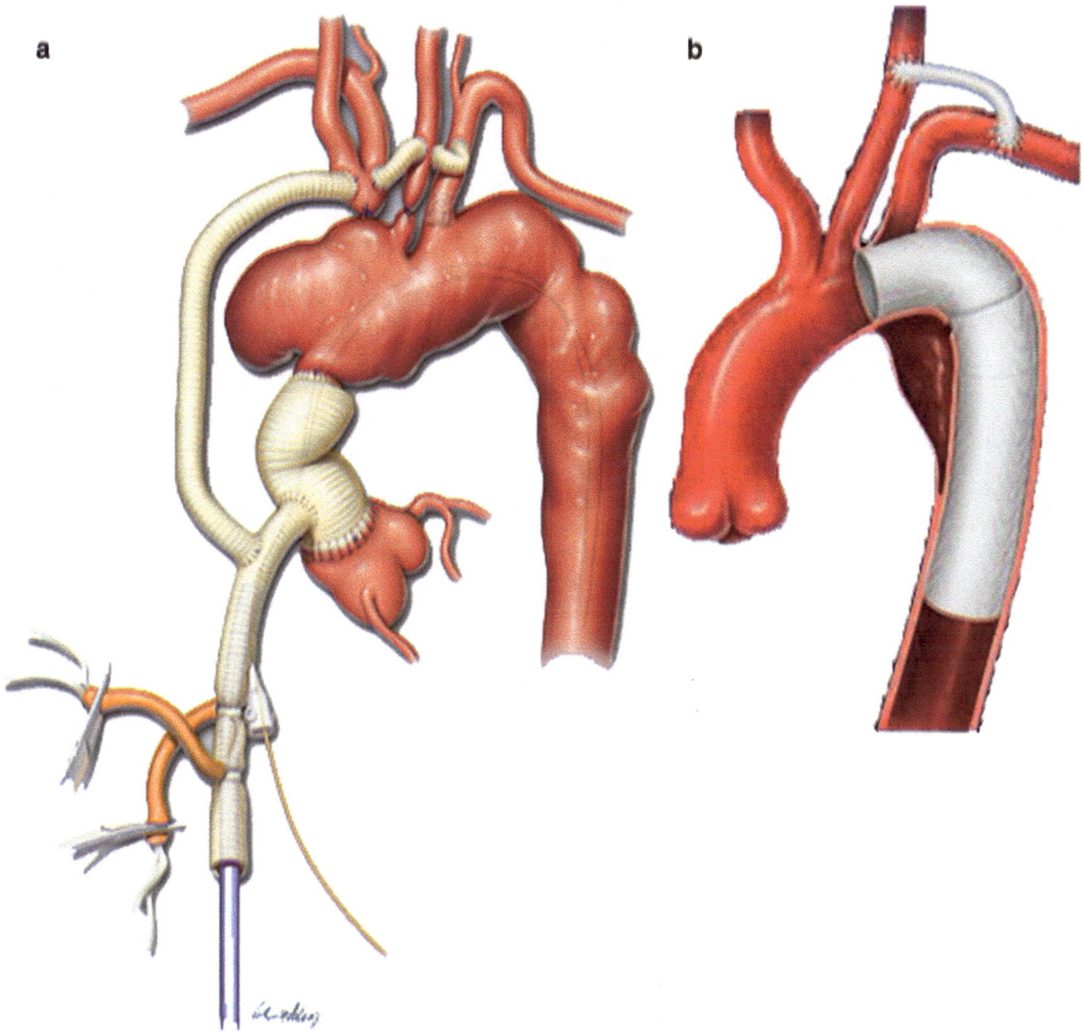

Fig. 7.3 (**a**) Extra-anatomic debranching of aortic arch vessels with replacement of ascending aorta and antegrade TEVAR via Dacron side branch. (**b**) Endograft repair of descending thoracic aortic aneurysm with occlusion of left subclavian artery requiring left common carotid-subclavian bypass

Minimally Invasive Hybrid Arch Repair

The alternative to a median sternotomy is a small anterior right thoracotomy and cervical incisions [31–34]. Our group has used a small right anterior thoracotomy as access for aortic valve replacement and find it provides good access to the ascending aorta [35]. A small incision at the lower sternocleidomastoid muscle on each side allows access for the right and left common carotid arteries. A small left supraclavicular incision allows exposure of the left subclavian artery. A 10-mm Dacron graft is presewn onto a 12-mm graft on the back table and tailored to fit the proximal ascending aorta. The 12-mm graft is attached to the proximal ascending aorta as described in the previous section. It is important that the graft attached to the aorta is angled toward the patient's feet. When the 24-Fr sheath used to deliver the stent graft is inserted into the aorta, it straightens the graft and applies stress to the toe of the anastomosis.

At the completion of this anastomosis, clamps are placed on the 12-mm and the 10-mm grafts,

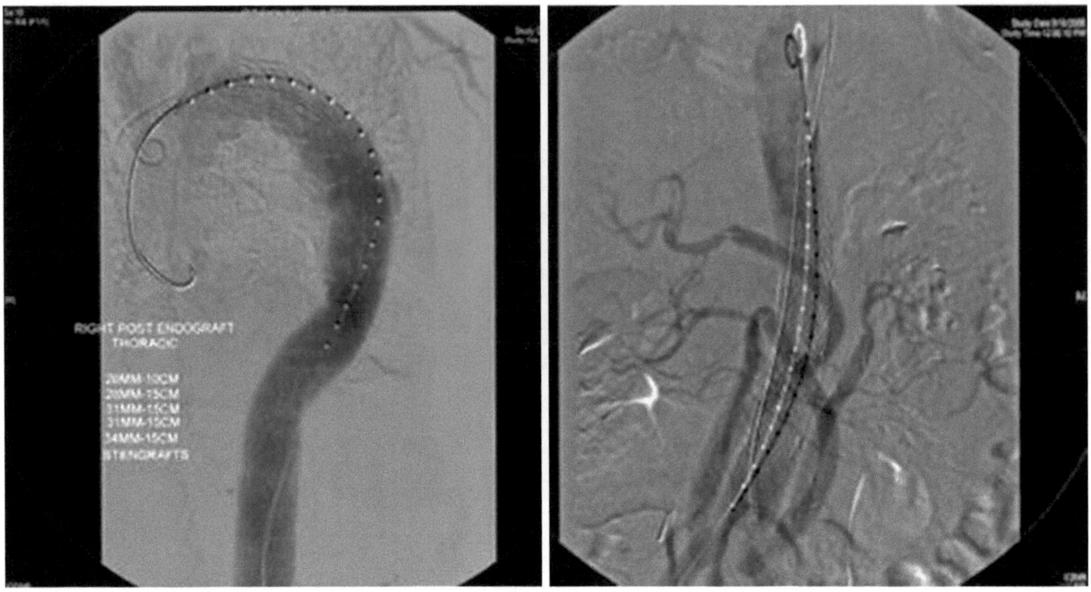

Fig. 7.4 Completion angiography after stent grafting in a patient that underwent arch and abdominal debranching shows the patency of bypass grafts and the exclusion on the aneurysm [9]

and the side-biting clamp is removed. Pledgeted sutures are again placed at the toe and heal of the ascending attachment and the anastomosis carefully inspected for any bleeding. At this point, the 10-mm graft is within the chest and next to the ascending aorta and would not be an easy anastomosis if not already done. The 10-mm graft must then be passed through the sternal outlet into the right cervical incision for anastomosis to the right common carotid artery. Great care must be exercised at this point to exit the sternum in the midline and against the posterior table of the sternum to avoid injury to the innominate vein. An 8-mm graft is then attached to this 10-mm graft and passed in a retro pharengeal path and attached to the left common carotid artery. A standard left carotid-subclavian bypass completes the arch debranching. The proximal left carotid is ligated to prevent a type II endoleak. The left subclavian is closed proximally with a coil or plug via the left arm to prevent endoleak while preserving the vertebral artery. Antegrade deployment of the stent graft can then be carried out via the original 12-mm graft attached to the ascending aorta. We prefer to do all our aortic arch hybrid cases as a single stage using antegrade deployment whenever possible, in contrast to visceral debranching and stent grafting for thoracoabdominal aortic aneurysm which we often prefer to do as a staged procedure with retrograde deployment [36] (Fig. 7.5).

Results

Hybrid arch procedures provide a safe and viable alternative to open traditional surgical repair. In general, hybrid approaches have a lower mortality and morbidity for high-risk older patients. Recently, such approaches have extended hybrid repair indications for complex arch pathology once thought to be prohibitively high risk for open arch surgical repair.

At the MDHVC, hybrid TAAA and arch repairs have become the preferred approach for patients that are poor condidates for surgery with open procedures performed only in younger good risk patients and if hybrid approaches are not possible for technical reasons. We reviewed our experience with hybrid aortic repair in patients who were denied open surgery due to preoperative comorbidities and low physiologic reserve. Fifty-five percent of cases were symptomatic on presentation and 83 % were done

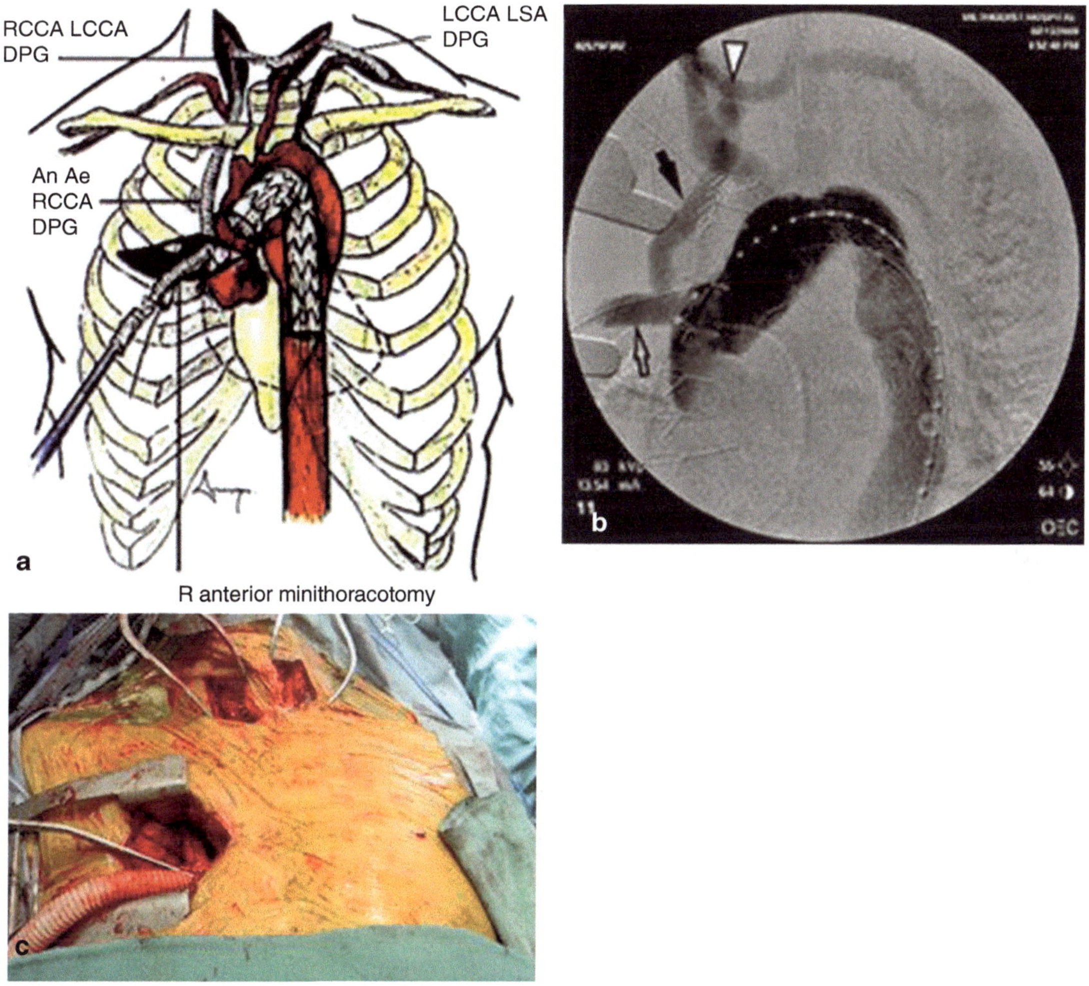

Fig. 7.5 (**a**) Schematic drawing showing the procedure. Via a 5-cm incision at the 3rd intercostal space to access the ascending arch, a 12–10-mm bifurcated hemashield Dacron graft is created. A partial occluding clamp is used on the ascending aorta to attach the 10-mm arm of the bifurcated 10/12-mm graft to the right common carotid or innominate artery. Remaining arch vessels are bypassed through carotid-carotid and left carotid-subclavian bypass. Antegrade stenting of the aortic arch is carried out through the RAM via the remaining 12-mm limb. (**b**) Intraoperative angiogram showed the ascending aorta to R common carotid artery BPG (*black arrow*), RCCA to LCCA BPG (*white arrow*), and the stent-graft deployment via a 12-mm limb (*hollow arrow*) through the anterior minithoracotomy and complete exclusion of the aneurysmal sac. (**c**) Intraoperative photograph

emergently. Seventy-six percent underwent debranching of the aortic arch, 17 % of the visceral vessels, and 7 % required both. Primary technical success was achieved in all cases, and of these, 43 % were staged. The 30-day mortality was 5 %. Myocardial infarction developed in 6 % and respiratory failure in 33 % (Table 7.1). These hybrid approaches, while initially performed mostly for very sick or emergent cases, proved the technical feasibility given the medical and anatomical complexity of these patients with encouraging results [8–11].

Milewski and coworkers compared a hybrid arch repair cohort with an open aortic arch repair cohort and found a trend for lower incidence of neurologic deficit of 4 % compared to 9 % per group, while the short-term/in-hospital mortality rate was 11 and 16 %, respectively. The only statistically significant difference was the mortality rate between age groups and not among surgical

Table 7.1 Comparison of the outcome of aneurysm and dissection (%) [9]

Complication	Hybrid aneurysm (n=33), %	Hybrid dissection (n=7), %	P value
MI	6	0	1
Respiratory failure	33	20	0.65
Renal failure	15	20	1
GI	24	0	0.38
SCI	15	0	0.56
CVA/TIA	18	40	0.61
Death (30 days)	24	0	0.31
Composite endpoint	13	0	0.07

Composite endpoint is the combined death and permanent paraplegia rate at 30 days
CVA cerebrovascular accident, *GI* gastrointestinal, *MI* myocardial infarction, *SCI* spinal cord ischemia, *TIA* transient ischemic attack

approaches; the older patients (more than 75 years old) had a higher mortality rate of 36 % [37].

In another series reported by Hughes and colleagues, 28 patients underwent hybrid arch repair with a 30-day/in-hospital rates of death, stroke, and permanent paraplegia/paresis at 0, 0, and 3.6 %, respectively. At a mean follow-up of 14 ± 11 months, there were no late aortic-related events. Two patients (7 %) required secondary endovascular reintervention for a type 1 endovascular leak. No patient has a type 1 or 3 endovascular leak at latest follow-up [38–40]. Similarly, Canaud reported a 6.8 % risk of stroke with an actuarial survival of 70 % at a mean follow-up of 29.9 months [41].

Regardless of the configuration used, hybrid approaches to arch repair are achieving similar or better short- and long-term outcomes compared to the open arch replacement procedures in most reported series.

Conclusion

In the future, branched endografts (Fig. 7.6) may play a role in the management of aortic arch pathology [42]. The technology for this, however, remains in the development phase. In the meantime, open aortic arch repair for aortic arch aneurysm can be carried out at reasonable but not insignificant risk in appropriate patients. Hybrid endovascular stent-graft approach has been developed in an attempt to decrease the mortality and morbidity of open arch repair and to allow extension of lifesaving therapy to high-risk patients who may not be reasonable candidates for open repair.

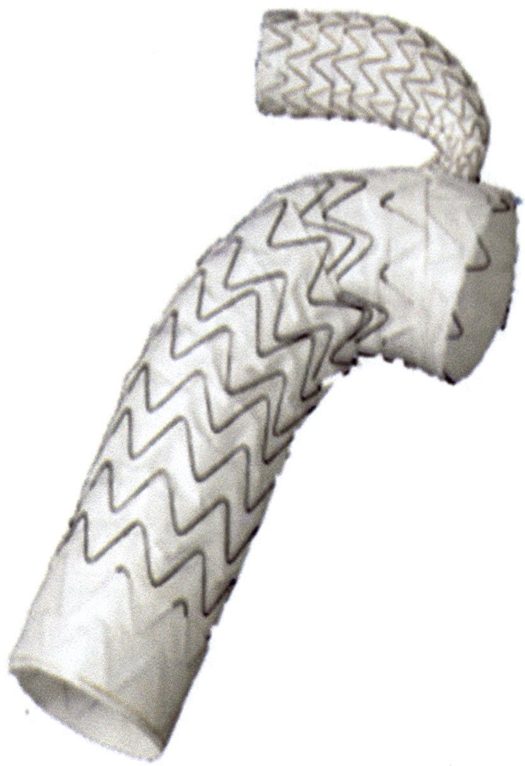

Fig. 7.6 Prototype of branched aortic endograft

References

1. Clouse WD, et al. Improved prognosis of thoracic aortic aneurysms: a population-based study. JAMA. 1998;280(22):1926–9.
2. Juvonen T, et al. Prospective study of the natural history of thoracic aortic aneurysms. Ann Thorac Surg. 1997;63(6):1533–45.
3. de Bakey ME, McCollum CH, Graham JM. Surgical treatment of aneurysms of the descending thoracic aorta: long-term results in 500 patients. J Cardiovasc Surg (Torino). 1978;19(6):571–6.

4. Griepp RB, et al. The superiority of aortic cross-clamping with profound local hypothermia for myocardial protection during aorta-coronary bypass grafting. J Thorac Cardiovasc Surg. 1975;70(6):995–1009.
5. Sundt 3rd TM, et al. Improving results of open arch replacement. Ann Thorac Surg. 2008;86(3):787–96; discussion 787–96.
6. Coselli JS, Buket S, Djukanovic B. Aortic arch operation: current treatment and results. Ann Thorac Surg. 1995;59(1):19–26; discussion 26–7.
7. Svensson LG, et al. Deep hypothermia with circulatory arrest. Determinants of stroke and early mortality in 656 patients. J Thorac Cardiovasc Surg. 1993; 106(1):19–28; discussion 28–31.
8. Mussa FF, et al. Novel technique for arch and visceral artery debranching using ascending aortic inflow. Vascular. 2008;16(5):275–8.
9. Younes HK, et al. Hybrid thoracic endovascular aortic repair: pushing the envelope. J Vasc Surg. 2010;51(1): 259–66.
10. Zhou W, et al. Hybrid approach to complex thoracic aortic aneurysms in high-risk patients: surgical challenges and clinical outcomes. J Vasc Surg. 2006; 44(4):688–93.
11. Zhou W, et al. Endovascular repair of a proximal aortic arch aneurysm: a novel approach of supra-aortic debranching with antegrade endograft deployment via an anterior thoracotomy approach. J Vasc Surg. 2006; 43(5):1045–8.
12. Di Eusanio M, et al. Brain protection using antegrade selective cerebral perfusion: a multicenter study. Ann Thorac Surg. 2003;76(4):1181–8; discussion 1188–9.
13. Kazui T, et al. Improved results of atherosclerotic arch aneurysm operations with a refined technique. J Thorac Cardiovasc Surg. 2001;121(3):491–9.
14. Keeling WB, Kerendi F, Chen EP. Total aortic arch replacement for the treatment of Kommerell's diverticulum in a Jehovah's witness. J Card Surg. 2010; 25(3):333–5.
15. Ogino H, et al. Aortic arch repairs through three different approaches. Eur J Cardiothorac Surg. 2001; 19(1):25–9.
16. Spielvogel D, et al. Aortic arch replacement using a trifurcated graft: simple, versatile, and safe. Ann Thorac Surg. 2005;80(1):90–5; discussion 95.
17. Ueda Y. Retrograde cerebral perfusion with hypothermic circulatory arrest in aortic arch surgery: operative and long-term results. Nagoya J Med Sci. 2001; 64(3–4):93–102.
18. Akhyari P, et al. Aortic dissection type A after supra-aortic debranching and implantation of an endovascular stent-graft for type B dissection: a word of caution. J Thorac Cardiovasc Surg. 2009;137(5):1290–2.
19. Chiesa R, et al. Hybrid approach to thoracoabdominal aortic aneurysms in patients with prior aortic surgery. J Vasc Surg. 2007;45(6):1128–35.
20. Donas KP, et al. Early and midterm outcome of a novel technique to simplify the hybrid procedures in the treatment of thoracoabdominal and pararenal aortic aneurysms. J Vasc Surg. 2009;50(6):1280–4.
21. Esposito G, et al. Hybrid treatment of thoracoabdominal aortic aneurysms with the use of a new prosthesis. Ann Thorac Surg. 2008;85(4):1443–5.
22. Greenberg RK, et al. Hybrid approaches to thoracic aortic aneurysms: the role of endovascular elephant trunk completion. Circulation. 2005;112(17):2619–26.
23. Kawaharada N, et al. Hybrid treatment for aortic arch and proximal descending thoracic aneurysm: experience with stent grafting for second-stage elephant trunk repair. Eur J Cardiothorac Surg. 2009;36(6): 956–61.
24. Rancic Z, et al. Floating aortic arch thrombus involving the supraaortic trunks: successful treatment with supra-aortic debranching and antegrade endograft implantation. J Vasc Surg. 2009;50(5):1177–80.
25. Szeto WY, et al. The hybrid total arch repair: brachiocephalic bypass and concomitant endovascular aortic arch stent graft placement. J Card Surg. 2007;22(2):97–102; discussion 103–4.
26. Bavaria JE, et al. Endovascular stent grafting versus open surgical repair of descending thoracic aortic aneurysms in low-risk patients: a multicenter comparative trial. J Thorac Cardiovasc Surg. 2007;133(2): 369–77.
27. Greenhalgh RM, et al. Endovascular versus open repair of abdominal aortic aneurysm. N Engl J Med. 2010;362(20):1863–71.
28. Makaroun MS, et al. Five-year results of endovascular treatment with the Gore TAG device compared with open repair of thoracic aortic aneurysms. J Vasc Surg. 2008;47(5):912–8.
29. Holt PJ, et al. Outcomes of the endovascular management of aortic arch aneurysm: implications for management of the left subclavian artery. J Vasc Surg. 2010;51(6):1329–38.
30. Wang S, et al. Endovascular treatment of arch and proximal thoracic aortic lesions. J Vasc Surg. 2008; 48(1):64–8.
31. Donas KP, et al. Hybrid open-endovascular repair for thoracoabdominal aortic aneurysms: current status and level of evidence. Eur J Vasc Endovasc Surg. 2007;34(5):528–33.
32. Saleh HM, Inglese L. Combined surgical and endovascular treatment of aortic arch aneurysms. J Vasc Surg. 2006;44(3):460–6.
33. Shimamura K, et al. Long-term results of the open stent-grafting technique for extended aortic arch disease. J Thorac Cardiovasc Surg. 2008;135(6): 1261–9.
34. Zierer A, Sanchez LA, Moon MR. Combined open proximal and stent-graft distal repair for distal arch aneurysms: an alternative to total debranching. Ann Thorac Surg. 2009;88(1):307–9.
35. Anaya-Ayala JE, et al. Hybrid thoracic endovascular aortic repair via right anterior minithoracotomy: brief technique report. J Thorac Cardiovasc Surg. 2011;142:314–8. Epub 2011 Feb 1.
36. Estrera AL, et al. Staged repair of extensive aortic aneurysms. Ann Thorac Surg. 2002;74(5):S1803–5; discussion S1825–32.

37. Milewski RK, et al. Have hybrid procedures replaced open aortic arch reconstruction in high-risk patients? A comparative study of elective open arch debranching with endovascular stent graft placement and conventional elective open total and distal aortic arch reconstruction. J Thorac Cardiovasc Surg. 2010; 140(3):590–7.
38. Hughes GC, et al. "Hybrid" repair of aneurysms of the transverse aortic arch: midterm results. Ann Thorac Surg. 2009;88(6):1882–7; discussion 1887–8.
39. Hughes GC, McCann RL. Hybrid thoracoabdominal aortic aneurysm repair: concomitant visceral revascularization and endovascular aneurysm exclusion. Semin Thorac Cardiovasc Surg. 2009;21(4):355–62.
40. Hughes GC, et al. Use of custom Dacron branch grafts for "hybrid" aortic debranching during endovascular repair of thoracic and thoracoabdominal aortic aneurysms. J Thorac Cardiovasc Surg. 2008;136(1):21–8. 28.e1–6.
41. Canaud L, et al. Endovascular repair of aortic arch lesions in high-risk patients or after previous aortic surgery: midterm results. J Thorac Cardiovasc Surg. 2010;140(1):52–8.
42. Chuter TA, et al. Branched stent-grafts: will these become the new standard? J Vasc Interv Radiol. 2008;19(6 Suppl):S57–62.
43. Anaya-Anyala JE et al. Hybrid thoracic endovascular aortic repair via right anterior minithoracotomy J. Thorac Cardiovasc Surg. 2011 Aug:142 (2):314–8.

Aortic Dissection

8

Vikas A. Pandey and M. Hamady

Abstract
Aortic dissection is an acute emergency requiring the interdisciplinary cooperation between vascular surgery, interventional radiology, cardiology, and cardiothoracic surgery to aggressively treat this condition that to this day carries a high mortality rate. Aortic dissection (AD) is part of the spectrum of acute aortic syndromes which also include intramural hematoma, penetrating atherosclerotic ulcer, aneurysmal leak, and aortic transection.

Keywords
Aorta • Surgery • Intervention • TEE • Stent

Introduction

Aortic dissection is an acute emergency requiring the interdisciplinary cooperation between vascular surgery, interventional radiology, cardiology, and cardiothoracic surgery to aggressively treat this condition that to this day carries a high mortality rate. Aortic dissection (AD) is part of the spectrum of acute aortic syndromes which also include intramural hematoma, penetrating atherosclerotic ulcer, aneurysmal leak, and aortic transection.

The reported incidence of AD is about 3.5 cases per 100 000 population per year [1]. There is an expectedly higher incidence among males in their fifth and sixth decade of life.

The process is characterized by the dissection of vessel wall along plane of the media together with formation of blood-filled channel along the aortic wall. Aortic dissection has two main causes: hypertension (over 90 % of all cases of aortic dissection) and connective tissue diseases (5 %—Marfan syndrome being the commonest). For reasons not clearly understood, there is also a higher incidence of aortic dissection in pregnancy. Recently, aortic dissection is an uncommon but recognized consequence of cocaine use (most likely due to the drug effect on blood pressure) [2].

V.A. Pandey, M.D., FRCS (✉)
Department of Vascular Surgery,
Imperial College London,
St. Mary's Hospital, London W2 1NY,
NY, UK
e-mail: v.pandey@imperial.ac.uk

M. Hamady, MBChB, FRCR
Consultant interventional radiologist,
Senior Lecturer - Imperial College,
St Mary's Campus W2 1NY, London, UK
e-mail: m.hamady@imperial.ac.uk

J.J. Hoballah, A.B. Lumsden (eds.), *Vascular Surgery*, New Techniques in Surgery Series,
DOI 10.1007/978-1-4471-2912-7_8, © Springer-Verlag London 2012

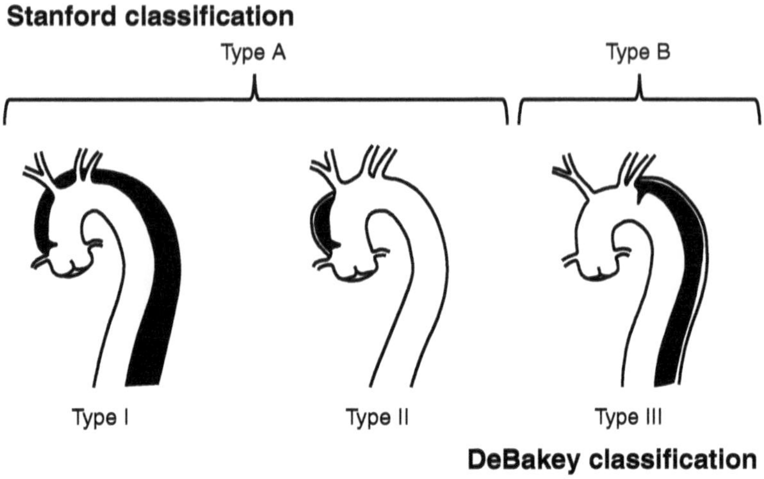

Fig. 8.1 DeBakey and Stanford classifications. Stanford *type A* encompasses both DeBakey types I and II. Stanford *type B* is equivalent to a DeBakey III aortic dissection (Illustration by Anne-Sophie Sillesen)

Classification

Dissections almost always originate from tears in the intima, although tears may be absent in 5 % of cases suggesting an alternative pathogenesis such as progression of an intramural hematoma or penetrating ulcer. Of all aortic dissections, 90 % are within 10 cm of the aortic valve. The second commonest location is the descending thoracic aorta, distal to the left subclavian artery. The Stanford classification is the most widely used classification system. Dissections proximal to the left subclavian artery are type A. Dissections distal to the left subclavian artery are type B. The DeBakey classification has three types. Type I originates in the ascending aorta and propagates to the aortic arch or beyond. A DeBakey type II dissection originates and is confined to the ascending aorta. A type III dissection originates in the descending thoracic aorta and extends distally (rarely extending proximally). A DeBakey type III dissection is equivalent to a Stanford type B (Fig. 8.1). More recently, the DeBakey type III classification has been subdivided into IIIa and IIIb with the abdominal aorta affected in the latter.

Dissections can further be classified acute or chronic if their presentation is before or after 2 weeks of onset of symptoms.

Pathogenesis

The entry tear may be longitudinal, oblique, or spiral but is typically 4–5 cm long. The flow of blood splits a cleavage plane in the media and propagates along the medial planes usually between the outer and middle third.

The dissection itself usually involves half to two-thirds of the circumference of the aorta and may extend either antegradely or retrogradely. Retrograde dissection along the aortic root risks coronary ischemia (the right coronary artery being commonly affected), pericardial effusion, or tamponade. The dissection may involve the origin of the great vessels leading to upper limb ischemia or stroke. Acute aortic valve incompetence is a recognized complication of retrograde dissection. These features give this grave condition a mortality rate of 1 % per hour if left untreated [3]. Standard treatment of dissections of the aortic root and valve can include transaction of affected aortic segment and repair. Aortic root repair with or without replacement of the aortic valve and total arch replacement are also used (Fig. 8.2). The management of type A aortic dissection is beyond the scope of this text and is not discussed further.

Antegrade propagation of dissection may involve branches of the aorta with loss of

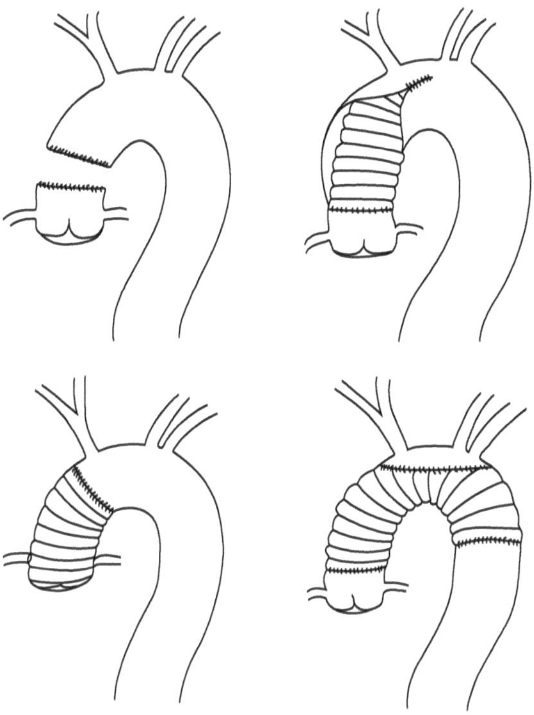

Fig. 8.2 Open repair in type A aortic dissection. *Top left*, transection of primary entry tear and end-to-end aortic anastomosis. *Top right*, aortic root replacement. *Bottom left*, aortic root and valve replacement, and *bottom right*, total arch replacement (Illustration by Anne-Sophie Sillesen)

intercostals and lumbar vessels risking paraplegia. The involvement of mesenteric or renal branches risks the possibility of gut or renal ischemia. Occasionally, the dissection propagates to the iliac arteries and occasionally to the lower limbs, threatening the viability of the legs.

Rupture of the restraining adventitia often leads to fatal hemorrhage and, if occurring within the pericardium, causes tamponade and, within the chest, a hemothorax. In long dissections, the hemorrhage may re-rupture back into the aortic lumen (reentry tear) to produce a false lumen. The reentry tears are usually multiple and at different levels.

Marfan syndrome, an autosomal dominant disease, has a strong association with aortic dissection. It is thought that genetic defects in fibrillin (a connective tissue protein involved with elastic tissue formation) cause cardiovascular, skeletal, and ocular manifestations all attributable to fibrillin mutations.

Clinical Features

The classical presentation of aortic dissection is one of "tearing" interscapular pain or anterior chest pain radiating to the back, the neck, the upper limbs, or the abdomen. Collapse is common. The patient may be hypertensive or hypotensive secondary to coronary complications or hemorrhage.

A differential of 20 mmHg between upper limb blood pressure measurements raises the possibility of aortic dissection. Cardiac auscultation may demonstrate the presence of a diastolic murmur suggestive of aortic regurgitation associated with valvular involvement in the dissection.

Radiographic Changes

Plain X-Ray

This is often performed in the emergency departments for patients presenting with chest pain and may show a widened mediastinum. The presence of a pericardial or pleural effusion may inform of the possibility of rupture into these cavities. Changes consistent with cardiac failure may be present in association of acute aortic incompetence. The separation of intimal calcium (where present) from the outer aortic wall is suggestive of dissection. Other radiographic associations included obliteration of the aortic knuckle, tracheal deviation, or depression of the left main stem bronchus. Overall, the chest X-ray is of little benefit in the diagnosis of aortic dissection.

Aortography

Once considered, the "gold standard" in the diagnosis of aortic dissection has all the complications

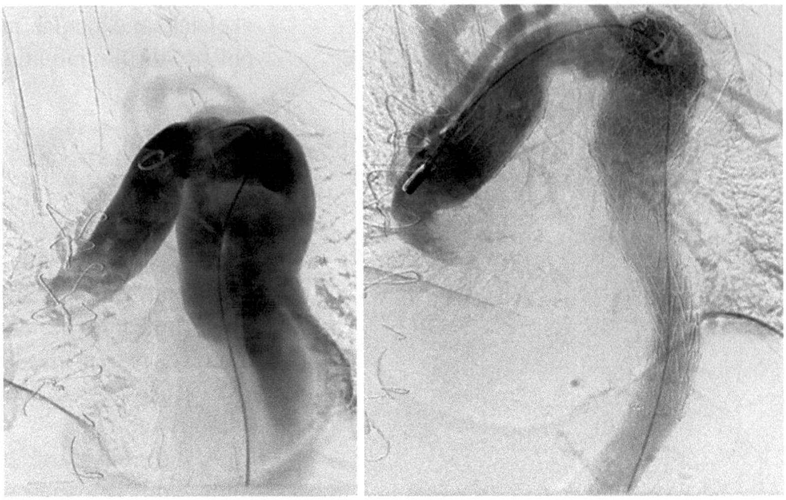

Fig. 8.3 A 47-year-old male with acute type B aortic dissection and hypertension. Arch angiography (*left*) outlines the dissected lumen and the landing zone. Completion angiogram (*right*) post stent graft deployment shows complete exclusion of the proximal false lumen and restoration of flow in the true lumen

of arteriography and has largely been superseded by noninvasive imaging modalities. Findings can be divided into direct and indirect. Direct findings identify the anatomy of the dissection and include visualization of the intimal flap or of two lumens in the aorta. Indirect findings include true lumen compression, aortic valve incompetence, aortic wall thickening, or abnormalities with aortic branches. Aortography in addition has a low specificity (a high false-negative rate) and cannot visualize the aortic wall as such cannot give accurate information on arterial size, the presence of intramural hematoma, or other intramural or extravascular complications. Occasionally, one lumen will opacify or both lumens will opacify equally preventing the diagnosis being made, one of the causes of the high false-negative rate. Although aortography has fallen out of favor as a diagnostic modality in aortic dissection, its therapeutic use is expanding rapidly in the endovascular era (Fig. 8.3).

Computed Tomography

The use of CT as an imaging modality in aortic dissection has grown exponentially over the last two decades. The introduction of multidetector CT improved the speed of acquisition, coverage area, and resolution of the images. Other benefits include a reduction of the intravenous contrast needed for aortic scanning and reduction of motion artifact. New multidetector CT scanners can now image the thoracoabdominal aorta and iliofemoral vessels in a matter of seconds, making this the ideal imaging modality for potentially unstable patients. CT has both a sensitivity and specificity of 96–100 % (Fig. 8.4).

Contrast-enhanced CT images can be displayed at different slice thicknesses but are typically displaced at 1–2-mm slices. These images can be viewed in a workstation with appropriate multiplanar imaging software or can be reformatted using a variety of post-processing algorithms such as volume rendering or maximum intensity projection. Although these post-processing techniques are time-consuming and have no added benefits in making the diagnosis, they are useful in planning for vascular and endovascular reconstruction. CT has additional advantages over aortography as it can allow the identification of alternative diagnoses if aortic dissection has been excluded [4].

The ability of CT scan to produce isotropic data, its high speed, and wide availability gives CT the advantage over MRI and places CT angiography as the first-line imaging technique in acute aortic dissection.

The greatest disadvantage of CT is the use of ionizing radiation, making it less attractive than other imaging modalities for the surveillance of chronic aortic dissections. Iodinated contrast

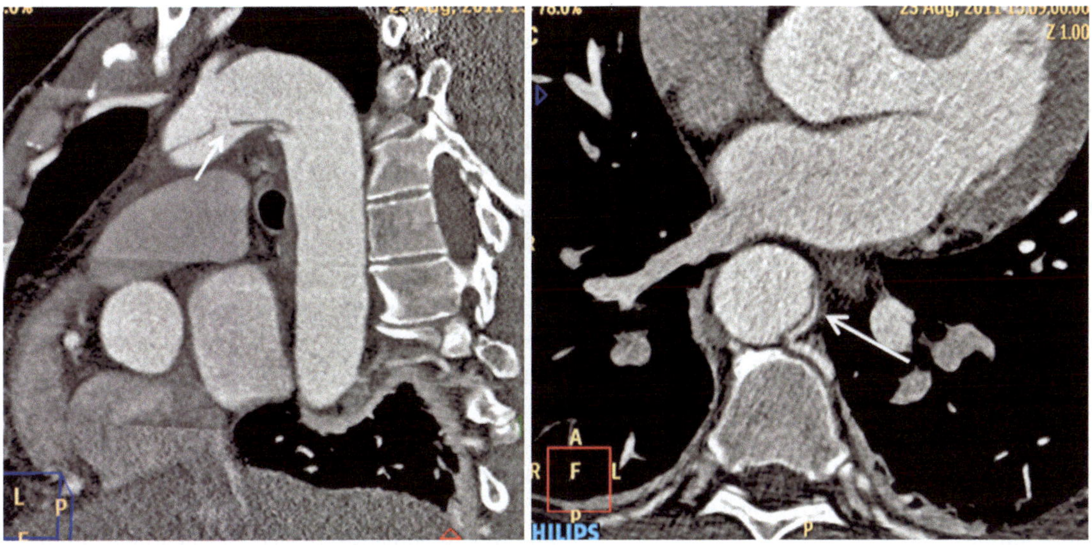

Fig. 8.4 Coronal (*left*) and axial (*right*) images of aortic dissection originating distal to the left subclavian artery. The coronal slice demonstrates retrograde extension of the dissection to the distal aortic arch

agents are nephrotoxic and could induce acute tubular necrosis in patients with borderline or impaired renal function. The iodine-based contrast is contraindicated in those with iodine allergy and should be used with caution in those patients with thyrotoxicosis, even those adequately treated, for risk of precipitating a thyroid storm. Artifacts may occur at the aortic root due to cardiac motion, although this may be limited in some of the new CT scanners that employ electrocardiographic gating (as in CT coronary angiography).

Magnetic Resonance Imaging (MRI)

From the early 1990s, MRI with or without contrast agent superseded the catheter angiography in diagnosis of aortic pathology. However, the acquisition time is longer than with CT but avoids the antecedent risks of ionizing radiation. Gadolinium-enhanced imaging techniques have increased the use of MRI in evaluating the thoracoabdominal aorta. The aorta is ideally imaged with gadolinium enhancement using multiple sequential acquisitions, and this is particularly useful in dissections with different flow rates within the true and false lumina. Images acquired at multiple sequential time points after administration of gadolinium can identify a patent false lumen that may not fill immediately as opposed to a thrombosed false lumen. With the popularity and advantages of CT, MRI is the least commonly performed imaging technique for the initial diagnosis of aortic dissection, but it has great value in the surveillance of chronic aortic dissection especially with the younger patient, reducing the lifetime exposure to ionizing radiation. There are also the obvious contraindications to MR imaging including cardiac pacemakers, aneurysm clips, and other ferrous materials. MRI is also less well tolerated than CT especially in those patients suffering with claustrophobia. Recent advances in MR technology, including blood pool contrast agents and 4D image acquisition, will probably renew the interest in this modality. Recent research has shown that the use of blood pool agents instead of the standard gadolinium contrast would enable the diagnosis of endoleaks and false lumen flow, which otherwise is not seen on CT angiography. Clough et al. showed, in a small series of patients, higher sensitivity for detecting flow in the false lumen when compared with standard CT angiography. This could have significant implication in decision making and management of chronic dissection. The same team, as well as others, also demonstrated the potential MR ability to predict sac growth by visualizing entry tear and velocity changes in dissected aorta [5, 6].

Transthoracic Echocardiography

TTE is noninvasive, readily available, and with some of the newer scanners, portable. It is an excellent tool for the identification and quantification of aortic valve incompetence, but its greatest restrictions are its lack of utility in visualizing the aorta beyond its root. TTE can be helpful in those patients with concurrent coronary ischemia by identifying regional wall motion abnormalities.

Transesophageal Echocardiography (TEE)

Visualization of the thoracic aorta with TTE is limited by the small acoustic windows. TEE was the obvious evolution of the transthoracic echocardiogram, eliminating restrictions of the acoustic window and allowing greater visualization of the thoracic aorta, but with the disadvantage of being more invasive. TEE has all the advantages of TTE but can also visualize extravascular complications such as acute hematomas at the site of intimal tears. A greater length of aorta is visualized, but the distal ascending aorta and proximal aortic arch is not visualized well due to the presence of the trachea at the opposite side of the aorta at that point. It is not possible to visualize the great vessels or the abdominal aorta beyond the midpoint. TEE like TTE is operator dependent but unlike TTE requires sedation and is not without complications, especially in patients with esophageal disease.

Intravascular Ultrasound

IVUS uses a miniaturized ultrasound probe attached to the end of an intra-arterial catheter, delivering a picture of the endothelium through the column of blood. Historically, IVUS's main role is visualization of atherosclerotic plaques; however, a few small studies attested to the benefits of using this technology in the endovascular management of aortic dissection [7, 8]. The potential advantages include identification of lumens, visualization of reentry tears, guidance for percutaneous fenestration, and aortic diameter measurements. Although researchers have shown superiority of IVUS over angiography in detecting reentry tear and helps catheter-guided fenestration, its exact role remains ill defined. Improvements in IVUS technology, including color, Doppler capabilities, gradient measurement, and 3D imaging, may reinvent interests in this modality.

Positron Emission Tomography

Fluorodeoxyglucose (FDG) is an analogue of glucose. The uptake of FDG administered is proportional to the metabolic activity of the tissue. This constitutes the basis for PET. PET produces a three-dimensional image of functional processes. The scanner detects gamma ray pairs emitted indirectly by a positron-emitting radionuclide tracer, which is introduced into the body on a biologically active molecule (in this case ^{18}F-FDG). Three-dimensional images of tracer concentration within the body are then constructed by computer analysis. With most modern PET scanners, the imaging is often co-registered with CT imaging performed on the patient in the same scanner (CT-PET). CT-PET has found applications in vascular diseases and in the diagnosis of vasculitis and graft infection. It was the hypothesis of Reeps et al. that suggested the diagnostic conundrum of confidently differentiating an acute and chronic dissection may be solved. The authors showed that the FDG uptake patterns and standardized uptake values (SUV) in patients with acute dissection were significantly greater than those in patients with chronic aortic dissection. However, the use of this modality remains limited.

Management of Type B Aortic Dissection

Initial Management

Stanford type A dissection carries a high mortality and on suspected or confirmed diagnosis, referral should be made to the nearest cardiothoracic unit. At present, the management of type A aortic dissection remains surgical with endovascular techniques not having as important a role. Some of the surgical options for the management of type A aortic dissection are outlined in Fig. 8.2. The management of type B aortic dissection is initially medical with strict control of the blood pressure and amelioration of pain by antihypertensives and opiate analgesia, respectively.

On diagnosis of a type B aortic dissection, patients should be managed on intensive care, a high dependency unit, or coronary care. After placement of a central venous and radial artery catheter and urinary catheter, intravenous antihypertensives are administered. The first-line agent in the absence of severe pulmonary airways disease is labetalol. Concomitant lower limb peripheral arterial disease is no longer seen as a contraindication to beta-blockade in this situation. Continuous blood pressure measurements from the arterial line are required, aiming for a blood pressure of 120/80 mmHg or less if tolerated. Urine output less than 30 ml/h or in association with a rising serum creatinine is suggestive of renal malperfusion. Similarly, a raised serum lactate is suggestive of visceral malperfusion.

Aortic dissection represents a spectrum of conditions that comprise the acute aortic syndrome. Other conditions in this category include penetrating atherosclerotic ulcers (PAU) and acute intramural hematoma (IMH). Some authors also include aneurysm rupture and aortic transaction among the acute aortic syndrome [9].

PAUs are focal intimal defects at the site of atherosclerotic plaques. Patients presenting from this group tend to be older than for aortic dissection and carry a greater cardiorespiratory burden. It most commonly affects the descending thoracic aorta. Eventually, intimal erosion may lead to pulsatile blood entering the media resulting in hemorrhage. This condition can progress to IMH or onto aortic dissection.

IMH is thought to account for 10–30 % of cases of acute aortic syndrome. It is a subtle variation of aortic dissection in that blood collects within the aortic media without the presence of an intimal flap. The rupture of the nutrient vasa vasorum or hemorrhage is within an atherosclerotic plaque. Unlike aortic dissection, the plane of cleavage of the vessel wall is closer to the adventitia, and this is said to account for the higher rate of rupture in IMH compared with aortic dissection. It may also advance toward the intima and progress to aortic dissection.

The mechanics between these three entities are different, but the management is similar. The management of aortic aneurysm leak and aortic transaction is not discussed further. Ahmad et al. describe a treatment algorithm for acute aortic syndromes (Fig. 8.5).

If the patient is hemodynamically stable and the lesion has remained unchanged on imaging 24–48 h apart, a conservative approach may be undertaken with the intention of substituting intravenous hypertensive agents to oral agents. The patient should be pain free with no evidence of end-organ ischemia. In particular, they should not have any abdominal pain or tenderness, and their lactate should be normal. A stable or declining creatinine level with good urine output is an indication that at least one kidney is well perfused. This approach has been used for decades with aortic dissection and more recently been applied to the other acute aortic syndromes [10, 11]. Despite the relatively benign nature of type B aortic dissection, there remains a small risk of rupture (4–8 %), and this rises to 45–50 % with PAU and IMH.

Indications for the early intervention in acute type B pathology include the following:

Aortic pain or blood pressure refractory to medical management

Increasing aortic wall thickness or increase in aortic diameter

Evidence of end-organ malperfusion

PAU greater than 20 mm in diameter or 10 mm in depth

Increasing volume or progression of IMH or bulging hematoma

Contrast seen outside the adventitia or increasing pleural effusion

IMH associated with PAU

Open Surgery

The indications for open surgery for complicated type B aortic dissection have diminished

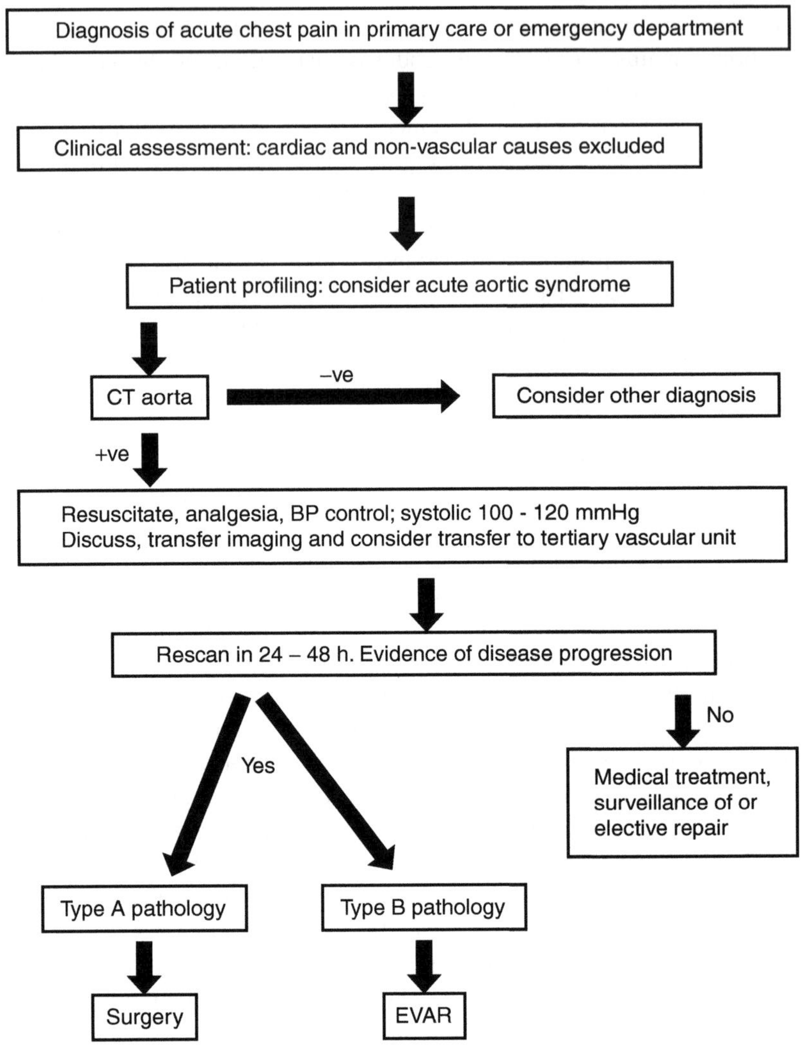

Fig. 8.5 A diagnostic and treatment algorithm for the management of acute aortic syndromes

significantly with the advances in aortic stent technology that have revolutionized the treatment of this condition. The results of open repair for aortic dissection are generally poor and relate to the advancing age of affected patients and also by the presence of renal or intestinal ischemia which are often the drivers for early surgery. Open aortic surgery also carries with it a significant cardiorespiratory morbidity in addition to the risk of renal failure and paraplegia, especially with surgery of the thoracic aorta. Open surgery still has a place with chronic type B dissections with aneurysmal degeneration of the infrarenal aorta in the younger patient or for those not anatomically suitable for endovascular aneurysm repair (EVAR).

Endovascular Intervention

The aims of endovascular therapy in aortic dissection are to cover the primary entry tear with a covered stent graft. This closure should lead to depressurization of the false lumen, re-expansion of a compressed true lumen, and control of the intimal flap to allow aortic remodeling. Covering the primary entry tear will in most instances treat the complications of aortic dissection. False lumen thrombosis reduces the risk of late rupture, and true lumen re-expansion will limit any visceral malperfusion in over three quarters of cases.

Endovascular stenting for thoracic aortic dissection is similar to that for thoracic aortic aneurysms except that graft oversizing is limited to or less than 10 % to reduce trauma to the potentially friable proximal aorta. For this reason, balloon dilatation at the end of the procedure is not encouraged.

The length of aortic coverage is also an important area of controversy. A short graft covering the entry tear relies on distal aortic remodeling to avoid false lumen perfusion in the lower thoracic aorta. A longer endograft reduces the likelihood of false lumen perfusion but with a higher risk of paraplegia as it has been shown that this risk increases with length of aorta covered [12].

Due to the aggressive nature of PAU and IMH, there is growing interest in stenting for these conditions, and their localized nature makes them ideal for an endoluminal approach. There have been a number of studies claiming technical success rates between 96 and 100 % with almost no reports of serious morbidity. Small studies comparing the morbidity and mortality of open versus endovascular repair have demonstrated significant reductions in both from endovascular repair [13].

The limitations of a totally endovascular approach to aortic dissection relate to the requirements of favorable anatomy, with normal aorta extending for at least 15–20 mm proximally to secure proximal landing zone. Excessive thrombosis, calcification, and vessel tortuosity also limit the application of this technology. Involvement of the great vessel segment may require arch hybrid open and endovascular procedures to reconstruct the aortic arch and create the needed landing zone.

Fenestrated and branched stent grafts have limited role in AD due to frequent severe compression of the true lumen and variable side vessel origin from true lumen [14].

Technique

The access is obtained in the groin through cutdown in the common femoral artery or conduit to the external/common iliac artery if the vessel diameter is less than 7 mm, as all thoracic stent grafts have relatively large profile of 22–26F. Selecting the true lumen is mandatory in order to push the super stiff wire into the normal segment of the aortic arch, over which the stent graft is introduced. Once the stent graft is positioned in the deployment segment, the blood pressure is lowered to 75–80 mmHg to avoid the windsock effect during stent deployment. Following graft deployment, the operator should check the effect on the distal true lumen and the status of aortic side branches. In the authors' experience, extending the stented segment into the diaphragmatic level can serve several purposes including better expansion of the true lumen, more chances of thrombosing the false lumen and thereby prompts aortic wall healing, and prevention of future aneurysmal dilatation.

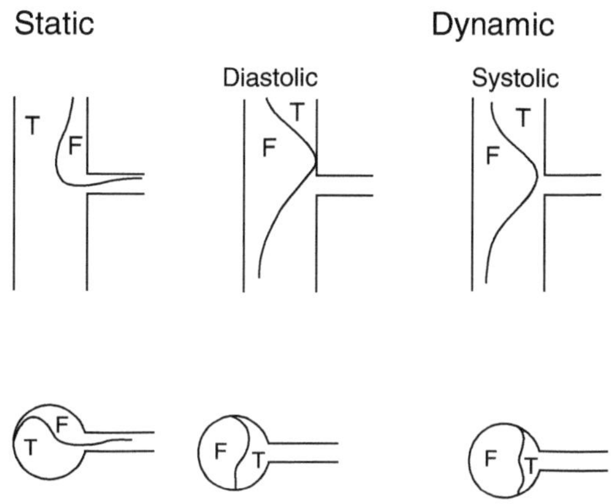

Fig. 8.6 Mechanisms of malperfusion in aortic dissection (Illustration by Anne-Sophie Sillesen)

Type B Aortic Dissection and Mechanisms of Malperfusion

Patients with complicated type B aortic dissection, malperfusion, impending rupture, intractable pain, and uncontrolled hypertension represent a high-risk group when compared with uncomplicated type B AD. The hospital mortality in this group of patients is greater than 50 %. The predictors of poor outcome are age over 70 years, hypotension, absence of chest/back pain, and visceral malperfusion as reported by the International Registry of Aortic Dissection (IRAD) [15]. It is generally agreed that intervention is indicated in complicated type B AD, as medical treatment alone can be associated with high mortality and morbidity [16].

There are three mechanisms of visceral and/or lower limb malperfusion in the setting of type B dissection [17] (Fig. 8.6). The first mechanism is

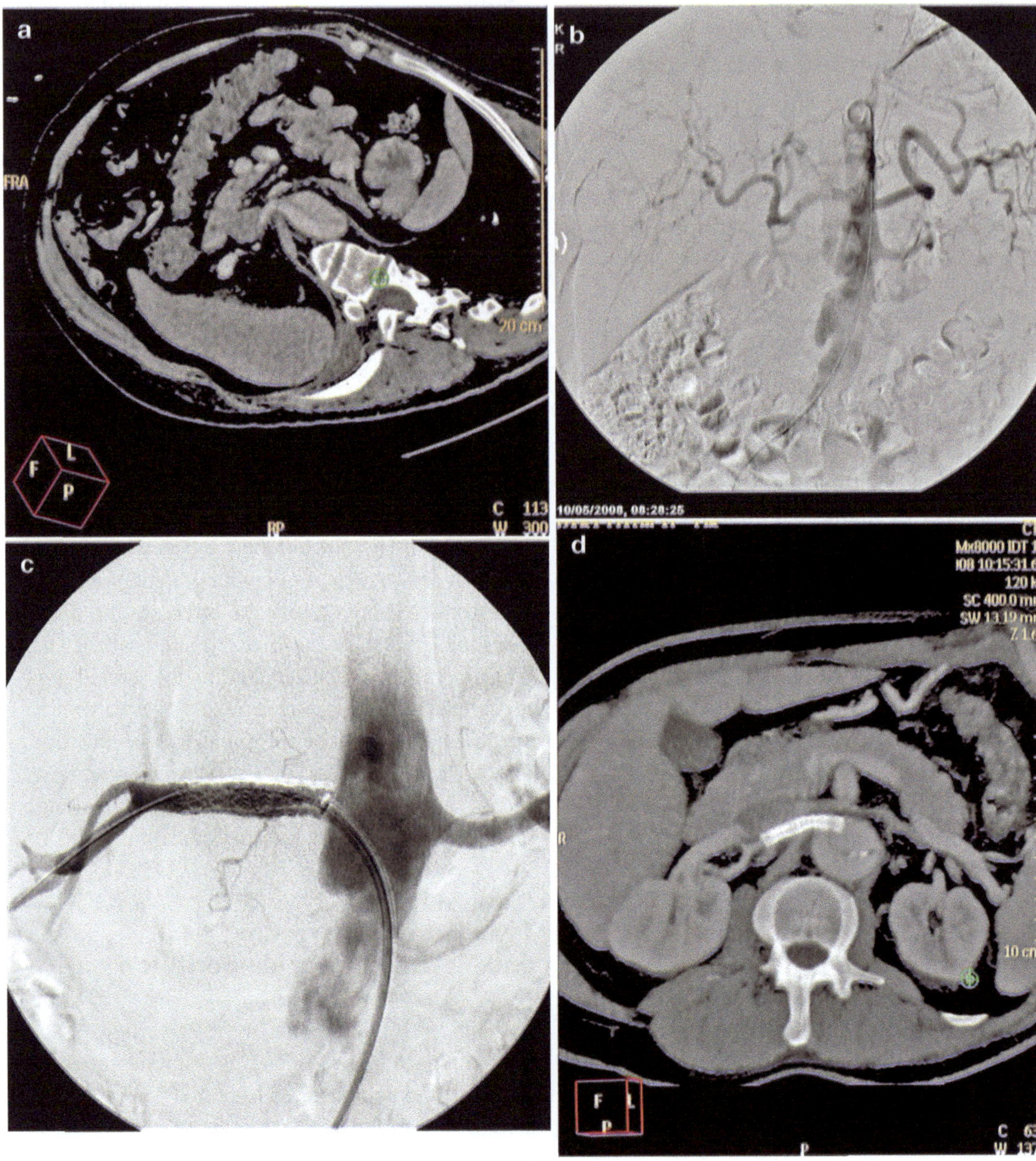

Fig. 8.7 A 68-year-old male with acute type B TAD and acute renal insufficiency, (**a**) CT angiogram shows the dissection flap extending into the right renal artery causing severe stenosis (static mechanism), (**b**) angiogram shows faint flow to the right renal artery despite thoracic stent graft deployment, (**c**) angiogram shows restored flow following renal artery stenting, and (**d**) completion CT

static occlusion of the side branch. The dissection flap extends into the side branch or iliac artery, causing severe stenosis (Fig. 8.7). The second mechanism is dynamic occlusion. In this type, the intimo-medial flap pushed intermittently throughout the cardiac cycle against the mouth of the branch vessel as a result of high pressure in the false lumen (Figs. 8.8 and 8.9). The most narrowed area could be at or above the vessel level. The third mechanism is combination of static and dynamic occlusion (Figs. 8.10 and 8.11). Dynamic compression of visceral arteries can result in the floating viscera sign. With the catheter placed in the true lumen in aortography, opacification of

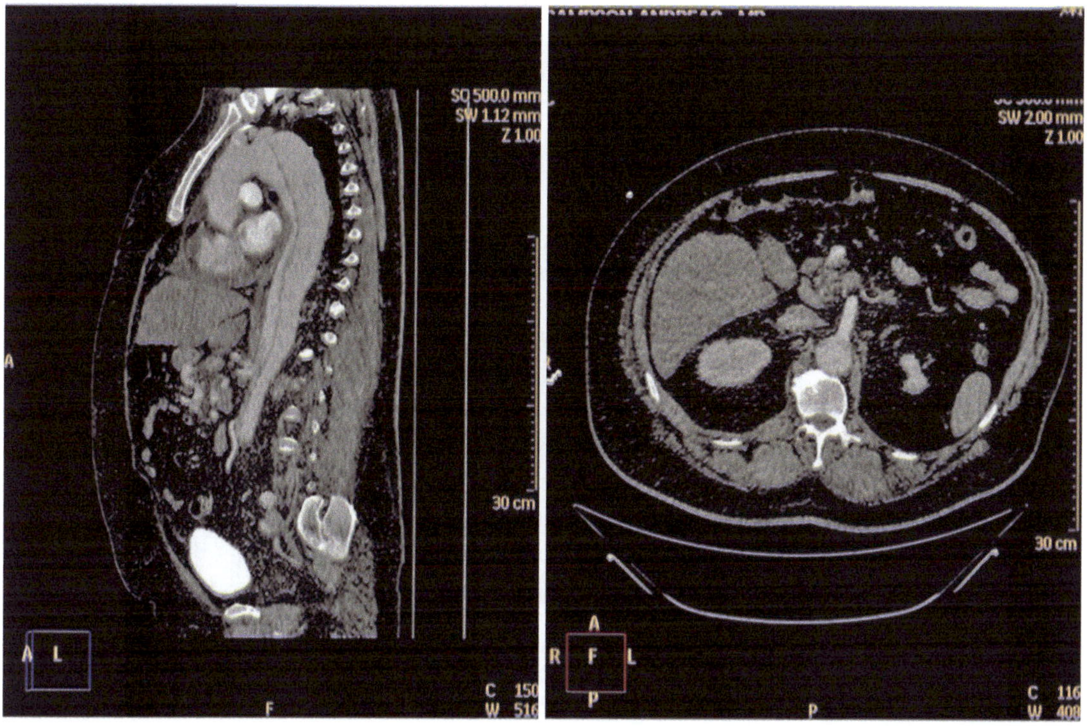

Fig. 8.8 A 56-year-old male with acute type B AD and elevated lactate. Oblique sagittal and axial CT angiogram confirms dissection and severe compression of the visceral arteries (dynamic compromise)

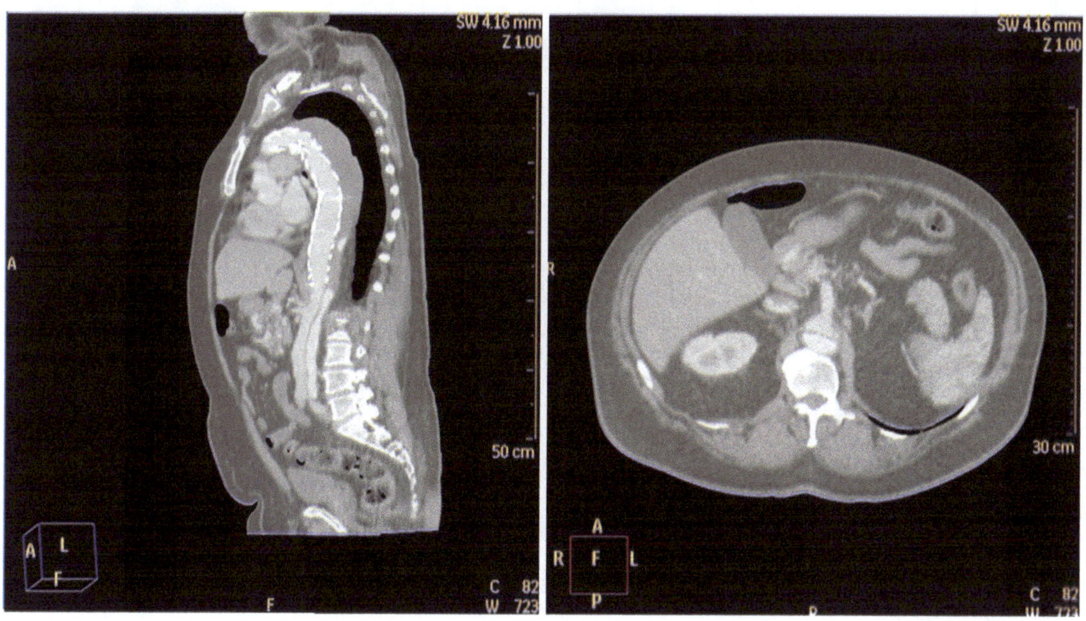

Fig. 8.9 Post stent graft deployment, note the expansion of the true lumen and improve flow to compromised SMA

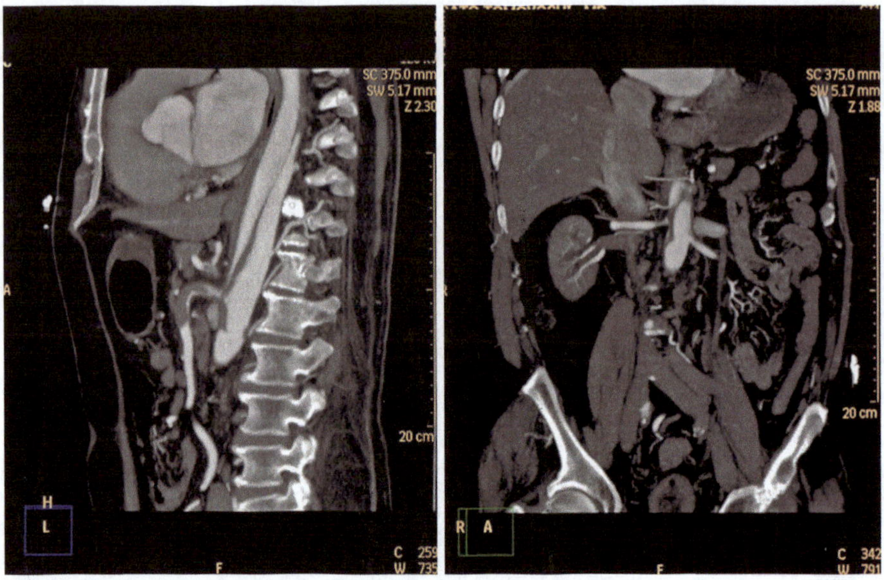

Fig. 8.10 A 60-year-old male with acute type B AD and lower limb ischemia. Sagittal and coronal images on CT angiography showing severe compression of the true lumen, combined static, and dynamic compression of the celiac trunk and SMA as well as complete occlusion of the infrarenal aorta

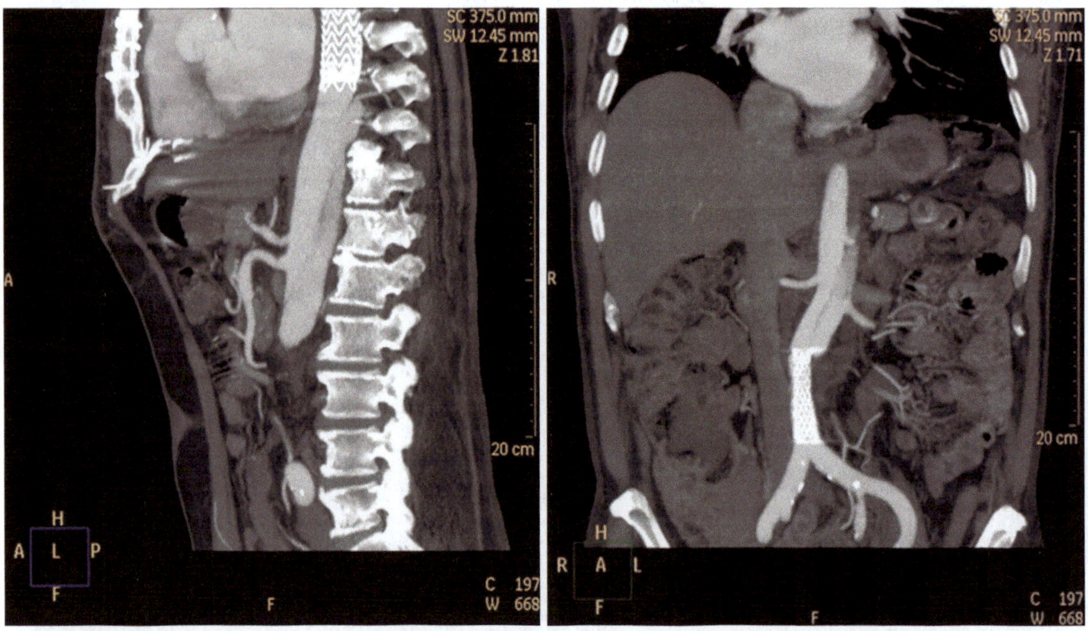

Fig. 8.11 CT angiogram post thoracic stent grafting (*left*) and bare stent deployment in the infrarenal aorta (*right*) showing complete expansion of the true lumen and revascularization of both lower limbs

aortic branches occurs with little or no antegrade opacification of the aortic true lumen. The sign occurs as a result of the dissection flap sparing origin of aortic branches but expanding false lumen compressing the aortic true lumen proximal to the visceral arteries (Fig. 8.12).

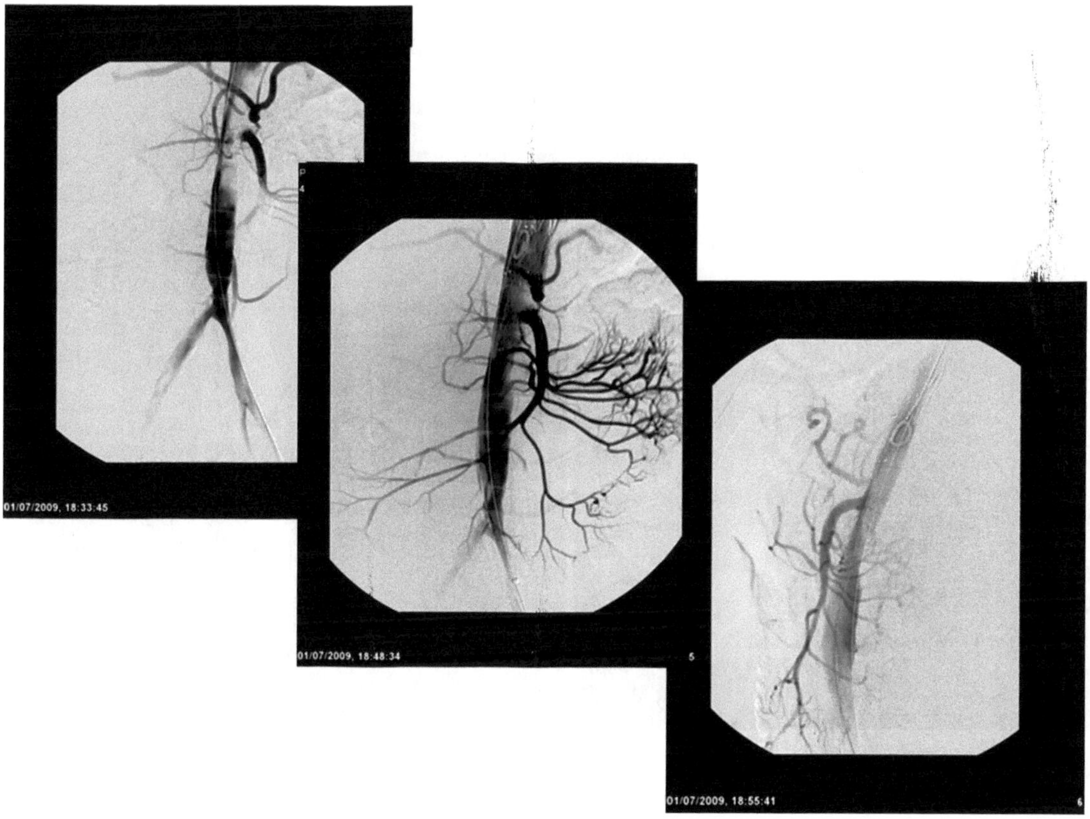

Fig. 8.12 A 70-year-old hypertensive male with acute type B AD and bowel ischemia. Angiogram shows floating viscera sign (*left*). Anterior-posterior (*middle*) and lateral angiogram (*right*) post uncovered stent across the vessel arteries confirm improved flow to the celiac trunk and SMA

It is important to understand the mechanism of malperfusion prior to intervention to tailor the management strategy accordingly.

The open surgery treatment of complicated type B dissection includes resection of the primary entry tear, bypass grafting of the compromised visceral or iliac artery, and open fenestration of the dissected flap. However, open approach is associated with significant morbidity and mortality with in-hospital death as high as 40 % [18].

The emerging endovascular techniques can provide effective treatment with better outcome for complicated type B AD. Historically, fenestration is considered the best adjuvant to open surgery or a bridge to open repair after stabilizing the patient. The principle of this treatment is equalizing pressure between the true and false lumen by creating a fenestration at the compromised level, followed by stenting the true lumen. Stenting of the renal or superior mesenteric artery is contemplated in cases of static compromise. The early and late outcome of this technique has been outlined in a largest single-center experience of 69 patients by Patel and colleagues [19]. The technical success rate of around 95 % has been achieved. The early mortality and morbidity are 17.4 and 22 %, respectively. The all-cause late mortality is reported at 36.2 %. However, the mean time to aortic ruptures or need for repair is 79.2 months. Nevertheless, beside percutaneous fenestration being technically demanding, it does not offer aortic remodeling and protection since the false lumen remains perfused.

As the experience with the stent graft is evolving, the need for percutaneous fenestration is diminishing. The stent graft covers the primary entry tear, reduces pressure and promotes thrombosis of the false lumen, and encourages aortic remodeling. Once the entry tear is covered by the

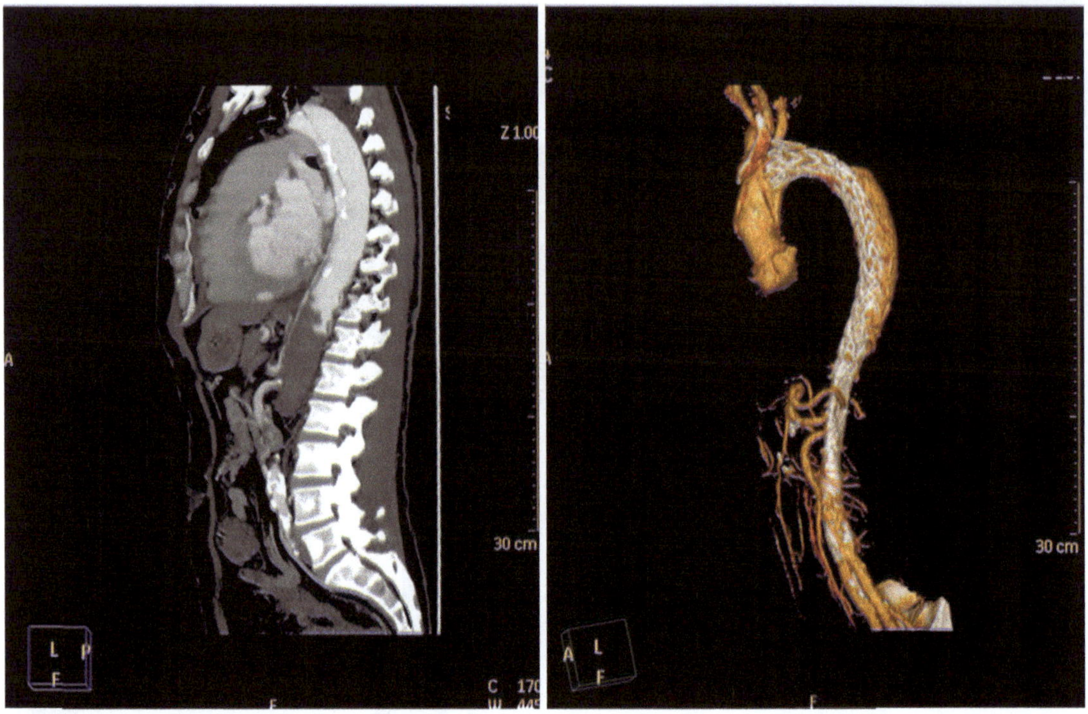

Fig. 8.13 A 61-year-old male with acute type B AD and visceral ischemia. *Left*: Oblique sagittal CT angiogram shows the dissection flap, severe compression of the true lumen, and partial thrombosis of the false lumen at the level of the visceral arteries. *Right*: Post stenting of the entire thoracic and proximal abdominal aorta (PETTICOAT) with restoration of flow to the celiac and superior mesenteric arteries

stent graft, the pressure in the false lumen decreases, the flap is pushed away from the side branch, and the flow pressure in the true lumen improves. On the other hand, the pure static type of malperfusion is not expected to resolve with stent graft alone. In those cases, additional side branch stenting with covered or uncovered balloon-expandable stent and/or bare stent in the infra-/suprarenal abdominal aorta (PETTICOAT – provisional extension to induce complete attachment) is still needed (Fig. 8.13) [20].

In the authors' experience, the overwhelming majority of cases of aortic dissection complicated by malperfusion can be resolved by aortic stenting with or without additional bare stenting to aortic side branches.

Although there is lack of sizable randomized controlled trials, there is growing body of evidence in the literature supporting the use of stent graft as the first-line management in complicated type B AD. Reported results from IRAD showed lower mortality rates following TEVAR than open surgery of 9.3 and 33.9 %, respectively [21]. Another large single-center series of 77 patients also showed low mortality rate following TEVAR of 4 % versus high mortality of 40 and 33 % following surgery and medical therapy [22]. Despite the overall good results of stent graft in complicated cases, the morbidity rate remains significant. Neurological injuries (stroke and paraplegia), stent-related complications, and failure to achieve false lumen thrombosis with subsequent need for long-term imaging follow-up represent hindrance to wider use of this technology.

Outcome for Treatment of Complicated Acute Aortic Dissection

Data from the International Registry of Acute Aortic Dissection (IRAD) [23] would suggest a satisfactory outcome for the medical management of acute type B aortic dissection (although the authors would argue, this should be in a tertiary unit capable of dealing with complications promptly). Other experienced units have found similar findings [24]. Needless to say, such management in the acute setting should be in the context of invasive monitoring in a high dependency or intensive care unit. The aims of pharmacological treatment are to reduce the incidence of adverse events associated with AD, in particular aortic expansion, proximal or distal extension of the dissection, or aortic rupture. The patient also needs to be closely monitored for the development of end-organ or lower limb ischemia that may prompt more aggressive management.

Early Results

In patients with uncomplicated type B AD, IRAD indicated a 30-day, 1-year, and 3-year survival of 91, 89, and 77 %, respectively [25]. Until the advent of aortic stenting in the early 1990s, open repair was the mainstay of treatment for complicated aortic dissection with notoriously high morbidity and mortality rates. Two landmark publications in 1999 sparked worldwide interest in the endovascular management of acute complicated type B aortic dissection [10, 13]. Nienaber et al. compared the results of endovascular stenting in 12 consecutive patients with complicated type B aortic dissection with 12 patients undergoing surgery. No morbidity or mortality was encountered in the endovascular group compared with four deaths and five adverse events within the 12-month period following treatment. Successful placement of the stent graft was confirmed by intraoperative transesophageal ultrasound which confirmed sealing of the primary entry tear. Completion angiography demonstrated the same findings. False lumen thrombosis was confirmed by magnetic resonance imaging in all 12 patients in the endovascular group after a mean of 3 months [13].

In Hagen's report from 2000, evaluating 464 patients with both type A ($n=289$) and type B ($n=175$) AD, mortality rates ranged from 58 % for the patients with type A aortic dissection treated medically compared with a mortality rate of 26 % of patients with type A dissection treated surgically. Conversely, the mortality rate for patients with type B aortic dissection treated surgically was higher than that for the medically managed patients (31.4 % vs. 10.7 %). Aortic rupture and cardiac complications were responsible for the majority of patients with type A dissection with visceral ischemia being responsible for the majority of deaths in patients with type B dissection. Of the patients with type B AD, 20 % underwent surgical therapy, and 4.3 % underwent endovascular management (percutaneous fenestration to depressurize the false lumen with or without aortic stenting). It is the management of visceral ischemia or the unusual complication of acute aortic dilatation that results in the early intervention for acute type B aortic dissection [23], the success of endovascular techniques especially within the thoracic aorta has resulted in endovascular techniques superseding open repair for the management for complications of acute type B AD.

Midterm Results

Dake et al. evaluated stent placement across the primary entry tear in 15 patients with type B (confined to the descending thoracic aorta) and 4 patients with type A aortic dissection. Aortic branches were involved in three quarters of patients, and symptomatic compromise of multiple branches was observed in over a third of patients. Technical success was achieved in all patients. Stenting resulted in complete thrombosis in 15 patients and partial thrombosis in the remaining four cases. Three of 19 patients died in the first 30 days; however, there were no deaths, aneurysmal dilation, or aortic rupture in the remaining 16 patients in the 13-month follow-up period [10].

Ehrlich et al. published the midterm results from a European unit, their indications for intervention included aortic rupture, malperfusion, intractable pain, and visceral malperfusion. All patients were treated by endovascular means. Technical success (the stent graft covering the primary entry tear) was accomplished in 87 %. The left subclavian artery was intentionally totally or partially covered in over a quarter of patients with no evidence of immediate post-procedural ischemic symptoms or subclavian steal, necessitating reintervention. Further intra-procedural stenting was required in one of five patients being treated including stenting of the renal, celiac, or mesenteric arteries. Patients were followed up for an average of 2 years with no endoleaks in the series. Survival at 1 and 5 years was 81 and 76 %, respectively. Freedom from treatment failure (requiring reintervention, aortic rupture, aortic-related death, or unexplained late death) was 78 and 61 %, respectively [26]

Long-Term Results

IRAD evaluated long-term survival of 242 patients from 21 units worldwide successfully treated for complicated type B aortic dissection over an 8-year period with a median follow-up time of 2.3 years. Only centers with over 80 % follow-up were included in the analysis. The in-hospital mortality rate was 12.3 %, and these patients were excluded from the outcome data. The mean age of the patient was 62.1, and 69 % of the patients were male. Patients receiving surgery or endovascular treatment were more likely to have complications in particular mesenteric ischemia, extension of the aortic dissection, and acute limb ischemia, compared with the medically treated group (this may however reflect the localized pattern of dissection with the medically managed group). Refractory pain and hypertension was the indication for intervention in over a quarter of cases. Limb and visceral ischemia was indications in 28 and 30 %, respectively. Predictors of mortality in those patients surviving their intervention for complicated AD included age over 70 years, patients with atherosclerosis (as opposed to patients with connective tissue disorders), prior aortic aneurysm repair, and in-hospital hypotension or shock [25]. Age-adjusted female gender was recognized as an independent predictor of death in this study. Absence of false lumen thrombosis was recognized as a significant predictor of aortic dilatation and aneurysmal expansion. False lumen enlargement by an average of 3.3 mm/year has been observed in uncomplicated, untreated AD associated with a patent false lumen [27].

Treatment of Uncomplicated Type B Aortic Dissection

The relative simplicity of thoracic aortic stenting and the need to avoid early and late complications of AD suggest that intervention may be beneficial in those patients with uncomplicated type B AD. The INSTEAD trial (Investigation of Stent Grafts in Aortic Dissection) was designed to test the hypothesis that endovascular treatment was beneficial compared to medical management alone in uncomplicated AD. This study was supported by industry (Medtronic Bakken Research Institute), and all patients were treated with the company's proprietary aortic stent (TALENT, Medtronic Inc., Santa Rosa, California, USA). Patients were selected on the basis to successfully treat the AD with this stent. Patients were excluded from randomization if they had any indications for emergent treatment of their AD or if anatomic exclusions for endovascular treatment existed (including 75–100 % false lumen thrombosis). Patients were enrolled after 14 days to identify complicated cases including acute aortic dilation and spontaneous false lumen thrombosis. Of 597 patients, 140 were enrolled to the study with 72 having stenting. Patient demographics and dissection morphology were evenly distributed, and the time from dissection to randomization was not significant between the two groups. Time from randomization to stenting was a median of 12 days (range 1–29 days), and thoracic stenting was successfully completed in all but two of the patients. Just under a quarter of patients had predetermined occlusion of the left subclavian artery without prior or perioperative revascularization. Survival probability was 88.9 % with TEVAR and 95.6 % with medical treatment (taking into account vascular injuries necessitating repair, secondary intervention, and one incidence of stroke). Analysis of fatalities included four patients that violated study protocol (acute malperfusion, renal dysfunction, and lower limb ischemia). There were two cases of spinal cord ischemia following thoracic stenting and one case following medical treatment; however, the differences between the two groups for this secondary end point were not significant. False lumen thrombosis was promoted by stent graft placement, and there was a statistically significant difference compared with best medical therapy alone. The authors concluded that the management of uncomplicated type B AD is best managed medically, but there is a prerequisite of tight surveillance and early intervention for the complications associated with AD. At present, there is no data on aneurysmal degeneration between the two groups.

Conclusion

Aortic dissection remains a challenging problem for vascular specialists. Improvements in imaging have led to increased awareness of this condition and decreased misdiagnosis. Prompt diagnosis and classification of aortic dissection along with better multidisciplinary cooperation will improve outcome for individual patients. MRI may have been considered the "gold standard," but CT is the most commonly used modality for initial imaging and has high sensitivity and specificity for the condition and is widely available. Open repair in the context of aortic dissection has always been fraught with difficulties and has been superseded by endovascular repair, which for lesions in the thoracic aorta have good results. The success of endovascular intervention in aortic dissection has been expanded for use with the other acute aortic syndromes which have a more aggressive course than aortic dissection again with excellent results. The prevalence of this condition is much lower than that for aneurysmal disease, and as a result, even the largest worldwide multicenter trials have relatively small numbers. TEVAR has a definite place in the management of complicated type B AD; its place in uncomplicated disease is less certain. Improvements in fenestrated stent graft technology that has expanded the role of endovascular treatment in aneurysmal disease will no doubt influence management of complicated AD. Needless to say, the management of the acute aortic syndromes requires close multidisciplinary cooperation and should take place in a specialist vascular unit.

References

1. Meszaros I, Morocz J, Szlavi J, Schmidt J, Tornoci L, Nagy L, et al. Epidemiology and clinicopathology of aortic dissection. Chest. 2000;117(5):1271–8.
2. Kumar V, Cotran RS, Robbins SL. Blood vessels. In: Basic pathology. 6th ed. Philadelphia: Saunders; 1997. p. 300–2.
3. Hirst Jr AE, Johns Jr VJ, Kime Jr SW. Dissecting aneurysm of the aorta: a review of 505 cases. Medicine (Baltimore). 1958;37(3):217–79.
4. Kapustin AJ, Litt HI. Diagnostic imaging for aortic dissection. Semin Thorac Cardiovasc Surg. 2005; 17(3):214–23.
5. Clough RE, Hussain T, Uribe S, Greil GF, Razavi R, Taylor PR, et al. A new method for quantification of false lumen thrombosis in aortic dissection using magnetic resonance imaging and a blood pool contrast agent. J Vasc Surg. 2011;54(5):1251–8.
6. Clough RE, Waltham M, Giese D, Taylor PR, Schaeffter T. A new imaging method for assessment of aortic dissection using four-dimensional phase contrast magnetic resonance imaging. J Vasc Surg. 2012; 55:914–23. Epub 2012 Mar 2.
7. Koschyk DH, Nienaber CA, Knap M, Hofmann T, Kodolitsch YV, Skriabina V, et al. How to guide stent-graft implantation in type B aortic dissection? Comparison of angiography, transesophageal echocardiography, and intravascular ultrasound. Circulation. 2005;112(9 Suppl):I260–4.
8. Bartel T, Eggebrecht H, Muller S, Gutersohn A, Bonatti J, Pachinger O, et al. Comparison of diagnostic and therapeutic value of transesophageal echocardiography, intravascular ultrasonic imaging, and intraluminal phased-array imaging in aortic dissection with tear in the descending thoracic aorta (type B). Am J Cardiol. 2007;99(2):270–4.
9. Ahmad F, Cheshire N, Hamady M. Acute aortic syndrome: pathology and therapeutic strategies. Postgrad Med J. 2006;82(967):305–12.
10. Dake MD. Aortic intramural haematoma: current therapeutic strategy. Heart. 2004;90(4):375–8.
11. Troxler M, Mavor AI, Homer-Vanniasinkam S. Penetrating atherosclerotic ulcers of the aorta. Br J Surg. 2001;88(9):1169–77.
12. Drinkwater SL, Bockler D, Eckstein H, Cheshire NJ, Kotelis D, Wolf O, et al. The visceral hybrid repair of thoraco-abdominal aortic aneurysms–a collaborative

approach. Eur J Vasc Endovasc Surg. 2009;38(5):578–85.
13. Nienaber CA, Fattori R, Lund G, Dieckmann C, Wolf W, von Kodolitsch Y, et al. Nonsurgical reconstruction of thoracic aortic dissection by stent-graft placement. N Engl J Med. 1999;340(20):1539–45.
14. Rodd CD, Desigan S, Cheshire NJ, Jenkins MP, Hamady M. The suitability of thoraco-abdominal aortic aneurysms for branched or fenestrated stent grafts–and the development of a new scoring method to aid case assessment. Eur J Vasc Endovasc Surg. 2011; 41(2):175–85.
15. Suzuki T, Mehta RH, Ince H, Nagai R, Sakomura Y, Weber F, et al. Clinical profiles and outcomes of acute type B aortic dissection in the current era: lessons from the International Registry of Aortic Dissection (IRAD). Circulation. 2003;108 Suppl 1:II312–7.
16. Hiratzka LF, Bakris GL, Beckman JA, Bersin RM, Carr VF, Casey Jr DE, et al. ACCF/AHA/AATS/ACR/ASA/SCA/SCAI/SIR/STS/SVM guidelines for the diagnosis and management of patients with thoracic aortic disease: executive summary. A report of the American College of Cardiology Foundation/American Heart Association Task Force on Practice Guidelines, American Association for Thoracic Surgery, American College of Radiology, American Stroke Association, Society of Cardiovascular Anesthesiologists, Society for Cardiovascular Angiography and Interventions, Society of Interventional Radiology, Society of Thoracic Surgeons, and Society for Vascular Medicine. Catheter Cardiovasc Interv. 2010;76(2):E43–86.
17. Williams DM, Lee DY, Hamilton BH, Marx MV, Narasimham DL, Kazanjian SN, et al. The dissected aorta: percutaneous treatment of ischemic complications–principles and results. J Vasc Interv Radiol. 1997;8(4):605–25.
18. Trimarchi S, Nienaber CA, Rampoldi V, Myrmel T, Suzuki T, Bossone E, et al. Role and results of surgery in acute type B aortic dissection: insights from the International Registry of Acute Aortic Dissection (IRAD). Circulation. 2006;114(1 Suppl):I357–64.
19. Patel HJ, Williams DM, Meerkov M, Dasika NL, Upchurch Jr GR, Deeb GM. Long-term results of percutaneous management of malperfusion in acute type B aortic dissection: implications for thoracic aortic endovascular repair. J Thorac Cardiovasc Surg. 2009;138(2):300–8.
20. Melissano G, Bertoglio L, Rinaldi E, Civilini E, Tshomba Y, Kahlberg A, et al. Volume changes in aortic true and false lumen after the "PETTICOAT" procedure for type B aortic dissection. J Vasc Surg. 2012;55(3):641–51.
21. Fattori R, Tsai TT, Myrmel T, Evangelista A, Cooper JV, Trimarchi S, et al. Complicated acute type B dissection: is surgery still the best option?: a report from the International Registry of Acute Aortic Dissection. JACC Cardiovasc Interv. 2008;1(4):395–402.
22. Zeeshan A, Woo EY, Bavaria JE, Fairman RM, Desai ND, Pochettino A, et al. Thoracic endovascular aortic repair for acute complicated type B aortic dissection: superiority relative to conventional open surgical and medical therapy. J Thorac Cardiovasc Surg. 2010; 140(6 Suppl):S109–15; discussion S42–6.
23. Hagan PG, Nienaber CA, Isselbacher EM, Bruckman D, Karavite DJ, Russman PL, et al. The International Registry of Acute Aortic Dissection (IRAD): new insights into an old disease. JAMA. 2000;283(7):897–903.
24. Estrera AL, Miller 3rd CC, Safi HJ, Goodrick JS, Keyhani A, Porat EE, et al. Outcomes of medical management of acute type B aortic dissection. Circulation. 2006;114(1 Suppl):I384–9.
25. Tsai TT, Fattori R, Trimarchi S, Isselbacher E, Myrmel T, Evangelista A, et al. Long-term survival in patients presenting with type B acute aortic dissection: insights from the International Registry of Acute Aortic Dissection. Circulation. 2006;114(21):2226–31.
26. Ehrlich MP, Dumfarth J, Schoder M, Gottardi R, Holfeld J, Juraszek A, et al. Midterm results after endovascular treatment of acute, complicated type B aortic dissection. Ann Thorac Surg. 2010;90(5):1444–8.
27. Sueyoshi E, Sakamoto I, Hayashi K, Yamaguchi T, Imada T. Growth rate of aortic diameter in patients with type B aortic dissection during the chronic phase. Circulation. 2004;110(11 Suppl 1):II256–61.

9 Endovascular Treatment of Traumatic Thoracic Aortic Rupture, Ruptured TAA and AAA

Manish Mehta, Philip S.K. Paty, Sean P. Roddy, and R. Clement Darling

Abstract

Treatment strategies for ruptured aortic aneurysms including traumatic thoracic transections have evolved significantly over the past decade from open surgical repair to minimally invasive endovascular repair using stent grafts. This change in paradigm requires not just the addition of endovascular skills but a change in infrastructures that enable hospitals to manage the complexities of these new endovascular procedures. This chapter will focus on endovascular repair of acute thoracic and abdominal aortic emergencies and highlight the importance of establishing standardized infrastructures that enable health care providers to provide comprehensive and up-to-date care for patients with these catastrophic emergencies.

Keywords

Aorta • EVAR • Imaging • Vascular surgery • Stent grafts

Introduction

The metamorphosis of abdominal aortic aneurysm (AAA) repair and thoracic aortic aneurysm repair (TAA) from open surgical to endovascular means has evolved substantially over the past two decades. Today, endovascular abdominal aneurysm repair (EVAR) and thoracic endovascular aortic aneurysm repair (TEVAR) are considered as the first choice of therapy for treatment of infrarenal AAA and descending TAA in patients with favorable morphology. Furthermore, in "real-world" clinical scenarios, with increasing physician experience and ability, the indications of EVAR and TEVAR have expanded from treatment of elective to emergent aneurysms and from favorable morphology to sometimes complex and unfavorable anatomy, particularly in high-risk patients [1–4]. When considering these endovascular techniques for treating ruptured abdominal and thoracic aortic aneurysms, or thoracic aortic transections, one has to prepare for the challenges of streamlining patient care from the emergency room to the operating room and subsequent endovascular procedure that often requires a multidisciplinary approach

M. Mehta, M.D., MPH (✉) • P.S.K. Paty, M.D.
S.P. Roddy, M.D. • R.C. Darling, M.D.
The Vascular Group PLLC, The Institute for Vascular Health and Disease, Albany Medical Center Hospital, The Center for Vascular Awareness, Inc,
43 New Scotland Ave, MC 157, Physicians Pavilion, 3rd Floor, Albany, NY 12208, USA
e-mail: mehtam@albanyvascular.com

J.J. Hoballah, A.B. Lumsden (eds.), *Vascular Surgery*, New Techniques in Surgery Series,
DOI 10.1007/978-1-4471-2912-7_9,

and a change in paradigm and local cultures. This chapter will focus on a comprehensive and standardized technical approach for treating patients presenting with ruptured abdominal and thoracic aortic aneurysms and traumatic thoracic aortic transections by endovascular means that can maximize our ability to offer this treatment of most patients and optimize outcomes.

EVAR for Ruptured AAA

Since the initial reports in mid-1990s [5, 6], EVAR for ruptured AAA has evolved from being performed selectively by a few centers in hemodynamically stable patients to being performed by many endovascular specialists in patients with varying degrees of hemodynamic instability [7]. As with most procedures, the reason for vast dissemination of these techniques and technology is due to its many advantages over the standard open surgical repair, the most important being its association with significant reduction in morbidity and mortality when compared to open surgical repair [8–11].

Today, the question is not whether patients with ruptured AAA should undergo EVAR, rather how to develop systems that allow for broader utilization of these complex procedures that have shown great benefit in high-risk patients with aneurysm rupture. There remain several fundamental concerns regarding EVAR for ruptured AAA that include the availability of preoperative imaging (CTA) in all patients with ruptured AAA to identify anatomical suitability for EVAR, the availability of dedicated staff and equipment to perform emergent EVAR at all hours, the feasibility of treating hemodynamically stable and unstable patients by EVAR, and the surgeon/interventionist ability to manage unexpected scenarios under emergent circumstances. Although one or more of the above-mentioned "limitations" might have some impact on one's ability to incorporate endovascular techniques in managing patients with ruptured AAA, the fundamentals for success begin from establishing an infrastructure of a standardized approach that is multidisciplinary and inclusive of the emergency room (ER) physicians, the anesthesiologists, the operating room (OR) nurses, the technologists, and the vascular surgeons.

To get started, the surgeon/interventionist should (1) become comfortable performing EVAR under elective circumstances; (2) obtain an inventory of standard equipment (wires, catheters, sheaths, balloons, particularly the compliant aortic occlusion balloons, and fluoroscopic equipment) that is needed to perform elective EVAR safely; (3) pick and choose the stent grafts that one is most comfortable using and acquire select stent graft sizes to match the largest aortic neck diameter and the shortest aneurysm length, with a variety of iliac extensions to treat most if not all AAA; (4) become comfortable with adjunctive procedures such as iliac interventions that might be needed to facilitate access, use of compliant aortic occlusion balloon, and placement of Palmaz stents at the aortic neck; and (5) only treat hemodynamically stable patients with preoperative CT scans. With increasing experience, one can easily modify their inclusion and exclusion criteria for EVAR of ruptured AAA that can accommodate even hemodynamically unstable patients.

EVAR for Ruptured AAA: A Standardized Approach

Treatment of ruptured AAA patients involves a multidisciplinary approach that is inclusive of ER staff, anesthesiologists, OR staff, radiology technologists, and the vascular surgeon/interventionist, and therefore requires a standardized approach that engages all parties and facilitates a seamless transition of the patient from the emergency room to the operating room for EVAR. Although the standardization of any approach will vary from hospital to hospital, the fundamentals are simple in that success depends on the early diagnosis of ruptured AAA, the ability to have an expeditious CT scan to evaluate the aortoiliac morphology, and the quick transition of patient from the emergency room to the operating room which is equipped to perform endovascular as well as open surgical repair under these emergent circumstances.

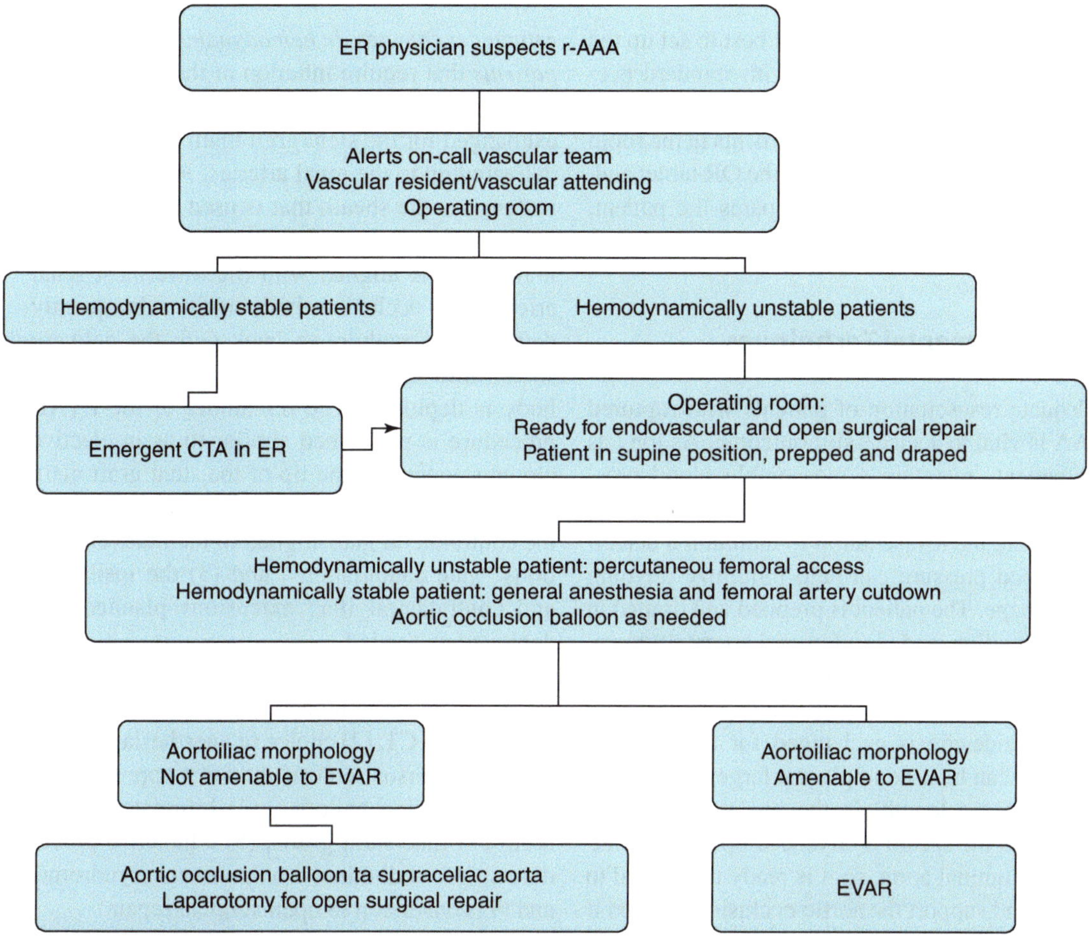

Fig. 9.1 Albany Vascular Group standardized protocol for endovascular aneurysm repair (EVAR) of ruptured abdominal aortic aneurysms (r-AAA). *BP* blood pressure, *CTA* computed tomographic angiography, *ER* emergency room

In 2002, at the Vascular Institute for Health and Disease in Albany, we developed a standardized approach [2] that has enabled us to use endovascular approach as the first line of therapy for all patients that present with ruptured AAA, and this has resulted in a significant improvement on patient survival (Fig. 9.1). The fundamentals of the protocol include a heightened awareness among the ER staff to suspect the diagnosis of ruptured AAA and notify the on-call vascular surgeon and the OR staff. In the emergency room, hemodynamically stable patients undergo expeditious CT scan and are subsequently transferred to the OR, and hemodynamically unstable patients are directly transferred to the OR without a preoperative CT scan for endovascular-first approach and conversion to open surgical repair as needed.

Operating Room Setup

Since not all patients with ruptured AAA can undergo endovascular repair, all OR/hybrid endovascular-OR suits should be set up to facilitate endovascular as well as open surgical repair. Depending on the size of the room and the fluoroscopic equipment which can be fixed or portable with viewing screens and power injectors, one has to customize the layout of the OR suite that is conducive for endovascular and open surgical repair; we have found it best to set up the room for endovascular repair with standard needles, wires, catheters, and sheaths open on a sterile table; have the surgical instruments in the room if needed; situate the patient on the OR table; and, as the anesthesiology team prepares the patient, set up the fluoroscopic equipment and supplies.

The Fundamental Techniques

Adequate resuscitation of patients with ruptured AAA is vital to a successful outcome. As long as the patients maintain a measurable blood pressure, the techniques of "hypotensive hemostasis" by limiting the resuscitation to maintain a detectable blood pressure can help minimize ongoing hemorrhage. The patient is prepped and draped in supine position, and via a femoral artery cutdown, ipsilateral access is obtained using a needle, a floppy guidewire, and a guiding catheter. The floppy guidewire is exchanged for a super-stiff wire that can be used to place a large sheath (12–14 Fr×45 cm length) in the ipsilateral femoral artery, and the sheath is advanced up to the juxtarenal abdominal aorta, so it is ready to be used to deliver and support the aortic occlusion balloon if needed. A compliant occlusion balloon should always be available in these procedures, and in hemodynamically unstable patients, the occlusion balloon is advanced through the ipsilateral sheath over the super-stiff wire into the supraceliac abdominal aorta under fluoroscopic guidance, and the balloon is inflated as needed. In our experience of over a hundred ruptured EVARs, the aortic occlusion balloon is needed in <25 % of cases. Access is subsequently obtained from contralateral femoral artery cutdown in similar fashion, and a "marker flush catheter" is advanced to the juxtarenal aorta for an arteriogram.

The placement of the stent graft main body is planned based on the aortoiliac morphology that is best suited for EVAR. Unless prohibitive, *in hemodynamically* stable patients, following the initial arteriogram, the aortic occlusion balloon is removed from the initial ipsilateral side, and the stent graft main body is advanced under fluoroscopic guidance; this limits the number of catheter exchanges. *In hemodynamically unstable patients* that require inflation of the aortic occlusion balloon, the "marker flush catheter" is exchanged for the stent graft main body which is delivered up to the renal arteries. An arteriogram is done via the sheath that is used to support the aortic occlusion balloon, the tip of the stent graft main body is aligned with the lowermost renal artery, the occlusion balloon is subsequently deflated and withdrawn back with the delivery sheath into the AAA, and the stent graft main body is deployed. The remainder of the EVAR procedure is performed similar to as in elective circumstances: (1) the tip of the stent graft main body aligned with the lowermost renal artery, (2) the contralateral gate aligned to facilitate expeditious "gate cannulation", and (3) the ipsilateral and contralateral iliac extensions planned and deployed as needed.

There are several important technical aspects that merit discussion, including (1) availability of preoperative CT, (2) choice of anesthesia and percutaneous versus femoral cutdown approach, (3) aortic occlusion balloons, (4) bifurcated versus aorto-uni-iliac stent grafts, (5) adjunctive procedures, (6) abdominal compartment syndrome, and (7) conversion to open surgical repair.

Availability of Preoperative CT Scan

The hemodynamic status of the ruptured AAA patient generally dictates the need for a preoperative CT scan, and although while planning for this emergent open surgical repair a preoperative CT is not considered a necessity, while planning an emergent EVAR, most would agree that we would like to have a CT scan for evaluating the feasibility of EVAR as well as for stent graft sizing. So the question is whether one has the time to get an emergent CT scan prior to EVAR, and if not, are there other tools available that might help us manage these hemodynamically unstable patients by endovascular means? Lloyd et al. published data on a time to death study in patients with ruptured AAA who did not undergo treatment [12]. Their findings indicated that 88 % (49 of 56) patients died >2 h after admission with the diagnosis of ruptured AAA. The median time interval from the onset of symptoms to admission to the hospital was 2.5 h, and the interval between hospital admission with the diagnosis of ruptured AAA and death was 10.5 h. This data would clearly suggest that majority of patients with ruptured AAA have the time to undergo an emergent CT scan, particularly if there is an established protocol that facilitates early diagnosis and transfer of patient from the ER to the OR. The obvious question that remains is how often are ruptured AAAs suitable for endovascular repair? Recently, we have tried to answer just that by evaluating CT scans of 50 consecutive patients that presented with ruptured AAA and had an available CT scan. The endovascular anatomical inclusion criteria was slightly modified from the standard "indications for use" defined by each of the FDA-approved devices and focused on feasibility of EVAR for ruptured AAA; this included aortic neck length ≥ 10 mm, aortic neck diameter ≤ 32 mm, aortic neck angulation ≤ 75°, and bilateral iliac artery diameter > 5 mm. Using the above-mentioned criteria, our findings indicated that 80 % of ruptured AAA patients could be considered anatomically suitable for EVAR, and this is comparable to our clinical findings of treating over 120 ruptured AAA patients by endovascular means. When evaluating patients with ruptured AAA, even if one were to adhere strictly to the stent graft IFU (indications for use) that were used during the pivotal trials that lead to FDA approval of the device, approximately 60 % of the patients would be considered anatomically suitable to undergo ruptured EVAR [13].

Choice of Anesthesia and Approach

Depending on one's comfort level and the logistics, EVAR for rupture can be performed under local anesthesia via percutaneous approach to general anesthesia and femoral artery cutdown. The potential benefits of local anesthesia and percutaneous approach is that it might avoid the loss of "sympathetic tone" in the compromised ruptured AAA patients [14]. The percutaneous techniques have several limitations since currently available stent grafts are delivered through large sheath sizes ranging from 18 to 24 Fr, and one has to be comfortable with obtaining percutaneous access and using closure devices in patients that might be hemodynamically unstable with difficult to palpate femoral pulses. One also needs to be comfortable in utilizing "preclose" techniques with ProStar XL and Perclose ProGlide Suture-Mediated Closure System (Abbott Vascular, Santa Clara, CA) [15]. In hemodynamically stable patients, particularly in the hands of experienced operators, these percutaneous procedures are quite feasible. However, it has been our standard approach to perform EVAR for rupture under general anesthesia with femoral artery cutdown. We have found that femoral access via cutdown can be accomplished within minutes, and this approach is easier to standardize than the percutaneous approach.

We have reserved the percutaneous approach for endovascular aneurysm repair of ruptured abdominal aortic aneurysm in select patients that are considered to be hemodynamically unstable, are conscious, and can cooperate with the anesthesiologist and the vascular surgeon/interventionist. In these patients, we prefer to access the femoral artery percutaneously *without* a closure device, advance an appropriately sized sheath 18–22 Fr as needed, and carry out the endovascular aneurysm repair procedure. At the completion of the endovascular procedure, the femoral sheaths are removed via femoral artery cutdown and direct femoral artery repair. Of course, the preclose technique for totally percutaneous EVAR for ruptured aneurysms is most certainly utilized. This approach needs to be individualized on the basis of the patients' hemodynamic status.

Aortic Occlusion Balloon

The appropriate use of aortic occlusion balloons in hemodynamically unstable patients is vital to the success of EVAR in these emergent circumstances. Our preferred method for placing aortic occlusion balloons is to use the femoral approach, and we have found this to have several advantages: (1) it allows the anesthesia team to have access to both upper extremities for arterial and venous access; (2) the patients who require the aortic occlusion balloon are often hypotensive, and in these patients, percutaneous brachial access can be difficult and more time-consuming than femoral cutdown; and (3) the currently available aortic occlusion balloons require at least a 12-Fr sheath, which requires a brachial artery cutdown and repair, and stiff wires and catheters across the aortic arch without prior imaging under emergent circumstances might lead to other arterial injuries and/or embolization causing stroke.

There are several important points to consider during procedures that require inflation of the aortic occlusion balloons to maintain hemodynamic stability. To facilitate stabilization of the balloon catheter during inflation and maintain aortic occlusion at the suprarenal/supraceliac level, the sheath supporting the balloon should be advanced and supported fully into the aortic neck prior to inflation of the occlusion balloon as this will prevent downward displacement and prolapse of the occlusion balloon into the AAA (Fig. 9.2). Inability to fully engage the sheath into the aortic neck due to the presence of significant aortoiliac stenosis, calcifications, or tortuosity might result in downward displacement of the inflated occlusion balloon; this often required forward traction on the inflated balloon catheter to maintain adequate position at the suprarenal/supraceliac aorta (Fig. 9.3).

If inflation of the aortic balloon is required to maintain a viable blood pressure, then the remainder of the EVAR should be conducted expeditiously to limit the time of aortic occlusion and further limit the development of complications of ongoing bleeding such as abdominal compartment syndrome and multisystem organ failure. During the procedure, just prior to deployment of the stent graft main body, the aortic occlusion balloon should be deflated from the suprarenal level and withdrawn. The stent graft main body is subsequently deployed; this will avoid trapping the compliant aortic occlusion balloon between the aortic neck and the stent graft. This temporary deflation of the aortic occlusion balloon rarely results in hemodynamic collapse and usually is of little consequence. In hemodynamically unstable patients, the occlusion balloon can be redirected into the aortic neck from the side ipsilateral to the stent graft main body and reinflated at the infrarenal aortic neck within the stent graft main body; this allows for aortic occlusion and does not interfere with the remainder of the endovascular procedure (Fig. 9.4a–c).

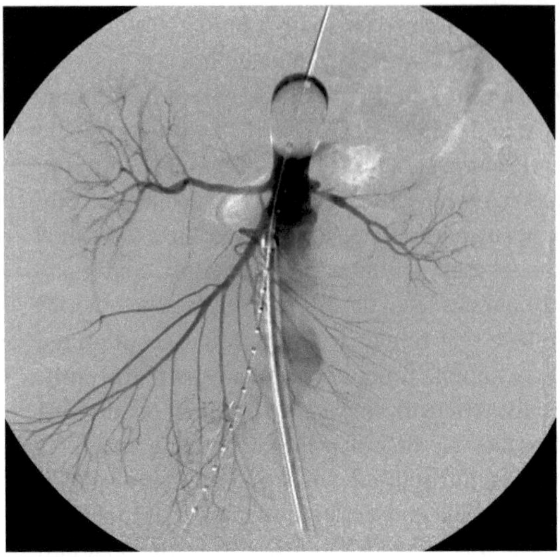

Fig. 9.2 The sheath supporting the aortic occlusion balloon should be advanced and supported fully into the aortic neck to prevent downward displacement and prolapse of the occlusion balloon into the AAA

Currently there are four different compliant occlusion balloons that are readily available, with subtle differences (Table 9.1). Occlusion balloons are composed of compliant materials such as polyurethane latex, or silicone, and have low burst pressures of <5 atm. Their primary function is not angioplasty but molding to the surrounding with gentle inflation and function in capacity of obtaining proximal aortic occlusion during EVAR for ruptured AAA and should be in the armamentarium of all vascular specialists treating AAA.

Bifurcated Versus Aorto-Uni-Iliac (AUI) Stent Grafts for Ruptured AAA

Although the decision to use a particular stent graft type and size is determined by the patient's aortoiliac morphology, there are several factors which

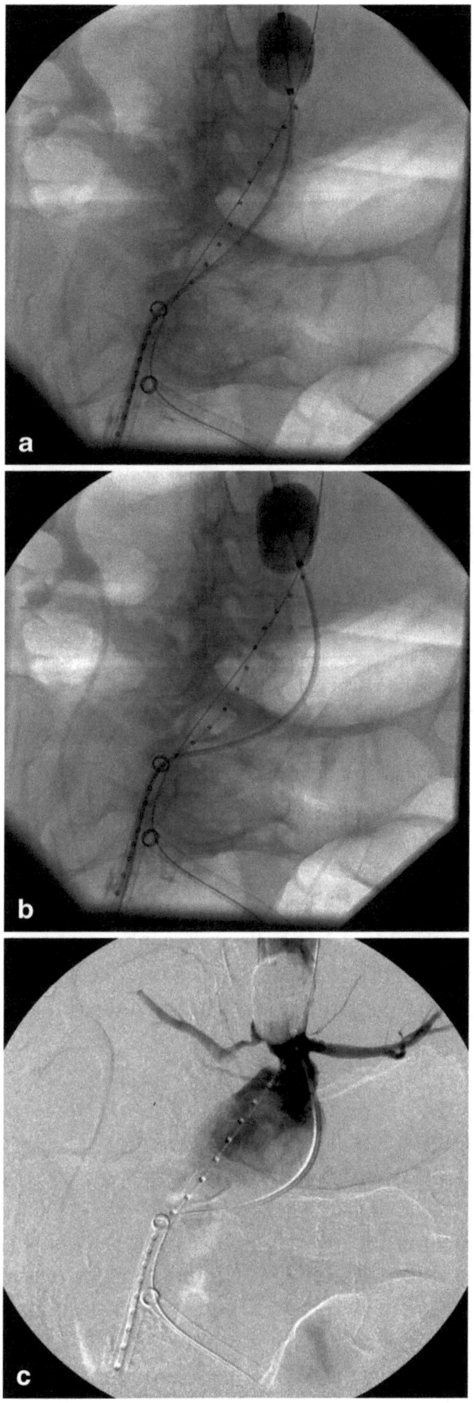

Fig. 9.3 Inability to fully engage the sheath into the aortic neck due to the presence of significant aortoiliac stenosis, calcifications, or tortuosity might result in downward displacement of the inflated occlusion balloon (**a**–**c**); this often required forward traction on the inflated balloon catheter to maintain adequate position at the suprarenal/supraceliac aorta

predispose our decisions to use bifurcated versus AUI stent grafts in these aortic emergencies: (1) inability to access the contralateral gate expeditiously and (2) inability to access the contralateral iliac artery due to significant occlusive disease and/or tortuosity. When using bifurcated stent grafts even in patients that maintain adequate hemodynamic status, there is the potential for ongoing bleeding until adequate proximal and distal fixation in the aortic neck and iliac arteries is obtained. During the procedure, if rapid gate cannulation is not obtained, particularly in hemodynamically unstable patients, the bifurcated stent grafts should be converted to AUI devices by using stent grafts such as the Renu device (Cook Inc) or placing aortic cuffs or a second stent graft main body across the stent graft flow divider to divert all blood flow to the ipsilateral iliac artery. This does require subsequent interruption of flow from the contralateral common iliac artery into the AAA via a stent graft occluder and a femoral-femoral bypass.

In our experience of over 120 EVARs for ruptured AAA, approximately 16 % require emergent conversion of bifurcated stent grafts into AUI devices. To facilitate contralateral gate cannulation during EVAR, we routinely cross the stent graft limbs to align them with the contralateral sheath which is usually crossed and anterior to the ipsilateral sheath in most cases. With this approach, gate cannulation can usually be achieved within minutes.

Adjunctive Procedures

Due to the obvious emergent nature of ruptured AAA, preoperative planning can be less than ideal, which can lead to the need for additional unexpected adjunctive procedures. To discuss all adjunctive procedures that might be needed during EVAR for ruptured AAA is beyond the scope of this chapter; however, the use of Palmaz stents at the aortic neck for treatment of type I endoleaks is a technique that should be in one's armamentarium [14]. Our standard approach includes the following: (1) a Palmaz 4,910 stent is hand crimped and centered onto a 20–25-mm noncompliant Maxi-LD balloon (Cordis), (2) both

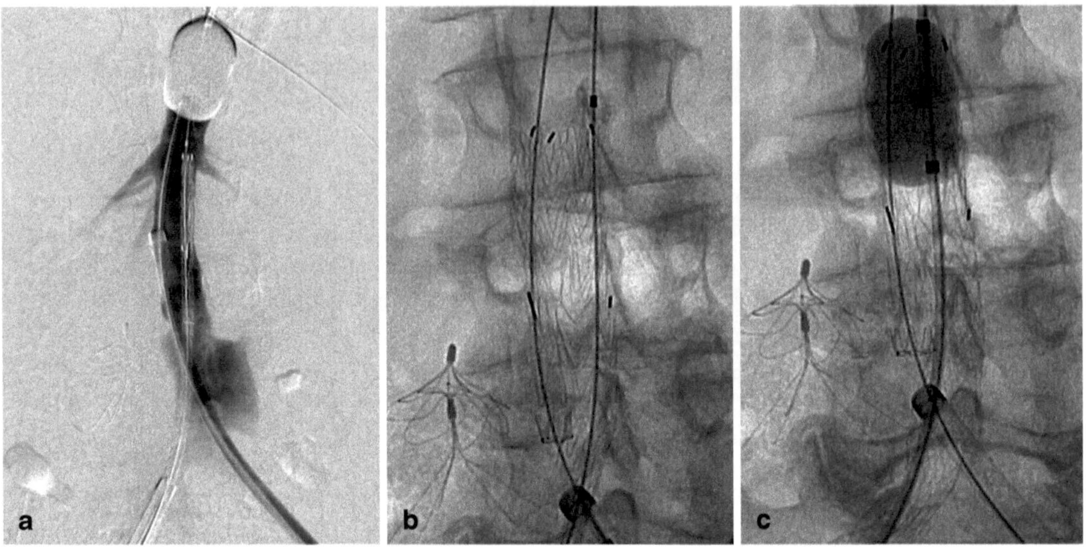

Fig. 9.4 (**a**) Managing the aortic occlusion balloon during stent graft deployment. Inflated suprarenal aortic occlusion balloon via left femoral approach, the stent graft main body via right femoral approach, and arteriogram done through the left femoral sheath supporting the occlusion balloon. (**b**) Managing the aortic occlusion balloon during stent graft deployment. The aortic occlusion balloon is deflated and retracted back from the aortic neck, and the stent graft main body subsequently deployed; this avoids trapping of the compliant aortic occlusion balloon between the aortic neck and the stent graft. (**c**) Managing the aortic occlusion balloon during stent graft deployment. In hemodynamically unstable patients, the occlusion balloon can be redirected into the aortic neck from the side ipsilateral to the stent graft main body and reinflated at the infrarenal aortic neck within the stent graft main body prior to contralateral gate cannulation

Table 9.1 Properties of compliant aortic occlusion balloons

Occlusion balloon	Sheath size (Fr)	Catheter length (cm)	Max. balloon diameter (mm)
Reliant (Medtronic Ave)	12	100	46
Coda (Cook Inc)	14	100–120	32, 40
Equalizer (Boston Scientific Corp)	14–16	65, 110	20, 27, 33, 40
Q-50	12	65	10–50

ends of the Maxi-LD balloon with the Palmaz stent are slightly inflated to avoid "watermelon seed" displacement of the Palmaz stent during deployment, (3) a 16–18-Fr delivery sheath is advanced into the straight and nontortuous main body of the stent graft, (4) the Palmaz stent loaded onto the balloon is delivered to the juxtarenal aorta and aligned for deployment partially in the stent graft main body and the native aortic neck and deployed under fluoroscopic guidance, and (5) the Maxi-LD balloon is exchanged for a compliant aortic occlusion balloon, described earlier, and the Palmaz stent is molded to anchor the stent graft to the aortic wall.

Assessing for Abdominal Compartment Syndrome

With increasing use of endovascular techniques for treating ruptured AAA, there is an increased recognition of new complications, such as abdominal compartment syndrome (ACS) [15]. The pathophysiology of ACS after EVAR for ruptured AAA is multifactorial: (1) the retroperitoneal hematoma is a space-occupying lesion and a significant factor contributing to intra-abdominal hypertension, (2) ongoing bleeding from lumbar and inferior mesenteric arteries into the disrupted aneurysm sac in the setting of severe coagulopathy might be a contributing factor, and (3) the shock state associated with ruptured AAA is associated with alterations in microvascular permeability that can lead to visceral and soft tissue edema.

Most published data would suggest that the incidence of ACS following EVAR for ruptured AAA varies and probably dependent on the hemodynamic status of the patients being treated. In our own series of EVAR for ruptured AAA in hemodynamically stable and unstable patients, the incidence of ACS was noted to be 18 %, and several variables were identified as significant contributing factors. These include (1) use of aortic occlusion balloon, (2) need for massive blood transfusions (mean 8 units PRBC), and (3) coagulopathy with elevated aPTT at completion of case. In our experience, patients that developed ACS had a significantly increased mortality (67 %) when compared to those without ACS (10 %). As a result of these observations, our protocol for the endovascular treatment of r-AAA has evolved. Systemic heparinization which was used earlier in our experience during EVAR for rupture is avoided, and coagulation studies are aggressively corrected during the perioperative period to help limit the ongoing bleeding from collateral vessels. Furthermore, bladder pressures are recorded on an hourly basis during the procedure as well as in the postoperative period. If the bladder pressures are increased, regardless of the presence of other associated factors, we emphatically recommend that patients undergo decompression laparotomy. However, the question is how many factors need to be present in the absence of increased bladder pressures to accurately predict ACS. In our clinical practice, regardless of the presence of increased bladder pressures, if patients have more than one risk factor for developing ACS (aortic occlusion balloon, massive blood transfusion, or coagulopathy), have abdominal distention, and manifest signs of end-organ dysfunction, they undergo on-table laparotomy. It is our belief that taking these measures might help identify and treat ACS and decrease the associated morbidity and mortality.

Conversion to Open Surgical Repair

Regardless of all the improvements in endovascular techniques, there are times when on-table conversion to open surgical repair is needed, and this approach should be in the armamentarium of all surgeons/interventionists involved in treating ruptured AAA patients. A comprehensive discussion of open surgical repair is beyond the scope of this chapter, but there are a few key points that need to be mentioned here. When on-table surgical conversion is needed, the use of aortic occlusion balloon can be extremely valuable in maintaining hemodynamic stability; the techniques of aortic occlusion balloon have been discussed above. In addition, during the time of laparotomy and open surgical conversion, it is crucial to maintain the position of the aortic occlusion balloon and its delivery sheath; failure to do so might result in aortic occlusion balloon prolapse into the AAA and loss of aortic occlusion. If open surgical conversion is needed subsequent to stent graft deployment, the exact approach should be tailored to the type of stent graft and the type of proximal and distal fixation including suprarenal versus infrarenal stents and barbs [16].

Relevant Outcomes

Today, the vascular literature has ample evidence that goes well beyond the feasibility of ruptured EVAR. Recent findings of the Albany Vascular Group indicate that ruptured EVAR is associated not only with a lower 30-day mortality but also a significant long-term survival advantage when compared to open surgical repair [17]. Mehta et al. evaluated 283 patients with ruptured AAA that underwent EVAR ($n = 120$, 42.4 %) and OSR ($n = 163$, 57.6 %) at Albany Medical Center. EVAR patients had a significantly lower 30-day mortality than OSR patients (29/120, 24.2 % vs. 72/163, 44.2 %; $p < 0.005$) and better cumulative 5-year survival (35 % vs. 25 %, $p < 0.005$). Men benefited more from EVAR (mortality 20.9 % for EVAR vs. 44.3 % for OSR, $p < 0.001$) than women (mortality 32.4 % vs. 43.9 %, $p = 0.39$). Age ≥80 years was a significant predictor of death for EVAR (OR 1.07, $p = 0.003$), but not for OSR (OR 1.04, $p = 0.056$). For r-AAA, EVAR reduces the 30-day mortality and improves long-term survival up to 5 years. However, women do not benefit as much as men and seem to do equally well from OSR. Older patients have higher mortality rates. Secondary interventions were required in 23 % of EVAR patients.

A meta-analysis of 23 published studies on endovascular versus open surgical repair of ruptured AAA analyzed outcomes in 7,040 patients that underwent EVAR (n=730, 10 %) or open surgical repair (n=6,130, 90 %). The findings indicated that ruptured EVAR was associated with a significant reduction in 30 day mortality, reduction in the mean intensive care unit length of stay by 4 days, and reduction in the mean hospital length of stay by 9 days [18]. A further analysis of the US NSQIP database, a prospective multicenter registry, that collectively evaluated 427 ruptured AAA patients from 2005 to 2007 that underwent either EVAR (23 %) or open surgical repair (77 %) also indicated that open surgical repair of ruptured AAA was associated with a significantly higher 30-day mortality (OR 1.9, p=0.006) when compared to EVAR [19]. Collected ruptured EVAR world experience with collaboration from 49 centers indicates the overall 30-day mortality after EVAR in 1,037 patients to be 21 % provided that they have favorable anatomy, adequate endovascular skills, facilities, and protocols available [20]. Regardless of dozens of reports indicating the benefits of ruptured EVAR, there is some controversy on this subject as three prospective trials, two randomized and one nonrandomized, have failed to demonstrate the benefits of EVAR to open surgical repair for ruptured AAA, and an additional two prospective RCTs evaluating endovascular versus open surgical repair of ruptured AAA are underway [21–25]. There are several limitations of the above-mentioned trials that failed to demonstrate the benefit of EVAR including a significant delay in treatment in an intent-to-treat study following the diagnosis of ruptured AAA that resulted in equally poor outcomes of EVAR when compared to open surgical repair (EVAR 53 % vs. open surgical 53 %). The findings of a recent Dutch multicenter randomized trial (AJAX) that evaluated death and severe complications as primary endpoints have indicated no difference between ruptured EVAR and open surgical repair. AJAX findings indicate that death and severe complications occur in 42 % of patients following ruptured EVAR and in 47 % following ruptured open surgical repair, and this difference is nonsignificant. Now there are several limitations of this study. The AJAX trial was conceived in 2003 and randomized 116 patients over nearly an 8-year period. Over this time period, 520 patients were enrolled in the trial, of which nearly 90 % were enrolled at a single trial center. Of the 520 patients, 395 (76 %) were evaluated by CT scan, of which 240 (61 %) were found to have unfavorable anatomy for EVAR and were excluded. Another 39 (10 %) patients were excluded for a variety of reasons. The remaining 116 (22 %) patients were randomized to EVAR (57) or open surgical repair (59). For a prospective randomized multicenter trial, this trial had a significant patient selection bias, rendering its outcomes questionable in the real world. In the real-world clinical scenarios, with currently available data on over a thousand patients demonstrating favorable outcomes of ruptured EVAR, one can argue whether randomized prospective trials on EVAR versus open surgical repair offer any benefit.

Over the past decade, the proportion of ruptured AAA patients being treated by endovascular means is steadily increasing, and ruptured EVAR is evolving from being performed in academic tertiary medical centers only to community hospital. Anain and colleagues were early adopters of a standardized EVAR-first approach for ruptured AAA in a community hospital setting; their findings indicate that regardless of the hemodynamic status, 75 % of ruptured AAA patients can undergo EVAR with a technical success of over 90 % and a marked improvement in survival (EVAR 83 % vs. open repair 60 %, $p<0.05$) [26]. Although earlier reports on Nationwide Inpatient Sample (NIS) database indicate that the mortality of ruptured EVAR continues to be significantly higher in nonteaching community hospitals when compared to academic medical centers (55 % vs. 21 %, $p<0.05$), with establishment of standardized ruptured EVAR protocols, current nationwide literature suggests wider adoption of ruptured EVAR approximating 25 % of all ruptured AAA with improved outcomes [27, 28]. Implementation of a standardized protocol for emergent ruptured EVAR has been demonstrated to improve outcomes and allow for emergent treatment of hemodynamically unstable patients in our experience as well as others. Moore et al. have demonstrated evidence of a significant reduction in mortality (17.9 % vs. 30 %, $p<0.05$) after introduction on an emergency endovascular therapy protocol for ruptured AAA [29]. Their findings also suggest that hemodynamically unstable patients show trends toward improved survival after ruptured EVAR when compared to open surgical repair. A significant percentage of ruptured AAA present with hemodynamic instability, and without a standardized protocol, these patients are often not considered suitable for EVAR and undergo open surgical repair [30]. It is these hemodynamically unstable patients that have the highest mortality of open surgical repair and might be the ones to experience the greatest benefit of EVAR, and further studies on hemodynamically unstable ruptured AAA patients are needed. Lastly, health care cost implications play a major role in evolution of treatments and technology, and a recent report by Hayes and colleagues in the cost-effectiveness analysis of endovascular versus open surgical repair of ruptured AAA based on worldwide experience indicates significant cost reduction and improvements in quality-adjusted life years in patients that undergo EVAR [31].

The Bottom Line

Endovascular repair of ruptured AAA is evolving and offers the potential for improved patient survival. Unlike elective EVAR, during emergent EVAR, the time for preoperative planning is limited, and often the preoperative imaging is less than ideal; under these circumstances, one often has to get creative and utilize more of a "problem-solving approach" to address challenging issues that might arise during these emergent circumstances. A standardized multidisciplinary approach can be instrumental in organizing pathways that can accommodate individual practices and hospital infrastructure and facilitate a seamless transition of these often hemodynamically unstable patients from the time of diagnosis to successful EVAR. There are several important technical aspects including the choice of anesthesia, percutaneous versus femoral cutdown approach, use of aortic occlusion balloons, use of bifurcated versus aorto-uni-iliac stent grafts, and adjunctive procedures that need to be well understood as one embarks on performing these procedures.

TEVAR for Ruptured Thoracic Aortic Aneurysms

The first report of TEVAR for ruptured TAA was in 1997 [32], and similar to EVAR over the past decade, TEVAR is clearly becoming the procedure of choice in patients with ruptured TAA and suitable proximal and distal stent graft landing zones. Today, there are three FDA-approved thoracic stent grafts (TAG: WL Gore & Ass, Flagstaff, AZ; TALENT: Medtronic Ave, Santa Rosa, CA; Zenith TX2: Cook Inc, Bjaeverskow, Denmark), another has completed US phase II clinical trial (RELAY: Bolton Medical Inc, Sunrise, FL), and clinical data for all approved devices indicates TEVAR to have a significantly lower morbidity and mortality when compared to open surgical repair [33–35]. TEVAR also has evolved from treatment of elective TAA to emergent acute thoracic aortic emergencies including ruptured TAA and traumatic thoracic aortic transections. Similar to ruptured AAA, ruptured TAA is a life-threatening emergency that has traditionally been associated with a significant mortality ranging from 35 to 90 % [36]. Similar to ruptured EVAR, the potential benefit of ruptured TEVAR in decreasing the morbidity and mortality is all too obvious; however, there are several limitations that surgeons/interventionists have to better understand to optimize outcomes of TEVAR for acute thoracic aortic emergencies, including advances and limitations of stent graft technology and imaging.

The incidence of ruptured TAA is far less than that of ruptured AAA, and hence, reports in literature comprise of most single centers reporting only a handful of cases each. Recently, Jasper et al. published a meta-analysis on worldwide experience of open versus endovascular repair of ruptured descending TAA as most studies evaluated indicate that TEVAR for ruptured TAA is associated with significantly lower 30-day mortality when compared to open surgical repair, and although the morbidity of myocardial infarction, stroke, and paraplegia tends to be lower with endovascular therapy, this difference is not statistically significant [37]. A meta-analysis of contemporary published reports on ruptured TEVAR evaluated 29 studies that included 224 patients (mean age 70 ± 5.6 years) with ruptured TAA, 143 (64 %) treated with TEVAR and 81 (36 %) treated with open surgical repair. The results indicated that when compared to open surgical repair, the 30-day mortality of ruptured TAA was significantly lower for TEVAR (19 % vs. 33 %, $p < 0.05$), and at 3 years, the estimated aneurysm-related survival was 71 % in the TEVAR group. Although the TEVAR patients had a trend toward lower morbidity, the differences in the immediate postoperative complications of myocardial infarction, stroke, or paraplegia among the two groups were not statistically significant.

Recent data would suggest that TEVAR for ruptured TAA is associated with significantly less mortality when compared to open surgical repair and, similar to EVAR for ruptured AAA, is being considered the first approach for managing ruptured TAA by centers with comprehensive endovascular capabilities. The complexities of ruptured TEVAR evolve around imaging, accessing, and dealing with the arch great vessels at the proximal stent graft landing zones and the visceral vessels at the distal stent graft landing zones [38]. Furthermore, complications of stroke and spinal cord ischemia are additional risks that one has to consider when treating ruptured TAA patients via endovascular techniques [39, 40]. Although there are no set guidelines for cerebrospinal fluid (CSG) drainage during ruptured TEVAR, we generally follow CSF drainage recommendations similar to those during elective TEVAR; CSF drainage is reserved for patients with prior abdominal aortic reconstructions (endovascular and open surgical) and if extensive thoracic aortic coverage is planned extending from the subclavian to the celiac artery.

When planning TEVAR, particularly in emergent circumstances, the surgeon/interventionist needs to have a comprehensive understanding of imaging; today, CTA is most frequently used to evaluate patients with thoracic aortic emergencies, and one has to be able to perform adequate measurements and select the appropriate stent grafts for TEVAR. Ruptured TAA limited to the descending thoracic aorta account for approximately one-third of all aortic emergencies and stent graft coverage of arch vessels, including the left subclavian and sometimes the left common carotid artery, which often require extra-anatomical carotid-subclavian and carotid-carotid bypasses. The details of this discussion are beyond the scope of this chapter. Suggest some edits to the following: Furthermore, in patients with ruptured TAA that have inadequate distal landing zones, the risks and benefits of celiac artery coverage to lengthen the distal stent graft landing zone need to be evaluated. Data is scarce on this subject, and recently we evaluated our single-center findings of outcomes of planned celiac artery coverage during TEVAR for elective and emergent repair [41]. The study analyzed 228 patients that underwent TEVAR under elective ($n = 162$, 71 %) and emergent circumstances ($n = 66$, 29 %), of which 31 (14 %) patients underwent planned celiac artery coverage during TEVAR. CTA was primarily used for a detailed evaluation of the gastroduodenal arcade and communicating collaterals between the celiac and the superior mesenteric artery (SMA). Intraoperative visceral arteriogram with selective celiac artery balloon occlusion was selectively used to identify the presence of these collaterals. The majority of patients had demonstrable collaterals between the celiac and the SMA ($n = 24$, 77 %), the mean age was 74 years (range 55–87 years), and the mean TAA size was 6.5 cm. Postoperative complications included visceral ischemia in 2 (6 %) patients, paraplegia in 2 (6 %) patients, and death in 2 (6 %) patients. All type 1b endoleaks ($n=2$, 6 %) and type 2 endoleaks vial retrograde flow from the celiac artery ($n=3$, 10 %) were successfully treated by transfemoral coil embolization. Over a mean follow-up of 15 months, there have been no other complications of mesenteric ischemia, spinal cord ischemia, SMA in-stent stenosis, or conversion to open surgical repair. Our findings suggest that celiac artery coverage to facilitate adequate distal sealing during TEVAR with complex TAA is relatively safe in the presence of SMA-celiac collaterals. Preexisting SMA stenosis can be successfully treated by balloon-expandable stents during TEVAR, and endoleaks arising from distal stent grafts' attachment site or via retrograde flow from the celiac artery can be successfully managed by transfemoral coil embolization.

TEVAR requires delivery sheaths ranging from 18 to 24 Fr, and these larger sheath sizes may pose access-related issues when planning TEVAR, particularly in emergent circumstances. The CTA should not only focus on the TAA but needs to be inclusive of imaging up to the femoral heads to evaluate the iliac and femoral arteries. Although iliac artery caliber of <7 mm is generally considered to be a limitation in passage of large sheaths, it is more than just the iliac artery diameter that needs to be considered during planning TEVAR; the presence of significant tortuosity, calcifications, prior iliac stents, and prior aortoiliac/femoral bypass using prosthetic conduits are variables that can impact on our ability to access these arteries, and in such instances, a prosthetic conduit (10-mm PTFE or Dacron) can be sewn to a larger common iliac artery via retroperitoneal exposure for access. Lastly, the use of aortic occlusion balloons during ruptured TEVAR is rarely if ever needed, and there are several reasons for that; the survivors of ruptured TAA that get to the ER often are stable enough for an expedited thorough workup and treatment, and patients that are hemodynamically unstable and require the need for aortic occlusion balloon need an aortic occlusion balloon landing zone in the descending thoracic aorta, since inflation of these occlusion balloons in the ascending thoracic aorta or the thoracic arch would generally be catastrophic.

TEVAR for Traumatic Thoracic Aortic Transections

Thoracic aortic transection is a morbid condition that historically was difficult to manage. The treatment involved open surgery and aortic cross clamping with its associated significant morbidity and mortality. These injuries are related to blunt trauma, and most are caused by deceleration related to motor vehicle accidents. Bleeding from thoracic aortic transections is the second most common cause of death from motor vehicle accidents (after head injury) with an overall mortality of over 90 % [42]. It is estimated that in the USA approximately 7,500–8,000 blunt aortic traumatic injuries occur yearly, only 25 % of patients are alive on arrival to the emergency rooms, and nearly half of these patients will die within the first 24 h [43]. Similar to the evolution of endovascular technology in treatment of ruptured AAA and TAA, over the past decade, TEVAR has also been used frequently for treatment of traumatic thoracic aortic transections.

Recently, the Society of Vascular Surgery issued guidelines for endovascular repair of traumatic thoracic aortic injury after a systemic review of literature that included 7,768 patients with traumatic thoracic aortic transections that underwent TEVAR, open surgical repair, and nonoperative conservative management [44]. The finding of this comprehensive review indicates that TEVAR when compared to open surgical repair was associated with significantly lower 30-day mortality (9 % vs. 19 %, $p<0.05$), complications of spinal cord ischemia (3 % vs. 9 %, $p<0.05$), and renal failure (5 % vs. 8 %, $p<0.05$), and nonoperative therapy was associated with a mortality of 46 %. There has been much debate as to the indications for cerebrospinal fluid (CSF) drainage during TEVAR, currently available data would indicate that patients with traumatic thoracic aortic injury require short-segment thoracic aortic coverage and have a low incidence of complications of spinal cord ischemia, and therefore, routine CSF drainage is not recommended.

Although these findings and the Society of Vascular Surgery recommendations indicate that TEVAR for traumatic thoracic aortic transections is associated with improved outcomes when compared to open surgical repair or nonoperative therapy, there are several important factors one needs to consider during endovascular management of these complex problems. Currently, there is no FDA-approved stent graft for treatment of traumatic thoracic aortic injuries, and use of stent grafts designed to treat TAA to accommodate the thoracic aortic of a younger patient population poses some inherent risks of limitations in access vessels, procedure-related complications that can result in stent graft collapse and endoleaks, coverage of left subclavian artery, and follow-up strategy via CTA that might have additional risks to the patients. The traumatic thoracic aortic injury is usually located at the isthmus just distal to the left subclavian artery. The proximal stent graft landing zone is the key component to successful endovascular repair, and since most stent grafts require 2 cm of proximal landing zone to obtain a seal, this can sometimes pose a challenge as nearly one-half of the patients with aortic rupture are within 1 to 2 cm of the left subclavian artery. However, the clinical experience suggests that this does not provide an acute risk of limb ischemia, and late "steal" phenomenon can be electively treated with carotid-subclavian bypass when the patient has stabilized [45]. Young patients with relatively normal thoracic aortas have acute angulation across the thoracic arch which adds complexity with sizing, tracking, and deployment of currently available thoracic stent grafts. Significant oversizing can lead to suboptimum conformation of these devices which can lead to device collapse, kinks, stent fractures, and other device-related issues that might require secondary interventions. Furthermore, it is often difficult to know when to intervene on these complications; currently, data on management of these device-related complications following TEVAR for traumatic thoracic aortic injury is scarce. The future TEVAR devices will have to incorporate improvements in stent graft design that allows improved trackability, deployment, lower profile, and ability to accommodate branch vessels.

References

1. Dgorova N, Giacovelli J, Greco G, et al. National outcomes of treatment of ruptured AAA: comparison of open versus endovascular repair. J Vasc Surg. 2008; 48(5):1092–100.
2. Mehta M, Taggert J, Darling III RC, et al. Establishing a protocol for endovascular treatment of ruptured abdominal aortic aneurysms: outcomes of a prospective analysis. J Vasc Surg. 2006;44:1–8.
3. Patel HJ, Williams DM, Upchurch Jr GR, Dasika NL, Deeb GM. A comparative analysis of open and endovascular repair for the acute rupture of the descending thoracic aorta. J Vasc Surg. 2009;50:1265–70.
4. Jonker FH, Giacovelli JK, Muhs BE, Sosa JA, Indes JE. Trends and outcomes of endovascular and open treatment of thoracic aortic injury. J Vasc Surg. 2010;51:565–71.
5. Yusuf SW, Whitaker SC, Chuter TA, et al. Emergency endovascular repair of leaking aortic aneurysms. Lancet. 1994;344:1645.
6. Marin ML, Veith FJ, Cynamon J, et al. Initial experience with transluminally placed endovascular grafts for the treatment of complex vascular lesions. Ann Surg. 1995;222:1–17.
7. Veith FJ, Lachat M, Mayer D, Malina M, Holst J, Mehta M. Collected world and single center experience with endovascular treatment of ruptured abdominal aortic aneurysms. Ann Surg. 2009;250(5):818–24.
8. Lee WA, Hirneise CM, Tayyarah M, et al. Impact of endovascular repair on early outcomes of ruptured AAA. J Vasc Surg. 2004;40:211–5.
9. Resch T, Malina M, Lindblad B, et al. Endovascular repair of ruptured abdominal aortic aneurysm: logistics and short-term results. J Endovasc Ther. 2003; 10(3):440–6.
10. Hechelhammer L, Lachat ML, Wildermuth S, et al. Midterm outcome of endovascular repair of ruptured abdominal aortic aneurysms. J Vasc Surg. 2005;41(5): 752–7.
11. Moore R, Nutley M, Cina CS, et al. Improved survival after introduction of an emergency endovascular therapy protocol for ruptured abdominal aortic aneurysms. J Vasc Surg. 2007;3:443–50.
12. Lloyd GM, Brown MJ, Norwood MGA, et al. Feasibility of preoperative computed tomography in patients with ruptured AAA; A time to death study in patients without operation. J Vasc Surg. 2004;39: 788–91.
13. Brandt M, Walluscheck KP, Jahnke T, et al. Endovascular repair of ruptured AAA: feasibility and impact on early outcomes. J Vasc Interv Radiol. 2005;16(10):1309–12.

14. Kim JK, Noll Jr RE, Tonnessen BH, et al. A technique for increased accuracy in the placement of the "giant" Palmaz stent for treatment of type 1A endoleak after EVAR. J Vasc Surg. 2008;48(3):755–7.
15. Mehta M, Darling III RC, Roddy SP, et al. Factors associated with abdominal compartment syndrome complicating endovascular repair of ruptured abdominal aortic aneurysms. J Vasc Surg. 2005;42(6):1047–51.
16. Mehta M, Paty PSK, Roddy SP, et al. Treatment options for delayed AAA rupture following endovascular repair. J Vasc Surg. 2011;53:14–20. Epub 2010 Sept 26.
17. Mehta M, Byrne J, Darling RC, et al. Endovascular repair of ruptured abdominal aortic aneurysms is associated with a lower 30-day mortality and a better 5-year survival rate s than open surgical repair. J Vasc Surg. In press.
18. Sadat U, Boyle JR, Walsh SR, Tang T, Varty K, Hayes PD. Endovascular vs open repair of acute abdominal aortic aneurysms – a systematic review and meta-analysis. J Vasc Surg. 2008;48:227–36.
19. Davenport D, O'Keeffe S, Minion D, et al. Thirty-day NSQIP database outcomes of open versus endoluminal repair of ruptured abdominal aortic aneurysms. J Vasc Surg. 2010;51:305–9.
20. Veith FJ, Lachat M, Mayer D, Kalina M, Holst J, Mehta M, et al. Collected world and single center experience with endovascular treatment of ruptured abdominal aortic aneurysms. Ann Surg. 2009;250(5):818–24.
21. Hinchliffe RJ, Bruijstens L, MacSweeney ST, Braithwaite BD. A randomized trial of endovascular and open surgery for ruptured abdominal aortic aneurysm-results of a pilot study and lessons learned for future studies. Eur J Vasc Endovasc Surg. 2006;32(5):506–13.
22. Peppelenbosch N, Geelkerken RH, Soong C, Cao P, Steinmetz OK, Tiejink JA. Endograft treatment of ruptured abdominal aortic aneurysms using the Talent aortouniilac system: an international multicenter study. J Vasc Surg. 2006;43(6):1111–23.
23. Powell JT, Thompson SG, Thompson MM, Grieve R, Nicholson AA, IMPROVE Trail, et al. The immediate management of the patient with rupture: open versus endovascular repair (IMPROVE) aneurysm trial. Acta Chir Belg. 2009;109(6):678–80.
24. Desgranges P, Kobeiter H, Castier Y, Senechal M, Majewski M, Krimi A. The endovascularie vs chirurgie dans les anevrysmes rompus PROTOCOL trial update. J Vasc Surg. 2010;51(1):267–70.
25. Acute endovascular treatment to improve outcome of ruptured aorto-iliac aneurysms (The AJAX Trial). Last edited: 27/01/2009. Available at: http://www.controlled-trials.com/ISRCTIN66212637. Accessed May 2012.
26. Anain PM, Anian Sr JM, Tiso M, et al. Early and mid-term results of ruptured abdominal aortic aneurysms in the endovascular era in a community hospital. J Vasc Surg. 2007;46(5):898–905.
27. Lesperance K, Andersen C, Singh N, et al. Expanding use of emergency endovascular repair for ruptured AAA: disparities in outcomes form nationwide perspective. J Vasc Surg. 2008;47(6):1165–70.
28. Devenport DL, O'Keeffe SD, Minion DJ, et al. Thirty-day NSQUIP database outcomes of open versus endoluminal repair of ruptured abdominal aortic aneurysms. J Vasc Surg. 2010;51(2):305–9.
29. Moore R, Nutley M, Cina CS, et al. Improved survival after introduction of an emergency endovascular therapy protocol for ruptured AAA. J Vasc Surg. 2007;45(3):443–50.
30. Coppi G, Silingardi R, Gennai S, et al. A single center experience in open and endovascular treatment of hemodynamically unstable and stale patients with ruptured abdominal aortic aneurysms. J Vasc Surg. 2006;44(6):1140–7.
31. Hayes PD, Sadat U, Walsh SR, et al. Cost-effectiveness analysis of endovascular versus open surgical repair of acute abdominal aortic aneurysms based on worldwide experience. J Endovasc Ther. 2010;17(2):174–82.
32. Semba CP, Kato N, Kee ST, Lee GK, Mitchell RS, Miller DC, et al. Acute rupture of the descending thoracic aorta: repair with use of endovascular stent-grafts. J Vasc Interv Radiol. 1997;8:337–42.
33. Makaroun MS, Killavou ED, Wheatley GH, Cambria RA. Give year results of endovascular treatment with gore TAG device compared to open repair of thoracic aortic aneurysms. J Vasc Surg. 2008;47:912–8.
34. Fairman RM, Criado F, Farber M, Kwolek CJ, Mehta M, White R, et al. Pivotal results of the Medtronic Vascular Talent Thoracic Stent Graft System for patients with thoracic aortic disease: the VALOR trial. J Vasc Surg. 2008;48:546–54.
35. Matsumura JS, Cambria RP, Dake MD, Moore RD, Svensson LG, Snyder S. International controlled clinical trial of thoracic endovascular aneurysm repair with the Zenith TX2 endovascular graft: 1-year results. J Vasc Surg. 2008;47:247–57.
36. Johansson G, Markstrom U, Swedenborg J. Ruptured thoracic aortic aneurysms: a study of incidence and mortality rates. J Vasc Surg. 1995;21:985–8.
37. Jonker FHW, Trimarchi S, Verhagen HJM, et al. Meta-analysis of open versus endovascular repair for ruptured descending thoracic aortic aneurysms. J Vasc Surg. 2010;51:1026–32.
38. Raghuveer V, Sanchez L. Open techniques for arc vessel reconstructions during thoracic endovascular aneurysm repair. J Vasc Surg. 2010;52:71S–6.
39. Buth J, Harris PL, Hobo R, van Eps R, Cuypers P, Duijm L, et al. Neurologic complications associated with endovascular repair of thoracic aortic pathology: incidence and risk factors. A study from the European Collaborators on Stent/Graft Techniques for Aortic Aneurysm Repair (EUROSTAR) registry. J Vasc Surg. 2007;46:1103–10;discussion 1110–1.
40. Hnath JC, Mehta M, Taggert JB, Sternbach Y, Roddy SP, Kreienberg PB, et al. Strategies to improve spinal cord ischemia in endovascular thoracic aortic

repair: outcomes of a prospective cerebrospinal fluid drainage protocol. J Vasc Surg. 2008;48:836–40.
41. Mehta M, Darling III RCD, Taggert JB, Roddy SP, Sternbach Y, Ozsvath KJ, et al. Outcomes of planned celiac artery coverage during TEVAR. J Vasc Surg. 2010;52:1153–8.
42. Feliciano DV, Mattox KL. Thoracic and abdominal vascular trauma. In: Veith FJ, Hobson RW, Williams RA, Wilson SE, editors. Vascular surgery: principles and practice. New York: McGraw-Hill; 1994. p. 947–66.
43. Fabian TC, Richardson JD, Croce MA, Smith Jr JS, Rodman Jr G, Kearney PA, et al. Prospective study of blunt aortic injury: multicenter trial of the American Association for the Surgery of Trauma. J Trauma. 1997;42:374–80.
44. Lee AW, Matsumura JS, Mitchell SR, Farber MA, Greenberg RK, Asissadeh A, et al. Endovascular repair of traumatic thoracic aortic injury: clinical practice guidelines of the Society for Vascular Surgery. J Vasc Surg. 2011;53(1):187–92.
45. Karmy-Jones RC, Salerno C. Thoracic vascular trauma. In: Zelenock GB, Huber TS, Messina LM, Lumsden AB, Moneta GL, editors. Mastery of vascular and endovascular surgery. Philadelphia: Lippincott Williams & Wilkins; 2006. p. 629–35.

Laparoscopic and Robotic Aortic Surgery

10

Jean Bismuth

Abstract

Minimally invasive approaches have taken the world of vascular surgery by storm, particularly endovascular techniques. Nevertheless, open surgical technique like the aortobifemoral bypass (AFB) remains an extremely efficacious and durable operation and is the procedure against which all other iliac procedures are benchmarked. However, if one thinks of an open procedure, like an endovascular procedure, as consisting of both a "delivery system" and a therapeutic component, the delivery system for aortobifemoral bypass remains unappealing and in many instances a very high-risk operation in patients with significant comorbidities. Consequently, endovascular management of aortoiliac disease has moved to the front line of the treatment algorithm. Being able to deliver the results of open surgical techniques in a more acceptable manner is possible today both by totally laparoscopic or robotic abdominal procedure. This not only reduces the convalescence period but also leads to fewer operative complications than standard techniques. This chapter discusses current minimally invasive laparoscopic and robotic techniques in aortic surgery.

Keywords

Robotic • Laparoscopic • Aortic • Aortoiliac • Minimally invasive

Introduction

Minimally invasive surgery has profoundly impacted the management of the surgical diseases across all specialties. Advances in endovascular technologies have fundamentally changed the practice of cardiovascular surgery, while the role for laparoscopy has remained limited. Management of the diseased aorta has been no exception. Large-scale trials have shown that patients benefit

J. Bismuth, M.D.
Department of Cardiovascular Surgery,
Methodist DeBakey Heart and Vascular Center,
The Methodist Hospital,
6550 Fannin, Suite 1401 Smith Tower,
Houston, TX 77030, USA
e-mail: jbismuth@tmhs.org

J.J. Hoballah, A.B. Lumsden (eds.), *Vascular Surgery*, New Techniques in Surgery Series,
DOI 10.1007/978-1-4471-2912-7_10, © Springer-Verlag London 2012

in the immediate postoperative period from minimally invasive endovascular interventions, while they have also confirmed the superiority of the open approach in terms of cost and durability over time [1, 2]. Laparoscopic and robotic aortic surgeries have the potential to provide surgeons with an option that diminishes short-term complications associated with open abdominal operations and at the same time maximizes long-term success by reducing surveillance requirements and re-intervention rates. Over the past 20 years, a number of vascular surgeons have demonstrated feasibility as well as good short- and midterm outcomes for laparoscopic and robotic aortic surgery. In this chapter, we will describe validated techniques, review outcomes, and examine the future of laparoscopy and robotics in aortic surgery.

Laparoscopic Aortic Surgery

Laparoscopy was introduced first into general surgery over 30 years ago and has been widely incorporated into surgical practice. Minimally invasive techniques have been shown to reduce postoperative cardiopulmonary complications, pain, and length of stay [3–5]. Vascular surgery has been slower to adopt laparoscopic techniques, as attention in the field has been focused on endovascular interventions and laparoscopy presents numerous technical challenges, particularly for surgeons who have not had advanced laparoscopic training. Despite important advances and widespread use of endovascular therapies, open repair of AAA and aortic occlusive disease remains superior with respect to decreased rates of re-intervention and diminished surveillance burden [6]. As such, options for laparoscopic and/or robotic approaches that capitalize on the known benefits of both minimally invasive surgery and open repair of the diseased aorta have continued to be explored. In 1993, Dion and colleagues described the first laparoscopic-assisted approach for management of aortoiliac disease [7]. Working alongside experienced laparoscopists, a minority of vascular surgeons have since developed a variety of approaches to minimally invasive aortic surgery.

Techniques

Laparoscopic surgery for aortoiliac occlusive disease and abdominal aortic aneurysms may be performed in a totally laparoscopic or hand-assisted fashion. The aorta is accessed by either a retroperitoneal or transperitoneal approach, and choice of approach is dictated by patient-specific factors (body habitus, previous abdominal operations), aneurysm-specific factors (relationship to renal arteries), and surgeon preference. Techniques for a transperitoneal approach that have been described include a retrocolic, prerenal approach; a retrocolic, retrorenal approach; and a direct transperitoneal approach [7–9]. The retrocolic, prerenal transperitoneal approach described by Coggia and colleagues is a modification of the technique originally performed by Dion for accessing the aorta and using peritoneum to retract bowel. It allows for access to the aorta by incising along the Toldt fascia lateral to the left colon. Dissection of the left mesocolon along the entire length of the descending colon and medially to the left renal vein allows for fixation of the mesocolon to the anterior abdominal wall, which forms an "apron" behind which bowel can be retracted for optimal exposure of the aorta (Fig. 10.1) [7, 9]. Coggia also described a transperitoneal retrorenal alternative to a purely retroperitoneal approach, which is useful in patients with juxtarenal lesions requiring suprarenal clamping or in patients who have undergone previous abdominal surgeries that would preclude straightforward dissection along the line of Toldt [8].

Hand-assisted laparoscopic surgery (HALS) is performed by making a 7–8-cm midline incision at the level of the presumed proximal anastomosis and introducing a specialized hand port that allows for maintenance of pneumoperitoneum. The surgeon's nondominant hand aids in retraction of bowel and provides tactile feedback during the dissection. The hand port may also be removed and the incision converted to a minilaparotomy, permitting the surgeon to hand sew the aortic anastomosis under direct vision [10]. In the laparoscopic-assisted approach, dissection is performed totally laparoscopically. Upon accessing the aorta, a minilaparotomy is performed, and in

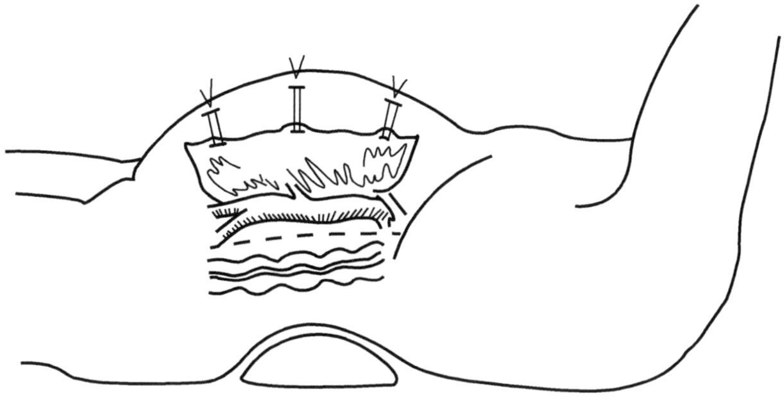

Fig. 10.1 Position of aorta and depiction of "apron" in laparoscopic exposure

a similar fashion to the HALS approach, the anastomosis is sewn within the incision [11].

Robotic Aortic Surgery

Surgical robotics was first utilized to facilitate neurosurgical biopsies in 1985 and has since found application in orthopedics, urologic, gynecologic, cardiothoracic, general, and vascular surgery [12]. Surgical assistance systems provide intelligent, versatile tools that augment the physician's ability to treat patients in a minimally invasive fashion, by eliminating hand tremor and enabling dexterous operation inside the patient's body. Surgical robotics systems have enabled surgeons to treat otherwise untreatable conditions, all while reducing morbidity and error rates, shortening operative times, reducing radiation exposure, and improving overall workflow [13]. These capabilities have begun to be realized in only a few centers in robot-assisted laparoscopic aortic surgery for occlusive and aneurysmal disease.

Robotic-Assisted Laparoscopic Surgery

Throughout surgical disciplines, the advantages of minimally invasive surgery have been demonstrated and have, in many cases, become the standard. However, the particular difficulty of performing vascular anastomoses has heretofore proved prohibitive for accomplishing timely and safe minimally invasive operations for patients requiring aortic repair. In 1995, Intuitive Surgical created the computer-enhanced robotic system known today as the da Vinci Surgical System. The goal of this device was to create familiar hand movements from open surgery while performing operations via a minimally invasive approach. In cardiovascular surgery, the advent of robotics made a minimally invasive approach to aortic surgery, a technically challenging procedure, more practicable. Key to the success of the robotic approach was the development of EndoWrist (Intuitive Surgical, Inc., Sunnyvale, CA) technology. EndoWrist attachments for da Vinci are modeled after the human wrist, which allows full range of motion, facilitates hand-eye coordination similar to the human brain, and provides dual-channel (3-dimensional) vision necessary for the more dexterous maneuvers required in creating vascular anastomoses [14].

Animal studies confirmed the benefits of the da Vinci Surgical System by showing that the time required to perform an anastomosis, clamp time, and total operative times were reduced [14–16]. We have had similar animal experience demonstrating both ease of dissection and anastomosis. Although we did not find the porcine model ideal, as far as the infrarenal aorta was concerned, it provides a good perspective on safe tissue handling, ideal placement of access ports, safe placement of aortic clamp, as well as accuracy and consistency of anastomosis configuration and timing. Wisselink and colleagues pioneered robotic-assisted surgical repair of aortic occlusive disease, publishing reports of the first two cases performed in humans and demonstrating feasibility of the operation [17]. They went on to publish promising results with respect to the steep learning curve of the operation in the initial series of 17 patients, demonstrating a 50 % reduction in clamp times for the later 9 patients as compared with the initial 8 [18]. Stadler and colleagues, the group with the largest experience with robot-assisted laparoscopic aortoiliac procedures, recently published results from a series of 150 patients. They reported a 97.3 % rate of successful completion, 2.7 % complication rate, and shortened anastomosis and clamp times (27 and 39 min, respectively) as compared to a purely laparoscopic approach [19]. Since this published series, Stadler's group has changed their combined laparoscopic dissection followed by robotic anastomosis to performing the entire procedure robotically, including the dissection. These results have not yet been compared to their original approach. Several groups in Europe have now demonstrated not only the feasibility of robot-assisted aortic reconstruction but also safety and shortened anastomosis times [17–19]. Our group has initiated an investigational device exemption (IDE) trial through which we aim to pave the way for the introduction of robotic vascular surgery in the USA. We have developed and participated in a training program that begins with work on inanimate models, thereafter advancing to pig models and ultimately cadavers. We have shown the effectiveness of this training insofar as having a great degree of preparedness for the cadaver labs, where we were able to perform aorto-bifemoral bypasses within 2 h. Inanimate and team training are probably the two elements that played the greatest role in the training paradigm. With the direct involvement and proctoring of Dr. Petr Stadler, we plan to perform robot-assisted repair of aortoiliac occlusive disease in humans in the USA later this year (2010).

Current Clinical Evidence

Laparoscopy

Reviewing the literature and developing a consensus on laparoscopic/robotic approaches to the aorta are a challenge due to not only a variety of approaches but also very small series. Taking the learning curve, as described by Wisselink, into consideration, we limited our evaluation of the literature to the series which included ≥20 cases. Outside of this, the criteria for inclusion comprised reporting of operative time, clamp time, length of stay, mortality, and conversion rates. For series reporting duplicate numbers for the same author, data from the more recent publication were retained. Outcomes for TLS, HALS, and lap-assisted surgery for the treatment of aortoiliac disease and abdominal aortic aneurysms are recorded in Tables 10.1 and 10.2, respectively. Operative times for TLS varied widely both within groups for aneurismal (180–600 for Edoga's group [30]) and occlusive (Di Centa et al. [26] 120–450) disease. In a meta-analysis of outcomes for aortoiliac disease, mean operative times for occlusive disease were 221 min for TLS and 197 min for HALS. Clamp times were also reduced in the HALS group (29 min) compared with the TLS group (70 min). Similarly, in patients with aneurysmal disease, the hand-assisted approach had reduced mean operative times (TLS = 275 min, HALS = 205 min) and clamp times (TLS = 99, HALS = 39). HALS also reduced the conversion rates for both aortoiliac and aneurismal disease from 8.9 % (AOID) and 12.6 % (AAA) for TLS to 4.4 % (AOID) and 2.2 % (AAA) for HALS. Hospital length of stay and mortality rates were similar between the two groups, in both occlusive and aneurysmal disease.

Robotic-Assisted Laparoscopic Surgery

Operative times for robotic-assisted surgery did not differ from those calculated for laparoscopic approaches (243 min). Clamp times (46 min) were more in line with those reported for HALS, suggesting that the improved dexterity of the robot allowed for the anastomosis to be sewn in a comparable time with conventional open techniques. The mortality, length of stay, and conversion rates were also comparable to those found in the laparoscopic group.

Table 10.1 Total laparoscopic and hand-assisted surgery for occlusive disease

Author	Patient no.	Operative time, min	Clamp time, min	Length of stay, day	Mortality, no. (%)	Conversion no. (%)
TLS						
Dion et al. [20]	51	290±62	99 ±28	5 (4–24)	1 (1.9 %)	5 (10 %)
Olinde et al. [21]	22	267 (198–365)	90±20	4 (2–7)	1 (4.5 %)	2 (9.1 %)
Lin et al. [22]	105	195 (125–250)	45 (25–115)	4 (3–22)	2 (1.9 %)	12 (11.4 %)
Rouers et al. [23]	30	244±11	85±32	5±3	0 (0 %)	6 (20 %)
Remy et al. [24]	21	240 (150–420)	60 (30–120)	7 (5–30)	0 (0 %)	1 (4.8 %)
Cau et al. [25]	72	216±50	57±21	8 (5–42)	0 (0 %)	2 (2.8 %)
Fourneau [36]	50	328 (205–490)	69 (20–173)	5 (3–29)	0 (0 %)	11 (22 %)
Di Centa et al. [26]	145	260 (120–450)	81 (36–190)	7 (2–57)	4 (2.7 %)	5 (3.4 %)
Totals	496	221	70	5.6	1.6 %	8.9 %
HALS						
Lin et al. [22]	87	165 (100–250)	25 (1–40)	6 (4–17)	3(3.4 %)	4 (2.1 %)
Wijtenburg [37]	25	180 (120–290)	37 (15–60)	7 (4–15)	1 (4 %)	2 (8 %)
Fourneau et al. [27]	46	208 (155–300)	28 (15–55)	6 (3–26)	2 (4.3 %)	1 (2.2 %)
Klem et al. [28]	33	281 (NR)	34.2 (NR)	8.83 (NR)	0 (0 %)	NR
Totals	191	197	29	7	3.14 %	4.4 %
Lap-assisted						
Alimi et al. [29]	58	238 (140–420)	54 (15–170)	8 (3–32)	2 (3.4 %)	1(1.7 %)

Table 10.2 Total laparoscopic and hand-assisted surgery for AAA

Author	Patient no.	Operative time, min	Clamp time, min	Length of stay, day	Mortality, no. (%)	Conversion no. (%)
TLS						
Edoga et al. [30]	22	391 (180–600)	146 (60–286)	6 (2–25)	2 (9.0 %)	2 (9.1 %)
Lin et al. [22]	131	265 (145–405)	95 (30=160)	5 (3–21)	4 (3 %)	23 (17.5 %)
Coggia et al. [31]	30	255 (170–410)	80 (35–110)	9 (5–37)	1 (3.3 %)	1 (3.3 %)
Cau [24]	23	251±57	101±15	6 (4–12)	1 (4.3 %)	0 (0 %)
Totals	206	275	99	5.8	3.9 %	12.6 %
51						
HALS						
Ferrari et al. [32]	271	228±66	26±6	4.2±1.9	0 (0 %)	0 (0 %)
Lin et al. [22]	215	175 (85–290)	55 (25–130)	7 (5–18)	4 (1.8 %)	11(5.1 %)
Totals	486	205	39	5.4	.8 %	2.2 %
Lap-assisted						
Kline et al. [11]	20	246±55	NR	6±2	0 (0 %)	2 (10 %)
Castronuovo et al. [33]	60	462 (90–690)	112 (43–286)	6 (1–25)	3 (5 %)	3 (5 %)
Alimi et al. [34]	24	238 (155–360)	76 (42–160)	7 (3–21)	1 (4.2 %)	4 (16.6 %)
Totals	104	368	101	6.2	(3.8 %)	(8.7 %)

Discussion

As we move toward more widespread utilization of minimally invasive techniques for aortic surgery, it is important to consider the relative advantages and drawbacks for conventional laparoscopy as compared to robotic surgery as techniques are adopted for either strict laparoscopy, pure robotic, or a combination approach to the aorta. Laparoscopy is a well-developed

Table 10.3 Robot-assisted laparoscopic aortic surgery

Author	Patient no.	Operative time, min	Clamp time, min	Length of stay, day	Mortality, no. (%)	Conversion no. (%)
Kolvenbach et al. [35]	10	242±42.5	95.9±21.6	7.5±6	NR	2 (20 %)
Diks [18]	17	370 (225–589)	82.7 (25–205)	5.6 (3–57)	1(5.88 %)	3 (17.6 %)
Stadler et al. [19]	150	228 (150–360)	39 (22–120)	5 (4–10)	0	4 (2.7 %)
Totals	177	243	46	5.2	N/A	(5.1 %)

technology with a proven track record for success. Its availability and affordability are also important considerations for its implementation in vascular surgery. However, this approach has failed to gain widespread acceptance, which is likely attributable to the technical challenges imposed by the laparoscopic approach (i.e., compromised dexterity, limited degrees of motion, amplification of physiologic tremors, and loss of 3-D visualization). Conversely, robotic surgery offers clear advantages from a technical standpoint, such as excellent maneuverability, dexterity, and elimination of physiologic tremors. The data from Stadler's group clearly demonstrate the importance of these technical advantages. Clamp times for robotic surgery were less than half as long as laparoscopic approaches, with comparable times to the HALS anastomosis performed in conventional open fashion within the "minilaparotomy" incision (Tables 10.1, 10.2, and 10.3). Nonetheless, the high initial and ongoing costs for equipment and staff training for a new technology with unproven benefit and known technical hurdles (loss of tactile feedback, poor haptic interface) may ultimately prove to create insurmountable barriers to the extensive utilization of robotic techniques. Furthermore, as this is, at least in the USA, not an approved procedure for the da Vinci robot, support is not given for training by Intuitive Surgical. This ultimately means that any procedures performed in the USA can only be performed under a research protocol approved by the Food and Drug Administration (FDA) and/or the local institutional review board (IRB). Beyond actually doing these procedures in a clinical setting, we firmly believe that adequate training is needed, and costs can be significant. We believe that a few pioneers and early adopters will push the techniques in the USA and pave the way for FDA approval and adoption by Intuitive Surgical and other device companies, paving the way for training and proctoring much like for robotic valve surgery. This is likely a few years away but can potentially open the door to other minimally invasive techniques to performing vascular surgery, by performing not only other intra-abdominal procedures but also performing hybrid operations (endovascular and surgical approaches).

Conclusion

Laparoscopic and robotic aortic surgery have the potential to provide surgeons with an option that maximizes the benefits of both endovascular and open vascular aortic reconstruction. Feasibility of the techniques has been well demonstrated, and outcomes in large prospective series show promising early and midterm results. The steep learning curve associated with the laparoscopic approach has hindered widespread acceptance, despite evidence showing that proficiency can be gained in 25–30 cases and patients do not suffer worse outcomes during the learning period [36]. Robotic technology is set to revolutionize cardiovascular surgery, and robotic surgery of the aorta is no exception. Some issues such as lack of haptics, tactile feedback, and interface in human-robotic interactions remain a significant safety concern and will add another safeguard when resolved. It remains to be seen whether or not the benefit of its usage overcomes its cost. To date, no prospective randomized trials evaluating efficacy and safety have been undertaken, and further research must evaluate cost-effectiveness or a true benefit over conventional therapy for minimally invasive surgery of the aorta to take full root.

References

1. The United Kingdom EVAR Trial Investigators. Endovascular versus open repair of abdominal aortic aneurysm. N Engl J Med. 2010;362:1863–71.
2. De Bruin JL, Baas AF, Buth J, Prinssen M, Verhoeven ELG, Cuypers PWM, van Sambeek MRHM, Balm R, Grobbee DE, Blankensteijn JD, for the DREAM Study Group. Long-term outcome of open of endovascular repair of abdominal aortic aneurysm. N Engl J Med. 2010;362:1881–9.
3. Schwenk W, Haase O, Neudecker J, Muller JM. Short term benefits for laparoscopic colorectal resection. Cochrane Database Syst Rev. 2005;20:CD003145.
4. Sauerland S, Jaschinski T, Neugebauer EA. Laparoscopic versus open surgery for suspected appendicitis. Cochrane Database Syst Rev. 2010;10: CD001546.
5. Bijen CB, Vermeulen KM, Mourits MJ, de Bock GH. Costs and effects of abdominal versus laparoscopic hysterectomy: systematic review of controlled trials. PLoS One. 2009;4:e7340.
6. Brewster DC, Cronenwett JL, Hallett JW, Johnston KW, Krupski WC, Matsumura JS. Guidelines for the treatment of abdominal aortic aneurysms. Report of a subcommittee of the Joint Council of the American Association for Vascular Surgery and Society for Vascular Surgery. J Vasc Surg. 2003;37:1106–17.
7. Dion YM, Katkhouda N, Rouleau C, Aucoin A. Laparoscopy-assisted aortobifemoral bypass. Surg Laparosc Endosc. 1993;3:425–9.
8. Barbera L, Mumme A, Metin S, Zumtobel V, Kemen M. Operative results and outcome of twenty-four totally laparoscopic vascular procedures for aortoiliac occlusive disease. J Vasc Surg. 1998;28:136–42.
9. Coggia M, Bourriez A, Javerliat I, Goeau-Brissonnière O. Totally laparoscopic aortobifemoral bypass: a new and simplified approach. Eur J Vasc Endovasc Surg. 2002;24:274–5.
10. Kolvenbach R, Da Silva L, Deling O, Schwierz E. Video-assisted aortic surgery. J Am Coll Surg. 2000; 190:451–7.
11. Kline RG, D'Angelo AJ, Chen MHM, Halpern VJ, Cohen JR. Laparoscopically assisted abdominal aortic aneurysm repair: first 20 cases. J Vasc Surg. 1998; 27:81–8.
12. Kwoh YS, Hou J, Jonckheere EA, Hayati S. A robot with improved absolute positioning accuracy for CT guided stereotactic brain surgery. IEEE Trans Biomed Eng. 1988;35(2):153–60.
13. Zorn KC, Gautam G, Shalhav AL, Clayman RV, Ahlering TE, Albala DM, et al. Training, credentialing, proctoring and medicolegal risks of robotic urological surgery: recommendations of the society of urologic robotic surgeons. J Urol. 2009;182(3):1126–32.
14. Riga CV, Cheshire NJW, Hamady M, Bicknell CD. Robotic endovascular catheters improve accuracy, reduce time and minimize radiation exposure in complex vascular procedures. Br J Surg. 2009;96(S1):7.
15. Riga CV, Bicknell CD, Cheshire NJW, Hamady M. Robotic endovascular catheters improve accuracy, reduce time and minimize radiation exposure for visceral vessel and fenestrated stent cannulation. Cardiovasc Intervent Radiol. 2009;32:S1–27.
16. Malhotra SP, Le D, Thelitz S, Hanley FL, Riemer RK, Suleman S, Reddy VM. Robotic-assisted endoscopic thoracic aortic anastomosis in juvenile lambs. Heart Surg Forum. 2002;6(1):38–42.
17. Wisselink W, Cuesta MA, Gracia C, Rauwerda JA. Robot-assisted laparoscopic aortobifemoral bypass for aortoiliac occlusive disease: a report of two cases. J Vasc Surg. 2002;36(5):1079–82.
18. Diks J, Nio D, Jongkind V, Cuesta MA, Rauwerda JA, Wisselink W. Robot-assisted laparoscopic surgery of the infrarenal aorta: the early learning curve. Surg Endosc. 2007;21(10):1760–3.
19. Stadler P, Dvoracek L, Vitasek P, Matous P. Robotic vascular surgery, 150 cases. Int J Med Robot. 2010;6: 394–8.
20. Dion YM, Griselli F, Douville Y, Langis P. Early and mid-term results of totally laparoscopic surgery for aortoiliac disease: lessons learned. Surg Laparosc Endosc Percutan Tech. 2004;14:328–34.
21. Olinde AJ, McNeil JW, Sam A, Hebert SA, Frusha JD. Totally laparoscopic aortobifemoral bypass: a review of 22 cases. J Vasc Surg. 2005;42:27–34.
22. Lin JC, Kolvenbach R, Schwierz E, Wassiljew S. Total laparoscopic aortofemoral bypass as a routine precedure for the treatment of aortoiliac occlusive disease. Vascular. 2005;13:80–3.
23. Rouers A, Meurisse N, Lavigne JP, Francart D, Quaniers J, Desiron Q, et al. Potential benefits of laparoscopic aorto-bifemoral bypass surgery. Acta Chir Belg. 2005;105:610–5.
24. Remy P, Deprez AF, D'hont CH, Lavigne JP, Massin H. Total laparoscopic aortobifemoral bypass. Eur J Vasc Endovasc Surg. 2005;29:22–7.
25. Cau J, Ricco JB, Marchand C, Lecis A, Habibeh H, Guillou M. Total laparoscopic aortic repair for occlusive and aneurysmal disease: first 95 cases. Eur J Vasc Endovasc Surg. 2006;31:567–74.
26. Di Centa I, Coffia M, Cerceau P, Javerliat I, Alfonsi P, Beauchet A, Goeau-Brissonnière O. Total laparoscopic aortobifemoral bypass: short- and middle term results. Ann Vasc Surg. 2008;22:227–32.
27. Fourneau I, Sabbe T, Daenens K, Nevelsteen A. Hand-assisted laparoscopy versus conventional median laparotomy for aortobifemoral bypass for severe aorto-iliac occlusive disease: a prospective randomised study. Eur J Vasc Endovasc Surg. 2006;32: 645–50.
28. Klem TM, van der Ham AC, de Smet AA, Hok Oei I, Wittens CH. Hand assisted laparoscopic surgery of aortoiliac occlusive disease: initial results. Eur J Vasc Endovasc Surg. 2006;32:639–44.
29. Alimi YS, De Cardi G, Hartung O, Bartheleby P, Aissi K, Otero A. Laparoscopy-assisted reconstruction to treat severe aortoiliac occlusive disease: early and midterm results. J Vasc Surg. 2004;39:777–83.

30. Edoga JK, Asgarian K, Singh D, James KV, Romanelli J, Merchant S. Laparoscopic surgery for abdominal aortic aneurysms. Technical elements of the procedure and a prelimanary report of the first 22 patients. Surg Endosc. 1998;12:1064–972.
31. Coggia M, Javerliat I, Di Centa I, Alfonsi P, Colacchio G, Ketzis M. Total laparoscopic versus conventional abdominal aortic aneurysm repair: a case-control study. J Vasc Surg. 2005;42:906–10.
32. Ferrari M, Adami D, Del Corso A, Berchiolli R, Pietrabissa A, Romagnanai F. Laparoscopy-assisted abdominal aortic aneurysm repair; early and middle-term results of a consecutive series of 122 cases. J Vasc Surg. 2006;43:695–700.
33. Castronuovo JJ, Resnikoff M, McLean ER, Edoga JK. Laparoscopic-assisted abdominal aortic aneurysmectomy. J Vasc Surg. 2000;32:224–33.
34. Alimi YS, De Molfetta L, Hartung O, Dhanis AF, Barthelemy P, Aissi K. Laparoscopy-assisted abdominal aneurysm endoaneurysmorraphy; early and mid-term results. J Vasc Surg. 2003;37:44–9.
35. Kolvenbach R, Schwierz E, Wasilljew S, Miloud A, Puerschel A, Pinter L. Total laparoscopically and robotically assisted aortic aneurysm surgery: a critical evaluation. J Vasc Surg. 2004;39:771–6.
36. Fourneau I, Lerut P, Sabbe T, Houthoofd S, Daenens K, Nevelsteen A. The learning curve of totally laparoscopic aortobifemoral bypass for occlusive disease. How many cases and how safe? Eur J Vasc Endovasc Surg, 2008;35(6):723–9. Epub 2008 Mar 4.
37. Wijtenburg E, Remy P, D'hont Ch, Vindevogel Ch, Blampain JP, Massin H. Hand-assisted laparoscopic aortoiliac surgery: preliminary report of 25 cases. Acta Chir Belg. 2003;103(5):493–6.

Popliteal Artery Aneurysm: Endovascular Surgery

11

Munier Nazzal and Viviane Kazan

Abstract

Popliteal artery aneurysms are the most common peripheral aneurysms. This chapter was written to provide the reader with background information regarding the popliteal artery aneurysm and its anatomy. A literature review is provided summarizing studies that have been done comparing endovascular treatment to open surgical repair. Endovascular treatment is discussed in-depth including stent types, progression of technology, advantages and disadvantages of stents, in addition to providing information in choosing patients for procedures. Empirical evidence for endovascular treatment is provided as well as information regarding the technique utilized by the author and colleagues.

Keywords

Popliteal artery aneurysm • Endovascular treatment • Stent grafts • Open surgery • Technique

Introduction

The popliteal artery's normal diameter ranges anywhere from 5 to 9 mm [1]. Studies have shown that differences exist in the arterial diameter between men and women. The mean popliteal artery diameter in women is 6.0±0.7 mm and 6.8±0.8 mm in men [2]. Galen (A.D. 131–200) was the first to define an aneurysm as "a localized pulsatile swelling which disappeared on pressure" [3]. A popliteal artery diameter that is greater than 15 mm is currently defined as aneurysmal [4]. A multicenter study conducted by Varga et al. [5] which included 200 popliteal arteries revealed a mean diameter of 2 cm for asymptomatic aneurysms and a mean of 3 cm for those presenting with limb-threatening ischemia. The popliteal artery aneurysm (PAA) is reported to be the most common peripheral aneurysm and comprises 70 % of all peripheral aneurysms [6–9] with a reported incidence rate ranging from 0.1 to 2.8 % [8]. Overall, the incidence increases from less than 0.1 % for the general population to 1 % for

M. Nazzal, M.D., FRCS, FACS (✉) • V. Kazan, M.D.
Division of Vascular and Endovascular Surgery,
Department of Surgery,
University of Toledo Medical Center,
3000 Arlington Avenue, Toledo, OH 43614, USA
e-mail: munier.nazzal@utoledo.edu,
munier.nazzal@yahoo.com

J.J. Hoballah, A.B. Lumsden (eds.), *Vascular Surgery*, New Techniques in Surgery Series,
DOI 10.1007/978-1-4471-2912-7_11, © Springer-Verlag London 2012

the age range of 65–80 years of age [10]. PAAs are associated with other arterial aneurysms and are bilateral in more than half of the cases [5, 11, 12] with an estimated 33–64 % experiencing an abdominal aortic aneurysm at the same time [12, 13]. PAAs also affect men significantly more than women. The majority of PAAs, 95–99 %, occur in men and are associated with other comorbidities such as ischemic cardiovascular disease, hypertension, diabetes, and smoking [5, 12, 14, 15].

Anatomy and Etiology

The popliteal artery can be divided into three sections labeled P1 to P3. Segment P1 is positioned between the adductor muscle hiatus to the superior edge of the patella. It then continues as segment P2 until it reaches the division of the knee articulation and becomes segment P3 extending to the origin of the crural arteries. The point at which the knee bends is positioned between segments P1 and P2 [1]. The distal part of the popliteal artery has been shown through radiological studies to be somewhat fixed at two points, near the origin of the anterior tibial artery and again near the origin of the descending genicular artery [16–18]. Flexion of the knee causes the popliteal artery to move dorsally between these two points and create flexures behind the knee [16, 17]. Previously, atherosclerosis was blamed as the underlying cause of aneurysm development, but views on this matter have evolved. Presently, knee flexion is believed to contribute to the development of popliteal artery aneurysms by causing the supra-articular popliteal artery to become more tortuous, while at the same time, the middle and lower segments of the artery remain fixed, curved, and retracted behind the knee joint [19, 20]. Repeated knee flexion and turbulent blood flow at arterial branches, in addition to wall fatigue, are all believed to contribute to aneurysm formation [7, 21]. Such mechanical forces exerted on the popliteal artery must be taken into consideration when dealing with intervention options. Stents placed in close proximity to the knee might be exposed to deformation and fracture casting doubt on the durability of such stents.

Other factors thought to play a role in popliteal aneurysm formation involve genetic predisposition, fragmented proteins, and immunological causes [12]. Jacob et al. [22] discovered breaks in the elastic lamellae as well as histological evidence of active proteolysis. Molecules usually associated with apoptosis were measured and found to be increased. CPP-32, Fas, and Bax levels were all increased in the vascular smooth muscle cells. As the inflammatory process proceeds and mediators are released, medial degradation and weakness of the vessel wall eventually will lead to dilatation [12] and lengthening of the artery [20]. Studies have shown this tortuosity to be more present in the elderly and persisting even upon knee extension [17].

The popliteal artery appears to become more convoluted with age as studies show low-grade tortuosity near the adductor hiatus while the knee is flexed in patients younger than 30 years old and becoming more extensive as it moves distal to the adductor hiatus to the popliteal fossa in those older than 45 years of age [17, 23].

Popliteal Artery Aneurysms

Popliteal artery aneurysm is a clinically important condition and warrants serious treatment consideration upon its discovery. It was described as a "sinister harbinger of sudden catastrophe" in 1953 [24, 25] with the "sudden catastrophe" referring to the possibility of thrombosis, embolization, rupture, and eventually an acutely ischemic limb with potential limb loss [3, 8]. Patients can present with compression of the tibial nerve [7, 21], causing neuropathy or compression of the popliteal vein resulting in limb edema, pain, or even deep venous thrombosis (DVT) [7]. Compressive symptoms usually have a vague onset, progress in severity, and are common in patients with previously diagnosed peripheral vascular occlusive disease. Symptoms of acute limb ischemia include "blue toe syndrome" that results from the repetitive embolization to the distal arteries. Blue toe syndrome is experienced by 4–12 % of patients with PAA [26, 27]. Patients that present with acute limb ischemia from thrombosis or embolism tend to have poorer outcomes due to runoff vessel occlusion resulting in an amputation rate of 15–30 % [8, 21]. Acute limb ischemia resulting from thrombosis or embolism comprises approximately 40 % of PAA diagnoses [8].

History of Treatment

Popliteal artery aneurysms were first documented over 4,000 years ago. The characteristics and treatment of PAAs were first described in 2000 B.C. in the Ebers Papyrus [28]. Treatment for popliteal artery aneurysms mainly consisted of inducing thrombosis until the twentieth century. Many different contraptions were created to flex the patient's leg for days until thrombosis was induced [3]. A Greek physician in the second century A.D., Antyllus, was the first to document and perform surgery by proximal and distal artery ligation and then evacuation of the aneurysm. Antyllus was known to have performed such surgeries on a variety of aneurysms caused by spear injuries; however, the specific vessels are not specified. (Was this for a popliteal aneurysm?) [29] John Hunter performed a proximal ligation in December 1785 for a PAA, and in 1888, Rudolph Matas, from New Orleans, executed a proximal and distal ligation of a brachial artery aneurysm. He then unsuccessfully attempted to remove the aneurysmal sac and eventually excluded it by suturing in layers from inside out. His procedure was aptly named an obliterative endoaneurysmorrhaphy. He later described two variants of this surgery named restorative and reconstructive endoaneurysmorrhaphy where clots were removed and the blood flow through the sac was closed off from the native artery or the blood flow was maintained by placing a stent over which the arteries were sewn in the proximal and distal communicating arteries, respectfully. The stent was then removed before the anastomosis was completed [3]. In 1969, PAA repair performed by Edwards utilized the saphenous vein as a bypass graft after arterial exclusion [30] paving the way for present-day treatment modalities.

Endovascular Versus Open Surgery

Open surgery continues to be the gold standard of treatment of PAA with secondary patency of 70 % and limb salvage rates greater than 85 % over a 5-year period [8]. Open surgical repair has been performed far longer than endovascular treatment with a large supporting body of evidence. Many different approaches and surgical techniques are employed in the treatment of PAA depending on the surgeons' preferences [31–33]. Surgical treatment of PAA does have drawbacks such as wound infection, graft thrombosis, longer operative and recovery times, large scars, and the utilization of the saphenous vein (thereby limiting graft options for cardiac bypass surgery).

Interest in endovascular treatment has grown significantly. Although there are a limited number of prospective trials which examine endovascular stent graft placement [34–39], a plethora of retrospective trials have been published [8, 40] as well as meta-analyses of the small cohort studies [12, 21, 41–43]. Some studies reported acceptable patency rates for endovascular stent graft placement [8, 12, 34–37, 39, 40, 44], while others found patency rates as good as [2, 19, 38, 41, 43] or inferior [7] to the gold standard of open surgery. Lovegrove et al. [41] performed a meta-analysis of studies comparing endovascular surgery with open surgery and found that overall the midterm results were comparable with open repair, but early graft thrombosis and reintervention rates were significantly higher for endovascular repair in comparison to open surgery. The meta-analysis showed that midterm patency rates for open surgery were 1.70 times greater than for endovascular surgery. Henke [7] reviewed multiple studies and reported a cumulative 5-year patency rate ranging from 47 to 74 % for endovascular stent grafts. Other researchers followed stent graft patients for approximately 36 months and reported initial primary patency rates of 92.9 % which gradually decreased to 74.5 % at the end of follow-up period. Nevertheless, these rates were considered to be comparable to open surgery [38]. A randomized prospective trial conducted in Italy directly compared 15 open procedure patients with 15 patients treated endovascularly

[19]. The follow-up period for open procedure patients was 46.1 months and 45.9 months in the endovascular group. At 12 months, the primary patency rate for the open procedure was 100 and 86.7 % for the endovascular procedure. The results between the two groups were comparable. The majority of studies comparing open and endovascular techniques for PAA repair involved small subject numbers, were mostly single-center studies, and had short follow-up periods. Larger, randomized, prospective studies need to be performed in order to concretely settle the dispute between these two treatment modalities.

Radiologic Evaluation

Planning for endovascular aneurysm repair starts at the time of diagnosis. Duplex scan of the popliteal artery is usually the initial diagnostic modality. It can be used to establish the size of the aneurysm, the adjacent arterial segment status, contents of the aneurysm, and calcification in the wall of the aneurysm (Fig. 11.1). Further evaluation may include CT scan of the popliteal arteries (Fig. 11.2), magnetic resonance angiography (MRA), and angiographic evaluation by digital subtraction. Both CT scans and digital subtraction angiography might be misleading in the presence of intraluminal thrombus leading to underestimation of the diameter of the arterial segments adjacent to the aneurysm. Reconstituted 3-D CT images might be of great help to define the extent of the aneurysmal disease in the adjacent arteries (Fig. 11.3).

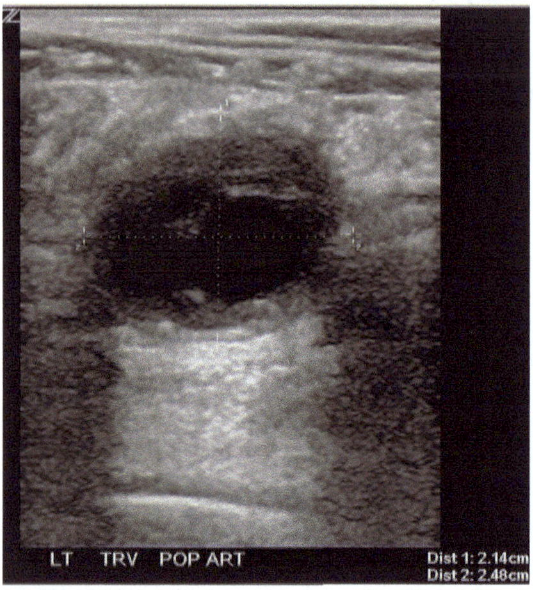

Fig. 11.1 Ultrasound showing PAA with thrombi within lumen

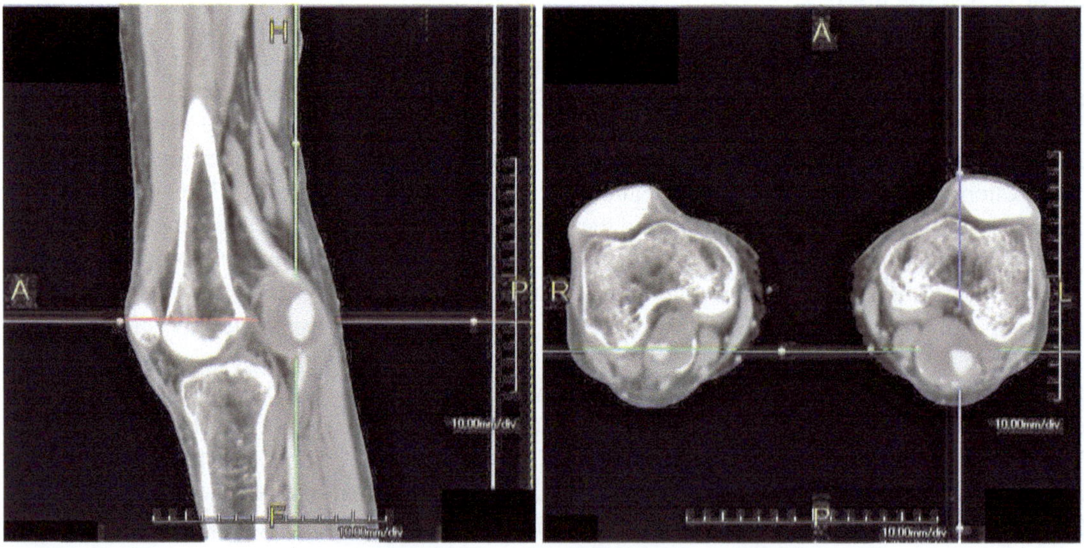

Fig. 11.2 Popliteal aneurysm, both saggital and transverse sections

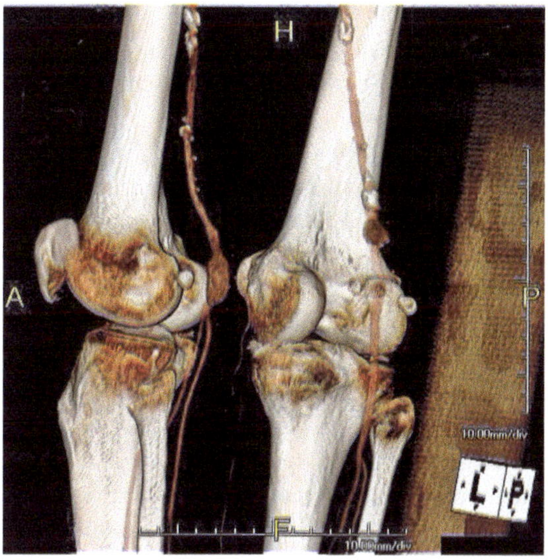

Fig. 11.3 3-D CT scan of popliteal artery segments

Endovascular Surgery

Stent Graft Types

The standard treatment of popliteal artery aneurysm continues to be open popliteal endoaneurysmorrhaphy with proximal and distal ligation of the aneurysm followed by bypass grafting or the use of interposition grafting [45]. More recently, however, there has been increasing interest in endovascular repair of PAAs with stent graft placement. In 1994, the first reported endovascular treatment of a popliteal aneurysm was performed by Marin et al. using a combination of Palmaz stents with a polytetrafluoroethylene graft establishing the feasibility of an endovascular approach [46]. The patient, a 63-year-old man with "advanced heart disease," was followed for 3 months with duplex ultrasound. During the follow-up period, the graft remained patent with no indication of any distal emboli. Since that time, interest in endovascular surgery has increased with the realization that an alternative treatment to open surgical bypass does exist [12]. Different types of stent grafts have been used in endovascular surgery, such as the Passager stent (Boston Scientific, Waterdown, MA, USA) or the AneuRx stent (Medtronic, Inc., Minneapolis, MN, USA) described by Mohan et al. [38]; however, the researchers noted the stiffness of these stent grafts made them less suitable for use in the popliteal artery. More recently, flexible stent designs have become more popular such as the Hemobahn and Viabahn stent grafts (W.L. Gore and Associates, Inc., Flagstaff, AZ, USA). These stents offer radial stiffness while at the same time maintaining flexibility [1]. The stents are self-expanding nitinol stents with an internal covering of ePTFE. The Hemobahn stent graft differs from the Viabahn stent graft in that it unfolds from a rolled position, while the Viabahn, an updated version of the Hemobahn stent graft [1], is packed with many concentric folds [38]. The rolled configuration of the Hemobahn stent graft poses a potential problem if the stent does not open fully in the artery and may go undetected by balloon dilatation [38]. The Gore Viabahn graft (W.L. Gore & Associates, Flagstaff, AZ) is now available with heparin covalently bound to the inner graft surface (Propaten Bioactive Surface Technology) [39]. The newer Viabahn stent grafts are available in a longer version (25 cm) and a smaller profile.

Advantages and Disadvantages of Endovascular Repair

As is the case with any medical procedure, endovascular stent graft placement has several potential advantages and disadvantages. Endovascular procedures take less time to perform, with less morbidity compared to an open approach. Endovascular repair may be a better option for those patients that are considered to be high surgical risk [26]. The surgery can be done without general anesthesia, through a small incision resulting in less blood loss, quicker recovery, and less potential for complications [12, 21]. Furthermore, the endovascular approach spares the saphenous vein or other autologous veins for cardiac or other bypass surgeries the patient may need in the future [12]. On the other hand, the procedure is not without disadvantages. One major concern associated with stent graft placement is early, midterm, and long-term patency. Some groups reported patency rates that were comparable with open surgery [1, 34, 37, 43]. In contrast, other groups suggested lower patency rates following stent graft placement [12, 35, 41]. The only cohort prospective study of endovascular grafts was performed by Tielliu and colleagues [35] in which 57 aneurysms were treated with Hemobahn and Viabahn stent grafts and were followed up for 24 months. Primary and secondary patency rates were 80 and 90 % at 1 year and 77 and 87 % at 2 years. It has been suggested that thrombosis occurs due to the repetitive stress on the device from constant bending [35, 47] as well as the development of kinks and stent fractures in the overlap zones when more than one stents were used [8, 35, 48]. Stent fractures were found to be more prevalent in younger patients but did not seem to affect patency in a significant way [48]. Other disadvantages include stent graft migration, component disconnection when several stent grafts were used, continued endoleak, and infection of the incision site [12]. Despite the aforementioned disadvantages of stent placement, better candidate selection for endovascular treatment could help to decrease complications and improve long-term patency rates.

Patient Selection

The anatomy of the popliteal artery and the aneurysmal segment help in the determination of whether endovascular surgery would be of benefit to the patient versus the traditional open surgery [12, 45]. The feasibility of endovascular repair is dependent upon a number of factors such as length of landing zones, distal runoff vessels, and angulations in addition to the presence of endovascular capabilities to safely do the procedure.

Current criteria include a symptomatic PAA or asymptomatic aneurysm greater than 2 cm in size, at least two patent runoff vessels, and appropriate proximal and distal landing zones for stent placement [12]. Midy et al. [8] recommend the proximal artery diameter to measure less than 12 mm with a distal neck of more than 5 mm in diameter and an aneurysmal sac with low-grade thrombosis. Others suggest a 3 cm length of proximal and distal landing zones in order to minimize the possibilities of endoleak and stent migration [35]. Success of endovascular PAA repair also involves proper treatment postoperatively with dual antiplatelet therapy [8]. Exclusion criteria for endovascular repair include a tortuous PAA [8], aneurysmal disease distal to the anterior tibial artery [12], and presentation with acute limb ischemia [42].

Deciding When to Treat

Gray areas still exist not only in the type of repair a patient must undergo but whether or not to even treat an aneurysm. Most agree that asymptomatic aneurysms require treatment once their diameter reaches 2 cm or if a significant mural thrombus is present as it could lead to acute limb ischemia with a high rate of limb loss (up to 20 %) [49, 50], increased mortality, and overall inferior results [14, 20, 26, 51–53]. Others suggest treatment in aneurysms with diameters ranging from 1.8 to 2 cm [26]. Etazadi et al. [40] recommended treatment with prophylactic anticoagulant therapy in those with asymptomatic aneurysms and no intervention. Lowell and colleagues [53] found that 18 % of their patients eventually became symptomatic when treated conservatively and found an association between aneurysmal size greater than 2 cm, mural thrombus, and poor distal runoff [20, 53]. (The researchers did not specify what conservative treatment entailed other than stating these patients were not surgically treated initially).

In a review to determine the applicability of endovascular repair of PAA, Zimmerman et al. [2] found that 59.4 % of all surgically repaired popliteal aneurysms were eligible for endovascular approach; in addition, 5.4 % of the cases were potentially eligible. In their study, they included all cases that had sufficient radiological images to determine eligibility. Criteria used to determine eligibility included sufficient proximal and distal landing zones of at least 2 cm, patency of the femoral vessels, and patency of at least one of the crural arteries. Choosing a 1–1.5-cm landing zone proximally and distally has been described by other authors.

This is expected to increase eligibility of endovascular approach in patients with PAA [2].

Durability of endovascular therapy for PAA is yet to be determined in long-term follow-up studies. Forces exerted on the femoropopliteal segments might compromise the long-term results. Repetitive stress forces of torsion, elongation, flexion-extension, and compression at the knee joint have been reported as a cause of stent fracture in the femoropopliteal segment. Although these reports were pertaining to occlusive disease with bare stents, similar effects are likely in covered stents used for PAA exclusion [54] as well.

Endovascular Popliteal Aneurysm Technique

In our patients, we use the Viabahn device which became available in 2003. It is made of a nitinol stent with ultrathin PTFE graft. The nitinol stent part is reported to improve resistance of the Viabahn device to fracture, but this is yet to be proven in long-term studies. The Viabahn device is available in many sizes (5–13 mm diameter) and lengths (25, 50, 100, 150, 250 mm) and can be deployed on a 0.035-in. wire. It deploys from tip to hub like many other nitinol stents. The deployment method is simple and consists of unsheathing the device by pulling on a string attached to the side of the delivery system once the device has been placed in the arterial segment to be excluded. Accuracy of deployment is crucial to proper exclusion of the PAA. With proper technique, it is unlikely to have significant displacement, or jumping of the graft. Other endoprostheses have been used in the endovascular treatment of PAA such as homemade covered stents, covered stents designed for abdominal aortic aneurysm, and an older version of the Viabahn with similar design called Hemobahn endoprosthesis. All such stent grafts are made of ePTFE with a nitinol skeleton. Other stents used include the Wallgraft (Boston Scientific/Meditech, Newton, MA), the Fluency stent graft (Bard Peripheral Vascular, Inc., Tempe, AZ), and a new endovascular stent made of polyester externally supported by separate nitinol rings (Anaconda limbs) (Vascutek, Renfrewshire, Scotland) [36, 37, 55]. In spite of claims of superiority, none of these endoprostheses were tested against other brands to prove such claims.

All procedures are done in the operating room in case a combined procedure will be needed. In addition, because of the large sheath size, we prefer to have an open access to a proximal artery in the ipsilateral leg. In patients with PAA, the ipsilateral superficial femoral artery is usually large in size and is thus chosen as the access site. Percutaneous access to the SFA or common femoral artery can be used in an antegrade fashion. In such case, closure of the access site should be the goal to avoid manual compression on the access site which theoretically carries the risk of thrombosis of the implanted graft. Procedures are done using local anesthesia and sedation with the patient in supine position. In open access cases, an 8-F sheath is inserted followed by an angiogram of the ipsilateral leg to evaluate the anatomy around the aneurysm. An adherent radiopaque measuring tape is placed on the leg to help plan the procedure for the diameter evaluation and for stent length.

In case of percutaneous access, all steps of planning and anatomical evaluation are done using a 5-F sheath. Once a decision is taken to proceed with the endovascular repair, the 5-F sheath is exchanged for an 8-F sheath. Part of the surgical evaluation should include the presence of large branches that might cause ischemia of the leg if covered or might continue to feed the excluded sac of the PAA. In the former situation, the endovascular procedure might not be a good option for the patient who should be treated by an open surgical approach, while in the latter situation, coil embolization of large branches should be considered before stent deployment.

For accurate evaluation of the surgical site, an intravascular ultrasound (IVUS) is used to evaluate the adjacent arterial segments. This is necessary to decide on the proper stent graft diameter and length. The IVUS will provide direct and accurate measurements of landing zone diameters, presence of thrombi, and calcification in the wall of the artery that might interfere with stent deployment. Accurate mapping of the sizes of the arterial segments at the fluoroscopic monitor screen should be done with an erasable marker. The anticipated areas of landing should be marked on the screen. This mapping step should be performed over a stiff wire to avoid any change in configuration when the stent delivery system is inserted, to eliminate redundancy in the wire for proper planning and stent delivery, and to avoid "wire jumping" when moving objects over the wire, thereby improving trackability over the wire. The distal end of the stiff wire should be parked in one of the tibial arties with the other end marked on the table to avoid migration of the wire tip distally and potentially injuring the hosting artery. We prefer a long wire (260 cm) to allow safe exchange of the devices with long delivery systems or shafts.

The next step will be to evaluate the length of the stent to be used. A catheter with markers is placed intra-arterially at the surgical site over the stiff wire. The length of the segment to be stented is determined, while both the catheter and stiff wire are in place. If a longer stent than the available stents is required, a decision should be made on the number of stents to be used, taking into consideration the requirement of a minimal 2-cm (Fig. 11.4) overlap between the stents. The most distal stent is deployed first to be followed by the more proximal stents. Once deployed, the position of the stent ends in relationship to the marked screen should be noted. A balloon of suitable size is inflated at the landing zone-stent transition areas and overlap areas. A completion angiogram is performed to evaluate for any leak around the endoprosthesis (type II) or into the sac from the transition zones (type I). One should note any folding of the endoprosthesis based on the radiological images and the completion IVUS. In case of an endoleak (type I), a noncompliant balloon, sized for the landing zone diameter, is inflated to correct the problem. In case it fails, stents should be extended to healthier zones.

A successful endovascular procedure should exclude the PAA sac, maintain blood flow to the crural arteries, and avoid any folding of the prosthesis.

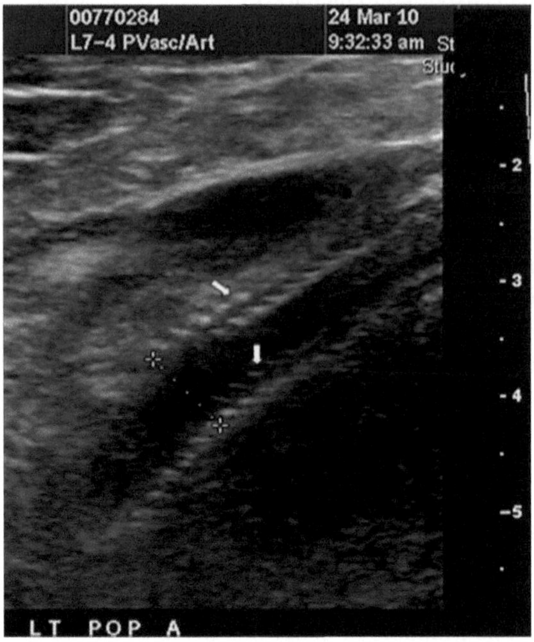

Fig. 11.4 Overlapping stents (*arrows*) in a popliteal artery aneurysm

The procedure should be done under full anticoagulation. All patients should be started on clopidogrel at least 48 h before the procedure. In those patients who were not taking clopidogrel, a loading dose of 300 mg should be given at the time of the procedure. Clopidogrel is continued for a minimum period of 3 months. After that, the patient should continue on lifelong aspirin. Dual antiplatelet therapy with aspirin and clopidogrel is given to patients with significant arterial disease or if the cardiac condition warrants that.

Both oversizing and undersizing of the Viabahn graft is likely to cause suboptimal results. With oversizing, infolding of the graft will occur causing both endoleak and an occlusive effect within the arterial segment. This can be partially corrected by balloon angioplasty or by deploying another stent graft to cover the transition zone from the stent graft to the adjacent arterial segment. However, selection of the proper stent graft size is the best assurance of avoiding such a problem.

Undersizing might result in a "floating" stent graft within the arterial segment causing incomplete exclusion of the PAA. This can be resolved by adding another Viabahn stent graft of larger size with at least 2-cm overlap with the first one.

We usually choose a stent graft diameter of approximately 10 % (approximately 1 mm) larger than the diameter of the landing zone. In the event of a discrepancy between both distal and proximal landing zones, two stent devices are used with at least 2-cm overlap between the stents. The most distal stent graft is deployed first followed by the proximal one.

Follow-Up

After endovascular repair, all patients should be followed up by looking for endovascular leak, stent fracture, and stenosis within and around the graft. This is achieved by duplex ultrasound, CT scan, and plain X-ray films. Follow-up should be done at 1, 3, 6, and 12 months and yearly after the procedure.

Conclusion

Popliteal artery aneurysms have been documented for centuries. Until the last two decades, the only surgical option for treatment involved open surgery. Even though open surgery remains the gold standard for therapy, the development of endovascular techniques has opened a new and exciting chapter in vascular surgery. It offers an alternative to those who are medically unable or unwilling to undergo the traditional open procedure. However, many unanswered questions remain, and more studies need to be done. Larger, prospective cohort studies need to evaluate these two procedures side by side for a longer period of follow-up. With more time and experience, newer stents can be produced. Researchers have already indicated the need for more flexible stents which are able to flex from within the vessel [12] without kinking or fracturing. Newer stents need also to address the size discrepancy between the proximal and distal landing zones perhaps by producing a tapered stent graft [40]. Newer stents such as the Fluency Plus stent graft are addressing some of the downfalls of the current stents being used such as improving the stent trackability to the target lesion site [1].

References

1. Ying H, Gloviczki P. Popliteal artery aneurysms: rationale, technique, and results of endovascular treatment. Perspect Vasc Surg Endovasc Ther. 2008;20(2):201–13.
2. Zimmermann A, Schoenberger T, Saeckl J, et al. Eligibility for endovascular technique and results of the surgical approach to popliteal artery aneurysms at a single center. Ann Vasc Surg. 2010;24(3):342–8.
3. Galland RB. History of the management of popliteal artery aneurysms. Eur J Vasc Endovasc Surg. 2008;35(4):466–72.
4. Belkin M, Rits Y, Erben Y, Ricotta JJ. Commentary on "endovascular repair of a ruptured popliteal artery". Perspect Vasc Surg Endovasc Ther. 2009;21(3):195.
5. Varga ZA, Locke-Edmunds JC, Baird RN. A multicenter study of popliteal aneurysms. Joint Vascular Research Group. J Vasc Surg. 1994;20(2):171–7.
6. Dawson I, Sie RB, van Bockel JH. Atherosclerotic popliteal aneurysm. Br J Surg. 1997;84(3):293–9.
7. Henke PK. Popliteal artery aneurysms: tried, true, and new approaches to therapy. Semin Vasc Surg. 2005;18(4):224–30.
8. Midy D, Berard X, Ferdani M, et al. A retrospective multicenter study of endovascular treatment of popliteal artery aneurysm. J Vasc Surg. 2010;51(4):850–6.
9. Moore RD, Hill AB. Open versus endovascular repair of popliteal artery aneurysms. J Vasc Surg. 2010;51(1):271–6.
10. Trickett JP, Scott RA, Tilney HS. Screening and management of asymptomatic popliteal aneurysms. J Med Screen. 2002;9(2):92–3.
11. Thompson MM, Bell PR. ABC of arterial and venous disease. Arterial aneurysms. BMJ. 2000;320(7243):1193–6.
12. Siauw R, Koh EH, Walker SR. Endovascular repair of popliteal artery aneurysms: techniques, current evidence and recent experience. ANZ J Surg. 2006;76(6):505–11.
13. Vermilion BD, Kimmins SA, Pace WG, Evans WE. A review of one hundred forty-seven popliteal aneurysms with long-term follow-up. Surgery. 1981;90(6):1009–14.
14. Anton GE, Hertzer NR, Beven EG, O'Hara PJ, Krajewski LP. Surgical management of popliteal aneurysms. Trends in presentation, treatment, and results from 1952 to 1984. J Vasc Surg. 1986;3(1):125–34.
15. Carpenter JP, Barker CF, Roberts B, Berkowitz HD, Lusk EJ, Perloff LJ. Popliteal artery aneurysms: current management and outcome. J Vasc Surg. 1994;19(1):65–72; discussion 72–3.
16. Avisse C, Marcus C, Ouedraogo T, Delattre JF, Menanteau B, Flament JB. Anatomo-radiological study of the popliteal artery during knee flexion. Surg Radiol Anat. 1995;17(3):255–62.

17. Wensing PJ, Scholten FG, Buijs PC, Hartkamp MJ, Mali WP, Hillen B. Arterial tortuosity in the femoropopliteal region during knee flexion: a magnetic resonance angiographic study. J Anat. 1995;187(Pt 1): 133–9.
18. Shiomi J, Takahashi T, Imazato S, Yamamoto H. Flexion of the knee increases the distance between the popliteal artery and the proximal tibia: MRI measurements in 15 volunteers. Acta Orthop Scand. 2001; 72(6):626–8.
19. Antonello M, Frigatti P, Battocchio P, et al. Open repair versus endovascular treatment for asymptomatic popliteal artery aneurysm: results of a prospective randomized study. J Vasc Surg. 2005;42(2):185–93.
20. Galland RB, Magee TR. Popliteal aneurysms: distortion and size related to symptoms. Eur J Vasc Endovasc Surg. 2005;30(5):534–8.
21. Hamish M, Lockwood A, Cosgrove C, Walker AJ, Wilkins D, Ashley S. Management of popliteal artery aneurysms. ANZ J Surg. 2006;76(10):912–5.
22. Jacob T, Ascher E, Hingorani A, Gunduz Y, Kallakuri S. Initial steps in the unifying theory of the pathogenesis of artery aneurysms. J Surg Res. 2001;101(1): 37–43.
23. Klein AJ, Chen SJ, Messenger JC, et al. Quantitative assessment of the conformational change in the femoropopliteal artery with leg movement. Catheter Cardiovasc Interv. 2009;74(5):787–98.
24. Gifford Jr RW, Hines Jr EA, Janes JM. An analysis and follow-up study of one hundred popliteal aneurysms. Surgery. 1953;33(2):284–93.
25. Guvendik L, Bloor K, Charlesworth D. Popliteal aneurysm: sinister harbinger of sudden catastrophe. Br J Surg. 1980;67(4):294–6.
26. Ascher E, Markevich N, Schutzer RW, Kallakuri S, Jacob T, Hingorani AP. Small popliteal artery aneurysms: are they clinically significant? J Vasc Surg. 2003;37(4):755–60.
27. Ebaugh JL, Morasch MD, Matsumura JS, Eskandari MK, Meadows WS, Pearce WH. Fate of excluded popliteal artery aneurysms. J Vasc Surg. 2003;37(5): 954–9.
28. Osler W. Unity, peace and concord: abstract of a farewell address to the medical profession of the United States. Cal State J Med. 1905;3(9):275–7.
29. Friedman SG, Friedman MS. Matas, Antyllus, and endoaneurysmorrhaphy. Surgery. 1989;105(6): 761–3.
30. Edwards WS. Exclusion and saphenous vein bypass of popliteal aneurysms. Surg Gynecol Obstet. 1969;128(4):829–30.
31. Beseth BD, Moore WS. The posterior approach for repair of popliteal artery aneurysms. J Vasc Surg. 2006;43(5):940–4; discussion 944–5.
32. Pulli R, Dorigo W, Troisi N, et al. Surgical management of popliteal artery aneurysms: which factors affect outcomes? J Vasc Surg. 2006;43(3):481–7.
33. Kropman RH, van Santvoort HC, Teijink J, et al. The medial versus the posterior approach in the repair of popliteal artery aneurysms: a multicenter case-matched study. J Vasc Surg. 2007;46(1):24–30.
34. Rajasinghe HA, Tzilinis A, Keller T, Schafer J, Urrea S. Endovascular exclusion of popliteal artery aneurysms with expanded polytetrafluoroethylene stent-grafts: early results. Vasc Endovascular Surg. 2006;40(6):460–6.
35. Tielliu IF, Verhoeven EL, Zeebregts CJ, Prins TR, Span MM, van den Dungen JJ. Endovascular treatment of popliteal artery aneurysms: results of a prospective cohort study. J Vasc Surg. 2005;41(4):561–7.
36. Cina CS, Moore R, Maggisano R, Kucey D, Dueck A, Rapanos T. Endovascular repair of popliteal artery aneurysms with Anaconda limbs: technique and early results. Catheter Cardiovasc Interv. 2008;72(5): 716–24.
37. Idelchik GM, Dougherty KG, Hernandez E, Mortazavi A, Strickman NE, Krajcer Z. Endovascular exclusion of popliteal artery aneurysms with stent-grafts: a prospective single-center experience. J Endovasc Ther. 2009;16(2):215–23.
38. Mohan IV, Bray PJ, Harris JP, et al. Endovascular popliteal aneurysm repair: are the results comparable to open surgery? Eur J Vasc Endovasc Surg. 2006; 32(2):149–54.
39. Dorigo W, Di Carlo F, Troisi N, et al. Lower limb revascularization with a new bioactive prosthetic graft: early and late results. Ann Vasc Surg. 2008;22(1): 79–87.
40. Etezadi V, Fuller J, Wong S, et al. Endovascular treatment of popliteal artery aneurysms: a single-center experience. J Vasc Interv Radiol. 2010;21(6):817–23.
41. Lovegrove RE, Javid M, Magee TR, Galland RB. Endovascular and open approaches to non-thrombosed popliteal aneurysm repair: a meta-analysis. Eur J Vasc Endovasc Surg. 2008;36(1):96–100.
42. Robinson 3rd WP, Belkin M. Acute limb ischemia due to popliteal artery aneurysm: a continuing surgical challenge. Semin Vasc Surg. 2009;22(1):17–24.
43. Cina CS. Endovascular repair of popliteal aneurysms. J Vasc Surg. 2010;51(4):1056–60.
44. Curi MA, Geraghty PJ, Merino OA, et al. Mid-term outcomes of endovascular popliteal artery aneurysm repair. J Vasc Surg. 2007;45(3):505–10.
45. Stone PA, Armstrong PA, Bandyk DF, et al. The value of duplex surveillance after open and endovascular popliteal aneurysm repair. J Vasc Surg. 2005; 41(6):936–41.
46. Marin ML, Veith FJ, Panetta TF, et al. Transfemoral endoluminal stented graft repair of a popliteal artery aneurysm. J Vasc Surg. 1994;19(4):754–7.
47. Ranson ME, Adelman MA, Cayne NS, Maldonado TS, Muhs BE. Total Viabahn endoprosthesis collapse. J Vasc Surg. 2008;47(2):454–6.
48. Roddy S. Stent fractures in the Hemobahn/Viabahn stent graft after endovascular popliteal aneurysm repair. J Vasc Surg. 2010;51:1581–2.
49. Galland RB, Magee TR. Management of popliteal aneurysm. Br J Surg. 2002;89(11):1382–5.

50. Mehta M, Champagne B, Darling 3rd RC, et al. Outcome of popliteal artery aneurysms after exclusion and bypass: significance of residual patent branches mimicking type II endoleaks. J Vasc Surg. 2004;40(5):886–90.
51. Dawson I, van Bockel JH, Brand R, Terpstra JL. Popliteal artery aneurysms. Long-term follow-up of aneurysmal disease and results of surgical treatment. J Vasc Surg. 1991;13(3):398–407.
52. Shortell CK, DeWeese JA, Ouriel K, Green RM. Popliteal artery aneurysms: a 25-year surgical experience. J Vasc Surg. 1991;14(6):771–6; discussion 776–9.
53. Lowell RC, Gloviczki P, Hallett Jr JW, et al. Popliteal artery aneurysms: the risk of nonoperative management. Ann Vasc Surg. 1994;8(1):14–23.
54. Schillinger M, Minar E. Past, present and future of femoropopliteal stenting. J Endovasc Ther. 2009;16 Suppl 1:I147–52.
55. Ferreira M, Medeiros A, Monteiro M, Laziutti L. A technical alternative for the endovascular treatment of popliteal artery aneurysms. J Vasc Bras. 2008;7(1):44–8.

Part II

Occlusive Disease

Carotid Artery Stenting: Current Status

12

Rabih A. Chaer and Michel S. Makaroun

Abstract

Severe carotid stenosis is traditionally treated by carotid endarterectomy (CEA), given that multicenter trials have shown a benefit in stroke reduction in symptomatic and asymptomatic patients. Carotid angioplasty and stenting (CAS) with cerebral protection has become an alternative to CEA in high-surgical-risk patients and the procedure of choice in patients with hostile neck anatomy or highly inaccessible lesions. This chapter summarizes and critically analyzes the existing data on CAS and the current indications for its use.

Keywords

Extracranial • Carotid stenosis • Angioplasty • Stenting • CAS

Introduction

The current management of carotid occlusive disease continues to evolve. While carotid endarterectomy (CEA), first introduced in the 1950s, was established as the gold standard for treatment of carotid stenosis [1–7], carotid angioplasty and stenting (CAS) is currently often used as a minimally invasive alternative. Several trials have aimed to determine the safety and efficacy of CAS and the indications for its use. Although CAS has proved feasible and relatively safe, the appropriate clinical setting for its preferential use over CEA continues to be refined and remains the subject of ongoing clinical trials. The purpose of this chapter is to review the literature and recent trials of CAS and to attempt to elucidate its proper role and indications in the therapeutic management of extracranial carotid artery occlusive disease.

Historical Overview

Percutaneous balloon angioplasty of the carotid artery was first described in the late 1970s as a proposed intervention for carotid artery stenosis [8]. It was initially promoted as a potentially safer alternative to CEA in medically high-risk patients

R.A. Chaer, M.D. (✉) • M.S. Makaroun, M.D.
Division of Vascular Surgery,
University of Pittsburgh Medical Center,
A-1011 PUH/200 Lothrop St.,
Pittsburgh, PA 15213, USA
e-mail: chaerra@upmc.edu; makarounms@upmc.edu

J.J. Hoballah, A.B. Lumsden (eds.), *Vascular Surgery*, New Techniques in Surgery Series,
DOI 10.1007/978-1-4471-2912-7_12,

and those with hostile neck anatomy. Early trials involving carotid angioplasty demonstrated feasibility of the technique but were not widely accepted because of small study size, relatively high complication rates, and random use of stenting, to name a few. Enthusiasm was further curtailed by the concern for embolic complications associated with the procedure. Gradually, however, CAS evolved to its current form with improvements in equipment and technique, increased operator experience, and the standard use of stenting and cerebral protection.

Cerebral Protection

The use of embolic protection devices (EPDs) for cerebral protection became standard practice in CAS trials after several articles suggested decreased risk of embolic complications with their use. These devices are based on three different approaches: distal filter placement, distal balloon occlusion, and proximal protection with flow reversal.

Filters are the most commonly used EPD and are positioned in the internal carotid artery distal to the target lesion. Antegrade cerebral flow is maintained through the filter during CAS. The embolic debris dislodged during the procedure are captured within the filter, which is then subsequently removed with retraction of the device. The filters typically retain fragments larger than their pore size, approximately 100 μm, but do allow passage of smaller particles. Filters are advantageous because they allow continued cerebral perfusion, particularly in patients who have inadequate collateral circulation to permit temporary carotid occlusion. Currently, several filters are FDA approved for use in the United States and include Accunet (Abbott Laboratories), Emboshield (Abbot Laboratories), FilterWire EZ (Boston Scientific Corporation), SpiderFx (ev3), and Angioguard XP (Cordis – Johnson & Johnson) [9–12].

In addition to filters, distal balloon occlusion can be used for embolic protection. The PercuSurge occlusion balloon (Medtronic) [13] is a component of an angiographic wire that is passed through the stenotic area and inflated in the distal internal carotid artery. After the CAS procedure, the standing column of blood containing particulate matter is aspirated. The balloon is then deflated and flow is restored to the cerebral circulation. Compared with filters, distal occlusion balloons have a lower device-crossing profile, but are disadvantageous in that they require temporary interruption of cerebral perfusion while the inflated balloon captures embolic debris. It was reported in one study that up to 23 % of patients had temporary neurologic intolerance to balloon occlusion, with a significant number of these patients exhibiting symptoms immediately after initial balloon inflation. Of note, however, is that all neurologic deficits were completely reversible with restoration of antegrade flow and did not recur with balloon reinflation [14].

Unlike both distal filters and balloons, proximal protection devices with flow reversal, such as the MO.MA device (Invatec) [15] and the Parodi Anti-Embolism System (Gore) [16], are beneficial because they do not require crossing of the stenosis. Such devices have only been recently tested and provide protection by occluding the common and external carotid arteries, after which collateral flow through the circle of Willis creates a back pressure that prevents antegrade flow into the internal carotid artery.

Despite the fact that EPDs likely provide additional cerebral protection, there is still a risk of stroke associated with CAS secondary to particle embolization from the aortic arch. In addition, EPDs have inherent risks and complications of their own, such as inability to cross the target lesion, failure to capture emboli through filter pores, and vasospasm or injury to the vessel wall [17]. In addition, it is still debatable whether the routine use of EPDs is required at all. A recent single-center randomized study found no demonstrable reduction of microemboli, as detected by diffusion-weighted MRI, as might be expected with filter use [18]. Nevertheless, there are no large-randomized trials to date that compare CAS with and without EPDs, and most data rely on historical comparison of results before widespread EPD usage. Nevertheless, EPD use has become standard and is currently mandated by the Centers for Medicare and Medicaid Services.

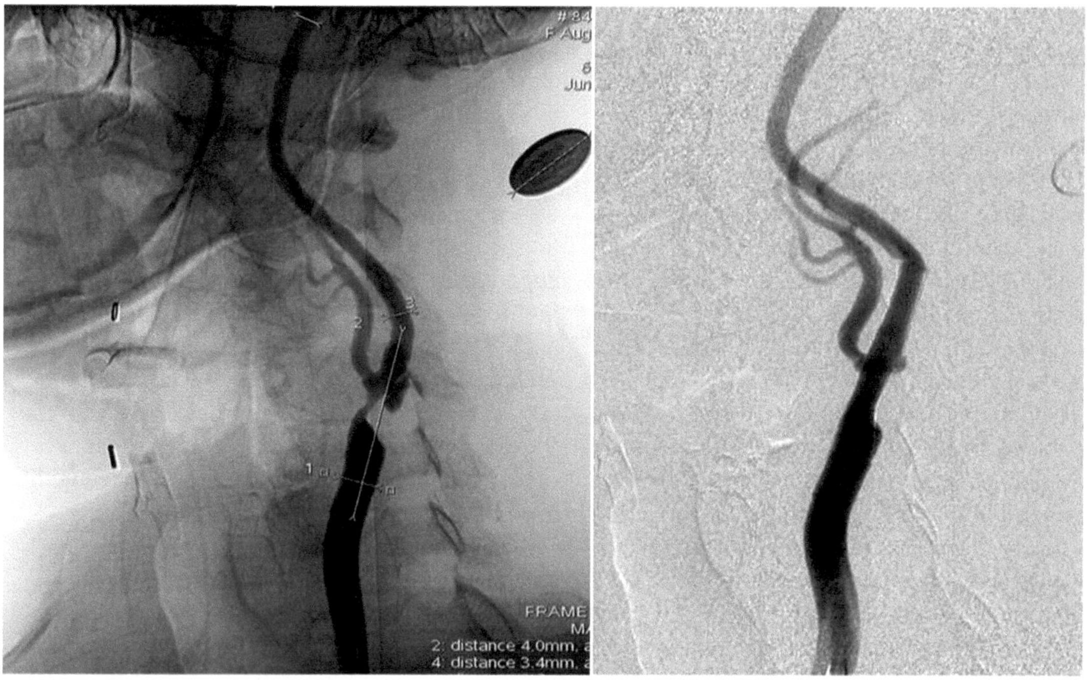

Fig. 12.1 CAS performed in the setting of restenosis post CEA

Carotid Artery Stenting Registry Trials

Initial CAS trial data was derived from industry-sponsored registry trials. Registry trials are non-randomized outcome trials evaluating the safety and efficacy of specific stents and EPDs, and most were performed in a predominantly asymptomatic population of patients who are all considered to be at high risk for conventional CEA (Fig. 12.1). Most registries are conducted to acquire initial device approval or as part of a required post-approval evaluation in a larger group of patients. Technical success was achieved in 97 % of patients in most studies. The combined incidence at 30 days of myocardial infarction, stroke, or death varied between 2.1 and 8.3 %, and stroke rate at 30 days ranged from 1.6 to 6.9 % [19–32].

Carotid Artery Stenting Randomized Trials

To date, several randomized controlled trials have been completed, and four other trials were all terminated before study completion [33–40].

The Carotid and Vertebral Artery Transluminal Angioplasty Study (CAVATAS) was designed to compare balloon angioplasty alone without embolic protection to CEA in symptomatic patients. Stents were incorporated once they became available but were used in only 26 % of patients in the endovascular arm. For the 504 patients enrolled, there was no significant difference found in the composite stroke or death rate at 30 days (10.0 % endovascular group vs. 9.9 % CEA group) or at 3 years (14.3 % endovascular group vs. 14.2 % CEA group) [33]. However, this study was criticized for a number of reasons. To name a few, the lack of embolic protection and 26 % stent usage are in contrast to current standard practice, and the substantially higher stroke rate of 9.9 % in the CEA arm makes comparison with other reports difficult.

The Wall stent trial followed; it was the first multicenter randomized trial designed to compare CAS and CEA equivalence but was stopped early after interim analysis revealed worse outcomes in the CAS arm with combined risk of stroke or death at 30 days of 12.1 % in the CAS group versus 4.5 % in the CEA group [38]. More encouraging were the results of the Kentucky trials, the first of which was published in 2001 and involved symptomatic patients, and the second of which was published in 2004 and involved asymptomatic patients [34, 35]. Extremely low-complication rates were observed in both arms, and the results of both trials suggested equivalence of CAS to CEA, but enthusiasm was appropriately guarded because these were small, single institution studies carried out by a highly select experienced team.

The Stenting and Angioplasty with Protection in Patients at High Risk for Endarterectomy (SAPPHIRE) trial demonstrated great promise for CAS. It was the first randomized trial to use mandatory distal embolic protection, and it was designed to demonstrate non-inferiority of CAS in a group of patients who were at high risk for conventional endarterectomy, and who turned out to be largely asymptomatic. The 30-day combined periprocedural adverse event rates were 4.8 % for CAS patients and 9.8 % for CEA patients. At 1 year, the combined major adverse event rates were 12.2 % for CAS patients and 20.1 % for CEA patients for non-inferiority analysis [36]. These data suggested non-inferiority of CAS for high-risk, largely asymptomatic patients. This trial, however, suffered from several biases in its design, investigator conflict of interest, and endpoints, which limited its generalizability.

Two multicenter randomized symptomatic European trials followed and included the Stent-Protected Angioplasty versus Carotid Endarterectomy (SPACE) and Endarterectomy Versus Stenting in Patients with Symptomatic Severe Carotid Stenosis (EVA-3S) trials. Both sought to establish non-inferiority in standard risk, symptomatic patients [39, 40].

The initial aim of the SPACE trial was to enroll 950 patients per group to achieve a power of 80 %. The final analysis, however, comprised 1,183 patients and reported a primary event rate of 6.84 % in the CAS group versus 6.34 % in the CEA group [39]. SPACE CAS patients were treated variably with embolic protection, but there were no significant differences found between those who were treated with and without. In addition, in most endpoints, there seemed to be a favorable trend toward the surgical arm, although none were statistically significant. After this interim analysis, the steering committee decided to terminate the study on the basis of both futility and financial constraints because it was revealed that 2,500 patients would be needed to adequately power the study to achieve trial endpoints. SPACE therefore failed to prove non-inferiority of CAS compared with CEA, and the authors concluded that CEA should remain the preferred treatment for patients with symptomatic stenosis. Subsequent subgroup analysis from SPACE revealed that this was particularly true for older patients, in whom CAS was associated with a worse outcome [41].

Similarly, the EVA-3S trial also failed to demonstrate non-inferiority of CAS in symptomatic patients. A variety of different stents were used at different centers, and cerebral protection was initially not required until the safety committee instituted a protocol change as a result of a 25 % 30-day rate of stroke or death in patients treated without EPDs [42]. The study randomized 527 patients and was subsequently ended prematurely for safety reasons after interim analysis revealed a significantly higher 30-day event rate in the CAS group (9.6 %) compared with the CEA group (3.9 %; $p=0.01$). These results persisted at 6 months, with an event rate of 11.7 % in the CAS arm versus 6.1 % in the CEA group ($p=0.02$) [40]. The EVA-3S results have been widely criticized for several reasons, namely, a significantly higher 30-day stroke rate observed in the CAS arm of the study as compared with other recently published results, namely, from the SAPPHIRE trial, and low operator experience in the CAS arm. Despite these claims, however, subgroup analysis failed to show any statistically significant difference between operators based on level of experience. The conclusion from the EVA-3S authors essentially supported the notion that CEA remains an excellent option for symptomatic carotid stenosis with low complication rates that are currently not outperformed by CAS.

The interim results of the ICSS trial were also recently released, comparing CEA to CAS in symptomatic patients with internal carotid stenosis [43]. The trial randomized 1,713 patients. The incidence of stroke, death, or procedural myocardial infarction was 8.5 % in the stenting group compared with 5.2 % in the endarterectomy group. Interestingly, the risks of any stroke and all-cause death were higher in the stenting group than in the endarterectomy group. Three procedural myocardial infarctions were recorded in the stenting group, all of which were fatal, compared with four, all nonfatal, in the endarterectomy group. Expectedly, there was one event of cranial nerve palsy in the stenting group compared with 45 in the endarterectomy group. There were also fewer hematomas of any severity in the stenting group than in the endarterectomy group.

The ICSS trial also evaluated the primary endpoint of the presence of at least one new ischemic brain lesion on diffusion-weighted imaging (DWI) on the posttreatment scan [44]. A total of 231 patients had MRI before and after treatment. Sixty-two (50 %) of 124 patients in the stenting group and 18 (17 %) of 107 patients in the endarterectomy group had at least one new DWI lesion detected on posttreatment scans done a median of 1 day after treatment (adjusted odds ratio [OR] 5.21; $p<0.0001$). At 1 month, there were also changes on fluid-attenuated inversion recovery sequences in 28 (33 %) of 86 patients in the stenting group and six (8 %) of 75 in the endarterectomy group (adjusted OR 5.93; $p=0.0003$). Moreover, the use of protection devices did not seem to be effective in preventing cerebral ischemia during stenting. Although the immediate and future clinical significance of these findings was not fully elucidated, and their impact on cognitive function is not well defined, they established DWI as a possible surrogate outcome measure in future trials of carotid interventions.

More recently, the results of the Carotid Revascularization Endarterectomy versus Stenting Trial (CREST) trial were published [45]. This trial randomly assigned patients with symptomatic or asymptomatic carotid stenosis to undergo carotid artery stenting or carotid endarterectomy. The primary composite endpoint was stroke, myocardial infarction, or death from any cause during the periprocedural period or any ipsilateral stroke within 4 years after randomization. In this trial, 2,502 patients were recruited and followed for a median follow-up period of 2.5 years. There was no significant difference in the estimated 4-year rates of the primary endpoint between the stenting group and the endarterectomy group. However, the 4-year rate of stroke or death was 6.4 % with stenting and 4.7 % with endarterectomy (hazard ratio, 1.50; $p=0.03$); the rates among symptomatic patients were 8.0 and 6.4 % (hazard ratio, 1.37; $p=0.14$), and the rates among asymptomatic patients were 4.5 and 2.7 % (hazard ratio, 1.86; $p=0.07$), respectively. Moreover, periprocedural rates of individual components of the endpoints differed between the stenting group and the endarterectomy group: for death (0.7 % vs. 0.3 %, $p=0.18$), for stroke (4.1 % vs. 2.3 %, $p=0.01$), and for myocardial infarction (1.1 % vs. 2.3 %, $p=0.03$). The main findings of this trial supported the notion that the risk of periprocedural stroke was higher with stenting, whereas the risk of myocardial infarction was higher with endarterectomy.

Hybrid Approaches

Combined surgical and endovascular approaches have become increasingly popular for patients with a hostile aortic arch and in patients undergoing CEA in the presence of a concomitant proximal common carotid stenosis (Fig. 12.2).

The aortic arch is clearly recognized as an embolic source during CAS, and this has been recently confirmed by interim data from the ICSS study demonstrating that greater than 10 % of strokes within 30 days of the procedure occurred contralateral to the target lesion after CAS [44]. Although the use of flow reversal is believed to reduce the incidence of contralateral cross embolization, this has not been widely accepted and is unlikely to circumvent embolization from manipulation in the aortic arch [46].

The transcervical technique via a small cut down or percutaneous access has been popularized and seems to result in a lower incidence of cerebral embolization, especially when used with a flow reversal technique [47]. Although not widely utilized, it may be an alternative option in patients with hostile access who are at high risk for surgery.

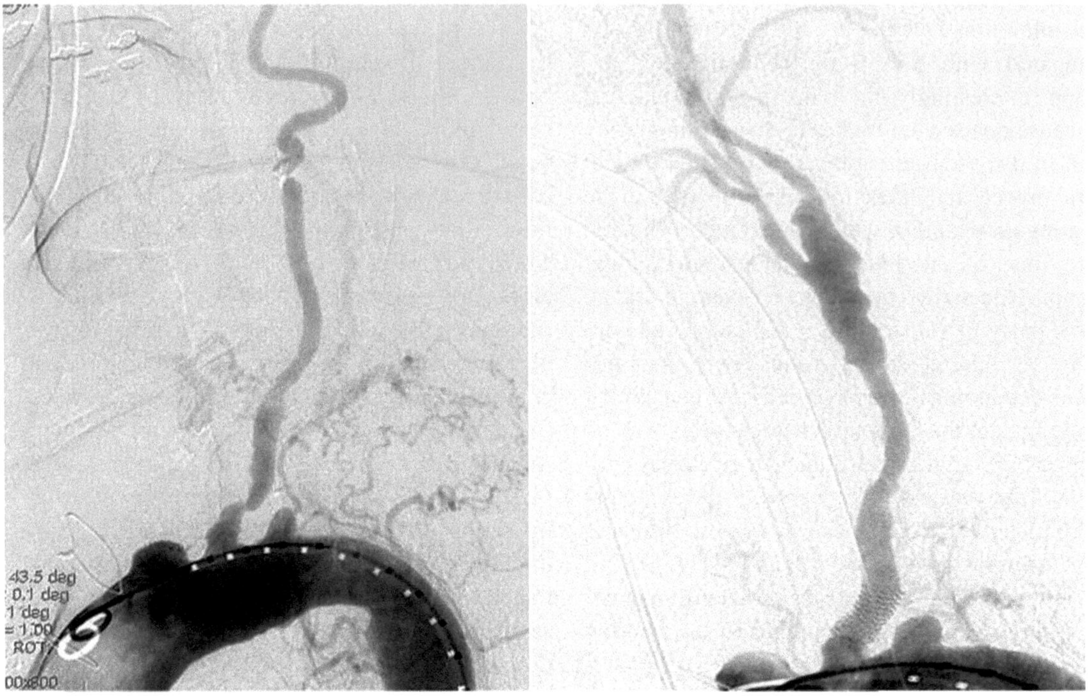

Fig. 12.2 Hybrid repair in a patient with bifurcation disease treated with CEA with patch closure, and concomitant retrograde stenting of a common carotid origin stenosis

High Risk for CAS

Overall, it had been challenging to collectively interpret the results of the randomized trials to date because they reached different conclusions about the safety and efficacy of CAS versus CEA. Current data, however, seems to define a subgroup of patient who are at high risk for CAS and who should be preferentially treated with CEA.

One clear limitation of CAS has become evident so far, namely, the higher rate of adverse outcomes in octogenarians. The CREST lead-in phase and other studies have shown increased rates for stroke and stroke and death in octogenarians [48]. Investigators in the CREST trial reported a 30-day stroke and death rate of 12 % for octogenarians compared with 3.23 % among non-octogenarians. Although this fact has been challenged, the observation has been repeated with such alarming regularity that age older than 80 years should be considered at least a relative contraindication to CAS [48–50]. The increased risk with age actually starts at 75 years and accelerates beyond the age of 80. The etiology remains obscure, but the increase in adverse outcomes seen with this population might be at least partly related to anatomic factors, such as adverse arch anatomy and vessel tortuosity (Table 12.1). Moreover, many unfavorable anatomic characteristics, such as arch elongation, calcification, lesion length, and vessel tortuosity, have been associated with increased risk of CAS anecdotally and seem to be more prevalent in the elderly [51–54].

Similarly, the European trials data seem to suggest that symptomatic patients may have to be

Table 12.1 Accepted high-risk criteria for CAS

Anatomic	Physiologic
Arch disease and anomalies	Octogenarians
Severe tortuosity	Symptomatic patients
Severe stenosis	Renal failure
Echolucent lesion	
Tandem lesions	
Calcified globular lesions	
Ostial lesions	
Long lesions (>15 mm)	

considered high risk for CAS, especially when associated with other risk factors, and may be best treated with CEA [39, 40]. These findings, however, have not been duplicated by the CREST trial data [45], and the differential outcomes may be biased by the shortcomings in each trial design and implementation.

Finally, plaque characteristics, such as echolucency on ultrasound or plaque hemorrhage, may be more common in symptomatic patients and the culprit in increasing risk of stroke with CAS more than with CEA. The soft plaque with low echogenicity scores seems to be associated with significant neurologic adverse events [55]. As such, unless high-risk factors mandate use of CAS, average-risk patients with symptoms and vulnerable plaque findings should be preferentially treated with CEA unless the patient is willing to enroll in a clinical trial [55].

Conclusion

The current indications for CAS continue to be better defined, with current data supporting its application in clinical trials or specific high-risk categories. While demonstrated to be relatively safer in patients with cardiac comorbidities, the neurologic outcomes with CAS continue to be suboptimal when compared to endarterectomy. Outcomes of CAS will continue to improve, however, and the approach to carotid disease is likely to evolve during the next several years with improved stenting and cerebral protection technology and a better understanding of plaque vulnerability. Ultimately, the benefit of CAS in terms of stroke prevention should depend on institutional outcomes and should be tailored to individual patient characteristics and comorbidities.

References

1. North American Symptomatic Carotid Endarterectomy Trial Collaborators. Beneficial effect of carotid endarterectomy in symptomatic patients with high-grade carotid stenosis. N Engl J Med. 1991;325:445–53.
2. Barnett HJ, Taylor DW, Eliasziw M, et al. Benefit of carotidendarterectomy in patients with symptomatic moderate or severe stenosis. North American Symptomatic Carotid Endarterectomy Trial Collaborators. N Engl J Med. 1998;339:1415–25.
3. European Carotid Surgery Trial Collaborators. Randomized trial of endarterectomy for recently symptomatic carotid stenosis: final results of the MRC European Carotid Surgery Trial (ECST). Lancet. 1998;351:1379–87.
4. Ferguson FF, Eliasziw M, Barr HW, et al. The North American Symptomatic Carotid Endarterectomy Trial: surgical results in 1415 patients. Stroke. 1999;30:1751–8.
5. Asymptomatic Carotid Surgery Trial Collaborative Group. Prevention of disabling and fatal strokes by successful carotid endarterectomy in patients without recent neurological symptoms: randomized controlled trial. Lancet. 2004;363:1491–502.
6. Executive Committee for the Asymptomatic Carotid Atherosclerosis Study. Endarterectomy for asymptomatic carotid stenosis. JAMA. 1995;273:1421–8.
7. Hobson RW, Weiss DG, Fields WS, et al. Efficacy of carotid endarterectomy for asymptomatic carotid stenosis. The Veterans Affairs Cooperative Study Group. N Engl J Med. 1993;328:221–7.
8. Mathias K. A new catheter system for percutaneous transluminal angioplasty of carotid artery stenosis. Fortschr Med. 1997;95:1007–11.
9. Accunet and emboshield filters. Available at: www.abbott.com. Accessed 4 July 2012.
10. Filter Wire EZ. Available at: www.bostonscientific.com. Accessed 4 July 2012.
11. SpiderFx. Available at: www.ev3.net. Accessed 4 July 2012.
12. Angioguard XP. Available at: www.cordis.com. Accessed 4 July 2012.
13. PercuSurge. Available at: www.medtronic.com. Accessed 4 July 2012.
14. Chaer RA, Trocciola S, DeRubertis B, et al. Cerebral ischemia associated with PercuSurge balloon occlusion during carotid stenting. J Vasc Surg. 2006;43:946–52.
15. MOMA. Available at: www.invatec.com. Accessed 4 July 2012.
16. Parodi anti-embolic system. Available at: www.goremedical.com. Accessed 4 July 2012.
17. Fanelli F, Bezzi M, Boatta E, et al. Techniques in cerebral protection. Eur J Radiol. 2006;60:26–36.
18. Barbato JE, Dillavou E, Horowitz MB, et al. A randomized trial of carotid artery stenting with and without cerebral protection. J Vasc Surg. 2008;47:760–5.
19. White CJ, Iyer SS, Hopkins LN, et al. Carotid stenting with distal protection in high surgical risk patients: the BEACH trial 30 day results. Catheter Cardiovasc Interv. 2006;67:503–12.
20. Gray WA, Hopkins LN, Yadav S, et al. Protected carotid stenting in high-surgical-risk patients: the ARCHeR results. J Vasc Surg. 2006;44:258–68.
21. Hopkins LN, Myla S, Grube E, et al. Carotid artery revascularization in high surgical risk patients with

the NexStent and the Filterwire EX/EZ: 1 year results in the CABERNET trial. Catheter Cardiovasc Interv. 2008;71:950–60.
22. Ramee S, Higashida R. Evaluation of the Medtronic self expanding carotid stent system with distal protection in the treatment of carotid artery stenosis. Am J Cardiol. 2004;94:61E.
23. CaRESS Steering Committee. Carotid Revascularization Using Endarterectomy or Stenting Systems (CaRESS) phase I clinical trial: 1-year results. J Vasc Surg. 2005;42:213–9.
24. Whitlow P. SECuRITY Investigators. SECuRITY: multicenter evaluation of carotid stenting with a distal protection filter. Unpublished data, presented by Patrick L Whitlow at the 2003 Transcatheter cardiovascular therapeutics meeting, Washington, D.C., 2003.
25. Coppi G, Moratto R, Silingardi R, et al. PRIAMUS – proximal flow blockage cerebral protection during carotid stenting. J Cardiovasc Surg (Torino). 2005;46: 219–27.
26. Safian RD, Bresnahan JF, Jaff MR, et al. Protected carotid stenting in high-risk patients with severe carotid artery stenosis. J Am Coll Cardiol. 2006;47:2384–9.
27. Gray WA, Yadav JS, Verta P, et al. The CAPTURE registry: predictors of outcomes in carotid artery stenting with embolic protection for high surgical risk patients in the early post-approval setting. Catheter Cardiovasc Interv. 2007;70:1025–33.
28. Reimers B, Sievert H, Schuler GC, et al. Proximal endovascular flow blockage for cerebral protection during carotid artery stenting. J Endovasc Ther. 2005;12:156–65.
29. Internet Stroke Center. Stroke Trials Registry. Available at: www.strokecenter.org/trials. Accessed 4 July 2012.
30. Gray WA. EXACT/CAPTURE-2: postmarketing carotid stent registry data. Presented at American College of Cardiology 2007. Scientific sessions: abstract 2409–5, New Orleans, 24–27 Mar 2007.
31. Katzen BT, Criado FJ, Ramee SR, et al. Carotid artery stenting with embolic protection surveillance study. Catheter Cardiovasc Interv. 2007;70:316–23.
32. Cremonesi A, Rubino P, Grattoni C, et al. Multicenter experience with a new "hybrid" carotid stent. J Endovasc Ther. 2008;15:186–92.
33. CAVATAS Investigators. Endovascular versus surgical treatment in patients with carotid stenosis in the Carotid and Vertebral Artery Transluminal Angioplasty Study (CAVATAS): a randomized trial. Lancet. 2001;357:1729–37.
34. Brooks WH, McClure RR, Jones MR, et al. Carotid angioplasty and stenting versus carotid endarterectomy. J Am Coll Cardiol. 2001;38:1589–95.
35. Brooks WH, McClure RR, Jones MR, et al. Carotid angioplasty and stenting versus carotid endarterectomy for treatment of asymptomatic carotid stenosis. Neurosurgery. 2004;54:318–25.
36. Yadav JS, Wholey MH, Kuntz RE, et al. Protected carotid-artery stenting versus endarterectomy in high-risk patients. N Engl J Med. 2004;351:1493–501.
37. Naylor AR, Bolia A, Abbott RJ, et al. Randomized study of carotid angioplasty and stenting versus carotid endarterectomy: a stopped trial. J Vasc Surg. 1998;28:326–34.
38. Alberts MJ. Results of a multicentre prospective randomized trial of carotid artery stenting vs carotid endarterectomy. Stroke. 2001;32:325.
39. The SPACE Collaborative Group. 30-day results from the SPACE trial of stent-protected angioplasty versus carotid endarterectomy in symptomatic patients. Lancet. 2006;368:1239–47.
40. Mas J-L, Chatellier G, Beyssen B, et al. Endarterectomy versus stenting in patients with symptomatic severe carotid stenosis. N Engl J Med. 2006;355:1660–71.
41. Stingele R, Berger J, Alfke K, et al. Clinical and angiographic risk factors for stroke and death within 30 days after carotid endarterectomy and stent-protected angioplasty: a subanalysis of the SPACE study. Lancet Neurol. 2008;7:216–22.
42. Mas JL, Chatellier G, Beyssen BL, EVA-3 S Investigators. Carotid angioplasty and stenting with and without cerebral protection: clinical alert from the Endarterectomy Versus Angioplasty in Patients With Symptomatic Severe Carotid Stenosis trial. Stroke. 2004;35:e18–20.
43. International Carotid Stenting Study investigators, Ederle J, Dobson J, Featherstone RL, Bonati LH, van der Worp HB, de Borst GJ, Lo TH, Gaines P, Dorman PJ, Macdonald S, Lyrer PA, Hendriks JM, McCollum C, Nederkoorn PJ, Brown MM. Carotid artery stenting compared with endarterectomy in patients with symptomatic carotid stenosis (International Carotid Stenting Study): an interim analysis of a randomised controlled trial. Lancet. 2010;375(9719):985–97.
44. Bonati LH, Jongen LM, Haller S, Flach HZ, Dobson J, Nederkoorn PJ, Macdonald S, Gaines PA, Waaijer A, Stierli P, Jäger HR, Lyrer PA, Kappelle LJ, Wetzel SG, van der Lugt A, Mali WP, Brown MM, van der Worp HB, Engelter ST, ICSS-MRI study group. New ischaemic brain lesions on MRI after stenting or endarterectomy for symptomatic carotid stenosis: a substudy of the International Carotid Stenting Study (ICSS). Lancet Neurol. 2010;9(4):353–62.
45. Brott TG, Hobson 2nd RW, Howard G, Roubin GS, Clark WM, Brooks W, Mackey A, Hill MD, Leimgruber PP, Sheffet AJ, Howard VJ, Moore WS, Voeks JH, Hopkins LN, Cutlip DE, Cohen DJ, Popma JJ, Ferguson RD, Cohen SN, Blackshear JL, Silver FL, Mohr JP, Lal BK, Meschia JF, CREST Investigators. Stenting versus endarterectomy for treatment of carotid-artery stenosis. N Engl J Med. 2010;363(1):11–23.
46. Leal JI, Orgaz A, Fontcuberta J, Flores A, Doblas M, Garcia-Benassi JM, Lane B, Loh C, Criado EA. Prospective evaluation of cerebral infarction following transcervical carotid stenting with carotid flow reversal. Eur J Vasc Endovasc Surg. 2010;39(6):661–6.
47. Palombo G, Stella N, Faraglia V, Rizzo L, Fantozzi C, Bozzao A, Taurino M. Cervical access for filter-protected carotid artery stenting: a useful tool to

reduce cerebral embolisation. Eur J Vasc Endovasc Surg. 2010;39(3):252–7.
48. Stanziale SF, Marone LK, Boules TN, et al. Carotid artery stenting in octogenarians is associated with increased adverse outcomes. J Vasc Surg. 2006;43:297–304.
49. Gray WA, Yadav JS, Verta P, et al. The CAPTURE registry: results ofcarotid stenting with embolic protection in the post approval setting. Catheter Cardiovasc Interv. 2006;69:341–8.
50. Roubin GS, New G, Iyer SS, et al. Immediate and late clinical outcomes of carotid artery stenting in patients with symptomatic and asymptomatic carotid artery stenosis: a 5-year prospective analysis. Circulation. 2001;103:532–7.
51. Lam RC, Lin SC, DeRubertis B, Hynecek R, Kent KC, Faries PL. The impact of increasing age on anatomic factors affecting carotid angioplasty and stenting. J Vasc Surg. 2007;45:875–80.
52. Faggioli GL, Ferri M, Freyrie A, et al. Aortic arch anomalies are associated with increased risk of neurological events in carotid stent procedures. Eur J Vasc Endovasc Surg. 2007;33:436–41.
53. Sayeed S, Stanziale SF, Wholey MH, Makaroun MS. Angiographic lesion characteristics can predict adverse outcomes after carotid artery stenting. J Vasc Surg. 2008;47:81–7.
54. Mathur A, Roubin GS, Iyer SS, et al. Predictors of stroke complicating carotid artery stenting. Circulation. 1998;97:1239–45.
55. Biasi GM, Froio A, Diethrich EB, et al. Carotid plaque echolucencyincreases the risk of stroke in carotid stenting: the Imaging in Carotid Angioplasty and Risk of Stroke (ICAROS) study. Circulation. 2004;110:756–62.

Mesenteric Artery Occlusive Disease 13

Panos Kougias

Abstract

Vascular occlusive disease of the mesenteric vessels is a relatively uncommon but potentially devastating condition that generally presents in patients over 60 years of age and has been recognized as an entity since 1936. The incidence of such a disease is low and represents 2 % of the revascularization operations for atheromatous lesions. The most common cause of mesenteric ischemia is atherosclerotic vascular disease. Autopsy studies have demonstrated splanchnic atherosclerosis in 35–70 % of cases. Other etiologies exist and include fibromuscular dysplasia, nodose panarteritis, arteritis, and celiac artery compression from a median arcuate ligament, but they are unusual and have an incidence of 1/9 compared to that of atherosclerosis.

Keywords

Embolic mesenteric ischemia • Thrombotic mesenteric ischemia • Occlusive disease • Surgical reconstruction • Mesenteric ischemia

Introduction

Vascular occlusive disease of the mesenteric vessels is a relatively uncommon but potentially devastating condition that generally presents in patients over 60 years of age and has been recognized as an entity since 1936 [1]. The incidence of such a disease is low and represents 2 % of the revascularization operations for atheromatous lesions. The most common cause of mesenteric ischemia is atherosclerotic vascular disease. Autopsy studies have demonstrated splanchnic atherosclerosis in 35–70 % of cases [2]. Other etiologies exist and include fibromuscular dysplasia, nodose panarteritis, arteritis, and celiac artery compression from a median arcuate ligament, but they are unusual and have an incidence of 1/9 compared to that of atherosclerosis.

Chronic mesenteric ischemia is related to a lack of blood supply in the splanchnic region and is caused by disease in one or more visceral arteries: the celiac trunk, the superior mesenteric

P. Kougias, M.D.
Department of Surgery, Baylor College of Medicine,
2002 Holcombe Blvd, Houston, TX 77030, USA
e-mail: pkougias@bcm.edu

J.J. Hoballah, A.B. Lumsden (eds.), *Vascular Surgery*, New Techniques in Surgery Series,
DOI 10.1007/978-1-4471-2912-7_13, © Springer-Verlag London 2012

artery, and the inferior mesenteric artery. Mesenteric ischemia is thought to occur when two of the three visceral vessels are affected with severe stenosis or occlusion; however, in as many as 9 % of cases, a single vessel is only involved (SMA in 5 % and celiac trunk in 4 % of cases) [3, 4]. This disease process may evolve in a chronic fashion, as in the case of progressive luminal obliteration due to atherosclerosis. On the other hand, mesenteric ischemia can occur suddenly, as in the case of thromboembolism. Despite recent progress in perioperative management and better understanding in pathophysiology, mesenteric ischemia is considered one of the most catastrophic vascular disorders with mortality rates ranging from 50 to 75 %. Delay in diagnosis and treatment are the main contributing factors in its high mortality. It is estimated that mesenteric ischemia accounts for 1 in every 1,000 hospital admissions in this country. The prevalence is rising due in part to the increased awareness of this disease, the advanced age of the population, and the significant comorbidity of these elderly patients. Early recognition and prompt treatment before the onset of irreversible intestinal ischemia are essential to improve the outcome.

Anatomy and Pathophysiology

Mesenteric arterial circulation is remarkable for its rich collateral network. Three main mesenteric arteries provide the arterial perfusion to the gastrointestinal system: the celiac artery (CA), the superior mesenteric artery (SMA), and the inferior mesenteric artery (IMA). In general, CA provides arterial circulation to the foregut (distal esophagus to duodenum), hepatobiliary system, and spleen; the SMA supplies the midgut (jejunum to mid-colon); and the IMA supplies the hindgut (mid-colon to rectum). The CA and SMA arise from the ventral surface of the infradiaphragmatic suprarenal abdominal aorta, while the IMA originates from the left lateral portion of the infrarenal aorta. These anatomic origins in relation to the aorta are important when a mesenteric angiogram is performed to determine the luminal patency. In order to fully visualize the origins of the CA and SMA, it is necessary to perform both an anteroposterior and a lateral projection of the aorta since most arterial occlusive lesions occurs in the proximal segments of these mesenteric trunks.

Because of the abundant collateral flow between these mesenteric arteries, progressive diminution of flow in one or even two of the main mesenteric trunks is usually tolerated, provided that uninvolved mesenteric branches can enlarge over time to provide sufficient compensatory collateral flow. In contrast, acute occlusion of a main mesenteric trunk may result in profound ischemia due to lack of sufficient collateral flow. Collateral network between the CA and the SMA exist primarily through the superior and inferior pancreaticoduodenal arteries. The IMA may provide collateral arterial flow to the SMA through the marginal artery of Drummond, the arc of Riolan, and other unnamed retroperitoneal collateral vessels termed meandering mesenteric arteries. Lastly, collateral visceral vessels may provide important arterial flow to the IMA and the hindgut through the hypogastric arteries and the hemorrhoidal arterial network.

Regulation of mesenteric blood flow is largely modulated by both hormonal and neural stimuli, which characteristically regulate systemic blood flow. In addition, the mesenteric circulation responds to the gastrointestinal contents. Hormonal regulation is mediated by splanchnic vasodilators, such as nitric oxide, glucagon, and vasoactive intestinal peptide. Certain intrinsic vasoconstrictors, such as vasopressin, can diminish the mesenteric blood flow. On the other hand, neural regulation is provided by the extensive visceral autonomic innervation.

Clinical manifestation of mesenteric ischemia is predominantly postprandial abdominal pain, which signifies that the increased oxygen demand of digestion is not met by the gastrointestinal collateral circulation. The postprandial pain frequently occurs in the mid-abdomen, suggesting that the diversion of blood flow from the SMA to supply the stomach impairs perfusion to the small bowel. This leads to transient anaerobic metabolism and acidosis. Persistent or profound mesenteric ischemia will lead to mucosal compromise with release of intracellular contents and by-products of anaerobic metabolism to the splanchnic and systemic circulation. Injured bowel mucosa allows unimpeded influx of toxic substances from the bowel lumen with systemic consequences. If full-thickness necrosis occurs in the bowel wall, intestinal perforation ensues which will lead to peritonitis. Concomitant atherosclerotic disease in cardiac or systemic circulation frequently compounds the diagnostic and therapeutic complexity of mesenteric ischemia.

Types of Mesenteric Artery Occlusive Disease

There are three major mechanisms of visceral ischemia involving the mesenteric arteries, which include: (1) acute mesenteric ischemia, which can be either embolic or thrombotic in origin; (2) chronic mesenteric ischemia, and (3) nonocclusive mesenteric ischemia. Despite the variability of these syndromes, a common anatomic pathology is involved in these processes. The superior mesenteric artery (SMA) is the most commonly involved vessel in acute mesenteric ischemia. Acute thrombosis occurs in patients with underlying mesenteric atherosclerosis, which typically involves the origin of the mesenteric arteries while sparing the collateral branches. In acute embolic mesenteric ischemia, the emboli typically originate from a cardiac source and frequently occur in patients with atrial fibrillation or following myocardial infarction. Nonocclusive mesenteric ischemia is characterized by a low-flow state in otherwise normal mesenteric arteries and most frequently occurs in critically ill patients on vasopressors. Finally, chronic mesenteric ischemia is a functional consequence of a long-standing atherosclerotic process which typically involves at least two of the three main mesenteric vessels. The gradual development of the occlusive process allows the development of collateral vessels that prevent the manifestations of acute ischemia but are not sufficient to meet the high postprandial intestinal oxygen requirements, giving rise to the classical symptoms of postprandial abdominal pain and the resultant food fear.

Several less common syndromes of visceral ischemia involving the mesenteric arteries can also cause serious debilitation. Chronic mesenteric ischemic symptoms can occur due to extrinsic compression of the celiac artery by the diaphragm, which is termed "the median arcuate ligament syndrome." Acute visceral ischemia may occur following an aortic operation due to ligation of the IMA in the absence of adequate collateral vessels. Furthermore, acute visceral ischemia may develop in aortic dissection which involves the mesenteric arteries or after coarctation repair. Finally, other unusual causes of ischemia include mesenteric arteritis, radiation arteritis, and cholesterol emboli.

Clinical Presentation

Abdominal pain out of proportion to physical findings is the classic presentation in patients with acute mesenteric ischemia and occurs following an embolic or thrombotic ischemic event of the SMA. Other manifestations include sudden onset of abdominal cramps in patients with underlying cardiac or atherosclerotic disease, often associated with bloody diarrhea, as a result of mucosal sloughing secondary to ischemia. Fever, nausea, vomiting, and abdominal distention are some common but nonspecific manifestations. Diffuse abdominal tenderness, rebound, and rigidity are late signs and usually indicate bowel infarction and necrosis.

Clinical manifestations of chronic mesenteric ischemia are more subtle owing to the extensive collateral development. However, when intestinal blood flow is unable to meet the physiological gastrointestinal demands, mesenteric insufficiency ensues. The classical symptoms include postprandial abdominal pain, "food fear," and weight loss. Persistent nausea and occasionally diarrhea may coexist. Diagnosis remains challenging, and most of the patients will undergo an extensive and expensive gastrointestinal tract work-up for the above symptoms prior to referral to a vascular service.

The typical patient who develops nonocclusive mesenteric ischemia is elderly patients and has multiple comorbidities, such as congestive heart failure, acute myocardial infarction with cardiogenic shock, hypovolemic or hemorrhagic shock, sepsis, pancreatitis, and administration of digitalis or vasoconstrictor agents such as epinephrine. Abdominal pain is only present in approximately 70 % of these patients. When present, the pain is usually severe but may vary in location, character, and intensity. In the absence of abdominal pain, progressive abdominal distention with acidosis may be an early sign of ischemia and impending bowel infarction.

Diagnostic Studies

The differential diagnosis of acute mesenteric ischemia includes other causes of severe abdominal pain of acute onset, such as perforated viscus, intestinal obstruction, pancreatitis, cholecystitis, and nephrolithiasis. Laboratory evaluation is neither sensitive nor specific in distinguishing these various diagnoses. In the setting of mesenteric ischemia, complete blood count (CBC) may reveal hemoconcentration and leukocytosis. Metabolic acidosis develops as a result of anaerobic metabolism. Elevated serum amylase may indicate a diagnosis of pancreatitis but is also common in the setting of intestinal infarction. Finally, increased lactate levels, hyperkalemia, and azotemia may occur in the late stages of mesenteric ischemia.

Plain abdominal radiographs may provide helpful information to exclude other causes of abdominal pain such as intestinal obstruction, perforation, or volvulus, which may exhibit symptoms mimicking intestinal ischemia. Pneumoperitoneum, pneumatosis intestinalis, and gas in the portal vein may indicate infarcted bowel. In contrast, radiographic appearance of an adynamic ileus with a gasless abdomen is the most common finding in patients with acute mesenteric ischemia.

Upper endoscopy, colonoscopy, or barium radiography does not provide any useful information when evaluating acute mesenteric ischemia. Moreover, barium enema is contraindicated if the diagnosis of mesenteric ischemia is being considered. The intraluminal barium can obscure accurate visualization of mesenteric circulation during angiography. In addition, intraperitoneal leakage of barium can occur in the setting of intestinal perforation, which can lead to added therapeutic challenges during mesenteric revascularization.

Diagnosis of chronic mesenteric ischemia can be more challenging. Usually, prior to the evaluation by a vascular service, the patients have undergone an extensive work-up for the symptoms of chronic abdominal pain, weight loss, and anorexia. Rarely, the vascular surgeon is the first to encounter a patient with the above symptoms. In this situation, it is advisable to keep in mind that mesenteric ischemia is a rare entity, and that a full diagnostic work-up that should include CT scan of the abdomen and evaluation by gastroenterologist should be performed. Mesenteric occlusive disease may coexist with malignancy, and symptoms of mesenteric vessel stenosis may be the result of extrinsic compression by a tumor.

Duplex ultrasonography is a valuable noninvasive means of assessing the patency of the mesenteric vessels. Moneta and associates evaluated the use of duplex ultrasound in the diagnosis of mesenteric occlusive disease in a blinded prospective study [5, 6]. A peak systolic velocity in the SMA > 275 cm/s demonstrated a sensitivity of 92 %, specificity of 96 %, and an overall accuracy of 96 % for detecting >70 % stenosis. The same authors found sensitivity and specificity of 87 and 82 %, respectively, with an accuracy of 82 % in predicting >70 % celiac trunk stenosis. Duplex has been successfully used for follow-up after open surgical reconstruction or endovascular treatment of the mesenteric vessels to assess recurrence of the disease. Finally, spiral computed tomography with 3D reconstruction as well as magnetic resonance angiogram (MRA) have been promising in providing clear radiographic assessment of the mesenteric vessels.

The definitive diagnosis of mesenteric vascular disease is made by biplanar mesenteric arteriography, which should be performed promptly in any patient with suspected mesenteric occlusion. It typically shows occlusion or near occlusion of the CA and SMA at or near their origins from the aorta. In most cases, the IMA has been previously occluded secondary to diffuse infrarenal aortic atherosclerosis. The differentiation of the different types of mesenteric arterial occlusion may be suggested with biplanar mesenteric arteriogram.

Mesenteric emboli typically lodge at the orifice of the middle colic artery, which creates a "meniscus sign" with an abrupt cutoff of a normal proximal SMA several centimeters from its origin on the aorta. Mesenteric thrombosis, in contrast, occurs at the most proximal SMA which tapers off at 1–2 cm from its origin. In the case of chronic mesenteric occlusion, the appearance of collateral circulation is typically present. Nonocclusive mesenteric ischemia produces an arteriographic image of segmental mesenteric vasospasm with a relatively normal-appearing main SMA trunk.

Mesenteric arteriography can also play a therapeutic role. Once the diagnosis of nonocclusive mesenteric ischemia is made on the arteriogram, an infusion catheter can be placed at the SMA orifice and vasodilating agents, such as papaverine, can be administered intra-arterially. The papaverine infusion may be continued postoperatively to treat persistent vasospasm, a common occurrence following mesenteric reperfusion. Transcatheter thrombolytic therapy has little role in the management of thrombotic mesenteric occlusion. Although thrombolytic agents may transiently recannulate the occluded vessels, the underlying occlusive lesions require definitive treatment. Furthermore, thrombolytic therapy typically requires a prolonged period of time to restore perfusion, during which the intestinal viability will be difficult to assess.

A word of caution would be appropriate here regarding patients with typical history of chronic intestinal angina who present with an acute abdomen and classical findings of peritoneal irritation. Arteriography is the gold standard for the diagnosis of mesenteric occlusive disease; however, it can be a time-consuming diagnostic modality. In this group of patients, immediate exploration for assessment of intestinal viability and vascular reconstruction is the best choice.

Open Surgical Treatment

Acute Embolic Mesenteric Ischemia

Initial management of patients with acute mesenteric ischemia includes fluid resuscitation and systemic anticoagulation with heparin to prevent further thrombus propagation. Significant metabolic acidosis not responding to fluid resuscitation should be corrected with sodium bicarbonate. A central venous catheter, a peripheral arterial catheter, and a Foley catheter should be placed for hemodynamic status monitoring. Appropriate antibiotics are given prior to surgical exploration. The operative management of acute mesenteric ischemia is dictated by the cause of the occlusion. It is helpful to obtain a preoperative mesenteric arteriogram to confirm the diagnosis and to plan appropriate treatment options. However, the diagnosis of mesenteric ischemia frequently cannot be established prior to surgical exploration, and, therefore, patients in a moribund condition with acute abdominal symptoms should undergo immediate surgical exploration, avoiding the delay required to perform an arteriogram.

The primary goal of surgical treatment in embolic mesenteric ischemia is to restore arterial perfusion with removal of the embolus from the vessel. The abdomen is explored through a midline incision, which often reveals variable degrees of intestinal ischemia from the midjejunum to the ascending or transverse colon. The transverse colon is lifted superiorly, and the small intestine is reflected toward the right upper quadrant. The SMA is approached at the root of the small bowel mesentery, usually as it emerges from beneath the pancreas to cross over the junction of the third and fourth portions of the duodenum. Alternatively, the SMA can be approached by incising the retroperitoneum lateral to the fourth portion of the duodenum, which is rotated medially to expose the SMA. Once the proximal SMA is identified and controlled with vascular clamps, a transverse arteriotomy is made to extract the embolus using standard balloon embolectomy catheters. In the event the embolus has lodged more distally, exposure of the distal SMA may be obtained in the root of the small-bowel mesentery by isolating individual jejunal and ileal branches to allow a more comprehensive thromboembolectomy. Following the restoration of SMA flow, an assessment of intestinal viability must be made, and nonviable bowel must be resected. Several methods have been described to evaluate the viability of the intestine, which include intraoperative intravenous fluorescein injection and inspection with a Wood's lamp and Doppler assessment of antimesenteric intestinal arterial pulsations. A second-look procedure should be considered in many patients and is performed 24–48 h following embolectomy. The goal of the procedure is reassessment of the extent of bowel viability, which may not be obvious immediately following the initial embolectomy. If nonviable intestine is evident in the second-look procedure, additional bowel resections should be performed at that time.

Acute Thrombotic Mesenteric Ischemia

Thrombotic mesenteric ischemia usually involves a severely atherosclerotic vessel, typically the proximal CA and SMA. Therefore, these patients require a reconstructive procedure to the SMA to bypass the proximal occlusive lesion and restore adequate mesenteric flow. The saphenous vein is the graft material of choice, and prosthetic materials should be avoided in patients with nonviable bowel due to the risk of bacterial contamination if resection of necrotic intestine is performed. The bypass graft may originate from either the aorta or iliac artery. Advantages from using the supraceliac infradiaphragmatic aorta as opposed to the infrarenal aorta as the inflow vessel include a more smooth graft configuration with less chance of kinking, and the absence of atherosclerotic disease in the supraceliac aortic segment. Exposure of the supraceliac aorta is technically more challenging and time consuming than that of the iliac artery, which unless calcified is an appropriate inflow. Patency rates are similar regardless of inflow vessel choice [7].

Chronic Mesenteric Ischemia

The therapeutic goal in patients with chronic mesenteric ischemia is to revascularize mesenteric circulation and prevent the development of bowel infarction. Mesenteric occlusive disease can be treated successfully by either transaortic endarterectomy or mesenteric artery bypass. Transaortic endarterectomy is indicated for ostial lesions of patent CA and SMA. A left medial rotation is performed, and the aorta and the mesenteric branches are exposed. A lateral aortotomy is performed encompassing both the CA and SMA orifices. The visceral arteries must be adequately mobilized so that the termination site of endarterectomy can be visualized. Otherwise, an intimal flap may develop, which can lead to early thrombosis or distal embolization.

For occlusive lesions located 1–2 cm distal to the mesenteric origin, mesenteric artery bypass should be performed. Multiple mesenteric arteries are typically involved in chronic mesenteric ischemia, and both the CA and SMA should be revascularized whenever possible. In general, bypass grafting may be performed either antegrade from the supraceliac aorta or retrograde from either the infrarenal aorta or iliac artery. Both autogenous saphenous vein grafts and prosthetic grafts have been used with satisfactory and equivalent success. An antegrade bypass also can be performed using a small-caliber bifurcated graft from the supraceliac aorta to both the CA and SMA, which yields an excellent long-term result [8].

Nonocclusive Mesenteric Ischemia

The treatment of nonocclusive mesenteric ischemia is primarily pharmacologic, with selective mesenteric arterial catheterization followed by infusion of vasodilatory agents such as tolazoline or papaverine. Once the diagnosis is made via mesenteric arteriography, intra-arterial papaverine is given at a dose of 30–60 mg/h. This must be coupled with the cessation of other vasoconstricting agents. Concomitant intravenous heparin should be administered to prevent thrombosis in the cannulated vessels. The treatment strategy thereafter is dependent on the patient's clinical response to the vasodilator therapy. If abdominal symptoms improve, mesenteric arteriography should be repeated to document the resolution of vasospasm. The patient's hemodynamic status must be carefully monitored during papaverine infusion, as significant hypotension can develop in the event that the infusion catheter migrates into the aorta, which can lead to systemic circulation of papaverine. Surgical exploration is indicated if the patient develops signs of continued bowel ischemia or infarction as evidenced by rebound tenderness or involuntary guarding. In these circumstances, papaverine infusion should be continued intraoperatively and postoperatively. The operating room should be kept as warm as possible, and warm irrigation fluid and laparotomy pads should be used to prevent further intestinal vasoconstriction during exploration.

Celiac Artery Compression Syndrome

Abdominal pain due to narrowing of the origin of the celiac artery (CA) may occur as a result of extrinsic compression or impingement by the median arcuate ligament. This condition is known as celiac artery compression syndrome, or median arcuate ligament syndrome. Angiographically, there is CA compression that augments with deep expiration and post-stenotic dilatation. The syndrome has been implicated in some variants of chronic mesenteric ischemia, but its diagnosis is one of exclusion. A decision to intervene is therefore based on both an appropriate symptom complex and the finding of celiac artery compression in the absence of other findings to explain the symptoms. The patient should be cautioned that relief of the celiac compression cannot be guaranteed to relieve the symptoms. Most patients are young females between 20 and 40 years of age. Abdominal symptoms are nonspecific, but the pain is localized in the upper abdomen and may be precipitated by meals. The treatment goal is to release the ligamentous structure that compresses the proximal CA and to correct any persistent stricture by bypass grafting. In a number of reports on endovascular management of chronic mesenteric ischemia, the presence of CA compression syndrome has been identified as a major factor of technical failure and recurrence. Therefore, angioplasty and stenting should not be undertaken if extrinsic compression of the CA by the median arcuate ligament is suspected based on preoperative imaging studies. Open surgical treatment should be performed instead [9–11].

Endovascular Treatment Strategies

Chronic Mesenteric Ischemia

Endovascular treatment of mesenteric artery stenosis or short segment occlusion by balloon dilatation or stent placement represents a less invasive therapeutic alternative to open surgical intervention, particularly in patients whose medical comorbidities place them at a high-operative-risk category. Endovascular therapy is also suited in patients with recurrent disease or anastomotic stenosis following previous open mesenteric revascularization. Prophylactic mesenteric revascularization is rarely performed in the asymptomatic patient undergoing an aortic procedure for other indications [12]. However, the natural history of untreated chronic mesenteric ischemia may justify revascularization in some minimally symptomatic or asymptomatic patients if the operative risks are acceptable, since the first clinical presentation may be acute intestinal ischemia in as many as 50 % of the patients, with a mortality rate that ranges from 15 to 70 % [13]. This is particularly true when the SMA is involved. Mesenteric angioplasty and stenting are particularly suitable for this patient subgroup, given its low morbidity and mortality. Because of the limited experience with stent use in mesenteric vessels, appropriate indications for primary stent placement have not been clearly defined. Guidelines generally include calcified ostial stenoses, high-grade eccentric stenoses, chronic occlusions, and significant residual stenoses >30 % or the presence of dissection after angioplasty. Restenosis after PTA is also an indication for stent placement [3, 13–16].

Endovascular Technique

To perform endovascular mesenteric revascularization, intraluminal access is performed via a femoral or brachial artery approach. Once an introducer sheath is placed in the femoral artery, an anteroposterior and lateral aortogram just below the level of the diaphragm is obtained with a pigtail catheter to identify the origin of the CA and SMA. Initial catheterization of the mesenteric artery can be performed using a variety of selective angled catheters, which include the RDC, Cobra-2, Simmons I (Boston Scientific/Meditech, Natick, MA), or SOS Omni catheter (AngioDynamics, Queensbury, NY). Once the mesenteric artery is cannulated, systemic heparin (5,000 IU) is administered intravenously. A selective mesenteric angiogram is then performed to identify the diseased segment, which is followed by the placement of a 0.035 or less traumatic 0.014–0.018 guidewire to cross the stenotic lesion. Once the guidewire is placed across the stenosis, the catheter is carefully advanced over the guidewire across the lesion. In the event that the mesenteric artery is severely angulated as it arises from the aorta, a second stiffer guidewire (Amplatz or Rosen Guidewire, Boston Scientific) may be exchanged through the catheter to facilitate the placement of a 6-Fr guiding sheath (Pinnacle, Boston Scientific).

With the image intensifier angled in a lateral position to fully visualize the proximal mesenteric segment, a balloon angioplasty is advanced over the guidewire through the guiding sheath and positioned across the stenosis. The balloon diameter should be chosen based on the vessel size of the adjacent normal mesenteric vessel. Once balloon angioplasty is completed, a post-angioplasty angiogram is necessary to document the procedural result. Radiographic evidence of either residual stenosis or mesenteric artery dissection constitutes suboptimal angioplasty results which warrants mesenteric stent placement. Moreover, atherosclerotic involvement of the proximal mesenteric artery or vessel orifice should be treated with a balloon expandable stent placement. These stents can be placed over a low-profile 0.014 or 0.018 guidewire system. It is preferable to deliver the balloon-mounted stent through a guiding sheath, which is positioned just proximal to the mesenteric orifice while the balloon-mounted stent is advanced across the stenosis. The stent is next deployed by expanding the angioplasty balloon to its designated inflation pressure. The balloon is then deflated and carefully withdrawn through the guiding sheath.

Completion angiogram is performed by hand injecting a small volume of contrast though the guiding sheath. It is critical to maintain the guidewire access until satisfactory completion angiogram is obtained. If the completion angiogram reveals suboptimal radiographic results, such as residual stenosis or dissection, additional catheter-based intervention can be performed through the same guidewire. These interventions may include repeat balloon angioplasty for residual stenosis or additional stent placement for mesenteric artery dissection. During the procedure, intra-arterial infusion of papaverine or nitroglycerine can be used to decrease vasospasm. Administration of antiplatelet agents is also recommended for at least 6 months or even indefinitely if other risk factors of cardiovascular disease are present [4, 14, 17].

Complications are not common and rarely become life threatening. These include access sites thrombosis, hematomas, and infection. Dissection can occur during PTA and is managed with placement of a stent. Balloon-mounted stents are preferred over the self-expanding ones because of the higher radial force and the more precise placement. Distal embolization has also been reported, but it never resulted in acute intestinal ischemia, likely due to the rich network of collaterals already developed [18].

Thrombolytic Therapy for Acute Mesenteric Ischemia

Catheter-directed thrombolytic therapy is a potentially useful treatment modality for acute mesenteric ischemia, which can be initiated with intra-arterial delivery of thrombolytic agent into the mesenteric thrombus at the time of diagnostic angiography. Various thrombolytic medications, including urokinase (Abbokinase, Abbott Laboratory, North Chicago, IL) or recombinant tissue plasminogen activator (Activase, Genentech, South San Francisco, CA), have been reported to be successful in a small series of case reports. Catheter-directed thrombolytic therapy has a higher probability of restoring mesenteric blood flow success when performed within 12 h of symptom onset. Successful resolution of a mesenteric thrombus will facilitate the identification of the underlying mesenteric occlusive disease process. As a result, subsequent operative mesenteric revascularization or mesenteric balloon angioplasty and stenting may be performed electively to correct the mesenteric stenosis. There are two main drawbacks with regard to thrombolytic therapy in mesenteric ischemia. Percutaneous catheter-directed thrombolysis does not allow the possibility to inspect the potentially ischemic intestine following restoration of the mesenteric flow. Additionally, a prolonged period of time may be necessary in order to achieve successful catheter-directed thrombolysis, due in part to serial angiographic surveillance to document thrombus resolution. An incomplete or unsuccessful thrombolysis may lead to delayed operative revascularization, which may further necessitate bowel resection for irreversible intestinal necrosis. Therefore, catheter-directed thrombolytic therapy for acute mesenteric ischemia should only be considered in selected patients under a closely scrutinized clinical protocol.

Nonocclusive Mesenteric Ischemia

The treatment of nonocclusive mesenteric ischemia is primarily pharmacologic with selective mesenteric arterial catheterization followed by infusion of vasodilatory agents, such as tolazoline or papaverine. Once the diagnosis is made on the mesenteric arteriography, intra-arterial papaverine is given at a dose of 30–60 mg/h. This must be coupled with the cessation of other vasoconstricting agents. Concomitant intravenous heparin should be administered to prevent thrombosis in the cannulated vessels. Treatment strategy thereafter is dependent on the patient's clinical response to the vasodilator therapy. If abdominal symptoms improve, mesenteric arteriography should be repeated to document the resolution of vasospasm. The patient's hemodynamic status must be carefully monitored during papaverine infusion as significant hypotension can develop in the event that the infusion catheter migrates into the aorta which can lead to systemic circulation of papaverine. Surgical exploration is indicated if the patient develops signs of continued bowel ischemia or infarction as evidenced by rebound tenderness or involuntary guarding. In these circumstances, papaverine infusion should be continued intraoperatively and postoperatively. The operating room should be kept as warm as possible, and warm irrigation fluid and laparotomy pads should be used to prevent further intestinal vasoconstriction during exploration.

Treatment of Celiac Artery Compression Syndrome

Abdominal pain due to narrowing of the origin of the CA may occur as a result of extrinsic compression or impingement by the median arcuate ligament. This condition is known as celiac artery compression syndrome, or median arcuate ligament syndrome. The celiac artery compression syndrome has been implicated in some variants of chronic mesenteric ischemia. Most patients are young females between 20 and 40 years of age. Abdominal symptom is nonspecific, but the pain is localized in the upper abdomen, which may be precipitated by meals. The treatment goal is to release the ligamentous structure which compresses the proximal CA and correct any persistent stricture by bypass grafting. In a number of reports on endovascular management of chronic mesenteric ischemia, the presence of CA compression syndrome has been identified as a major factor of technical failure and recurrence. Therefore, angioplasty and stenting should not be undertaken if extrinsic compression of the CA by the median arcuate ligament is suspected based on preoperative imaging studies. Open surgical treatment should be performed instead [9–11].

Results from Clinical Series

The first successful percutaneous angioplasty of the SMA was reported in 1980 [19]. Since 1995, 11 series and multiple scattered case reports have reported results from endovascular management of mesenteric occlusive disease. In a recent literature review, AbuRahma et al. [18] showed that endovascular intervention had overall technical success rate of 91 %, early and late pain relief 84 and 71 %, respectively, and 30-day morbidity and mortality rates of 16.4 and 4.3 %, respectively. The average patency was 63 % during an average 26-month follow-up.

In our review of the literature [7] from series since 1995, restenosis was developed in 22 % of patients during 24.5 months of average follow-up. The long-term clinical relief without re-intervention was 82 %. Among the patients that had a technical failure, 15 were ultimately diagnosed with median arcuate ligament syndrome and underwent successful surgical treatment, an observation that emphasizes the need for careful patient selection. Interestingly, the addition of selective stenting after PTA was started in 1998; while it slightly increases the technical success rate, it is not correlated with any substantial overall clinical benefit or improved long-term patency rates.

In contrast to the endovascular treatment, open surgical techniques have achieved an immediate clinical success that approaches 100 %, surgical mortality rate from 0 to 17 %, and an operative morbidity rate of that ranges from 19 to 54 % in a number of different series [2, 6, 12, 13, 20–27]. AbuRahma and colleagues reported their experience of endovascular interventions of 22 patients with symptomatic mesenteric ischemia due to either SMA or CA stenosis [18]. They noted an excellent initial technical and clinical success rate, which were 96 % (23/24) and 95 % (21/22), respectively, with no perioperative mortality or major morbidity. During a mean follow-up of 26 months (range 1–54), the primary late clinical success rate was 61 %, and freedom from recurrent stenosis was 30 %. The freedom from recurrent stenosis at 1, 2, 3, and 4 years were 65, 47, 39, and 13 %, respectively. The authors concluded that mesenteric stenting, which provides excellent early results, is associated with a relative high incidence of late restenosis [18].

Several studies have attempted to compare the endovascular to standard open surgical approach [12, 13]. The results of the open surgery appear to be more durable but tend to be associated with higher morbidity and mortality rates and an overall longer hospital stay. In one study which compared the clinical outcome of open revascularization with percutaneous stenting for patients with chronic mesenteric ischemia, 28 patients underwent endovascular treatment and 85 patients underwent open mesenteric bypass grafting [12]. With both patient cohorts having similar baseline comorbidities and symptom duration, there was no difference in early inhospital complication or mortality rate. Moreover, both groups had similar 3-year cumulative recurrent stenosis and mortality rate. However, patients treated with mesenteric stenting had a significantly higher incidence of recurrent symptoms. The authors concluded that operative mesenteric revascularization should be offered to patients with low surgical risk [12].

Based on the above results, one could argue that mesenteric angioplasty and stenting demonstrate an inferior technical and clinical success rate. Long-term patency rates appear to also be superior with the open technique. There is a general consensus, however, that the endovascular approach is associated with lower morbidity and mortality rates and is therefore more suitable for high-risk patients. One should also keep in mind that practices representing standard of care for stent placement today were absent in the early era of endovascular experience. These include perioperative heparinization and short-term antiplatelet therapy, use of stents with higher radial force, routine use of postoperative surveillance with arterial duplex and early re-intervention to prevent a high-grade stenosis to progress to occlusion, and placement of drug-eluting stents.

Conclusion

Mesenteric ischemia is a rare but life-threatening condition. Open surgical reconstruction was traditionally considered the treatment of choice. Endovascular strategies have recently emerged and offer a viable alternative, associated with decreased morbidity and mortality. It is anticipated that improving technical skills, advances in technology and refinement of stent characteristics, as well as introduction of drug-eluting stents will broaden the indications for stent placement, improve the overall efficacy and patency rates, and finally redefine the role of the endovascular approach.

References

1. Dunphy J. Abdominal pain of vascular origin. Am J Med Sci. 1936;192:109–12.
2. Zelenock GB, Graham LM, Whitehouse Jr WM, et al. Splanchnic arteriosclerotic disease and intestinal angina. Arch Surg. 1980;115(4):497–501.
3. Maspes F, Mazzetti di Pietralata G, Gandini R, et al. Percutaneous transluminal angioplasty in the treatment of chronic mesenteric ischemia: results and 3 years of follow-up in 23 patients. Abdom Imaging. 1998;23(4):358–63.
4. Allen RC, Martin GH, Rees CR, et al. Mesenteric angioplasty in the treatment of chronic intestinal ischemia. J Vasc Surg. 1996;24(3):415–21; discussion 421–3.
5. Moneta GL, Yeager RA, Dalman R, et al. Duplex ultrasound criteria for diagnosis of splanchnic artery stenosis or occlusion. J Vasc Surg. 1991;14(4):511–8; discussion 518–20.
6. Moneta GL, Lee RW, Yeager RA, et al. Mesenteric duplex scanning: a blinded prospective study. J Vasc Surg. 1993;17(1):79–84; discussion 85–6.
7. Kougias P, Lau D, El Sayed HF, et al. Determinants of mortality and treatment outcome following surgical interventions for acute mesenteric ischemia. J Vasc Surg. 2007;46(3):467–74.
8. Kougias P, El Sayed HF, Zhou W, et al. Management of chronic mesenteric ischemia. The role of endovascular therapy. J Endovasc Ther. 2007;14(3):395–405.
9. Park WM, Gloviczki P, Cherry Jr KJ, et al. Contemporary management of acute mesenteric ischemia: factors associated with survival. J Vasc Surg. 2002;35(3):445–52.
10. Park WM, Cherry Jr KJ, Chua HK, et al. Current results of open revascularization for chronic mesenteric ischemia: a standard for comparison. J Vasc Surg. 2002;35(5):853–9.
11. Sheeran SR, Murphy TP, Khwaja A, et al. Stent placement for treatment of mesenteric artery stenoses or occlusions. J Vasc Interv Radiol. 1999;10(7):861–7.
12. Kasirajan K, O'Hara PJ, Gray BH, et al. Chronic mesenteric ischemia: open surgery versus percutaneous angioplasty and stenting. J Vasc Surg. 2001;33(1):63–71.
13. Rose SC, Quigley TM, Raker EJ. Revascularization for chronic mesenteric ischemia: comparison of operative arterial bypass grafting and percutaneous transluminal angioplasty. J Vasc Interv Radiol. 1995;6(3):339–49.
14. Nyman U, Ivancev K, Lindh M, et al. Endovascular treatment of chronic mesenteric ischemia: report of five cases. Cardiovasc Intervent Radiol. 1998;21(4):305–13.
15. Matsumoto AH, Angle JF, Spinosa DJ, et al. Percutaneous transluminal angioplasty and stenting in the treatment of chronic mesenteric ischemia: results and long term follow up. J Am Coll Surg. 2002;194(1 suppl):S22–31.
16. Pietura R, Szymanska A, El Furah M, et al. Chronic mesenteric ischemia: diagnosis and treatment with balloon angioplasty and stenting. Med Sci Monit. 2002;8(1):PR8–12.
17. Hallisey MJ, Deschaine J, Illescas FF, et al. Angioplasty for the treatment of visceral ischemia. J Vasc Interv Radiol. 1995;6(5):785–91.
18. AbuRahma AF, Stone PA, Bates MC, et al. Angioplasty/stenting of the superior mesenteric artery and celiac trunk: early and late outcomes. J Endovasc Ther. 2003;10(6):1046–53.
19. Furrer J, Gruntzig A, Kugelmeier J, et al. Treatment of abdominal angina with percutaneous dilatation of an arteria mesenterica superior stenosis. Preliminary communication. Cardiovasc Intervent Radiol. 1980; 3(1):43–4.
20. Derrow AE, Seeger JM, Dame DA, et al. The outcome in the United States after thoracoabdominal aortic aneurysm repair, renal artery bypass, and mesenteric revascularization. J Vasc Surg. 2001;34(1):54–61.
21. Mateo RB, O'Hara PJ, Hertzer NR, et al. Elective surgical treatment of symptomatic chronic mesenteric occlusive disease: early results and late outcomes. J Vasc Surg. 1999;29(5):821–31; discussion 832.
22. Foley MI, Moneta GL, Abou-Zamzam Jr AM, et al. Revascularization of the superior mesenteric artery alone for treatment of intestinal ischemia. J Vasc Surg. 2000;32(1):37–47.
23. Johnston KW, Lindsay TF, Walker PM, et al. Mesenteric arterial bypass grafts: early and late results and suggested surgical approach for chronic and acute mesenteric ischemia. Surgery. 1995;118(1):1–7.
24. McAfee MK, Cherry Jr KJ, Naessens JM, et al. Influence of complete revascularization on chronic mesenteric ischemia. Am J Surg. 1992;164(3):220–4.
25. Cunningham CG, Reilly LM, Stoney R. Chronic visceral ischemia. Surg Clin North Am. 1992;72(1):231–44.
26. Rheudasil JM, Stewart MT, Schellack JV, et al. Surgical treatment of chronic mesenteric arterial insufficiency. J Vasc Surg. 1988;8(4):495–500.
27. McMillan WD, McCarthy WJ, Bresticker MR, et al. Mesenteric artery bypass: objective patency determination. J Vasc Surg. 1995;21(5):729–40; discussion740–1.

Treatment of Renal Artery Stenosis and Fibromuscular Dysplasia

14

Daynene Vykoukal, Javier E. Anaya-Ayala, and Mark G. Davies

Abstract
Interventions for renal arterial disease are primarily driven by functional consequences of the disease. These are poorly controlled hypertension, increasing renal dysfunction (often associated with loss of renal mass), and, more recently, control of congestive heart failure. The dominant causes are atherosclerotic stenosis and fibromuscular dysplasia. Good interventional technique allows for precise definition of the lesions, safe intervention, and appropriate interpretation of the end result. Strict adherence to the gold standard indications for intervention results in good long-term functional results.

Keywords
Renal angioplasty • Renal stenting • Atherosclerosis • Fibromuscular dysplasia • Technique • Outcomes • Complications

Atherosclerotic Renal Artery Stenosis

Epidemiology

Renal artery stenosis (RAS) is an important underlying cause of secondary hypertension and causes chronic renal failure in 10–20 % of the cases [1]. With the aging of the patient population, the prevalence of renovascular disease as a cause of hypertension has also increased during the past 25 years [2]. Although RAS is often seen in patients with hypertension, all types of major renal artery stenoses can be found in both normotensive and hypertensive patients. The prevalence of renovascular hypertension in the general population is between 4 and 33 % [3]. However, in angiographic studies, this disease was found in 32–49 % of normotensive elderly patients with atherosclerosis [4, 5]. The prevalence of RAS ranges from 4 to 50 % in autopsy studies of unselected patients. The association of RAS and extrarenal atherosclerosis (peripheral, coronary, or carotid artery disease) ranges from 5 to 40 %

D. Vykoukal, Ph.D. • J.E. Anaya-Ayala, M.D.
M.G. Davies, M.D., Ph.D., M.B.A. (✉)
Department of Cardiovascular Surgery,
Methodist DeBakey Heart and Vascular Center,
The Methodist Hospital,
6550 Fannin, Smith Tower, Suite 1401,
Houston, TX 77030, USA
e-mail: mdavies@tmhs.org

J.J. Hoballah, A.B. Lumsden (eds.), *Vascular Surgery*, New Techniques in Surgery Series,
DOI 10.1007/978-1-4471-2912-7_14, © Springer-Verlag London 2012

[6, 7]. In patients with peripheral or coronary artery disease undergoing abdominal aortography, the prevalence of unsuspected renal artery stenosis ranges from 14 % to as high as 49 %. Elevated serum cholesterol concentration [8, 9], impaired renal function [9], a history of coronary artery disease [7, 10], and a history of smoking [7, 8] are associated predictors of renal artery stenosis. The cumulative incidence of RAS progression was 35 % at 3 years and 51 % at 5 years. The 3-year cumulative incidence of renal artery disease progression stratified by baseline disease classification was 18, 28, and 49 % for renal arteries initially classified as normal, <60 % stenosis, and ≥60 % stenosis, respectively ($P=0.03$, log-rank test) [11]. There were only 9 renal artery occlusions in 295 kidneys intervened on during the study, all of which occurred in renal arteries having ≥60 % stenosis at the examination before the detection of occlusion. The risk of renal artery disease progression during follow-up was linked to systolic blood pressure ≥ 160 mmHg, diabetes mellitus, and high-grade (>60 % stenosis or occlusion) disease in either the ipsilateral or contralateral renal artery [11]. The 2-year cumulative incidence (CI) of renal atrophy was 5.5, 11.7, and 20.8 % in kidneys with a baseline renal artery disease classification of normal, <60 % stenosis, and ≥60 % stenosis, respectively [12]. Factors associated with a high risk of renal atrophy included a systolic blood pressure > 180 mmHg, a renal artery peak systolic velocity > 400 cm/s, and a renal cortical end diastolic velocity ≤ 5 cm/s. The occurrence of renal atrophy is well correlated with changes in the serum creatinine concentration [12].

Indications

In general, the standard indications for intervention on renal artery stenosis are the presence of hypertension poorly controlled on four medications, a rising serum creatinine, and/or a decrease in renal mass measured by pole-to-pole length. A newer indication is poorly controlled congestive heart failure and flash pulmonary edema.

Outcomes

Mortality and Morbidity

Renal artery stenting has a low mortality rate and a relatively high complication rate that can be separated into local complications at the access site in the arm or groin and those at the site of intervention and within the parenchyma of the kidney. Martin et al. reviewed complication rates from two large series and two meta-analyses to determine weighted complication rates [13]. Periprocedural complication rates ranged from 12 to 36 %, the majority of which were related to the access site. The incidence of secondary nephrectomy is <1 %, and 30-day mortality rates are reported up to 3 % [14]. Nephrectomy may be required in instances of uncontrollable renal artery bleeding, occlusion, or dissection that cannot be managed with endovascular techniques. Common causes of mortality with renal artery stenting include hemorrhage, acute renal failure, cholesterol embolization, sepsis, and aortic dissection [14].

Anatomic

Technical success of angioplasty and/or stenting runs between 82 and 100 %. In studies of angioplasty, success is higher for nonostial lesions (72–82 %) than for ostial lesions (60–62 %). We recently demonstrated that renal interventions have 82 % primary patency and a 100 % primary assisted patency at 5 years [15].

Functional

Renal artery stenosis is an independent predictor of mortality. At 7 years, 73 % of patients with renal artery stenosis are dead [16]. The 7-year mortality in this study for patients with a solitary kidney was 66 %, which is equivalent to untreated disease and was significantly higher than those patients with two kidneys (32 % at 7 years). Similar to the current study, immediate and long-term postprocedure creatinine deterioration and dialysis dependency have been associated with increased mortality [15, 17, 18]. Elevated creatinine has already been shown to affect survival after therapy for renal artery stenosis despite adequate revascularization [15, 17, 18]. After simple angioplasty in all comers, improvement or cure of the blood pressure has been reported as 66–100 %, and improvement or stabilization of the renal functions was reported as 38–100 % [19–22]. In contrast, after primary stent placement, improvement or cure of the blood pressure was reported as 44–100 %, and improvement or stabilization of the renal functions was reported as 24–100 % [23–29]. Metabolic syndrome is associated with markedly reduced renal clinical benefit and increased progression to hemodialysis following endovascular intervention for atherosclerotic renal artery stenosis [30]. The recent ASTRAL trial has questioned the role of percutaneous transluminal renal angioplasty (PTRA) for symptomatic renal disease with the randomized study showing no significant benefit over best medical therapy. A review of the results of multiple clinical reports, which used accepted reporting standards, is shown in Table 14.1.

Recurrent Disease

Restenosis following renal angioplasty remains a considerable drawback of both angioplasty and primary stenting of renal artery stenosis, with rates of restenosis ranging from 15 to 20 % [13, 15, 17, 31–36]. Restenosis is strongly correlated with recurrent symptoms. Restenosis is more frequent in females, and about 80 % of cases are associated with recurrent symptoms. Patients with diabetes and prior restenosis have a higher rate of in-stent restenosis [37], and there is a correlation with prolonged in-stent thrombus and hyperglycemia [38]. Risk factors for late stent thrombosis include penetration of necrotic core, malapposition, overlapping stent placement, excessive stent length, and bifurcation lesions. In the Single Operator, Single Center, Renal Stent Retrospective Study (SOCRATES), 10 % of the vessels required reintervention, and this was best predicted by patient age ≤ 67 years, stent diameter ≤ 5.0 mm, solitary functioning kidney, history of lower extremity peripheral artery disease, and antecedent history of stroke [35]. Reintervention is safe and technically effective. At 5 years, anatomic and functional outcomes are equivalent. Outcomes in recurrent lesions are influenced by statins, contralateral kidney size (>9 cm), and a ≥20 % improvement in baseline creatinine within 3 months [39].

Solitary Kidney

Up to one-third of renal interventions are for solitary kidneys. At the present time, there are no unique established criteria for endovascular treatment of renal artery stenosis in a solitary functioning kidney. One criterion suggested has been kidney size, as it is reported that a pole-to-pole length of less than 8 cm is a significant predictor that revascularization will not help in improving renal function [40]. A second criterion is the anatomic location of the stenosis as an ostial localization, which has a more favorable outcome than a peripheral lesion [23, 41]. A third criterion is the degree of stenosis present, with >70 % having a better outcome. A final criterion is the state and rate of decline of the renal insufficiency [42–45]. There were no significant differences in mortality or morbidity between solitary kidney and dual kidney patients. There was a significant difference in the long-term survival with 55 ± 8 % patients with a normal contralateral kidney vs. 27 ± 7 % patients with a solitary functioning kidney alive at 10 years. Clinical benefit is equivalent at 10 years between solitary functioning kidney and normal contralateral groups. Predictors of long-term clinical benefit are ipsilateral kidney size (>9 cm), no immediate deterioration in function, and an eGFR > 30 mL/min/1.73 m^2 [46].

EVAR

Renal artery revascularization during endovascular aortic aneurysm repair (EVAR) should be considered higher risk than primary renal interventions for atherosclerotic disease. There were no significant differences in mortality or morbidity compared to the isolated renal artery stenting procedure. There is a higher incidence of procedural complications, early functional injury, and early occlusion rates. However, the long-term sequelae and benefits are similar to those of renal revascularization procedure in the absence of EVAR [47]. As a result, a cautious approach

Table 14.1 Treatment outcomes: percutaneous intervention for atherosclerotic renal artery stenosis

Author	Year	*n*	Bilateral treatment (%)	Preoperative renal dysfunction (%)	Renal function response (%)			Hypertension response (%)			Perioperative outcome (%)	
					Improved	Unchanged	Worsened	Cured	Improved	Failed	Death	Morbidity
Burke	2000	127	NR	29	43	57	NR	NR	NR	NR	2	4
Lederman	2001	300	41	37	9	78	14	70	NR	30	<1	2
Bush	2001	73	16	68	23	51	14	NR	NR	NR	1.4	9
Yutan	2001	76	41	65	10	76	26	18	53	29	3.8	5
Rocha-Singh	2002	51	55	100	77	18	5	91	NR	9	0	14
Kennedy	2003	361	NR	36	61	NR	39	NR	NR	NR	NR	NR
Gill	2003	100	36	75	31	38	31	4	79	17	2	18
Zeller	2003	215	23	52	52	48		76		24	0	5
Henry	2003	56	14	32	14	66	13	18	59	23	1.8	NR
Sivamurthy	2004	146	37	55	11	75	0	13	39	48	0.7	4
Zeller	2004	456	NR	52	34	39	27	46		54	1	NR
Nolan	2005	82	NR	59	23	53	24	NR	81	NR	0	7
Kayshap	2007	125	36	100	42	23	25	NR	NR	NR	1.6	6
Holden	2006	63	32	100	97	NR	3	0	55	45	NR	NR
Corriere	2008	99	11	75	78	65	7	1	21	78	0	5.5
Davies	2009	418	37	42	8	80	12	5	35	60	0	2
		Median	*36*	*57*	*33*	*55*	*14*	*18*	*54*	*30*	*1.2*	*5.5*

NR not reported

should be taken when faced with asymptomatic renal artery stenosis. Unless there are appropriate symptoms and indications, renal artery stenting should not be prophylactically performed. If there is concern for ostial compromise with placement of the EVAR device due to atherosclerotic disease, then stenting should be considered. Renal stenting in the presence of aneurysm is associated with parenchymal injury, and, therefore, staging renal stenting before aneurysm repair appears to be less beneficial than fixing the aneurysm first and dealing with the renals at an interval from the EVAR. There is no current data on the use of renal distal protection devices and EVAR.

Fibromuscular Dysplasia

Epidemiology

Fibromuscular dysplasia (FMD) can result in significant hypertension in women between 15 and 50 years of age but only accounts for less than 10 % of cases of renovascular hypertension [48]. First described in 1938 [49], FMD frequently involves the distal main renal artery and its branches [48]. While FMD has been shown to affect multiple arterial beds, the frequency of involvement in renal arteries is 60–70 %, with bilateral disease occurring in 35 % of patients. The natural history of renal FMD is progression in up to 37 % of patients [50], but this progression only rarely results in occlusion of the renal artery [51]. Patients with FMD do demonstrate a significant decrease in mean cortical thickness and reduced renal length compared to comparable patients with essential hypertension. While up to 63 % of patients with FMD experience a loss of renal mass, the incidence of renal failure remains remarkably low [50, 52].

Indications

The main impetus for the treatment of FMD is control of hypertension and its attendant complications. The majority of patients can be primarily managed medically. Revascularization is reserved for those patients who have recent onset of hypertension with the primary goal to cure the hypertension, those in whom blood pressure control has proved difficult, those intolerant of antihypertensive therapy, those who are not compliant with their antihypertensive medication, and those who have demonstrated a loss of renal volume leading to a diagnosis of ischemic nephropathy [53]. The primary mode of intervention is by balloon angioplasty, with surgery reserved for recalcitrant lesions.

Outcomes

Mortality and Morbidity

Interventions for FMD are associated with a very low procedural mortality rate and a relatively low major morbidity rate. The majority of complications occur at the access site in the arm or groin. Rates of atheroembolism into the kidney or during the procedure are relatively low because of the nature of the disease. The most common renal-related morbidity is dissection and rupture of the renal artery due to the nature of the disease.

Anatomic

Percutaneous transluminal renal angioplasty has become the treatment of choice for patients with renal artery FMD, with the literature reporting technical success rates ranging from 83 to 100 % [54–60]. Success rates with open revascularization range from 89 to 97 % [61–63]. Restenosis rates after PTRA for FMD range from 7 to 27 % in the literature [54–60]. Clinical factors associated with restenosis following initial PTRA include increased body mass index and duration and degree of hypertension [64]. Oertle et al. [65] have shown that about one-third of patients treated by PTRA for FMD who subsequently return during follow-up with deterioration of/or recurrent arterial hypertension have no angiographic demonstrable restenosis, whereas 15 % of patients without deterioration of/or recurrent arterial hypertension have angiographic demonstrable restenosis. In the one study, dyslipidemia (low HDL and high triglycerides), low eGFR

Table 14.2 Treatment outcomes: percutaneous intervention for renal artery fibromuscular dysplasia

Author	Year	*n*	Technical success (%)	Hypertension response (%)				Perioperative outcome (%)	
				Cured/ improved	Cured	Improved	Failed	Death	Morbidity
Sos	1983	31	87	93	59	34	7	0	6
Baert	1990	22	83	79	58	21	21	0	NR
Tegtmeyer	1991	66	100	98	39	59	2	0	3
Borrelli	1995	105	89	85	22	63	15	0	NR
Jensen	1995	30	97	86	39	47	14	0	15
Davidson	1996	23	100	74	52	22	26	0	13
Klow	1998	49	98	70	26	44	30	0	0
Birrer	2002	27	100	93	NR	NR	7	0	7.4
Mounier-Vehier	2002	20	100	97	NR	NR	3	NR	NR
Surowiec	2003	14	95	74	NR	NR	26	0	28.5
deFraissinette	2003	70	94	88	14	74	12	0	11
Alhadad	2005	67	95	84	NR	NR	16	0	32
Davies	2008	29	100	73	NR	NR	27	0	8
Kim	2008	16	79	80	7	73	20	0	16
Barrier	2010	60	82	74	NR	NR	26	0	30
		Median	*95*	*84*	*39*	*47*	*16*	*0*	*12*

NR not reported

(<30 mL/min/1.73 m^2), and patients older than 55 years were factors associated with the development of restenosis.

Functional

A review of the results of multiple clinical reports, which used accepted reporting standards, is shown in Table 14.2. Hypertension cure rates of 14–59 % and hypertension improvement rates of 21–63 % have been reported [54–60]. The incidence of "no effect" with endoluminal intervention ranges from 7 to 30 % [50]. With open surgery, cure of hypertension can be obtained in 33–63 % of patients with improvements in hypertension noted in 24–57 % of patients. The incidence of failure (i.e., "no effect" on hypertension) ranges from 3 to 33 %. Successful outcome appears to be associated with an age <50 years, the absence of associated coronary and carotid stenosis, and duration of hypertension less than 8 years. In the current study, we also identified the duration of hypertension as a significant factor related to successful outcome. However, we also identified an association with decreased long-term clinical benefit and a cluster of variables associated with metabolic syndrome—a fasting blood sugar > 110 mg/dL, triglycerides > 150 mg/dL, and HDL ≤ 50 mg/dL.

Techniques

Preoperative

Preoperative preparation for a renal angiogram should consist of prehydration with normal saline (0.9 %) and the use of a mucomyst (*N*-acetylcysteine) or bicarbonate infusion protocol if the creatinine is >1.5 mg/dL or eGFR < 60. Antihypertensives should be reviewed and the dose reduced. Oral hypoglycemics should also be reviewed and held as appropriate. If intervention is intended, then loading with clopidogrel 150–330 mg is advisable.

Approach

A femoral or a brachial approach is acceptable for renal intervention and is dictated by the preference of the physician, the anatomy of the access sites, and the orientation of the renal artery. Care should be taken when traversing the aortic arch and placing catheters to avoid atheroembolism.

Diagnostic

A flush abdominal aortogram should be performed using a right oblique view, and then selective catheterization of the renal can be performed using either a contact or no contact technique. The renal angiogram should display the entire renal and the parenchyma and be allowed to clear to demonstrate the late filling of the renal venous system. In the setting of significant renal insufficiency, CO_2 angiography can be performed to outline the renal ostium and gain entry and identify the lesion. 3D fusion imaging is now available in certain imaging systems to allow overlay preoperative studies using anatomic landmarks to guide the intervention. Intravascular ultrasound (IVUS) can be used to assess and define the lesion prior to intervention. Access to the ostium can be performed using a touch or no-touch technique to avoid scraping the wall and dislodging plaque.

Intervention

When an appropriate atherosclerotic lesion is found, the operator should determine the severity with pullback pressures or IVUS. Thereafter, the operator has the option of primary stenting with a balloon-mounted stent or predilating to allow the stent platform and delivery system to traverse the stenosis. Femoral or brachial approaches may be used, and the operators' preferential system (0.035-, 0.018-, or 0.014-in. guidewire) can be utilized to deliver a stent or a balloon (Figs. 14.1, 14.2, and 14.3). Very tight lesions are best predilated to avoid displacing a stent from the balloon. Stenting is important for ostial lesions as this reflects aortic disease. Balloon-expandable stents are typically utilized for renal arteries. Closed-cell stent designs are preferred, as they provide more radial strength at the renal ostium. Stent-to-artery ratio should be kept to 10 % of the reference renal artery diameter to ensure apposition and avoid complications. Care should also be taken so that 1–2 mm of the stent extends into the aorta in order to ensure that the ostium of the renal artery is covered. Balloon angioplasty or stenting is appropriate for proximal middle and distal renal artery lesions. Balloon angioplasty is the primary mode of intervention in FMD.

Distal Protection Devices

Renal protection is advised in management of renal artery stenosis in the solitary kidney, where any atheroembolism carries significant morbidity. In the presence of two kidneys, distal protection should be considered in patients with renal insufficiency. In such cases, endovascular intervention using distal protection devices resulted in 4- to 6-week postintervention renal function results approximating those of surgical revascularization [66].

Completion Studies

Completion studies should be performed which consist of two-dimensional or rotation angiography, repeat pullback pressures, or completion IVUS to ensure appropriate lesion correction and apposition of the stent to the wall.

Postoperative Care

The patient should be monitored for access-site complications and hydration maintained. Blood pressure should be monitored to ensure no rebound hypotension and remaining medications should be restarted.

Management of Complications

Arterial

Occlusion

The incidence of renal artery occlusion rates is between 0.8 and 2.5 % [13]. Surgical bypass or renal vessel reimplantation are traditional approaches that have been used, based upon a few reports in the literature, to salvage a threatened kidney [67, 68]. In recent years, however, thrombolysis has gained significant favor. A few reports relay the success of thrombolytic therapy in cases of acute renal artery occlusion following failed endovascular intervention [68, 69]. Generally, the presence of a normal contralateral kidney will lessen the need for surgical action. Surgery is mandatory, however, in the case of bilateral renal artery occlusion or when a solitary kidney is affected [70].

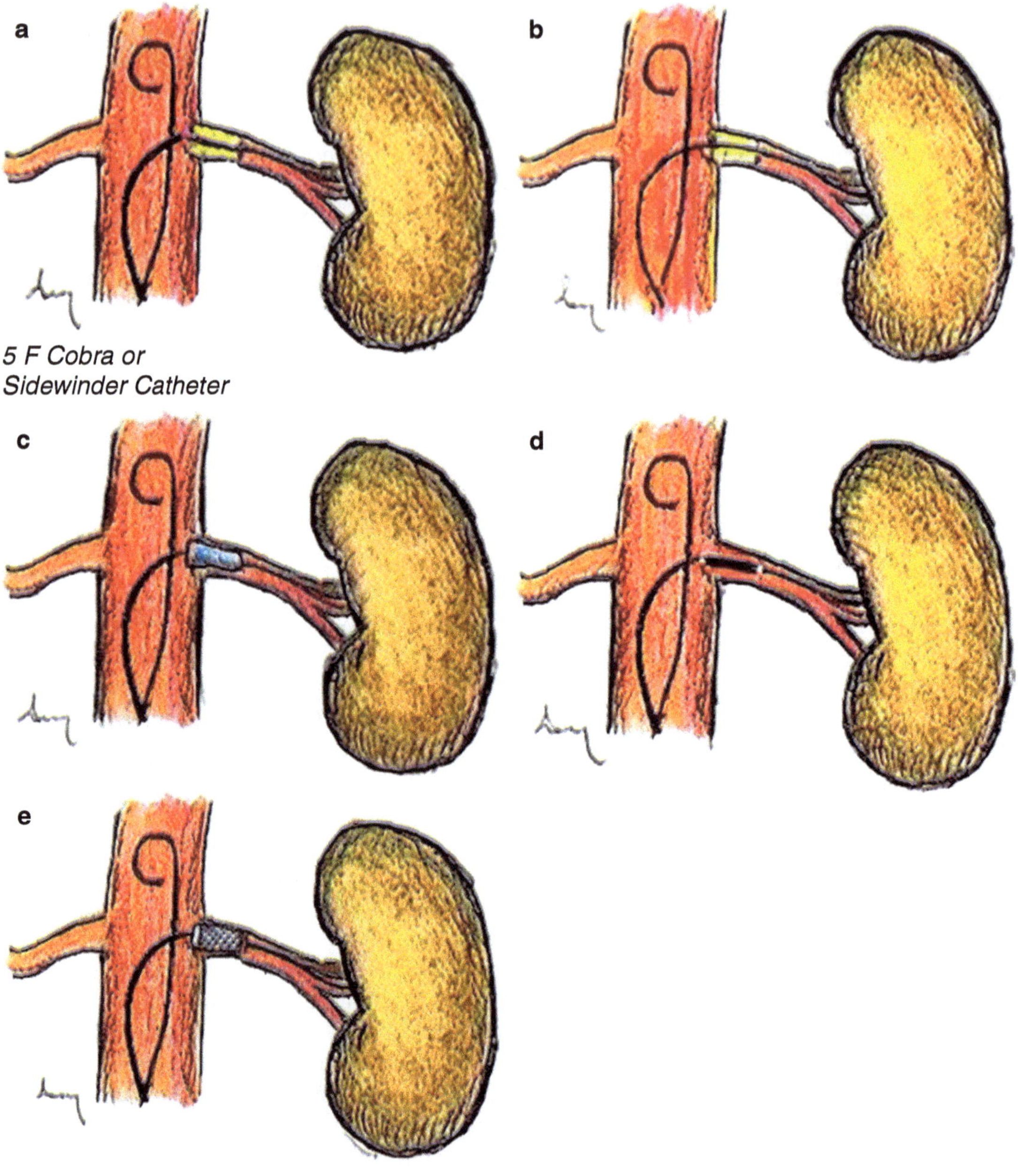

Fig. 14.1 Renal artery stenting using the guidewire technique. (**a**) A standard guidewire is advanced into the aorta from a femoral approach. The shape, type, and diameter of the wire will depend on the operator's preferences and the therapeutic platform to be used. An angled catheter is used to engage the renal. A pigtail catheter may be positioned cranial to the renal artery orifice via the right groin to confirm device position during the following steps: (**b**) guidewire and pigtail catheter in position and diagnostic catheter withdrawn, (**c**) predilation of the stenosis, (**d**) stent positioned at the stenosis, and (**e**) final angiogram via the pigtail catheter, showing the stent implanted and the balloon withdrawn (Adapted from Zeller T, J Endovasc Ther. 2004;11(Suppl 2):II96–106. Illustrations used with permission from the Department of Cardiovascular Surgery, Methodist DeBakey Heart & Vascular Center)

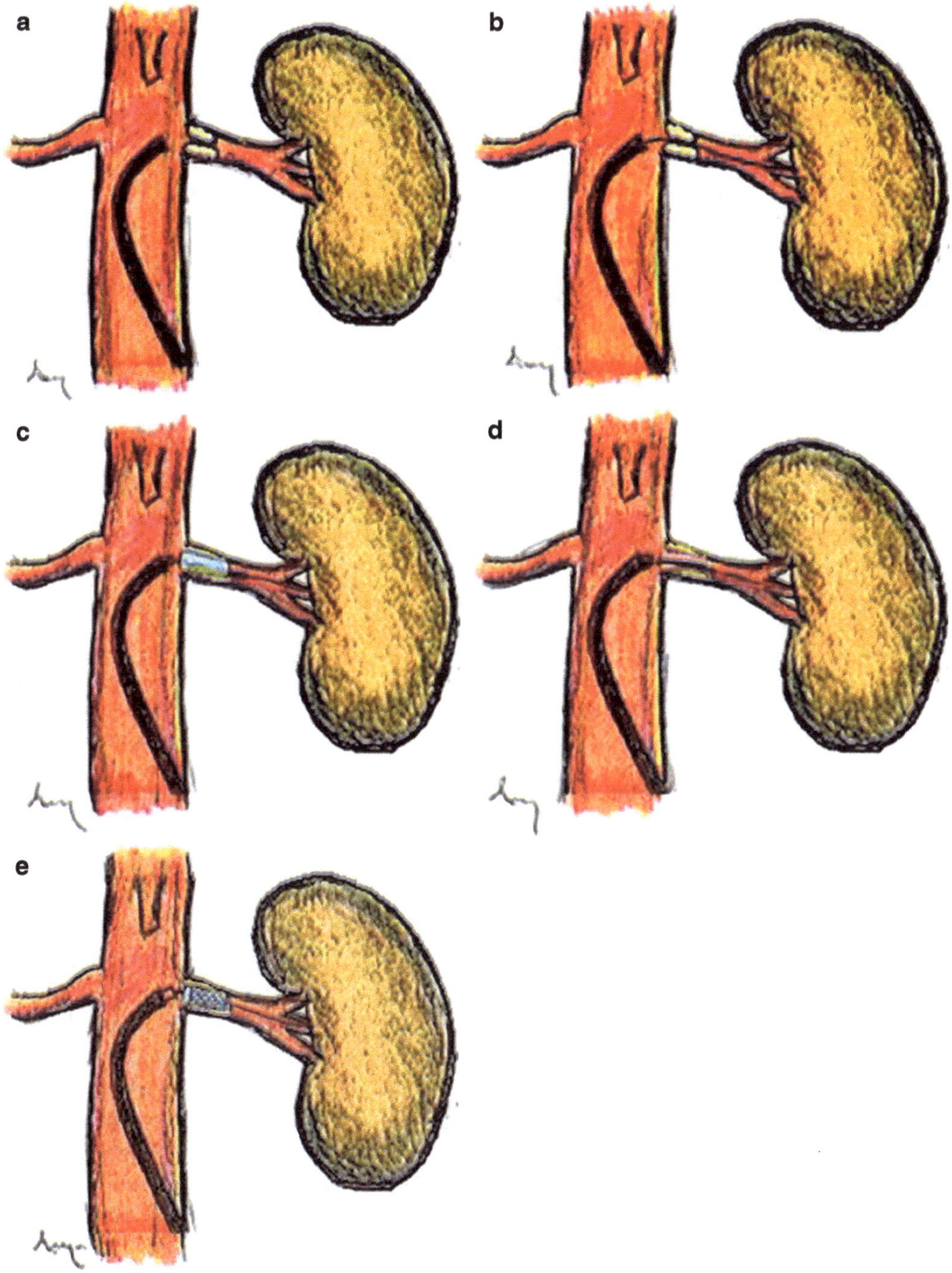

Fig. 14.2 Renal artery stenting using the guiding catheter technique. A catheter may be introduced with a guiding sheath to gain access to the renal artery. A straight, stiff wire placed in the guiding sheath will help to keep it off the wall and allow an angled catheter to freely engage the ostium and avoid scraping atheroma. (**a**) The renal artery is selectively catheterized with a guiding catheter. (**b**) The lesion is crossed with a 0.014- or 0.018-in. guidewire. (**c**) The lesion is predilated if there is concern that a stent will not easily pass through the lumen. (**d**) After the stent is delivered, the guiding catheter is pulled back into the aorta to check for correct stent position. (**e**) With the stent properly deployed, the proximal stent struts protrude 1–2 mm into the aorta and can be overdilated to flare the end (Adapted from Zeller T, J Endovasc Ther. 2004;11(Suppl 2):II96–106. Illustrations used with permission from the Department of Cardiovascular Surgery, Methodist DeBakey Heart & Vascular Center)

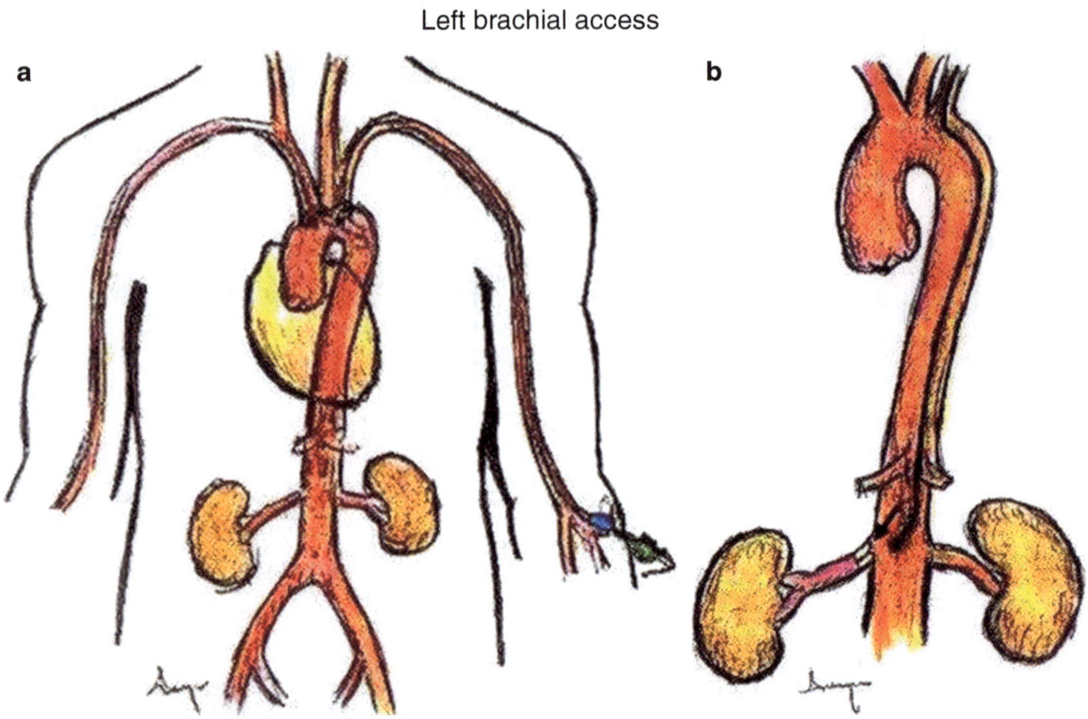

Fig. 14.3 Renal stenting from a brachial access. (**a**) With a 6-F sheath placed into the right or left brachial artery, a guiding catheter is advanced over a stiff wire until it reaches the aortic arch, where the catheter is rotated and the guidewire directed into the descending aorta. (**b**) A guidewire is then placed into the renal artery and is used as the platform to allow predilation (if necessary) or primary stenting (Adapted from Zeller T, J Endovasc Ther. 2004;11(Suppl 2):II96–106. Illustrations used with permission from the Department of Cardiovascular Surgery, Methodist DeBakey Heart & Vascular Center)

Dissection

A renal artery dissection during a percutaneous renal intervention that results in a change in management of the patient is unusual. In published series, this complication has been reported to occur in 1–18 % of cases [71, 72]. Beek et al. report three instances of renal artery dissection, two of which were of no clinical significance but resulted in loss of the kidney in the third [73]. The cause for significant dissection of the renal artery is typically the subintimal passage of the guidewire during the initial catheterization. However, it might also arise from other manipulations, including predilatation prior to stent deployment, oversizing the stent, or aggressive balloon dilatation of the stent. Regardless of the cause, dissection of the renal artery occurs more often in heavily calcified lesions. Technical error may be the cause when the initial guidewire placement takes a subintimal course and goes unrecognized. The resulting subintimal false channels are reported to occur in up to 18 % of cases [73]. If unrecognized, balloon inflation or stenting within the false channel may lead to acute renal artery occlusion or renal artery perforation. Though sometimes unavoidable, there are some techniques that may reduce the incidence of this complication. Aortic dissection is a rare, but potentially serious, complication of renal artery stenting that occurs with reported incidence of up to 2.2 % [72]. Though the precise cause of the development of aortic dissection in this situation is not known, it is postulated to be a consequence of the application of multidirectional forces on the aortic wall at the level of the renal ostium [74]. Prevention may not always be possible, but it does seem likely that overdilating a stent within the renal artery orifice may be a contributing factor. This is illustrated in a recently reported case where a dissection of the perirenal aorta developed after increasing the diameter of a balloon-expandable stent from 6 to 7 mm while treating a renal ostial stenosis [75]. At the time of the second balloon dilatation, the patient complained of severe chest and back pain, and the diagnosis of aortic dissection was confirmed during aortography. The diagnosis of aortic dissection should be considered whenever a patient develops severe chest, back, or abdominal pain following renal artery stent placement [74]. This may be confirmed angiographically, or the patient may be sent for cross-sectional imaging. Any imaging should include the thoracic aorta to determine the extent of the dissection, specifically whether it has extended into the chest to involve the aortic arch. Management will be similar to the management for an idiopathic aortic dissection. Pharmacologic management should be promptly instituted; if the blood pressure is elevated, it should be aggressively lowered.

Rupture

Renal artery rupture is one of the most feared, though fortunately, rare complications associated with renal artery stenting, with a reported incidence of only 0–1.7 % [19]. The clinical manifestation is often not subtle: there is immediate back or flank pain with bleeding into the retroperitoneum. The patient may become hypotensive and tachycardic. Contrast extravasation into the retroperitoneum is visible with angiography evident by an amorphous collection of contrast emanating from the renal artery. Balloon tamponade with or without covered stent placement is successful in the majority of cases [76]. Rarely, renal artery rupture may present several hours after the procedure [77]. Guidewire perforation of a distal renal artery branch is a rare but potentially serious complication of renal artery stent placement [76, 78]. Nephrectomy for main renal artery injury has outcomes similar to those of vascular repair, and it does not worsen posttreatment renal function in the short term. Nonoperative management for segmental renal artery injury results in excellent outcomes [79].

Renal Stent Fracture

There are six renal artery stent fracture cases that developed in-stent stenosis that resulted from stent fracture [80]. Two major anatomy features of renal artery stenosis were suggestive for development of stent fracture: (1) renal artery entrapment by diaphragmatic crus and (2) mobile kidney with acute angulation at the proximal segment of the renal artery. It is important to detect this etiology of renal artery stenosis because stenting in these vessels may contribute to in-stent restenosis or stent fracture. Management of renal artery stent fracture, including endovascular treatment or aortorenal bypass, should be considered on a case-by-case basis in relation to clinical settings.

Parenchymal

Parenchymal Injuries

Renal subcapsular hemorrhage may be a life-threatening problem that requires early detection and immediate angiographic intervention. A computed tomography (CT) scan with arterial phase will detect active hemorrhage and aid in planning the appropriate intervention. Superselective segmental renal artery catheterization and embolization is a safe and efficient method for the treatment of patients with severe renal hemorrhage. Technical and clinical success is approximately 85 and 65 %, respectively [81]. The derived CT angiographic images can closely mimic the "watering-can" appearance of multiple bleeding sites described angiographically and may indicate that embolization of the primary bleeding cortical artery alone may be insufficient to control hemorrhage and that nephrectomy is required. Iatrogenic injuries of the intrarenal arterial system include pseudoaneurysms and fistulas, and the majority can be successfully treated with transarterial embolization with Gelfoam with or without hydrogel particles, steel coils with Gelfoam, hydrogel particles, SURGICEL, silk with Gelfoam, or glue (*n*-butyl-2-cyanoacrylate) [82, 83].

Parenchymal Dysfunction

Acute functional renal injury occurs in approximately 20 % of patients undergoing percutaneous renal artery intervention and is more likely in the presence of an unrepaired abdominal aortic aneurysm (AAA), diabetes, and with preexisting renal disease. Transient acute renal dysfunction occurs in approximately 10 % of patients with peripheral arterial disease within 24 h after angioplasty; persistent renal failure or end-stage renal disease is rare. Predictors of acute renal failure were hypertension and congestive heart failure [84]. Other factors associated with transient renal dysfunction after any contrast-based intervention are preexisting renal insufficiency, non-insulin-dependent diabetes mellitus (NIDDM), hypoglycemic agents, and dehydration. The incidence of renal artery embolization varied from 1 to 8 %, with renal artery occlusion rates between 0.8 and 2.5 % [13]. Another series by Beutler reported that 8 % of patients showed clinical signs of cholesterol emboli, with at least 20 % of these patients experiencing a decrease in renal function [85]. Acute functional renal injury is a negative predictor of survival and is associated with subsequent renal failure, need for dialysis, and death [86].

Conclusion

Renal interventions for symptomatic arterial disease require a conscientious effort to apply stringent criteria to identify the patient that will respond. Careful technique and choice of intervention increase technical success and decrease perioperative events. While the procedures carry a relatively low mortality and morbidity, many complications have significant impact on survival and renal function. Functional benefit is presenting symptom dependent, and durability remains high for selected patients treated for hypertension and relatively low for those patients presenting with decreased renal function.

References

1. Conlon PJ, Athirakul K, Kovalik E, et al. Survival in renal vascular disease. J Am Soc Nephrol. 1998;9:252–6.
2. Rossi GP, Rossi A, Zanin L, et al. Excess prevalence of extracranialcarotid artery lesions in renovascular hypertension. Am J Hypertens. 1992;5:8–15.
3. Louie J, Isaacson JA, Zierler RE, et al. Prevalence of carotid and lower extremity arterial disease in patients with renal artery stenosis. Am J Hypertens. 1994;7:436–9.
4. Valentine RJ, Myers SI, Miller GL, et al. Detection of unsuspected renal artery stenoses in patients with abdominal aortic aneurysms: refined indications for preoperative aortography. Ann Vasc Surg. 1993;7:220–4.
5. Zierler RE, Bergelin RO, Polissar NL, et al. Carotid and lower extremity disease in patients with renal artery atherosclerosis. Arch Intern Med. 1998;158:761–7.
6. Choudhri AH, Cleland JGF, Rowlands PC, et al. Unsuspected renal artery stenosis in peripheral vascular disease. Br Med J. 1990;301:1197–8.
7. Olin JW, Melia M, Young JR, et al. Prevalence of renal artery stenosis in patients with atherosclerosis elsewhere. Am J Med. 1990;88:46N–51.
8. Miralles M, Corominas A, Cotillas J, et al. Screening for carotid and renal artery stenoses in patients with aortoiliac disease. Ann Vasc Surg. 1998;12:17–21.
9. Eyler WR, Clarck MD, Garman JE, et al. Angiography of the renal arteries including a comparative study of renal artery stenoses inpatients with and without hypertension. Radiology. 1962;78:879–92.
10. Holley KE, Hunt JC, Brown AL, et al. Renal artery stenosis. A clinical-pathologic study in normotensive and hypertensive patients. Am J Med. 1964;37:14–22.
11. Caps MT, Perissinotto C, Zierler RE, Polissar NL, Bergelin RO, Tullis MJ. Prospective study of atherosclerotic disease progression in the renal artery. Circulation. 1998;98(25):2866–72.
12. Caps MT, Zierler RE, Polissar NL, et al. Risk of atrophy in kidneys with atherosclerotic renal artery stenosis. Kidney Int. 1998;53(3):735–42.
13. Martin LG, Rundback JH, Sacks D, Cardella JF, Rees CR, Matsumoto AH. Quality improvement guidelines for angiography, angioplasty, and stent placement in the diagnosis and treatment of renal artery stenosis in adults. J Vasc Interv Radiol. 2003;14:S297–310.
14. Zeller T, Frank U, Muller C, et al. Technological advances in the design of catheters and devices used in renal artery interventions: impact on complications. J Endovasc Ther. 2003;10:1006–14.
15. Sivamurthy N, Suroweic SM, Culakova E, et al. Divergent outcomes after percutaneous therapy for symptomatic renal artery stenosis. J Vasc Surg. 2004; 39:565–74.
16. Zierler RE, Bergelin RO, Davidson RC, Cantwell-Gab K, Polissar NL, Strandness Jr DE. A prospective study of disease progression in patients with atherosclerotic renal artery stenosis. Am J Hypertens. 1996;9:1055–61.
17. Yutan E, Glickerman DJ, Caps MT, Hatsukami T, Harley JD, Davies MG. Percutaneous transluminal revascularization for renal artery stenosis: Veterans Affairs Puget Sound Health Care System experience. J Vasc Surg. 2001;34:685–93.
18. Galaria II, Surowiec SM, Rhodes JM, et al. Percutaneous and open renal revascularizations have equivalent long-term functional outcomes. Ann Vasc Surg. 2005;19(2):218–28.

19. Leertouwer TC, Gussenhoven EJ, Bosch JL, et al. Stent placement for renal arterial stenosis: where do we stand? A meta-analysis. Radiology. 2000;216:78–85.
20. Plouin PF, Chatellier G, Darne B, Raynoud A. Blood pressure outcome of angioplasty in atherosclerotic renal artery stenosis: a randomized trial. Essai Multicentrique Medicaments vs Angioplastie (EMMA) Study Group. Hypertension. 1998;31:823–9.
21. Hoffman O, Carreres T, Sapoval MR, et al. Ostial renal artery stenosis angioplasty: immediate and mid-term angiographic and clinical results. J Vasc Interv Radiol. 1998;9:65–73.
22. Jensen G, Zachrisson BF, Delin K, Volkmann R, Aurell M. Treatment of renovascular hypertension: one year results of renal angioplasty. Kidney Int. 1995;48:1936–45.
23. Chatziioannou A, Mourikis D, Agroyannis B, et al. Renal artery stenting for renal insufficiency in solitary kidney in 26 patients. Eur J Vasc Endovasc Surg. 2002;23:49–54.
24. Cioni R, Vignali C, Petruzzi P, et al. Renal artery stenting in patients with a solitary functioning kidney. Cardiovasc Intervent Radiol. 2001;24(6):372–7.
25. Taylor A, Sheppard D, MacLeod MJ, et al. Renal artery stent placement in renal artery stenosis: technical and early clinical results. Clin Radiol. 1997;52:451–7.
26. Lederman RJ, Mendelsohn FO, Santos R, Phillips HR, Stack RS, Crowley J. Primary renal artery stenting: characteristics and outcomes after 363 procedures. Am Heart J. 2001;142:314–23.
27. Dorros G, Jaff M, Mathiak L. Four-year follow-up of Palmaz-Schatz stent revascularization as treatment for atherosclerotic renalartery stenosis. Circulation. 1998;98:642–7.
28. Rocha-Singh KJ, Ahuja RK, Sung CH, Rutherford J. Long-term renal function preservation after renal artery stenting in patientswith progressive ischemic nephropathy. Catheter Cardiovasc Interv. 2002;57:135–41.
29. Hennequin LM, Joffre FG, Rousseau HP, et al. Renal artery stent placement: long-term results with the Wallstent endoprosthesis. Radiology. 1994;191:713–9.
30. Davies MG, Bismuth J, Saad WE, Naoum JJ, Peden EK, Lumsden AB. Impact of metabolic syndrome on the outcomes of percutaneous renal angioplasty and stenting. J Vasc Surg. 2010;51:926–32.
31. Dejani H, Eisen TD, Finkelstein FO. Revascularization of renal artery stenosis in patients with renal insufficiency. Am J Kidney Dis. 2000;36(4):752–8.
32. Beek FJ, Kaatee R, Beutler JJ, van der Ven PJ, Mali WP. Complications during renal artery stent placement for atherosclerotic ostial stenosis. Cardiovasc Intervent Radiol. 1997;20:184–90.
33. Boisclair C, Therasse E, Oliva VL, et al. Treatment of renal angioplasty failure by percutaneous renal artery stenting with Palmaz stents: midterm technical and clinical results. Am J Roentgenol. 1997;681(1):245–51.
34. White CJ. Catheter-based therapy for atherosclerotic renal artery stenosis. Circulation. 2006;113:1464–73.
35. Bates MC, Rashid M, Campbell JE, Stone PA, Broce M, Lavigne PS. Factors influencing the need for target vessel revascularization after renal artery stenting. J Endovasc Ther. 2006;13(5):569–77.
36. Blum U, Krumme B, Flügel P, et al. Treatment of ostial renal-artery stenoses with vascular endoprostheses after unsuccessful balloon angioplasty. N Engl J Med. 1997;336(7):459–65.
37. Abizaid A, Kornowski R, Mintz GS, et al. The influence of diabetes mellitus on acute and late outcomes following coronary stent implantation. J Am Coll Cardiol. 1998;32:584–9.
38. Carter AJ, Bailey L, Devries J, Hubbard B. The effects of uncontrolled hyperglycemia on thrombosis and formation of neoinitma after coronary stent placement in a novel diabetic porcine model of restenosis. Coron Artery Dis. 2000;11:473–9.
39. Davies MG, Saad WE, Bismuth J, Peden EK, Naoum JJ, Lumsden AB. Outcomes of endoluminal re-intervention for restenosis after percutaneous renal angioplasty and stenting. J Vasc Surg. 2009;49:946–52.
40. Rees CR, Palmaz JC, Becker GJ, et al. Palmaz stent in atherosclerotic stenoses involving the ostia of the renal arteries: preliminary report of a multicenter study. Radiology. 1991;181:507–14.
41. Baumgartner I, von Aesch K, Do DD, Triller J, Birrer M, Mahler F. Stent placement in ostial and nonostial atherosclerotic renal arterial stenoses: a prospective follow-up study. Radiology. 2000;216:498–505.
42. Pearce JD, Craven BL, Craven TE, et al. Progression of atherosclerotic renovascular disease: a prospective population-based study. J Vasc Surg. 2006;44(5):955–63.
43. Cherr GS, Hansen KJ, Craven TE, et al. Surgical management of atherosclerotic renovascular disease. J Vasc Surg. 2002;35(2):236–45.
44. Hansen KJ, Cherr GS, Craven TE, et al. Management of ischemic nephropathy: dialysis-free survival after surgical repair. J Vasc Surg. 2000;32(3):472–82.
45. Oskin TC, Hansen KJ, Deitch JS, Craven TE, Dean RH. Chronic renal artery occlusion: nephrectomy versus revascularization. J Vasc Surg. 1999;29(1):140–9.
46. Davies MG, Saad WE, Bismuth JX, Peden EK, Naoum JJ, Lumsden AB. Endovascular revascularization of renal artery stenosis in the solitary functioning kidney. J Vasc Surg. 2009;49:953–60.
47. Protack CD, Bakken AM, Saad WE, Davies MG. Renal artery interventions during EVAR: a greater potential of subsequent failure? J Vasc Interv Radiol. 2010;21(4):459–64.
48. Safian RD, Textor SC. Renal-artery stenosis. N Engl J Med. 2001;344(6):431–42.
49. Leadbetter WF, Burkland CE. Hypertension in unilateral renal disease. J Urol. 1938;39:611.
50. Slovut DP, Olin JW. Fibromuscular dysplasia. N Engl J Med. 2004;350:1862–71.
51. Ekelund L, Gerlock J, Molin J, Smith C. Roentgenologic appearance of fibromuscular dysplasia. Acta Radiol Diagn. 1978;19(3):433–46.
52. Goncharenko V, Gerlock AJJ, Shaff MI, Hollifield JW. Progression of renal artery fibromuscular dysplasia in 42 patients as seen on angiography. Radiology. 1981;139:45–51.

53. Fernando D, Garasic J. Percutaneous intervention for renovascular disease rationale and patient selection. Curr Opin Cardiol. 2004;19:582–8.
54. Birrer M, Do DD, Mahler F, et al. Treatment of renal artery fibromuscular dysplasia with balloon angioplasty: a prospective follow-up study. Eur J Vasc Endovasc Surg. 2002;23(2):146–52.
55. Sos TA, Pickering TG, Sniderman K, et al. Percutaneous transluminal renal angioplasty in renovascular hypertension due to atheroma or fibromuscular dysplasia. N Engl J Med. 1983;309:274–9.
56. Surowiec SM, Sivamurthy N, Rhodes JM, et al. Percutaneous therapy for renal artery fibromuscular dysplasia. Ann Vasc Surg. 2003;17(6):650–5.
57. Davidson RA, Barri Y, Wilcox CS. Predictors of cure of hypertension in fibromuscular renovascular disease. Am J Kidney Dis. 1996;28:334–8.
58. Bonelli FS, McKusick MA, Textor SC, et al. Renal artery angioplasty: technical results and clinical outcome in 320 patients [see comment]. Mayo Clinic Proc. 1995;70:1041–52.
59. Tegtmeyer CJ, Selby JB, Harlwell GD, Ayers C, Tegtmeyer V. Results and complications of angioplasty in fibromuscular disease. Circulation. 1991; 83(2 Suppl):I155–61.
60. Baert AL, Wilms G, Amery A, Vermylen J, Suy R. Percutaneous transluminal renal angioplasty: initial results and long-term follow-up in 202 patients. Cardiovasc Intervent Radiol. 1990;13:22–8.
61. Holden A, Hill A. Renal angioplasty and stenting with distal protection of the main renal artery in ischemic nephropathy: early experience. J Vasc Surg. 2003; 38(5):962–8.
62. Holden A, Hill A, Jaff MR, Pilmore H. Renal artery stent revascularization with embolic protection in patients with ischemic nephropathy. Kidney Int. 2006; 70(5):830–2.
63. Edwards MS, Corriere MA, Craven TE, et al. Atheroembolism during percutaneous renal artery revascularization. J Vasc Surg. 2007;46(1):55–61.
64. Kane GC, Textor SC, Schirger A, et al. Factors associated with restenosis in women following percutaneous renal artery revascularization for hypertension. Am J Hypertens. 2003;16:252A–3.
65. Oertle M, Do DD, Baumgartner I, Triller J, Mahler F. Discrepancy of clinical and angiographic results in the follow-up of percutaneous transluminal renal angioplasty. Vasa. 1998;27:154–7.
66. Edwards MS, Craven BL, Stafford J, et al. Distal embolic protection during renal artery angioplasty and stenting. J Vasc Surg. 2006;44:128–35.
67. Novick AC. Management of renovascular disease: a surgical perspective. Circulation. 1991;83:167–71.
68. Louden JD, Leen GLS, Cove-Smith R. Systemic thrombolysis for bilateral atherosclerotic renal artery occlusion resulting in prolonged recovery of renal function. Nephrol Dial Transplant. 1998;13: 2924–6.
69. Olin JW, Graor RA, Young JR. Thrombolytic therapy for renal artery occlusions: a preliminary report. Cleve Clin J Med. 1989;56(4):432–8.
70. Buri P. Acute renal artery occlusion. Origin, diagnosis, possibilities of treatment. Schweiz Med Wochenschr. 1975;105(30):941–8.
71. Fiala LA, Jackson MR, Gillespie DL, et al. Primary stenting of atherosclerotic renal artery ostial stenosis. Ann Vasc Surg. 1998;12:128–33.
72. Ivanovic V, McKusick M, Johnson III CM, et al. Renal artery stent placement: complications at a single tertiary care center. J Vasc Interv Radiol. 2003;14:217–25.
73. Beek FJ, Kaatee R, Beutler JJ, et al. Complications during renal artery stent placement for atherosclerotic ostial stenosis. Cardiovasc Intervent Radiol. 1997;20:184–90.
74. Bloch MJ, Trost DW, Sos TA. Type B aortic dissection complicating renal artery angioplasty and stent placement. J Vasc Interv Radiol. 2001;12:517–20.
75. Haesemeyer SW, Vedantham S, Braverman A. Renal artery stent placement complicated by development of a type B aortic dissection. Cardiovasc Intervent Radiol. 2005;28:98–101.
76. Morris CS, Bonnevie GJ, Najarian KE. Nonsurgical treatment of acute iatrogenic renal artery injuries occurring after renal artery angioplasty and stenting. AJR Am J Roentgenol. 2001;177:1353–7.
77. Peterson RA, Baldauf CG, Millward SF, et al. Outpatient percutaneous transluminal renal artery angioplasty: a Canadian experience. J Vasc Interv Radiol. 2000;11:327–32.
78. Axelrod DJ, Freeman H, Pukin L, et al. Guidewire perforation leading to fatal perirenal hemorrhage from transcortical collaterals after renal artery stent placement. J Vasc Interv Radiol. 2004;15:985–7.
79. Elliott SP, Olweny EO, McAninch JW. Renal arterial injuries: a single center analysis of management strategies and outcomes. J Urol. 2007;178(8):2451–5.
80. Chua SK, Hung HF. Renal artery stent fracture with refractory hypertension: a case report and review of the literature. Catheter Cardiovasc Interv. 2009;74(1): 37–42.
81. Breyer BN, McAninch JW, Elliott SP, Master VA. Minimally invasive endovascular techniques to treat acute renal hemorrhage. J Urol. 2008;179(6):2248–52.
82. Phadke RV, Sawlani V, Rastogi H, et al. Iatrogenic renal vascular injuries and their radiological management. Clin Radiol. 1997;52(2):119–23.
83. Cimsit NC, Baltacioglu F, Cengic I, Akpinar IN, Ilker Y, Turkeri L. Transarterial glue embolization in iatrogenic renovascular injuries. Int Urol Nephrol. 2008;40(4):875–9.
84. Schillinger M, Haumer M, Mlekusch W, Schlerka G, Ahmadi R, Minar E. Predicting renal failure after balloon angioplasty in high-risk patients. J Endovasc Ther. 2001;8(6):609–14.
85. Beutler JJ, Van Ampting JMA, van de Ven PJG, et al. Long-term effects of arterial stenting on kidney function for patients with ostial atherosclerotic renal artery stenosis and renal insufficiency. J Am Soc Nephrol. 2001;12:1475–81.
86. Davies MG, Saad WE, Peden EK, Mohiuddin IT, Naoum JJ, Lumsden AB. Implications of acute renal injury following percutaneous renal artery intervention. Ann Vasc Surg. 2008;22(6):783–9.

Aortoiliac Occlusive Disease

15

George Pisimisis and Carlos F. Bechara

Abstract

Treatment of aortoiliac occlusive disease has evolved over the past 10 years. Endovascular intervention is becoming more popular than aortobifemoral bypass, even for total aortoiliac artery occlusions. Endovascular angioplasty and stenting is now the first line of therapy in many if not all hospitals depending on the extent of the atherosclerotic disease as well as the experience of the interventionalists. This popularity is due to high technical success, early return to activity, and short hospital stay. Aortobifemoral bypass has excellent long-term patency. This procedure is being performed less due to the increase in either total endovascular intervention or hybrid procedures. Typically, these hybrid procedures involved open femoral reconstruction with retrograde iliac stenting. These procedures will be discussed in detail in this chapter.

Keywords

Aortobifemoral bypass • Aortoiliac occlusive disease • Hybrid procedures Stent graft • Stenting and angioplasty • Bare-metal stent • Stent graft Recanalization

Introduction

Aortoiliac occlusive disease (AIOD) results from atherosclerosis affecting the distal aorta and iliac arteries. Patients with AIOD are typically in their 50s and typically present with buttock and thigh claudication. When these patients present with buttock claudication, impotence, and diminished femoral pulses, this is referred to as Leriche syndrome [1]. Large collateral pathways develop in chronic aortic occlusion leading to claudication. The inflow for these collateral pathways comes from the superior mesenteric artery, lumbar, intercostals, and epigastric arteries (Fig. 15.1). Any compromise to these collateral pathways could lead to acute limb ischemia [2]. There are three types of AIOD patterns. Type 1 is confined to the aorta and proximal iliacs (5–10 %) of the cases. Type 2 extends to above the inguinal ligament (25 %), and type 3

G. Pisimisis, M.D. • C.F. Bechara, M.D., M.S. (✉)
Division of Vascular Surgery and Endovascular Therapy, Michael E. DeBakey Department of Surgery, Baylor College of Medicine and the Michael E. DeBakey VA Medical Center, Houston VAMC (112), 2002 Holcomb Blvd, Houston, TX 77030, USA
e-mail: bechara@bcm.edu

J.J. Hoballah, A.B. Lumsden (eds.), *Vascular Surgery*, New Techniques in Surgery Series, DOI 10.1007/978-1-4471-2912-7_15,

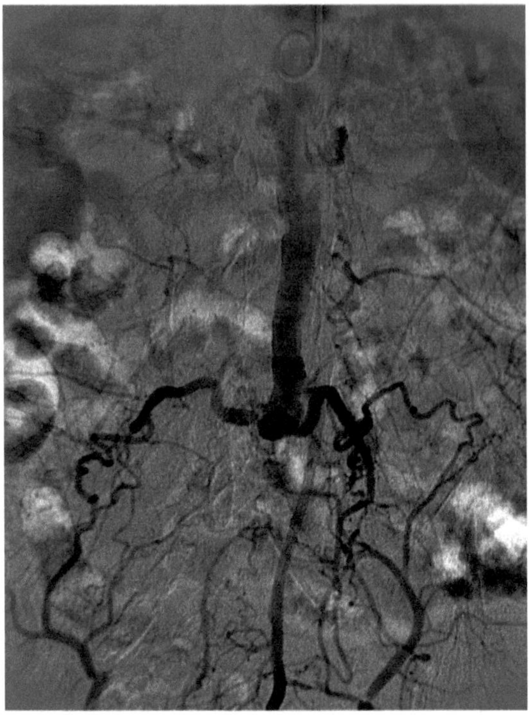

Fig. 15.1 Chronic distal aortic occlusion with large collaterals resulting in claudication

extends below the inguinal ligament. Type 3 is the most common type occurring in more than 60 % of the cases with 6:1 male to female ratio. These patients due to the extensive atherosclerotic disease also have atherosclerotic disease in other vascular beds like the coronary and cerebral arteries and have poorer 10-year life expectancy compared to other patients with type 1 or 2.

Pathophysiology

The majority of risk factors associated with the development and progression of AIOD can be modified, except for age. Approximately 10 % of patients over 70 years have peripheral arterial disease (PAD). Other risk factors are cigarette smoking, hyperlipidemia, hypertension, and diabetes. Quitting smoking is the cornerstone of nonoperative therapy for AIOD. Continued smoking leads to progression of disease and amputation [3], as well as cardiovascular disease progression [4].

Like mentioned earlier, the majority of these patients present with claudication due to either AIOD or high-grade stenosis. Some patients present with blue toe syndrome due to distal embolization. Others might present with an acute or chronic picture. Low-flow state or disruption of the collaterals could result in acute ischemia.

Diagnosis

History and physical exam provides tremendous information about the location, severity, and extent of the vascular disease. Patients with AIOD will have diminished or absent pulses with buttock and/or thigh claudication. Initial investigation, in most patients, is the vascular laboratory exam with segmental arterial pressure and ankle-brachial index. Some patients with palpable pulses but a convincing history for AIOD should undergo either exercise treadmill testing or other noninvasive testing to further elucidate the pathology.

Angiography is still widely used in evaluating and treating patients with AIOD. It also helps in determining if the patient is best served by an endovascular procedure, open procedure, or both (hybrid procedure). Angiography has become a part of the therapeutic intervention rather than a diagnostic test. This has shifted mainly due to the enhancement in magnetic resonance angiography (MRA) and computed tomographic angiography (CTA). Both MRA and CTA are noninvasive and can provide enough information in preparing the patient for intervention. In a recent study, contrast-enhanced MRA was comparable to digital subtraction angiography in detecting hemodynamically significant stenosis in patients with known AIOD. The contrast-enhanced MRA had a sensitivity of 80–88 % and specificity of 73–92 %. Mean acquisition time was less than 1 min [5]. In another study, MRA was able to show a patent and suitable pedal target for bypass in 38 % of cases not seen during conventional angiography [6]. The disadvantage for MRA is it cannot be used in patients with metallic implants like pacemakers and patients with claustrophobia. In addition, gadolinium should be avoided in patients with renal insufficiency due to the risk of nephrogenic systemic fibrosis.

With the recent advances with the multidetector scanners, currently 128 and 256, CTA has been used more frequently as a noninvasive diagnostic tool. It takes few minutes to scan from the aorta to the feet. A meta-analysis comparing CTA to conventional angiography [7] revealed CTA as an adequate diagnostic tool in assessing arterial disease, especially in AIOD patients. Pooled sensitivity was 92 % and specificity of 93 % in detecting stenosis >50 %. The main drawback of CTA is the ionizing radiation and the approximate use of 100 cc of contrast per CTA study that could cause contrast nephropathy.

Intravascular ultrasound (IVUS) is a modality used during an intervention rather than as an initial diagnostic tool. In a study where IVUS was used as an adjunctive tool in treating AIOD endovascularly, IVUS was shown to improve long-term patency of treated iliac arterial lesions. The main benefit was in identifying the appropriate angioplasty diameter as well as identifying the adequacy of stent deployment [8].

Treatment

Indication for surgery is disabling or life-limiting claudication, rest pain, limb-threatening ischemia, and embolization. Otherwise aggressive medical management with graduated exercise program is recommended.

The decision to pursue an open or an endovascular approach to treat AIOD depends on the extent of the atherosclerotic disease. A classification to help with this decision was put by the Transatlantic Intersocietal Commission (TASC) [9]. TASC A lesions are better treated with a catheter-based intervention, whereas TASC D lesions are best treated with a bypass. TASC lesions B and C remain controversial whether they should undergo stenting or surgical intervention. New TASC guidelines recommend endovascular intervention to be the first line of therapy for all AIOD. Surgical revascularization should be used for endovascular failures and unfavorable anatomy for endovascular intervention. These TASC IIb recommendations are still debated and remain unpublished at the time this chapter was written.

Balloon Angioplasty and Stenting

Technical Aspects

The technological advancement in percutaneous balloon angioplasty (PTA) balloon engineering has introduced a variety of options to choose from based on the lesion characteristics. Compliant balloons allow for even pressure distribution along the dilated segment. The availability of noncompliant and high-pressure balloons, in various lengths and diameters, offers a wide number of choices to treat long lesions and heavily calcified or occluded vessels.

For common iliac artery (CIA) lesions, retrograde ipsilateral approach is usually the first choice, unless there is occlusion with short stump or the lesion abuts the aortic bifurcation in which case contralateral approach is indicated to protect that proximal CIA side and obtain angiographic evaluation. Another option is bilateral femoral access and retrograde iliac artery stenting using the "kissing" technique. Occasionally, brachial approach would offer superior sheath support and "pushability" for flush occlusions at the aortic bifurcation or very calcified lesions. When there is a common iliac artery stump, "burying" the sheath and dilator in the stump seems to help facilitate wire entry into the occluded vessels.

Contralateral approach is also favorable for lesions extending to the distal external iliac artery (EIA), since the secure placement of a short sheath using ipsilateral retrograde approach would be challenging.

At our institution, we perform subintimal recanalization for most if not all chronic iliac occlusions using a Glidewire (Terumo Interventional Systems, Somerset, NJ) and an angled catheter for support. By tackling iliac occlusion from a brachial approach (antegrade) and/or femoral (retrograde) approach, we are able to achieve technical success in most cases and very rarely require the use of "reentry" devices.

The availability of various "reentry" devices can be of great importance in recanalization of chronic, sclerotic arterial occlusions. These devices are designed to facilitate luminal reentry under fluoroscopy or intravascular ultrasound and decrease the risk of dissection in the normal vessel that would complicate the procedure. However, not all hospitals carry these devices on their shelves because of their rare use, and they can be expensive.

The use of bare-metal stents to scaffold the vessel wall is applied in cases of residual stenosis (>30 %), rest gradient (>10 mmHg), flow-limiting dissection, ulcerative plaques showering distal emboli, and recanalization of occluded vessels. The two main categories of bare-metal stents are balloon-expandable and self-expandable. The first are premounted on a balloon and introduced into the lesion through sheath coverage to avoid dislodgment of the stent. The sheath is pulled back once positioning is satisfactory, and the stent is deployed under fluoroscopic guidance. Self-expanding stents (stainless steel or nitinol alloy) are already covered with a sheath and, thus, can be introduced into the lesion directly. Pulling back the sheath allows the stent to deploy in a coil-like fashion causing slight foreshortening of the stent. This difference in deployment and the mechanical characteristics of the two stent types render the balloon-expandable stents more precise in placement, more visible under fluoroscopy, and apply better radial force while treating short, orificial lesions. These balloons could cause rupture in tortuous vessels like the external iliac artery. On the other hand, self-expandable stents are flexible and available in longer sizes, therefore, are preferable in treating long lesions and tortuous vessels (Figs. 15.2 and 15.3).

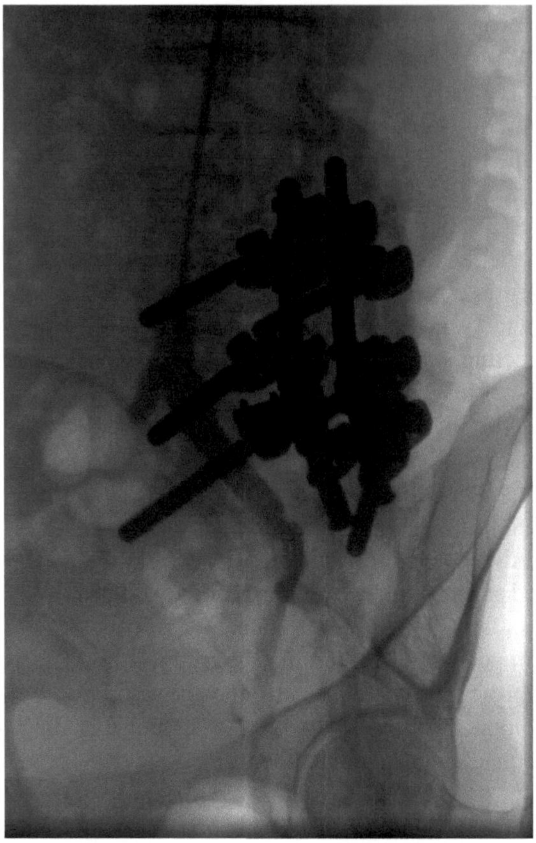

Fig. 15.2 This patient presented with disabling right leg claudication that was treated with bare-metal stent to preserve the right internal iliac artery (Fig. 15.3) via brachial approach

Results

The therapeutic dilemma whether to perform PTA alone or PTA with stenting was addressed in a meta-analysis by Bosch and Hunink [10]. The authors reviewed the results of studies reported in the literature (total of 2,116 patients) and found that technical success was higher for stenting, with comparable complication and 30-day mortality rates. In patients with claudication, 4-year primary patency rates after PTA were 65 % for stenoses versus 54 % for occlusions and were 53 % for stenoses versus 44 % for occlusions to treat critical limb ischemia. Following stent placement, these rates were 77 % for stenoses versus 61 % for occlusions to treat claudication and 67 % for stenoses versus 53 % for occlusions to treat critical ischemia. Overall, the risk of long-term failure was reduced by 39 % after stent placement compared with PTA.

Stenting alone was compared to PTA with selective stenting in a prospective randomized multicenter study [11]. Outcomes between the two methods were similar with 2-year reintervention rates of 7 and 4 % for PTA and primary stenting, respectively. At 5 years, the outcomes between primary stenting and PTA with selective stenting were also similar with 18 and 20 % of

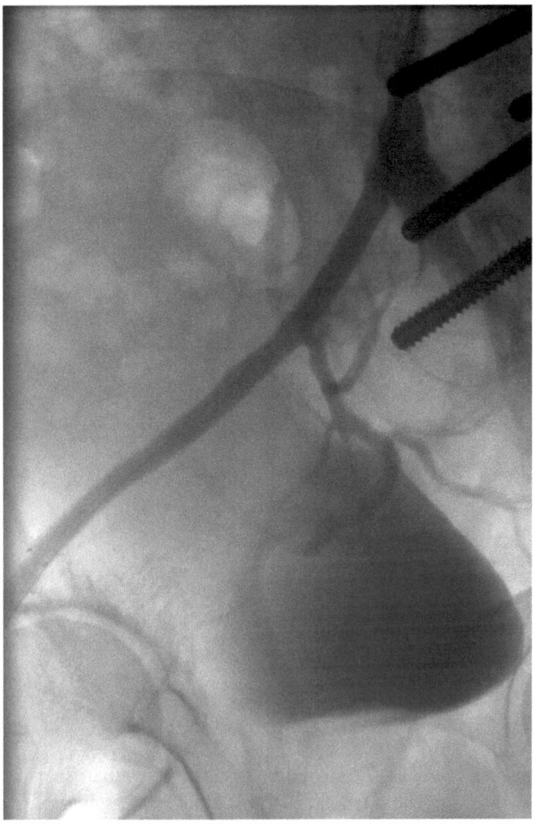

Fig. 15.3 Patient had palpable bilateral pedal pulses at the end of the case

the treated iliac artery segments, respectively, in need of reintervention [12]. Risk of cardiovascular complication and death was also similar in both groups.

In a retrospective study, Leville and colleagues presented their experience with PTA/stenting treatment for complex aortoiliac disease [13]. The authors reported three-year primary patency, secondary patency, and limb salvage rates at 76, 90, and 97 %, respectively. They concluded that TASC C and D lesions could be safely treated via endovascular approach with good midterm patency rates and low morbidity.

Stent Grafts

There has been increasing interest in the application of stent grafts beyond aneurysmal disease to include selected aortoiliac occlusive cases. High-risk patients with combination of aneurysmal and occlusive disease, small-diameter or severely calcified vessels, symptomatic aortic or iliac ulcerations, and patients that had endovascular intervention complicated with perforation and arteriovenous fistulae or frank extravasation. In the USA, available devices include balloon-expandable or self-expandable stents covered with polytetrafluoroethylene (PTFE) or Dacron material [14–16].

Technical Aspects

After crossing the area of stenosis and verifying luminal reentry in cases of obstruction, as described earlier in this chapter, device selection is made based on the location, extent, and anatomy of the area treated. For orificial lesions involving the CIA, there is a preference for balloon-expandable covered stents due to the superior radial force and precision in deployment of these devices. For long occlusive lesions located in rather tortuous vessels, i.e., EIA, self-expandable stent grafts are preferable due to the flexibility and length of available devices. In cases of more extensive occlusive segments involving the aortic bifurcation or infrarenal aorta, the use of bifurcated stent grafts has emerged as a viable alternative to open surgery. Selection of bifurcated devices is made based on the same anatomic criteria and limitations used for aneurysmal disease, keeping in mind that the limited diameter of distal infrarenal aorta might pose a technical challenge for the contralateral gate cannulation required in modular bifurcated device. In such cases, using the Powerlink unibody bifurcated endograft (Endologix, Inc., Irvine, California) simplifies the procedure since there is no need for gate cannulation (Figs. 15.4 and 15.5).

A variety of techniques have been described, both endovascular and open, to facilitate the introduction of aortic stent grafts [17]. Angioplasty alone may be successful in patients with isolated iliac artery stenoses but may not be enough in patients with diffusely stenotic and calcified arteries. In heavily diseased vessels, the risk of rupture is increased. At this stage, the methods of relining the iliac arteries with covered stents prior to aggressive

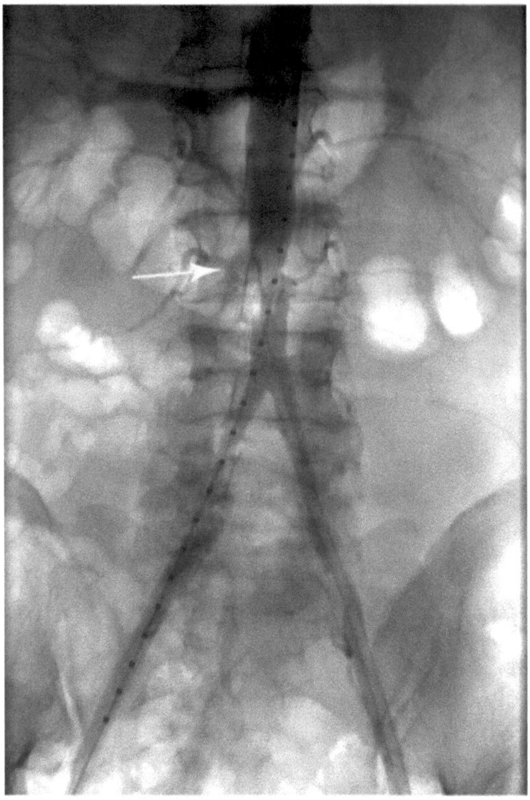

Fig. 15.4 Patient with symptomatic aortic and iliac atherosclerotic disease with 25 mmHg gradient across the aortic lesion (*arrow*). Resolution of aortoiliac stenosis and symptoms after deploying Powerlink endograft (Fig. 15.5) percutaneously

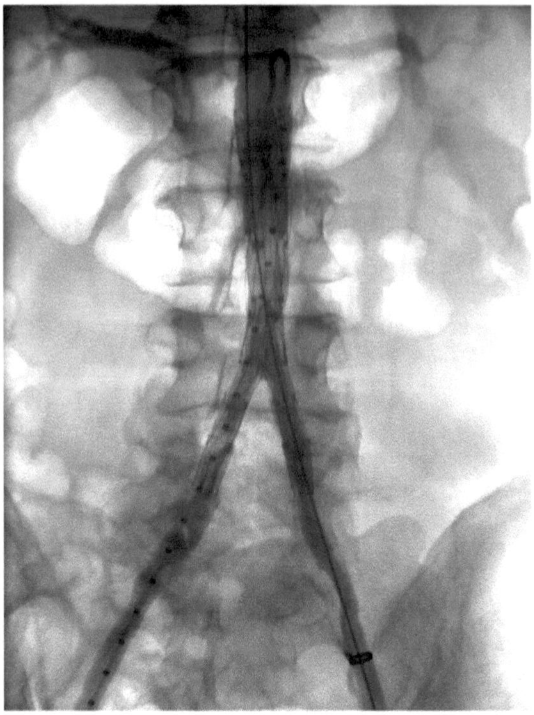

Fig. 15.5 Successful resolution of aortoiliac atherosclerotic disease. The advantage of this stent graft is snaring the contralateral limb rather than trying to cannulate the gate when using a modular bifurcated graft

dilatation may be a safer approach. Once the covered stents are deployed along the length of the diseased iliac arteries, angiography should be performed to assess patency and possible extravasation. In addition, the introduction of larger delivery systems for bifurcated devices is now possible, if needed, to treat more proximal lesions.

Results

The role of endovascular grafts has been studied by Ali et al. in high-risk patients with TASC C and D aortoiliac disease [18]. The authors reported 84 % primary patency at 2 years and 95 % limb salvage rate. All patients had hemodynamic improvement, and there was no mortality at 30 days. In 6 out of 22 patients, a concomitant infrainguinal outflow procedure was performed.

Short-term results have been reported by Rzucidlo et al. in patients with TASC C and D lesions [14]. One-year primary and primary-assisted patencies were 70 and 88 %, respectively, with hemodynamic and clinical improvement in all patients. Also, patients that underwent concomitant common femoral endarterectomy had improved one-year primary patency rate. Lammer and colleagues [19] reported their experience with self-expanding stent grafts in iliac arteries, with primary patency rates at 98 and 91 % at 6 and 12 months, respectively. Secondary patency rates were 95 % at 12 months after treatment.

In a prospective randomized trial, covered stents were evaluated in treatment of severe iliac stenoses and occlusions. Primary patency rates for iliac arteries were 94.3 % at 6 months and 90.7 % at 12 months [20]. In another prospective study, the 2-year patency of covered balloon-expandable kissing stents for atherosclerotic aortic bifurcation occlusive disease was superior to bare-metal balloon-expandable stents [15].

Bifurcated endoprosthesis was evaluated for treatment of TASC C or D iliac disease [21]. All aortoiliac reconstructions were patent at 17 months, and no mortality or amputation occurred during that time.

Long-term results for the treatment of aortoiliac occlusive disease using stent grafts and common femoral endarterectomy have been reported [22]. At 5 years after intervention, the primary, primary-assisted, and secondary patencies were 60, 97, and 98 %, respectively. The authors concluded that the use of stent grafts compared with bare stents is associated with improved primary patency.

Hybrid Procedures

The combination of open and endovascular approach termed as hybrid technique has been used to treat aortoiliac lesions combined with significant common femoral artery (CFA), profunda femoris artery (PFA), and superficial femoral artery (SFA) disease. In such cases, endarterectomy and patch angioplasty of the femoral arteries follows successful endovascular treatment of aortoiliac stenoses or occlusions. Based on preoperative imaging, these are selected patients that would benefit from additional infrainguinal procedure to improve outflow. Occasionally, an infrainguinal bypass may be needed at the same time with the endovascular iliac procedure in patients with critical limb ischemia.

Technique

Longitudinal exposure of the CFA, PFA, and SFA is usually required depending on the extent of disease and planned reconstruction. Retrograde puncture of the CFA and crossing of the ipsilateral iliac lesion is attempted first, using the techniques described previously. Alternatively, contralateral percutaneous femoral or brachial approach could be used in challenging lesions, bringing out the guidewire through the exposed CFA. All exposed vessels are controlled, and standard endarterectomy of the involved segments is performed followed by patch angioplasty as needed. The endarterectomy should extend as proximal to the inguinal ligament as possible via the current exposure to facilitate the stent placement in the EIA and sometimes into the femoral patch angioplasty. The wire is protected medially as it comes out of the proximal lumen to facilitate the endarterectomy procedure. Prior to completing the patch closure, all outflow vessels are flushed along with the inflow if not occluded from disease. The wire is brought out through the patch, closure is completed, and all clamps released. A sheath is passed over the wire through the patch, and the inflow is treated in an endovascular fashion as described previously. The stent is positioned to end at the proximal endarterectomy endpoint, without crossing the inguinal ligament.

Another technique would be to perform an EIA to PFA bypass and stent the CIA lesion into the bypass to establish in-line flow (Figs. 15.6 and 15.7).

An additional infrainguinal bypass procedure can be carried out at the same or later time, with or without femoral endarterectomy, based on the extent of outflow disease, the clinical condition of the patient, and the clinical condition of the treated limb.

Results

Hybrid revascularization procedures for lower extremity occlusive disease have been compared to both endovascular and open alternatives [23]. The authors reported comparable patency rates at 36 months follow-up between all three groups but higher limb salvage rates for the hybrid group in patients with critical limb ischemia. Although overall survival was similar in all groups, the patients in the hybrid group had significantly higher 30-day myocardial infarction/death rate, possibly because that group had higher-risk patients.

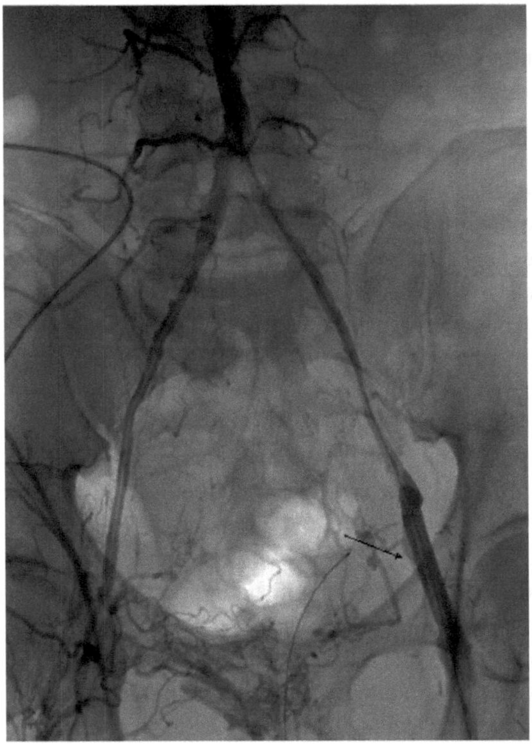

Fig. 15.6 This patient was referred for aortobifemoral bypass due to severe iliac disease and bilateral common femoral artery occlusion and L big toe ulcer. He was treated utilizing a hybrid approach and in a staged fashion, left leg first. This angiogram shows an interposition graft from the external iliac artery to the profunda artery (*arrow*). Then a retrograde stent graft was placed from the iliac artery into the bypass, and another bypass was performed to the above-knee popliteal artery (Fig. 15.7)

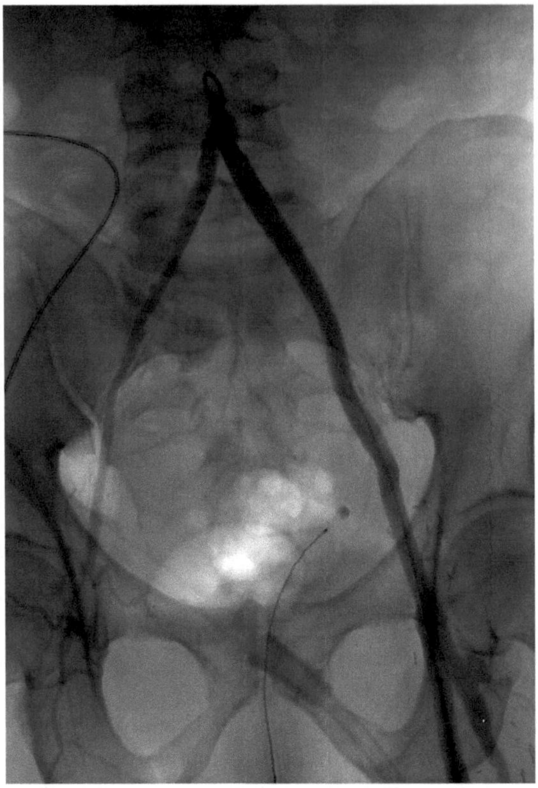

Fig. 15.7 Successful resolution of the iliac disease with establishment of in-line flow to the foot to help heal the big toe ulcer

Early results of combined common femoral endarterectomy and iliac artery stenting have also been reported [24]. In this retrospective series, the rates for 1-year primary patency and primary-assisted patency were 84 and 97 %, respectively, without any perioperative mortality.

Encouraging midterm results for hybrid procedures in patients with TASC D lesions have also been reported [25]. Primary patency rates were 94, 70, and 70 % at 6, 12, and 24 months, respectively, with primary-assisted patency rates up to 94 % and limb salvage rate of 100 % at 24 months. Survival was 88 % at 2 years. The authors reported better primary patency rates in patients with intermittent claudication compared to patients with critical limb ischemia.

Ideal Stent

The ideal stent is the stent that results in no acute and long-term restenosis. It is the stent that can be delivered and deployed with minimal intimal trauma resulting in minimal thrombogenic response. Biodegradable and bioabsorbable stents are gaining popularity over metallic stents with or without drug elution. As important are proper stent to artery sizing and wall apposition, which are crucial to improve long-term stent patency [8].

Conclusion

Historically, aortobifemoral bypass has been the gold standard for treating AIOD. Due to the advances in endovascular technology, the number of these bypasses has trended down due to an increase in endovascular intervention [26]. In order to achieve excellent long-term assisted patency of iliac stenting, a careful consideration of geometric variables related to the aortoiliac anatomy, the pathology, as well as the stenting configuration is beneficial [27]. Even though iliac stenting has excellent short- and long-term results and can be combined with hybrid procedures, aortobifemoral bypass is still considered an excellent alternative in treating AIOD [26]. A particular subgroup of the AIOD patients, flush aortic occlusion at the level of the renal arteries, remains a challenge for interventionalists. This group of patients is not necessarily technically challenging but more so the risk of renal artery embolization or pushing the thrombus into the renal orifice during stenting and angioplasty.

References

1. Leriche R, Morel A. The syndrome of thrombotic obliteration of the aortic bifurcation. Ann Surg. 1948;127:193–206.
2. Dietzek AM, Goldsmith J, Veith FJ, et al. Interruption of critical aortoiliac collateral circulation during non-vascular operations: a cause of acute limb-threatening ischemia. J Vasc Surg. 1990;12:645–51.
3. McGrath MA, Graham AR, Hill DA, et al. The natural history of chronic leg ischemia. World J Surg. 1983;7: 314–8.
4. Violi F, Criqui M, Longoni A, et al. Relation between risk factors and cardiovascular complications in patients with peripheral vascular disease. Results from the A.D.E.P. study. Atherosclerosis. 1996;120: 25–35.
5. Bui BT, Miller S, Mildenberger P, et al. Comparison of contrast-enhanced MR angiography to intraarterial digital subtraction angiography for evaluation of peripheral arterial occlusive disease: results of a phase III multicenter trial. J Magn Reson Imaging. 2010;31: 1402–10.
6. Kreitner KF, Kalden P, Neufang A, et al. Diabetes and peripheral arterial occlusive disease: prospective comparison of contrast-enhanced three-dimensional MR angiography with conventional digital subtraction angiography. AJR Am J Roentgenol. 2000;174: 171–9.
7. Heijenbrok-Kal MH, Kock MC, Hunink MG. Lower extremity arterial disease: multicenter CT angiography meta-analysis. Radiology. 2007;245:433–9.
8. Buckley CJ, Arko FR, Lee S. Intravascular scanning improves long-term patency of iliac lesions treated with balloon angioplasty and primary stenting. J Vasc Surg. 2002;35:316–23.
9. Norgern L, Hiatt WR, Dormandy JA, et al. Inter-society consensus for the management of peripheral arterial disease (TASC II). J Vasc Surg. 2007;45:S5–67.
10. Bosch JL, Hunink MG. Meta-analysis of the results of percutaneous transluminal angioplasty and stent placement for aortoiliac occlusive disease. Radiology. 1997;204:87–96.
11. Tetteroo E, Van der Graaf Y, Bosch JL, et al. Randomised comparison of primary stent placement versus primary angioplasty followed by selective stent placement in patients with iliac-artery occlusive disease. Dutch Iliac Stent Trial Study Group. Lancet. 1998;351:1153–9.
12. Klein WM, Van der Graaf Y, Seegers J, et al. Long-term cardiovascular morbidity, mortality, and reintervention after endovascular treatment in patients with iliac artery disease: the Dutch Iliac Stent Trial Study. Radiology. 2004;232:491–8.
13. Leville CD, Kashyap VS, Clair DG, et al. Endovascular management of iliac artery occlusions: extending treatment to TransAtlantic Inter-Society Consensus class C and D patients. J Vasc Surg. 2006;43:32–9.
14. Rzucidlo EM, Powell RJ, Zwolak RM, et al. Early results of stent-grafting to treat diffuse aortoiliac occlusive disease. J Vasc Surg. 2003;37:1175–80.
15. Sabri SS, Choudhri A, Orgera G, et al. Outcomes of covered kissing stent placement compared with bare metal stent placement in the treatment of atherosclerotic occlusive disease at the aortic bifurcation. J Vasc Interv Radiol. 2010;21:995–1003.
16. Schurmann K, Vorwerk D, Uppenkamp R, et al. Iliac arteries: plain and heparin-coated Dacron-covered stent- grafts compared with noncovered metal stents – an experimental study. Radiology. 1997;203:55–63.
17. Hinchliffe RJ, Ivancev K, Sonesson B, et al. "Paving and cracking": an endovascular technique to facilitate the introduction of aortic stent-grafts through stenosed iliac arteries. J Endovasc Ther. 2007;14:630–3.
18. Ali AT, Modrall JG, Lopez J, et al. Emerging role of endovascular grafts in complex aortoiliac occlusive disease. J Vasc Surg. 2003;38:486–91.
19. Lammer J, Dake MD, Bleyn J, et al. Peripheral arterial obstruction: prospective study of treatment with a transluminally placed self-expanding stent-graft. International Trial Study Group. Radiology. 2000;217:95–104.
20. Wiesinger B, Beregi JP, Oliva VL, et al. PTFE-covered self-expanding nitinol stents for the treatment of severe iliac and femoral artery stenoses and occlusions: final results from a prospective study. J Endovasc Ther. 2005;12:240–6.
21. Maynar M, Zander T, Qian Z, et al. Bifurcated endoprosthesis for treatment of aortoiliac occlusive lesions. J Endovasc Ther. 2005;12:22–7.
22. Chang RW, Goodney PP, Baek JH, et al. Long-term results of combined common femoral endarterectomy and iliac stenting/stent grafting for occlusive disease. J Vasc Surg. 2008;48:362–7.
23. Dosluoglu HH, Lall P, Cherr GS, et al. Role of simple and complex hybrid revascularization procedures for symptomatic lower extremity occlusive disease. J Vasc Surg. 2010;51:1425–35.

24. Nelson PR, Powell RJ, Schermerhorn ML, et al. Early results of external iliac artery stenting combined with common femoral artery endarterectomy. J Vasc Surg. 2002;35:1107–13.
25. Nishibe T, Kondo Y, Dardik A, et al. Hybrid surgical and endovascular therapy in multifocal peripheral TASC D lesions: up to three-year follow-up. J Cardiovasc Surg (Torino). 2009;50:493–9.
26. Burke CR, Henke PK, Hernandez R, et al. A contemporary comparison of aortofemoral bypass and aortoiliac stenting in the treatment of aortoiliac occlusive disease. Ann Vasc Surg. 2010;24:4–13.
27. Sharafuddin MJ, Hoballah JJ, Kresowik TF, et al. Long-term outcomes following stent reconstruction of the aortic bifurcation and the role of geometric determinants. Ann Vasc Surg. 2008;22:346–57.

Femoropopliteal Endovascular Interventions

16

Melhem J. Sharafuddin, Parth B. Amin, Rachael M. Nicholson, and Jamal J. Hoballah

Abstract

The treatment of peripheral arterial disease (PAD) has witnessed a remarkable evolution in the past two decades. While endovascular therapy has become well established as a primary treatment modality in aortoiliac occlusive disease, transcatheter treatment of infrainguinal occlusive disease remains controversial. The availability of a wide range of therapeutic options and devices applicable to infrainguinal interventions has resulted in a dramatic increase in the number of peripheral endovascular procedures over the past decade, with a staggering reported 979 % growth in peripheral vascular interventions reported since 1995. Despite this remarkable growth and increasing acceptance, many questions remain unanswered regarding the indications, choice of device/technique, clinical efficacy, long-term outcome, and cost-effectiveness of the available competing modalities. These decisions are also compounded by intense and often conflicting marketing efforts by the industry in the current competitive market. With the scarcity of randomized controlled trials, much of the published reports for newer endovascular technologies rely primarily on immediate angiographic outcomes and target limb revascularization (TLR) data. The following text

M.J. Sharafuddin, M.D. • P.B. Amin, M.D.
R.M. Nicholson, M.D.
Division of Vascular Surgery, Department of Surgery,
University of Iowa Hospitals and Clinics,
Iowa City, IA, USA
e-mail: mel-sharafuddin@uiowa.edu;
parth-amin@uiowa.edu; rachael-nicholson@uiowa.edu

J.J. Hoballah, M.D., M.B.A., FACS (✉)
Division of Vascular Surgery, Department of Surgery,
American University of Beirut Medical Center,
Cairo Street, AUBMC C456, Beirut, Lebanon

Division of Vascular Surgery, Department of Surgery,
University of Iowa Hospitals and Clinics,
Iowa City, IA, USA
e-mail: jh34@aub.edu.lb

J.J. Hoballah, A.B. Lumsden (eds.), *Vascular Surgery*, New Techniques in Surgery Series,
DOI 10.1007/978-1-4471-2912-7_16, © Springer-Verlag London 2012

is meant to provide an overview over current treatment options, technologies, and devices based on available evidence and the experience and opinions of the authors. The endovascular surgeon must be familiar with all the available treatments for PAD in order to continue to manage these patients amidst the increasingly complex health-care environment.

Keywords
Angioplasty • Vessel • Stents • CTO • Cryoplasty

Introduction

The treatment of peripheral arterial disease (PAD) has witnessed a remarkable evolution in the past two decades. While endovascular therapy has become well established as a primary treatment modality in aortoiliac occlusive disease, transcatheter treatment of infrainguinal occlusive disease remains controversial. The availability of a wide range of therapeutic options and devices applicable to infrainguinal interventions has resulted in a dramatic increase in the number of peripheral endovascular procedures over the past decade, with a staggering reported 979 % growth in peripheral vascular interventions reported since 1995 [1]. Despite this remarkable growth and increasing acceptance, many questions remain unanswered regarding the indications, choice of device/technique, clinical efficacy, long-term outcome, and cost-effectiveness of the available competing modalities. These decisions are also compounded by intense and often conflicting marketing efforts by the industry in the current competitive market. With the scarcity of randomized controlled trials, much of the published reports for newer endovascular technologies rely primarily on immediate angiographic outcomes and target limb revascularization (TLR) data. The following text is meant to provide an overview over current treatment options, technologies, and devices based on available evidence and the experience and opinions of the authors. The endovascular surgeon must be familiar with all the available treatments for PAD in order to continue to manage these patients amidst the increasingly complex health-care environment.

Prevalence and Clinical Manifestation of PAD

Although PAD is a common disease, symptoms vary and the majority of patients do not need treatment [2]. Thorough clinical and noninvasive evaluation of patients prior to angiography is important. Treatment should not only be based on anatomic criteria (i.e., the presence of occlusive disease) but more importantly on clinical ground as well as the anticipated treatment outcome. Patients who initially present with symptomatic PAD will likely return again with another vascular event [3]. It could not be overemphasized that once a patient presents with PAD, an effort should be made to reduce associated cardiovascular risk factors. The two most common risk factors for PAD are smoking and presence of diabetes. Unfortunately, it is often uncommon for patients to get appropriate risk factor modifications, treatment, and follow-up [4].

The prevalence of PAD based on noninvasive testing is age-dependent (2.5 % in patients <60 years of age, 13 % at ages 65–69, 16 % at ages 70–74, and 22 % at age > 75 [5]). In the USA, five million people suffer from intermittent claudication, the most common clinical disease presentation of PAD. The underlying mortality due to the cardiovascular risk profile in this patient population is close to 50 % in 10 years [6, 7]. Multisegment arterial involvement is present in 20 % of patients with intermittent claudication, and intermittent claudication is five times more common in diabetics than in nondiabetics. Since many patients are asymptomatic, the prevalence of PAD is higher than the prevalence of claudication or other signs of PAD [7].

Chronic critical limb ischemia (CLI) is the progression of intermittent claudication with persistently recurring rest pain for more than 2 weeks, ulceration, or gangrene at the foot, with an ankle systolic pressure less than 50 mmHg (Fontaine III and IV, Rutherford 4–6) [8]. In this stage, multilevel arterial disease involvement is common. Approximately 5 % of patients with IC will progress to CLI over the next 5 years, and the incidence of CLI is estimated at 1 new patient per 1,000 population per year [9]. The majority of patients with CLI will undergo some form of revascularization procedure, and 50 % will eventually require major amputation. The mortality rate of patients with CLI is up to 70 % at 5 years [10].

Patient Selection and Clinical Indications

The ideal management of patients with intermittent claudication remains controversial. Randomized clinical trials comparing revascularization with bypass surgery or percutaneous transluminal angioplasty (PTA) to exercise found benefit of supervised exercise programs with or without revascularization [11, 12]. Risk factor control with smoking cessation and a monitored exercise program can yield improvement or stabilization of their walking distance within 6–12 months in 75 % of patients [13, 14]. The remaining 25 % of these patients will usually deteriorate to severe chronic ischemia, with the likelihood for amputation in 5 or more years being approximately 10 %. The best predictor of deterioration of PAD is an ABI < 0.5. Supervised exercise programs have a definite advantage. The Cochrane Central Register of Controlled Trials reported an analysis of eight studies which showed statistically significant and clinically relevant differences in improvement of maximal treadmill walking distance with supervised exercise therapy compared with nonsupervised exercise therapy regimens [15] which translated to a difference of approximately 150 m increase in walking distance. This has been confirmed by a recent randomized controlled trial comparing supervised exercise, angioplasty, and combined therapy in patients with intermittent claudication [16].

Percutaneous treatment of infrainguinal disease in the claudicant depends on severity of symptoms, age, comorbidities, cardiovascular risk factors, and other issues [17–19]. Any proposed intervention should be associated with minimal risk and provide acceptable durability.

The incidence of patients with CLI is increasing, and approximately 50 % will indeed receive some type of revascularization. These patients often have severe multilevel atherosclerotic and infrapopliteal disease. The TransAtlantic Inter-Society Consensus of management of peripheral arterial disease (TASC) working group recommendation on the management of PAD is a comprehensive document and should be referred to as an important reference on patient selection and a guide for the various treatment modalities [19]. The TASC II document reflects an increased role for endovascular therapy in the infrainguinal segment including longer and more calcified lesions.

Procedural Considerations

Anatomic Considerations

In femoropopliteal segments, the TASC II document introduces useful guidelines for selecting between percutaneous and surgical treatment as follows (Fig. 16.1).

Recently, another clinical practice guideline for the diagnosis and treatment of patients with PAD has been completed by the American College of Cardiology (ACC) and American Heart Association (AHA) Task Force, with input from the Society for Vascular Surgery and Society of Interventional Radiology, and includes recommendations with different levels of scientific evidence. The goal of this comprehensive document is to significantly improve the care for patients with PAD. The final version can be downloaded at www.ACC.org/clinical/guidelines/PAD/index.pdf [18].

Procedure Planning

Careful planning is critical before undertaking an infrainguinal intervention. Unlike aortoiliac

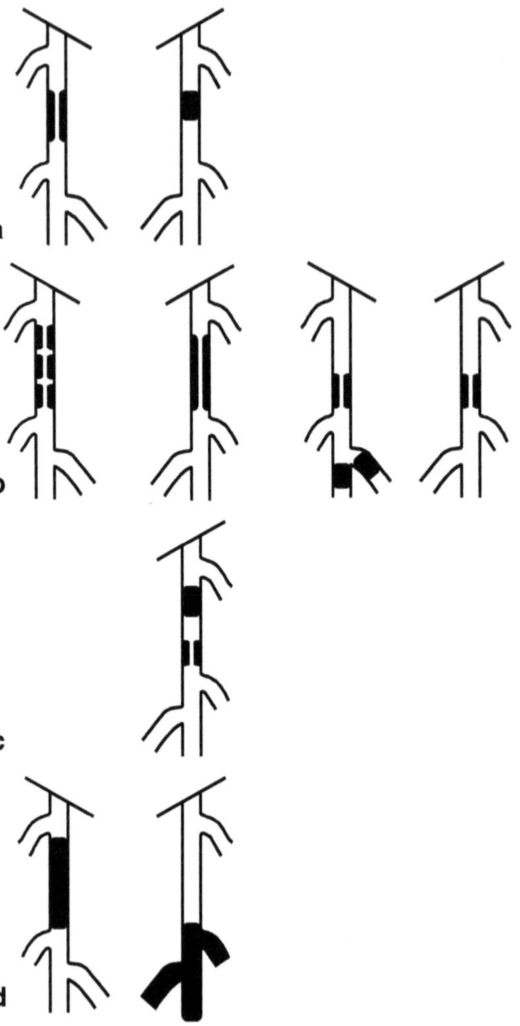

a b c d

Fig. 16.1 TASC-II recommendation based on lesion location and type for the femoropopliteal segment (Class **a**: endovascular therapy is treatment of choice; Class **b**: endovascular therapy is preferred; Class **c**: surgical therapy should be considered for low-risk patients; Class **d**: surgery is the treatment of choice)

interventions which can usually be planned "on the go," femoropopliteal interventions require prior knowledge of the patient's unique vascular anatomy to allow selection of approach and puncture site (antegrade, retrograde, or brachial) or the need for a hybrid approach (e.g., combination with an open common femoral artery repair). Prior knowledge of the presence of a chronic total occlusion (CTO) is important because it mandates a strategy for recanalization. Important anatomic features include proximal and distal levels of the occlusion, caliber and proximity of the proximal and distal stumps to important side branches such as the profunda femoris and popliteal trifurcation, proximity to joints and known flexion points, and quantity and quality of calcifications. Distal run-off baseline status as well as the exact pattern of collaterals is also very important to assess. Knowledge of the patient's prior vascular history and prior procedures/operations is mandatory as well as his/her general cardiovascular health. It is also crucial to be aware of the patient-specific body habitus and location of the common femoral artery bifurcation as it pertains to the bony landmark as this could impact the safety of the intervention. The need for a device closure strategy should usually be established periprocedurally.

Vessel and Device Sizing

Vessel sizing is an important component of planning infrainguinal interventions and may, in fact, further improve outcome [20]. Oversizing of the angioplasty balloon or stent can result in thrombosis and vessel injury including dissection. Stent undersizing is equally problematic because of the high risk of thrombosis and restenosis due to lack of wall opposition and decreased overall lumen diameter. Stent oversizing of 10–20 % is considered optimal in the SFA. Excessive sizing should be avoided with stent grafts due to the risk of fabric infolding which can result in early failure or edge restenosis [21]. Stent oversizing is also problematic with devices of higher radial strength, such as the SUPERA stent (IDEV, Webster, TX) which should not be oversized at all, whereas oversizing other devices such as Zilver (Cook, Bloomington, IN) or Control (Cordis, Miami, FL) may be better tolerated (do we need a reference for this). With plain PTA, proper oversizing is also an important key to success although it requires a delicate balance in order to avoid overdilation and vessel injury. In general, 10–25 % overdilation relative to adjacent "normal" segment is desired. Less overdilation is usually used with cutting balloons (up to 10 %) [22]. When sizing a vessel, a variety of approaches are valid, including the use of external radiopaque ruler or the now widely available automatically calibrated measuring tools available in most modern angiographic equipment. We have also found sizing on CTA and MRA source images quite helpful. Another way to size vessels in difficult anatomy is the use of the predilation balloon diameter as a reference. Inaccurate sizing can be due to inexperience of the operator, use of excessive magnification, poor filling on the angiogram, excessive calcification, and reliance on single projection angiography. IVUS is perhaps one of the most accurate and reliable sizing methods which also provides valuable information about the plaque burden and morphology [23]. Other helpful sizing tools include the small-vessel-sizing balloon Libra (Neovasc, British Columbia, Canada) capable of sizing vessels from 1.8 to 4.0 mm to the 100th mm [24].

Traversal of the Stenotic Lesion

Traversal of stenotic, not totally occlusive, lesions is best accomplished using a roadmap fluoroscopy technique or an overlay option. It requires careful navigation using a high-torque directional catheter-guidewire system and relies on constant tactile feedback by the operator. Gentle and controlled technique is paramount while attempting to traverse a stenosis, especially when irregular and complex in morphology, in order to avoid embolization, dissection, or perforation. The temptation to use a hydrophilic guidewire system first must be avoided because of the propensity of subintimal passage. Stenotic lesions can be traversed using a 0.014- to 0.035-in. guidewire introduced through a curved-tip catheter of an appropriate length. Our preferred choice is a 100-cm multipurpose curve (MPA) with a coaxial TAD II or Wholey 0.035-in. wire (Mallinckrodt, St Louis, MO), although we have also used 0.014- and 0.018-in. systems.

Chronic Total Occlusions (CTO)

Chronic total occlusions (CTOs) are a common occurrence in peripheral arterial disease. SFA and popliteal disease is one of the most prevalent patterns of infrainguinal involvement, especially in nondiabetics and nonelderly patients [25–27]. SFA interventions are challenging for a number of reasons: The SFA is one of the longest vessels in the body, has relatively few collaterals, courses through a narrow and restrictive adductor hiatus, is subjected to repetitive complex axial and rotational stresses (compression, contraction, distraction, torsion, flexion), has nonlaminar flow dynamics, and often has stenoses characterized by heavy calcifications and elastic recoil. This translates into higher rates of recurrence after endovascular interventions. In patients presenting with symptomatic PVD, SFA occlusions, usually longer than 10 cm, are twice more common than stenosis [19, 25]; therefore, familiarity in the management of CTO of SFA is crucial. Moreover, CTOs in the SFA are more prone to dissection and failure to reenter the true lumen especially in the presence of heavy calcifications. Other problems are flush occlusion of the SFA without a visible stump or presence of severe disease of the SFA ostium. The TransAtlantic Inter-Society Consensus (TASC) II guidelines classify CTOs of the femoropopliteal arteries and proximal trifurcation vessels as TASC II type C or D [28]. Although surgery has been the traditional recommendation for the treatment of TASC II type C and D lesions, many "vascular specialists" have adopted a more aggressive approach benefiting from improved technology and devices allowing a high success rate in traversal of CTOs, with recanalization rates of up to 97 % achieved in limbs with TASC II type femoropopliteal C and D occlusions [29]. Recent data suggest that claudicating patients with femoropopliteal TASC II C and D lesions will benefit from the endovascular treatment, although patients presenting CLI have a worse outcome [29].

Careful planning is crucial for success in the endovascular management of infrainguinal diseases especially when femoropopliteal CTO is present. The length of the occlusion, proximal and distal stump diameters, presence of calcification, collaterals, and status of the runoff are determined. The presence of a stump has to be confirmed on the proper steep oblique

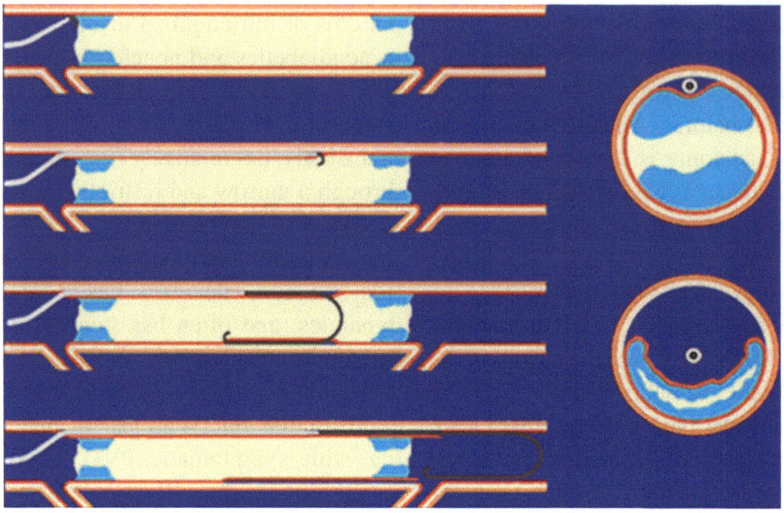

Fig. 16.2 Basic technique of percutaneous intentional extraluminal recanalization (PIER) also referred to as subintimal recanalization. The distal glide-wire is formed into a loop in the subintimal space. It is advanced firmly, acting as an endarterectomy dissector. Successful reentry into the true lumen usually occurs at the area of transition into a relatively disease-free lumen. Rapid drop in resistance can be immediately appreciated, and the loop then sails into the reconstituted distal lumen. The importance of experience and tactile feedback cannot be overemphasized

position. Certain anatomic variants must be excluded such as a large medial profunda branch that can arise from the medial aspect of the SFA and may overlap with the SFA on shallow projections. This greatly limits the options for therapy. In our practice, the need to cage the profunda or a major profunda branch during SFA stenting is considered a contraindication. One option in those cases is to resort to a hybrid procedure where the CFA-profunda disease is treated with endarterectomy/patch angioplasty. During that procedure, we create a 2–3-cm landing zone in the proximal SFA by eversion endarterectomy following which stenting could be undertaken without compromising the profunda.

There are two primary strategies for CTO crossing: intraluminal and subintimal. Careful pre-procedural planning is important to determine whether an intraluminal or subintimal strategy should be selected for the traversal of the lesion. For example, dense femoral calcification can serve as a relative contraindication for subintimal stenting because this can affect the eventual result (Fig. 16.2). Revascularization should also take into account the size and pattern of distal filling of collaterals, and when a stent-graft treatment plan is chosen, it should be planned to limit collateral compromise to avoid catastrophic ischemia in the event of interventional failure or reocclusion.

Percutaneous Intentional Extraluminal Recanalization

The technique of percutaneous intentional extraluminal recanalization (PIER) also sometimes referred to as subintimal recanalization was first described and popularized by Bolia et al. [30]. This technique can be used primarily or as a bailout in the case of failed intraluminal recanalization. PIER involves the following steps: (1) entry into the subintimal space proximal to an occlusion, (2) creation of a tissue plane within the arterial wall, (3) reentry into the patent arterial lumen at the point of reconstitution beyond the occlusion, and (4) balloon dilatation to pressurize the lumen created in the subintimal space to bridge the true lumen proximal and distal to the lesion. Successful subintimal revascularization is dependent on the effective traversal of the lesion, reentry into the true lumen at the most proximal, disease-free portion of the vessel, and the subsequent ability of balloon angioplasty to establish antegrade flow through the newly created lumen.

Despite increasing familiarity with this technique in name, the way it is described is often vague, and hence its application is quite variable among operators, which likely explains the variable success rates with it. The technique draws striking similarity to the surgical technique of endarterectomy in that the key to success is being in the proper plane. Surgeons who perform endarterectomy recognize this plane as an outer medial layer where the plaque simply peels off. During endovascular recanalization, this is also the plane where one gets to, either intentionally or unintentionally; the looped wire sails forward with relative ease. A looped glide-wire in the subintimal space acts much like the freer elevator-dissector, and successful reentry into the lumen depends upon the presence of rapid transition between heavy disease burden and relatively disease-free segment. Much like one can terminate the endarterectomy at this transition point during open carotid (most other endarterectomies like common femoral may end with a shelf distally) endarterectomy, one can force through the thin plaque covering the edge of the plaque with coiled wire loop (Fig. 16.2).

Reentry into the true lumen too distal to the occlusion can present a number of problems by compromising patency of important collaterals or side branches, or traversing flexion points or joints, which may limit surgical options for treatment. It is important to carefully review pre-procedural vascular imaging, as well as to obtain delayed angiographic images, to ascertain the actual point of reconstitution through collaterals to prevent overestimation of the lesion length. In cases where true lumen reentry is not feasible, such as in heavily calcified vessels, poor subintimal plane, or extensive plaque at the desired reentry location, one might try reentering at a different location in the hope of achieving a better transition point that enables breakthrough into the true lumen. If this fails, then the remaining options consist of sharp reentry techniques using either homemade systems or the more expensive reentry devices [31]. False channel balloon dilatation to allow breakthrough into the lumen can occasionally be helpful. Another option may be to attempt retrograde transpopliteal or transcrural recanalization [32, 33] which can also be accomplished using a micro-wire system with a snare docking technique. It is crucial when performing CTO recanalization to have a stable access that limits recoil. Antegrade access is ideal but not always feasible. If over-the-horn access is chosen, a stable, long, kink-resistant platform is desired, such as a 6-French 70-cm long Raabe sheath (Cook) or a similar product. In case of difficult anchoring with the sheath, a coaxial guide catheter technique or anchoring balloon technique may be used. Avoiding excessive forward pressure during PIER is important for preventing unintentional extraluminal passage of the guidewire into the perivascular space or fascial planes. If this occurs, it may be difficult or impossible to regain an intraluminal position for traversal of the lesion.

PIER is a particularly viable primary technique in patients with CLI who have long-segment (>30 cm) occlusions of infrainguinal vessels, including ostial disease, and occlusions extending to tibial vessel origins (TASC-D). Clinically, the biggest impact of subintimal angioplasty is in chronic critical limb ischemia (CLI). Subintimal angioplasty is at some centers the first-line treatment in CLI for up to 65 % of patients can be managed with this method without the need for surgery and reported 5-year limb salvage rates of 72.9 % comparing well to bypass surgery [34]. Initial technical success rates of 80–85 % have been reported using PIER with 50–58 % primary patency at 3 years for lesions of a mean length of 11–15 cm [35]. The length of occlusion does not have a major influence on the technical success or reocclusion rates. The lack of randomized trials to compare PIER to surgical bypass or conventional PTA and the requirement for advanced technical skills and experience by the operator limit this technique to select centers and mostly to patients with CLI who are nonsurgical candidates. The ability of this technique to achieve limb salvage in CLI is remarkable, and it may also serve as a bridge prior to electively planned surgery. Collective review of 23 studies reporting on a total of 1,549 patients treated with PIER was recently published. The technical success rates ranged from 80 to 90 %, with lower rates for crural lesions compared with femoral lesions. Complications were mostly minor and ranged from 8 to 17 %. Outcomes at 1 year were favorable with sustained clinical response between 50 and 70 %, primary patency around 50 %, and limb salvage rate from 80 to 90 % [36]. The most common complication during PIER was perforation of the arterial wall, which can occur in 3 % of cases [37, 38] and is usually of little significance other than the fact that the PIER procedure usually will have to be abandoned. If perforation complicated balloon dilation following recanalization, this can normally be managed by prolonged balloon tamponade, or adjunct stenting or stent grafting. Although guidewire perforations will generally seal, the unrecognized passage of a catheter or balloon outside of the artery may result in serious extravasation and/or compartment syndrome. Therefore, prompt recognition of extraluminal positioning is important so that the arterial channel can be coil embolized if needed or a stent graft placed across the perforation once true lumen reentry is achieved. The perforation may be tamponaded with an inflated balloon catheter while maintaining access for continued wire negotiation across the occlusion.

True Lumen Reentry Devices

A number of commercially available true lumen reentry devices can be used either primarily or to bail out PIER with inability to reenter. The Outback catheter (*Cordis Corporation, Miami, Florida*) uses a single-wire lumen and a directionally controlled, deployable, platinum-coated radiopaque 27-gauge needle (extendable cannula) for reentry, through which a 0.014-in. guidewire is passed into the disease-free vessel segment [39–41]. Its main mode of guidance is fluoroscopic triangulation. The Pioneer device (Medtronic, Inc., Santa Rosa, CA) which is used in conjunction with a dedicated intravascular ultrasound (IVUS) system (Volcano, San Diego, CA) is a popular true lumen reentry device because of its reliability and real-time image guidance [42, 43]. It has two wire lumens (one of which is monorail). IVUS is used in the ChromaFlow mode to identify blood flow in the true lumen [44]. The 25-gauge integrated nitinol reentry needle is then guided to the true lumen. As with PIER, reentry very distal to the end of the occlusion should be aggressively avoided when using reentry devices in order not to jeopardize patency of vital side branches or effectively converting the occlusion from an above-the-knee CTO to a below-the-knee CTO. This not only may adversely affect patency but also compromises future surgical options for bypass ("burning bridges"). In the event that reentry cannot be achieved at a more proximate reconstituted patent segment, either the subintimal tract should be coiled to allow a redirected attempt at reentry or the patient should be considered for a different approach.

Intraluminal Recanalization

The other approach in CTO is intraluminal recanalization where subintimal passage of the wire is avoided. Given the typically long length of CTO in femoropopliteal disease and high prevalence of calcifications which limit the ability to reenter into the true lumen, there has been an increasing interest in direct intraluminal recanalization without subintimal passage [45]. Proponents of this approach cite the low success rate of PIER in long-segment occlusions and in the presence of extensive calcifications. A direct approach is felt to lower the risk of both perforation and too-distal reentry. Current treatment modalities such as blunt microdissection, mechanical atherectomy, and subintimal reentry devices have improved the success rate in these often challenging cases. Importantly, maintaining an intraluminal course may also allow the use of debulking approaches of the commonly encountered heavily calcified lesions, which may allow a satisfactory outcome with atherectomy alone or atherectomy with adjunct balloon angioplasty without the need to stent.

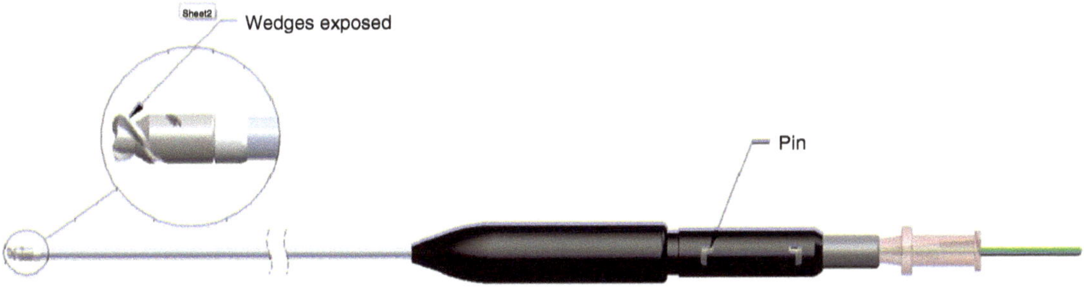

Fig. 16.3 The Avinger Wildcat-W500 support catheter (*Avinger, Inc., Redwood City, CA*). It is a guidewire-compatible catheter that acts like a corkscrew, wedging through the CTO. The deflectable, drill-like tip enables incremental advancement of the coaxial guidewire to pass through the occluded area. It is mainly intended to be used to support steerable guidewires in directly negotiating the occlusive plaque material

Intraluminal recanalization can occasionally be achieved with standard coaxial guidewire-catheter approach using a 4- or 5-French gentle-angle catheter with a 0.035-in. Our preferred approach for that is a floppy spring coil wire such as LLT (Cook, Bloomington, IN), although a straight glide-wire can also be used. However, rough "snow plow"-like technique is often required which may cause distal embolization and perforation. Often, a subintimal plane is entered, and the technique will then have to be changed to a PIER approach. As a result, a number of CTO-specific micro-guidewire systems have evolved originally for the coronary circulation but have been adopted to the periphery, especially in the infrageniculate segments.

Modern intraluminal recanalization requires the use of specialty CTO guidewires which are stiffer, coated wires with a tapered tip available in a variety of designs, specifications, and characteristics. Some of the popular designs are the ASAHI line (Abbott, Abbott Park, IL), Cross-It (Abbott, Abbott Park, IL), ChoICE PT (Boston Scientific/Scimed, Inc., Maple Grove, MN). A number of non-specialty wires that have good pushability, trackability, torquability can also prove quite successful in navigating CTOs at lower cost such as Hi-Torque Whisper (Abbott, Abbott Park, IL), Crosswire (Terumo Medical Corporation, Somerset, NJ), Persuader (Medtronic, Minneapolis, MN), and V-18 Control (Boston Scientific, Natick, MA), especially when used through a stable steerable microcatheter such as the Transit and Prowler lines (Cordis, Miami, FL), Excelsior (Boston Scientific), and FineCross and Progreat (Terumo Medical Co.).

It should be kept in mind that a catheter-guide combination approach can work best if high-support catheter platform system is used. The 4-French hydrophilic catheter works well in softer lesions but has limited pushability in fibrotic calcified subintimal recanalizations. The technique of anchoring balloon has been described and may allow a stable platform to enable traversal of the CTO with a wire [46]. High-support catheters have been recently developed that assist in this task. The CXI Support Catheter (Cook) is one example, available from in various profiles (2.6–4 French) with straight- and angle-tip configurations and compatible with 0.014–0.035-in. guidewires. The Quick-Cross support catheter line (Spectranetics, Colorado Springs, CO) is a possible CTO support catheter system.

The ASAHI Tornus specialty catheter (Abbott) is a novel over-the-wire stainless steel penetration catheter designed to provide greater support and assist with penetration of the CTO. It is constructed of eight individual 0.007-in. wires stranded together to form the catheter, with a silicone coating on the inner and outer surfaces and a tapered tip. The device works via a screw-like mechanism through counterclockwise rotation. The Avinger Wildcat support catheter (*Avinger, Inc., Redwood City, CA*) is a similar system. It is a 135 cm long, 0.035-in. compatible catheter with the key feature of distal tip with retractable bilateral wedges (Fig. 16.3).

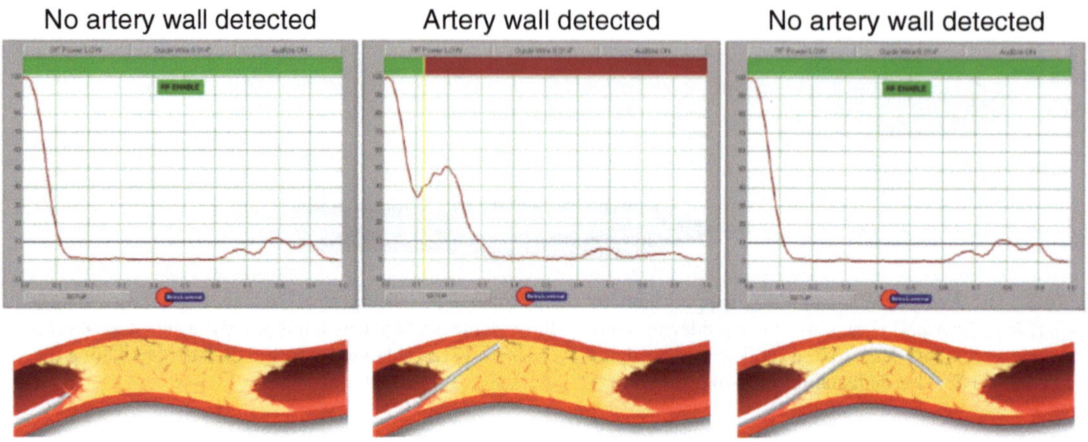

Fig. 16.4 Safe-Cross AP RF system: Dual function wire system that uses forward-looking OCT to guide RF application into the plaque

Another useful class of specialty devices include deflecting tip guidewires like the Steer-It (Cordis). Another related approach for controlled guidewire passage is "wire control" catheters (Venture, St. Jude Medical, St. Paul, MN). Another paradigm that is being currently evaluated is the use of a magnetic navigation system (Stereotaxis, St. Louis, MO) to assist in navigating a specialty guidewire across CTOs. Early results in coronary applications seem promising, but data remains limited [47]. Other interesting pharmacologic approaches (directed fibrinolysis, demineralization, or collagenase delivery into the occlusion) are also being studied.

In cases where occlusion cannot be traversed using conventional catheter-guidewire techniques, intraluminal recanalization may still be achieved with a number of specialized devices through an "ablative" approach. The Frontrunner XP CTO (*Cordis*, Warren, NJ) has actuating jaws that create a channel through occlusions via blunt microdissection with more pushability and control than traditional 0.035-in. guidewires. It theoretically relies on the differential elastic properties of adventitia versus the fibrocalcific plaque to create fracture planes. This technique may be advantageous in penetrating hard fibrous caps of the SFA occlusions. The Crosser catheter (BARD, Murray Hill, NJ) is an over-the-wire system that produces high-frequency mechanical vibrations that propagate through its tip. The resulting cavitational effects aid in the recanalization of the proximal core or edge of the occlusion, allowing the guidewire to incrementally traverse the occlusion. The PowerWire radio-frequency guidewire (*Baylis Medical Company, Montreal, QC, Canada*) delivers focused RF energy through a nitinol core wire with PTFE coating. The Safe-Cross AP RF system (IntraLuminal Therapeutics, Menlo Park, CA) is a marriage of the optical coherence reflectometry (OCR) forward-looking guidance technology and controlled radio-frequency energy (Fig. 16.4). The wire's integrated optical fiber relays light reflections to the console to distinguish plaque and blood vessel wall by OCT. The wire is coupled with radio-frequency energy that is delivered from the tip if the reflective signal obtained by the near-infrared sensor identifies a luminal position, signified by a green indicator. Radio frequency is not deliverable if the reflective signal is red, suggesting wire proximity to the endoluminal wall [48].

Excimer laser is another approach that has witnessed a revival in the past years. Its use in occlusive disease is discussed elsewhere in this chapter. The principle behind the use of excimer laser in CTO recanalization is based on the fact that CTO is usually composed of a focal proximal cap followed by a long segment of gelatinous debris culminating in another distal fibrous cap.

Various excimer laser catheters are available each with various specific features, including the Turbo Elite, Turbo-Booster, and Turbo-Tandem (Spectranetics Co., Colorado Springs, CO). The 308-nm excimer catheter is used to penetrate the fibrous cap of the chronic total occlusion. Once the proximal cap is crossed, it may be advantageous to directly interact with the platelet and coagulated material. Absorption of excimer laser energy within the target biologic tissue creates effects on the nonaqueous components of the irradiated atherosclerotic plaque and its accompanying thrombus. It accounts for development of plaque-specific photochemical and photomechanical reactions including formation of gas vapor and acoustic shock waves. The vaporization of plaque content and concomitant propagation of acoustic resonance waves ultimately lead to debulking and removal of the treated occlusive tissue. Underlying occlusive disease is then balloon dilated or stented as needed. The specific technique used to recanalize CTO excimer laser is the "step-by-step" technique [49]. The laser catheter and guidewire are advanced in tandem through the occlusion until access to the true lumen beyond the occlusion is achieved.

Plain Old Balloon Angioplasty (POBA)

Percutaneous transluminal angioplasty (PTA) is currently more "trendily" referred to as plain old balloon angioplasty (POBA). While angiographic results of POBA are often immediate, the long-term success of femoropopliteal POBA varies and is not clearly defined. Furthermore, the difficulty in assessing rapidly changing technological improvements is compounded by inconsistencies in the literature in regard to patient risk factors, lesion characteristics, indications for intervention, and follow-up. In addition, a number of technical factors such as dilation pressure, duration of PTA, and balloon to vessel ratio are rarely accounted for. Nevertheless, there are some common themes that warrant discussion.

The multicenter STAR registry prospectively examined predictors of long-term patency of femoropopliteal PTA in 219 limbs in 205 patients in the mid-1990s [50]. The presence of diabetes or renal failure conferred a four to fivefold increased risk of restenosis compared to matched controls. While this data examined patients in the early experience of PTA, more recent work confirms that diabetes leads to a decreased primary patency with PTA in both the subset of patients with a stent and those with PTA alone [51]. Interestingly, both these studies note that there was significant improvement in primary patency of PTA with at least one relatively disease-free tibial vessel. Patients with three patent runoff vessels may have an eightfold increase in patency when compared with those with a single, diseased (50–90 % stenosis) runoff vessel. The relationship between diabetes and the presence of extensive runoff disease may confer a large portion of diabetic risk of restenosis.

The overriding importance of clinical indications for intervention can be seen in a recent meta-analysis demonstrating a 3-year patency rate of 60 % for femoropopliteal angioplasty when done for claudication and 40 % when performed for limb salvage [52]. This data is further clarified by Johnston et al. who correlated improvement of lower extremity runoff as an indicator of 5-year PTA success [53]. Similarly, chronic total occlusions (CTO) with good runoff had a clinical success rate of 36 % at 5 years versus 16 % with poor runoff.

One recent comparative review of 112 peripheral PTA studies summarizes these points and denotes the importance of lesion characteristics in regard to PTA for femoropopliteal lesions [54]. The analysis revealed mean weighted primary patency ranging from 69 % at 1 year to 48 % at 5 years, which were dependent on lesion morphology, lesion length, patency of runoff vessels, and presence of diabetes. It is important to stress that the ultimate goal of any intervention in PAD is limb salvage. The standard surgical bypasses have 5-year (secondary) patency rates of 80 % when autologous vein grafts are used and 38 % with synthetic PTFE, with accordingly higher limb salvage rates [55, 56]. Similarly, long-term patency for PTA might not be necessary once the primary goal of tissue healing is accomplished.

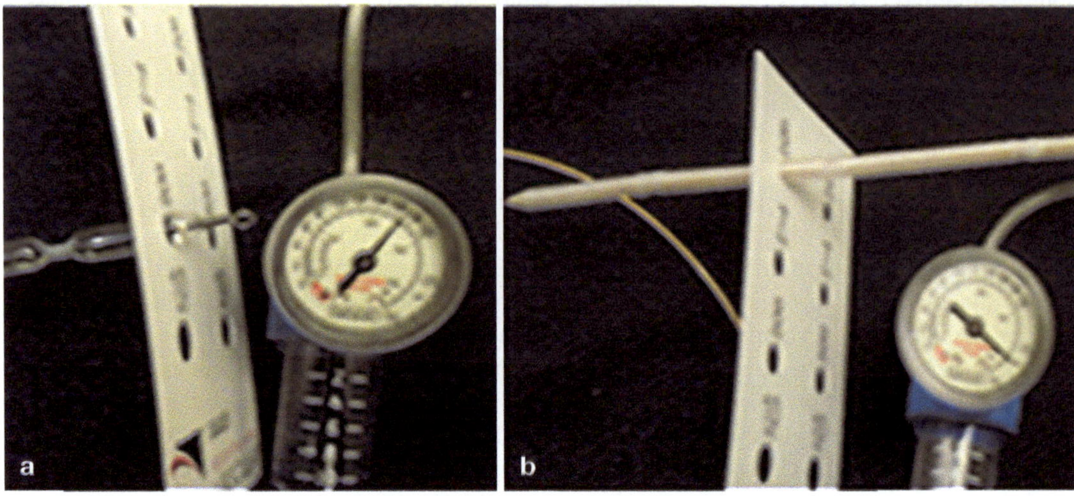

Fig. 16.5 The impact of balloon compliance and high-pressure expansion on the dilation of difficult lesions. (**a**) Standard nylon PTA balloon. At supranominal pressure, despite persistence stenosis, over-dilatation has occurred at both ends of the balloon. The 8×60 nylon balloon could not be inserted through the 8-mm hole. (**b**) Properly sized wrapped balloon (Dorado, BARD) used to treat three consecutive lesions. At 27 atm, the lesions are effaced with NO over-dilatation of intervening healthy tissue. The 6×200 balloon can be easily inserted through a 6-mm hole

Limb salvage rates following infrainguinal endovascular intervention at 2–3 years vary from 44 to 85 % [57–63]. However, the only randomized study to date comparing PTA and surgical bypass recommends infrainguinal PTA for rest pain and tissue loss in only those patients with a life expectancy less than 2 years [64].

A newer paradigm in PTA seems to be evolving based on the observation that high atmospheric inflation of current semi-compliant balloons is not efficient in dilating the target lesion and instead results in excessive injury to adjacent less diseased vessel segment, thereby contributing to restenosis [65]. This phenomenon is probably more significant in resistant, heavily calcified, or fibrotic lesions that are unlikely to be effaced at nominal balloon inflation pressures (Fig. 16.5). The new paradigm calls for the use of the newer "wrapped balloons" which have the combined features of strength, true noncompliance, and high atmospheric rating. The prototype wrapped balloon is the Dorado balloon line (BARD), which is also available in long balloon lengths allowing treatment of long lesions without overlapping. This achieves uniform inflation without overdilation and may translate into both better initial success and lower rates of restenosis. However, most importantly the use of such a strategy may obviate the need for secondary stenting for unsatisfactory angioplasty results. Although attractive in principle, this theory has not yet been supported with objective data from well-designed comparative trials.

Another closely related concept is the use of lesion remodeling prior to angioplasty, or effectively changing the compliance of the lesion favorably. This usually calls for reducing acute recoil by debulking of calcifications and other forms of resistant stenosis with atherectomy or excimer laser prior to low atmospheric balloon angioplasty. Along the same line, cutting balloon angioplasty using the longer balloon length devices may accomplish the similar goal without the need for supranominal balloon inflations. In light of the mounting evidence for long-term problems with stents in the SFA and popliteal segments, one additional important gain from such a strategy may be reducing the need for stenting in the infrainguinal segments [66]. One unpublished study reported significant reduction in the need to use stents following atherectomy in femoropopliteal disease (*Reduced stent utilization with SilverHawk atherectomy versus balloon angioplasty in patients undergoing peripheral vascular interventions: A randomized trial. Presented at CRT 2008* (*was this ever published*)) [67]. Although not directly related, another recently published randomized comparison of cryoplasty with POBA in the SFA demonstrated a significant reduction in the need for secondary stenting from 73 % in the POBA group to 22 % in the cryoplasty group [68], which is a testimony to the value of these approaches in higher up-front technical success rates without the use of stents.

For example, when a highly resistant lesion is treated with a standard nylon PTA balloon, inflation to a supranominal pressure despite persistence of the "resistant" stenosis will result in over-dilatation at both ends of the balloon which could result in significant damage to the normal segments of the vessel. In contrast, when a properly sized wrapped balloon (e.g., Dorado, BARD) is used to treat highly resistant disease, the lesions are effaced with no over-dilatation of adjacent or intervening healthy segments.

Special Balloon Angioplasty Techniques

Brachytherapy

Progression of neointimal proliferation and hyperplasia can be reduced by endovascular brachytherapy in the peripheral vascular bed [69]. Devices may include either a radioactive liquid-filled balloon or a radioactive wire placed into the diseased vessel for times ranging from 5 to 20 min [70, 71]. Research in this area for peripheral vasculature continues, although no FDA-approved devices are marketed at this time.

In the PARIS pretrial, 40 patients received high-dose radiation after conventional PTA in SFA lesions resulting in low 1-year restenosis rates [72]. The subsequent study which randomized 203 patients showed no difference in restenosis rates or clinical response when compared to PTA alone [73]. Similarly, the 5-year follow-up from the prospective Vienna-2 trial showed that there was no difference at in those patients receiving femoropopliteal PTA alone or those receiving adjuvant iridium-192 radiation using wire delivery [74]. It is important to note that in all studies done using brachytherapy for infrainguinal disease, none have dealt with treatment of recurrent stenosis, but instead have used brachytherapy at the time of initial intervention [75].

Thus, despite initial encouraging results, brachytherapy might not have the desired long-lasting effect. Furthermore, the significant logistical ramifications for instituting a brachytherapy program will likely not propel this therapeutic option into mainstream therapy.

Endovascular Cryotherapy (Cryoplasty)

Cryoplasty involves the application of cold thermal energy to balloon angioplasty and addresses two major challenges of conventional balloon angioplasty: early technical failure by intimal dissection or elastic recoil and late restenosis caused by neointimal proliferation. Early experience suggests that targeted delivery of cryotherapy within vessels may have the effect of altering the biologic vascular response, resulting in a more benign healing following balloon injury in a nonproliferative fashion [76]. Balloon inflation in cryoplasty is achieved with nitrous oxide cooling the balloon to −10°C. The balloon has an automated inflation time of 20 s at 8 ATM. As nitrous oxide is vaporized in the balloon, it delivers the inflation pressure in addition to cooling temperatures to the arterial wall. Standard balloon diameters (2.5–8 mm) and balloon lengths of 20, 40, and 60 mm are available.

In a study of 102 patients with claudication from 16 participating centers, femoropopliteal lesions (TASC type A, B, or C) were treated with a technical success rate of 85.3 % [77]. For all lesion types in this series (stenoses and occlusions), there was a 9-month clinical patency rate of 82.2 %. Multiple smaller series confirmed these early results.

While results from the POLAR randomized trial are awaited, analysis of the more recent literature on cryotherapy is disappointing. In one large single-center patient cohort, freedom from restenosis in successfully treated lesions was strikingly lower from the previous experience reported by the same investigators: 57 % at 12 months and 49 % at 24 months compared to 82.2 % (12 months) [78]. In particular, cryoplasty performed poorly in heavily calcified lesions, vein graft lesions, and in-stent restenotic lesions. Excluding these challenging lesion subtypes from the analysis resulted in a freedom-from-restenosis rate of 61 % at 12 months and 52 % at 24 months. Intention-to-treat analysis further weakened the results to 47 and 38 % at 12 and 24 months, respectively. This was particularly disappointing since the mean lesion length in the study was 3.9 cm (TASC A) which should have resulted in much better patency rates. Another retrospective review looking at 71 patients showed no difference in primary patency, assisted primary patency, or secondary patency between conventional PTA and cryoplasty [79]. A recent single-center study randomized 50 diabetic patients with femoropopliteal disease to cryoplasty or conventional PTA with the cryoplasty arm having significantly higher restenosis rates and lower primary patency rates and at 3 years, with no difference in limb salvage [80]. However, one recently published study demonstrated the potential benefits to using cryoplasty first approach compared to POBA in terms of reduction in the need for provisional stenting which was significantly lowered from 73 % in the POBA group to 22 % in the cryoplasty group, although patency rates were comparable for the two groups (56 and 49 % for cryoplasty vs. 61 and 56 % for POBA, respectively, at 1 and 3 years) [68].

Cutting Balloon Angioplasty

Cutting balloons are PTA balloons that contain a series of thin microtomes attached to a noncompliant balloon. When inflated, these microtomes expand longitudinally into the plaque and vessel wall and deliver a controlled incision resulting in plaque disintegration. In theory, CB has advantages in fibrotic or thick-walled vessels that are resistant to conventional PTA. Also less force is necessary compared to conventional PTA resulting in theoretical decrease in a neoproliferative response. Limited clinical data are available on the use of cutting balloons in infrainguinal interventions.

Although multiple early reports purport excellent results of CB [81, 82], a more recent prospectively randomized single-center trial comparing cutting balloons to PTA in short-segment de novo SFA lesions showed no benefit [83]. Notably, the restenosis rate at 6 months was significantly higher in the cutting balloon group compared to PTA (62 % vs. 32 %). Furthermore, one study evaluating the value of CB in the treatment of failing infrainguinal vein grafts shows no improvement when compared to PTA [84].

Newer cutting balloons have entered the market with proposed improvements over past designs. The AngioSculpt Scoring Balloon Catheter (AngioScore, Inc., Fremont, CA) initially developed for the treatment of complex coronary artery lesions combines a semi-compliant balloon with laser-cut nitinol scoring wire encircling the balloon in a helical pattern. Current devices are available in 2- to 6-mm diameter and 10- to 40-mm lengths and mainly used in the infrageniculate vessels. Case series have documented angiographic success in small numbers of patients with this device, although comparisons with conventional PTA are lacking [85].

Similarly, the VascuTrak PTA Dilatation Catheter (BARD Peripheral Vascular, Inc., Tempe, AZ) has two longitudinal wires which, in theory, lead to a focused plaque fracture and reduction in balloon pressure. Another important advantage of this line of balloons is availability in very long lengths which allows treating the target lesion without multiple overlaps. These devices are available ranging from 2 to 7 mm in diameter with lengths ranging from 20- to 300-mm lengths. There are no randomized or long-term data for either of these new devices at the present time.

Drug-Coated Balloon Angioplasty

Neointimal hyperplasia is a proliferative biological process that is triggered during PTA and is the main cause of lumen loss leading to restenosis following PTA. Being a primarily biologic process, pharmacological modulation of neointimal proliferation has been proposed as a means to inhibit neointimal hyperplasia and forms the basis also for drug-coated balloons to achieve long-term patency. Initial trials with paclitaxel-coated balloons in coronary in-stent restenosis were followed by two trials investigating treatment of de novo and restenotic lesions in the SFA and popliteal arteries. The initial multicenter randomized trial comparing paclitaxel-coated and uncoated balloons (THUNDER) demonstrated that patients in the paclitaxel-coated balloon group had far less late lumen loss and less target lesion revascularization compared to the control group [86]. This difference was maintained over the 2-year follow-up period (15 % vs. 52 %). In the second study, late lumen loss in the control group was less, and the difference to the group treated with the coated balloon smaller [87]. The PTA procedure itself does not differ from conventional PTA with similar inflation pressures and inflation times. Drug-eluting balloons are not at present commercially available in the USA for peripheral vascular beds.

Atherectomy

Atherectomy devices represent a new technology which removes plaque from lesions of any length. It has potential for the treatment of lesions in difficult anatomic locations such as across joints or folding points (common femoral artery, popliteal artery) and ostial lesions (such as the ostium of the SFA). It holds promise as an adjunct therapy for "prepping" heavily calcified lesions prior to another adjunct endovascular modality although enthusiast proponents have hailed this technique as a stand-alone treatment for long diseased segments. Although not approved for this indication, it has also been used for the treatment of in-stent restenosis, despite conflicting data [88].

The first broad group of devices evolved from the Simpson AtheroCath (Devices for Vascular Intervention, Redwood City, CA) and is extirpative in nature. The prototype device is the SilverHawk™ plaque excision system (ev3 Endovascular, Plymouth, MN). The newer generation devices, RockHawk and TurboHawk, are marketed by the same manufacturer and have a better profile with respect to treatment of heavily calcified lesions.

Approved by the FDA in June 2003 for use in lower extremity arteries ranging from 3 to 7 mm in diameter, the SilverHawk device consists of a flexible monorail catheter designed to track over a 0.014-in. guidewire. Directional plaque excision is accomplished with a cutting assembly located at the distal end of the catheter, comprised of a battery-operated cutting disc rotating at 8,000 rpm contained within a tubular housing with a lateral window. Atheromatous plaque is stored in a distal nose cone compartment, and focal lesions can be treated in a small amount of time. Once the storage compartment is full, the SilverHawk device has to be removed over the 0.014-in. wire, and the atheromatous tissue is removed from the nose cone. Theoretically, the SilverHawk catheter minimizes stretching of the vessel and reduces barotrauma to its wall.

No randomized studies are available to compare the results of SilverHawk atherectomy with other well-established endovascular treatments. The Treating Peripherals with SilverHawk Outcomes Collection (TALON) registry is a multicenter, prospective, nonrandomized, observational database. Recent data from this registry included analysis of 728 patients and 1,517 lesions treated with the SilverHawk catheter. Lesion lengths were approximately 6.3 cm for femoropopliteal and 3.5 cm for tibioperoneal vessels. Approximately 17 % of patients required additional therapy including stenting. At 6 and 12 months, the target lesion revascularization was 10 and 21 %, respectively, with a durable improvement of the ankle-brachial index [89]. Zeller et al. reported on the use of the SilverHawk device in 52 patients with femoropopliteal disease and stable chronic lower limb occlusive disease [90]. Additional PTA or stenting was needed in 58 and 6 % of cases, respectively. More than 80 % of their patient population was free of symptoms after 6 months of follow-up. A prospective, multicenter registry involving 160 lesions in 74 limbs treated with atherectomy was also published [91]. The treated segments included the femoropopliteal as well as the trifurcation vessels. Eleven percent of patients had to undergo adjunctive angioplasty and 6 % adjunctive stent placement. The target limb revascularization (TLR) rate was only 4 % at 6 months. However, following initial enthusiasm, a series of reports not relying on TLR as a means of follow-up revealed a disappointing mid- and long-term patency with this device [92–94]. In our own experience with the SilverHawk utilizing intensive duplex surveillance, the primary and assisted primary patency rates at 1 year were a dismal 10 % in a predominantly CLI patient population, although a 74 % limb salvage rate was maintained through secondary interventions, predominantly stenting and bypass surgery [93].

The main limitation to the use of the SilverHawk catheter is the presence of extensive or dense calcification of the arterial wall. It is difficult to cut these in part bulky plaques with the risk of distal embolization. This risk was highlighted in a report on ten consecutive patients treated with atherectomy of the femoropopliteal artery in the presence of a distal embolic protection device. The investigator reported debris retrieval in each case [95]. The clinical consequence of these atheroemboli and comparison to other endovascular techniques remain unclear. Treatment of longer lesion can add time to the treatment since intermittent evacuation of the collected atherosclerotic material from the device is necessary. Although a newer generation of extirpative atherectomy devices, *TurboHawk* and *RockHawk*, have been released, no substantive data has been published on their effectiveness or superiority compared to their predecessor. Expense is also an issue in particular for the cases where additional PTA or stenting is necessary and the need for secondary stenting following atherectomy has been repeatedly highlighted in many of the atherectomy series [93].

The second broad class of atherectomy devices is ablative in nature and conceptually related to the *Rotablator* (Boston Scientific, Natick, MA). These include the *Diamondback 360° Orbital Atherectomy System* (OAS, Cardiovascular Systems, Inc., St. Paul, MN) and the *Jetstream revascularization system* (Pathway Medical, Kirkland, WA).

Orbital atherectomy with the *Diamondback 360°* is similar to rotational atherectomy with the *Rotablator* with exception of using an orbital path around the periphery of the lumen, thereby minimizing the risk of deep vascular injury. In essence, the device debulks atheroma by using a sanding action of an orbiting diamond-coated crown mounted on the end of a flexible drive shaft and placed over a .014″ guidewire. Marketed as an effective way to debulk challenging calcified lesions in the femoropopliteal and infrageniculate vessels with any plaque morphology, comparative data are lacking. Recently, the prospective nonrandomized multicenter study to evaluate the efficacy and safety of the Diamondback 360° device in peripheral intervention (OASIS trial) was completed. In 201 lesions (50 % calcified) in 124 patients, a 4 % device-related complication rate and a 2.4 % TLR at 6 months were reported. Adjunctive therapy (PTA, stent) was necessary in 42 %. The study was designed as a noninferiority trial with no further conclusive data, save that of immediate angiographic success [96].

The *Pathway Jetstream revascularization system* is also a new rotational atherectomy device that includes a flushing and aspiration mechanism to retrieve atheromatous debris and avoid distal embolization. It is marketed to be used in 5–7-mm diameter vessels. The results of a prospective multicenter study were recently presented enrolling 172 patients with <10-cm femoropopliteal lesions. The technical success rate was 99 %, and TLR at 6 months was 14 %. Almost 70 % received adjunctive PTA or stent placement, and long-term data are not present [33]. The value of debulking atherectomy still has to be defined simply because no comparison trials exist and the majority of the data uses the device as an adjunct to conventional interventions.

Laser Angioplasty

Prior reports on laser-assisted angioplasty showed no benefit compared to conventional PTA which led to its abandonment [97, 98]. However, the recent advent of excimer laser-assisted PTA which consists of intense, short pulses of ultraviolet light to achieve penetration, atheroablation, and recanalization has led to renewed interest in laser technology for the treatment of PAD. The advantage of pulsed laser is the low risk of thermal injury compared to the historical hot-tip lasers. The 308-nm excimer laser uses flexible fiber-optic catheters. Tissue is ablated only if in contact with the laser with no significant surrounding thermal injury. These advances have led to increased utilization of laser treatment in complex peripheral arterial disease [99].

The prototype excimer laser device is the Spectranetics CVX-300 excimer laser system (Spectranetics Co., Colorado Springs, CO). Due to the small channel size created by the laser (2.5-mm maximal diameter), adjuvant PTA and stenting are usually necessary to achieve adequate lumen.

The LACI multicenter trial was a prospective registry of 155 limbs in 145 patients treated with laser-assisted angioplasty, all of which had critical limb ischemia. Sixty percent of limbs had complete, long-segment occlusions with a median total length of 11 cm. Adjunctive balloon angioplasty was performed in 96 %, and adjunctive stenting was required in 61 % of all lesions. The initial procedural success was 85 %, although limb salvage was not examined beyond a 6-month interval [100]. A more recent report using excimer laser ablation in the treatment of chronic total occlusions in diabetic patients who failed initial attempts at standard PTA or stenting was also promising. Most lesions were in the femoropopliteal segment (80 %) with a smaller number of crural lesions [101]. The study reported an extrapolated 1-year limb salvage rate for CLI of 94 %. Other promising data from CELLO registry was recently published showing safe treatment of SFA in-stent restenosis with TLR in only 23 % at 1 year [102].

Vascular Stents in the SFA

Early experience with stenting in the SFA was disappointing, which is likely attributable to the ill fit between the early designs that were used, which were primarily designed for the biliary system and iliac arteries. Balloon-expanded stents were highly susceptible to crush and the Wallstent which, although quite effective in the iliac segments, performed poorly in the SFA. This early disappointing experience changed with the introduction of tubular nitinol stents which over the past decade demonstrated good intermediate patency rates compared to POBA. This has in fact subsequently resulted in an almost "epidemic" adoption of stenting in the SFA. Despite its widespread use, stenting in SFA and popliteal segments remains controversial. To complicate matters further, several classes of devices have emerged, including next-generation iterations of previous designs of stents, stent grafts, high-pressure balloons, cutting balloons, cryoplasty balloons, atherectomy catheters, laser catheters, and so on. None of these technologies have yet proven to be a perfect fit for the SFA. The availability of various options, however, does allow for individualized selection of treatment modality based on the individual patient to better suit the anatomy and lesion morphology. The plethora of available devices is contrasted by the striking lack of evidence-based data comparing these often competing designs.

The main challenge facing stenting in the femoropopliteal arteries is the inherent complexity of the extrinsic forces exerted on this segment, the unique disease patterns that afflict this segment as well as the effect of stents on the arterial physiology. Complex repetitive stresses due to the complexity of the motions demanded by both the hip and knee joints result in chronic irritation that incites plaque buildup as well as intimal hyperplasia. It can also produce positional kinking, distraction, twisting, and luminal narrowing which can reduce flow, induce turbulence, and incite thrombosis. The stiff nature of metallic stents predisposes them to fracture which is a cause of restenosis and thrombosis.

Perhaps the most challenging lesion types in for femoropopliteal intervention are the higher TASC-grade lesions (TASC B through D), which include long-segment stenosis and occlusions. Balloon angioplasty often fails due to recoil or intimal dissection, and stents in these cases are valuable to convert early PTA failure into success.

The importance of proper sizing in the SFA cannot be overemphasized. One can draw an analogy with femoral-popliteal prosthetic bypass grafting where conduits less than 6 mm in diameter have a significantly higher propensity for occlusion [103]. The importance of a sufficient diameter is also demonstrated in a prospective study using self-expandable stents in the femoral-popliteal segment: Arteries with a diameter less than 5 mm had a significantly lower long-term patency rate both in bare stents and in stent grafts [104, 105]. The other factor related to proper sizing is ensuring adequate wall apposition. Poor apposition not only inhibits endothelialization which is crucial for long-term patency but also predisposes to thrombus formation which can result in reocclusion [104, 106]. Wall apposition is also related to lesion anatomy, with eccentric lesions, especially when heavily calcified and fibrotic which prevents adequate wall apposition. It is important to also achieve the desired expansion of the device which can at time be challenging in the presence of heavy calcifications, highly fibrotic lesions, and in-stent restenosis that are resistant to dilation. Given the wide availability of intravascular ultrasound (IVUS), this goal can be ascertained and every effort should be made to ensure adequate apposition when using bare stents [107]. In those cases, the use of debulking adjunctive "vessel-prep" techniques such as atherectomy and excimer laser have been reported to help achieve a better stent expansion and wall conformability and may lead to improved patency [108]. It should be made clear that fluoroscopy often underestimates the extent and configuration of intravascular calcification, whereas IVUS can also distinguish whether the calcium is in a superficial or deep location. Efforts to evaluate the lesion and to prepare the implantation site with rotational atherectomy or by cutting balloons will be well rewarded. Post-dilation with a properly sized (both diameter-wise and length-wise), noncompliant balloon is another important step.

Bare Metal Nitinol Stents

Stents initially used in the SFA prior to the nitinol era were designed for biliary and iliac use (e.g., Wallstent, Palmaz, Strecker), proved ill-suited for this application with very disappointing delayed outcomes noted in most series due to intimal hyperplasia in the stent or at stent edges. Introduction of laser slotted-tube nitinol stents reenergized the field of SFA stenting. The landmark study by Sabeti et al. demonstrated the significant improvement in patency of nitinol stents compared to Wallstents in the SFA [109]. Nitinol stents offer low profile, better wall apposition, improved radial strength, and generally more precise deployment due to minimal dynamic shortening. There are several attributes to the design of a nitinol stent that confer its specific characteristics, related to the alloy-specific characteristics, the manufacture process, and the geometric design. The most obvious feature of slotted-tube nitinol stents is the strut, characterized by its geometric shape, cross-sectional area, length, and angle. Other determinants include the number of struts per circumference and number and configuration of connecting bridges. Additional very important attributes include electropolishing of the struts surface and use of passive coating. Newer nitinol stent designs have departed from the traditional slotted-tube manufacture process. The SUPERA stent (IDEV) is manufactured from a single interwoven wire, a structure somewhat reminiscent of the Wallstent. Another newer, highly flexible design is the alternating helical design exemplified in the newer NovoStent, Inc. designs (HYPERION and SAMBA).

Since their introduction a decade ago, slotted-tube nitinol stents witnessed major evolutions. First-generation nitinol stents [Luminexx (BARD), Absolute and Dynalink (Abbott), SMART (Cordis), Zilver (Cook)] share in their design the features of interconnected or nested V pattern struts, resulting in a stiffer prosthesis and also limiting radial expansion strength. Second-generation stents [LifeStent (BARD), Protégé EverFlex (eV3)] have in common a helical pattern of strut interconnections and represented a major leap in terms of radial strength, flexibility, and fracture resistance compared to first-generation nitinol stents. A growing body of clinical experience with these newer stents in the femoropopliteal arteries shows encouraging mid-term results, with 3-year primary patency rates up to 76 % for SFA lesions [110].

The SIROCCO phase I study is one of the earliest randomized trials of nitinol stenting in the SFA. Interestingly, this study did not compare nitinol stenting with another standard of therapy;

instead, it was a randomized double-blind comparison of bare metal versus drug-eluting SMART stents. Patency of bare metal SMART stents was a remarkable 80 % at 6 months [106].

The ABSOLUTE trial is another early randomized trial comparing nitinol stenting with PTA in the SFA. This was a single-center study that compared 51 patients with SFA disease randomized to primary implantation of nitinol stents (Absolute, Abbott) with 53 patients. The restenosis rate at 12 months using duplex sonographic criteria was significantly lower in the nitinol stent group (37 % vs. 63 %) [111].

The femoral artery stenting trial (FAST) is a multicenter European trial which randomized 244 patients to either PTA or stenting using the Luminexx stent (BARD). This study contrasts with most other studies comparing nitinol stents and PTA in the SFA in that it showed no significant patency or TLR with stenting at 12 months, although longer occlusion did fair better with stenting [112]. This can be largely attributed to specific design and flexibility features of the Luminexx stent which makes it less desirable in the SFA.

A number of well-designed randomized, multicenter trials with independent core lab evaluation have become available or are currently underway to better define the use of self-expandable nitinol stents in the treatment of infrainguinal occlusive disease in the hope of providing level 1 evidence. Data from the RESILIENT trial was recently published [113]. This multi-institutional trial randomized a total of 206 patients from 24 centers in the USA and Europe with intermittent claudication due to femoropopliteal disease with lesion length < 150 mm to either PTA or LifeStent. Angiographic success, defined as <30 % residual stenosis, was superior for the stent group compared with the angioplasty group (95.8 % vs. 83.9 %), and 40 % of patients in the angioplasty group underwent bailout stenting because of a suboptimal angiographic result. Primary patency at 12 months (assessed by duplex sonography) was far better in the stent group (81.3 % vs. 36.7 %; $p<0.0001$). Fractures occurred in 3 % of stents implanted, and none resulted in loss of patency or target lesion revascularization.

The ASTRON trial is recently published randomized, multicenter European trial which randomized 34 patients to primary stent implantation and 39 patients to PTA with optional secondary stenting. The study used a second-generation design (Astron, Biotronik, Germany). In the PTA group, secondary stenting was performed in 10 of 39 patients (26 %) due to a suboptimal result after balloon dilation. Sonographic restenosis rates at 12 months were 34 % in the stent group compared to 61 % in the PTA group [114].

Reports of nitinol stent fractures were first noticed in the SFA in the SIROCCO phase I study, occurring in 18.1 % of the used stents (SMART, Cordis). A strong association was first noted between the placement of multiple overlapping stents in long lesions and development of fractures [106]. Scheinert et al. subsequently demonstrated that stent fracture rate can be as high as 37 % with some designs and is highly correlated with stent occlusion (four- to sixfold higher in the fracture group) [115]. To further evaluate the impact of multiple stent deployment, a nonrandomized multicenter trial assessed the utilization of single up to 15 cm long stents [Protégé (eV3)] in the SFA; the results demonstrated a 12-month primary patency rate of 72.2 % , but the stent fracture rate remained high at 8.1 % (DURABILITY I trial) [116]. A recent meta-analysis of the current literature confirmed the cumulative incidence of stent fractures ranging from 6 to 100 per 1,000 person-months [117]. Stent fractures occurred more frequently in the distal superficial femoral artery and were more common when multiple stents are deployed and overlapped. Stent fractures are progressive over time, associated with a higher risk of in-stent restenosis and reocclusion [117]. Thus, these fractures are not inconsequential.

The DURABILITY II trial is a uniquely designed study that was recently concluded. This is a prospective, multicenter, single-arm study evaluating the Protégé EverFlex® (eV3) Self-Expanding Stent System for the treatment of SFA and proximal popliteal lesions using a single long nitinol stent (up to 200 mm). The study is designed to test the hypothesis that single stent therapy may translate into a reduced incidence of stent fractures and, therefore, a reduced 12-month TLR rate. Enrollment into the DURABILITY II trial enrolled a total of 287 patients at 44 centers in the USA and Europe and was completed in April 2010, and publication of the results is awaited.

Despite continued uncertainty in the role of stents in the infrainguinal segment, the initial recommendation of TASC to reserve stent placement for PTA failure might have to be revisited in light of improved stent technology. Better understanding of biomechanical forces exerted on the SFA, salvage of stent failure, and cost benefit evaluations, however, need to be considered when using a permanently implantable device in the femoropopliteal segment. This has resulted in a number of very innovative, next-generation stents designed specifically for the SFA and popliteal segments. Each of these possesses advantages and drawbacks but overall allows the interventionist to customize the type of stent used to the specific demands of each clinical situation.

The SUPERA™ (IDEV Technologies, Inc.) stent represents a new class of self-expanding nitinol stents designed specifically for the SFA. The interwoven design allows for superior radial force, flexibility, durability, and vessel conformity compared to traditional laser-cut nitinol tube stent designs. Prior reports have demonstrated that fractures rarely occur with coil stent designs, suggesting that they are more compatible with the biomechanical forces present in the SFA [117]. Although no published studies are available on this stent, a number of case reports and cases studies in popular open-access publications report excellence performance in areas of high mobility, and its remarkable strength and resistance to fracture make it ideal for managing heavily calcified lesions. Data from the Leipzig SUPERA registry was presented at the meeting showing 12- and 24-month primary patency rates of 90 and 87 % in the SFA and 85 and 73 % in the popliteal artery (*S. Bräunlich* et al. *Leipzig Interventional Course-LINC, 2010*). The SUPERB trial (sponsored by IDEV Technologies, Inc.) is currently underway to evaluate the performance of the SUPERA stent to PTA.

Another next-generation stent concept is exemplified in the HYPERION and SAMBA stent designs (NovoStent Corporation). The design is that of a nitinol helical platform with a closed cell pattern. The design is extremely flexible yet has a very strong radial force and has high durability due to the lack of axial connectors. Clinical experience remains scant with these stents.

Yet, another promising femoropopliteal-specific stent design is the FlexStent (Flexible Stenting Solutions, Inc., Eatontown, NJ). The proprietary helical design is fully interconnected to prevent "fish scaling," which offers high flexibility, radial strength, conformability, and fracture resistance. The design also has the advantage of straightforward and reconstrainable deployment system. Although no publications exist, interim clinical results with the FlexStent in the SFA from two pooled European sites were recently presented, with a 6-month patency rate of 92.3 and 0 % fracture rate (*A. Holden* et al. *VIVA-2010 conference*).

Stent Grafts

Covered stents in the femoropopliteal segment have the potential advantage of decreased cellular ingrowth and decreased intimal hyperplasia and are in structure closest to surgical grafts. The initial experience, however, utilizing an expandable nitinol stent covered with woven polyester, Cragg EndoPro System, demonstrated substantial complication rates and limited patency [118]. The early stent designs have progressed to more durable and biocompatible devices. To date, the Viabahn (GORE) end graft, an expanded polytetrafluoroethylene (ePTFE) with an external nitinol stent is the only endograft with FDA approval for use in the SFA. Data from a single center that took part in the Hemobahn multicenter randomized registry was published, comparing PTA to an early generation Viabahn design demonstrated high technical success rates and patency benefit at 12 months for the endograft [21]. Others reported mixed results with the device. Lammer et al. in a mixed patient population including treatment of iliac and femoropopliteal arteries mostly TASC A or B lesions reported acute thrombosis rate of 4 % and reocclusion rates at 1 year of 20 % [119].

The primary patency rate was 90 % at 6 months and 79 % at 12 months, respectively. Deutschmann et al., on the other hand, published disappointing results with primary patency rates at 3 and 6 months of 61 and 49 % [120]. Twenty-two percent of patients had early reocclusions at less than 1 month, and an additional 49 % of all grafts were occluded at 7 months. Significant intimal hyperplasia was seen at the leading and trailing edges of the stent and the highest reocclusion rate in stents over 10 cm in length. Saxon more recently reported on the long-term follow-up [105], with 2-year patency rates in the Viabahn group of 87 % compared to 25 % in the PTA group. Remarkably, at 4-year follow-up, a primary patency of 55 % and secondary patency of 79 % were maintained without evidence of stent fractures. Notably, devices of 5-mm diameter (was it only diameter 5 or 5 and smaller) had a significantly lower patency, while neither total stented length nor extension of the stent graft across the knee joint had no impact on patency.

One important, recent, prospective randomized study compared a single-center experience with the Viabahn endograft compared to prosthetic femoral to above-knee popliteal bypass grafting in 86 patients with claudication [121]. Primary patency at 1 year was identical at 74 %, demonstrating comparability of the two techniques at 1 year in a head-to-head comparison.

The VIBRANT multicenter randomized trial comparing the Viabahn stent graft to nitinol bare metal stents in patients with long-segment lesions (TASC C, D). Interim 12-month data was presented at the 2010 New Cardiovascular Horizons meeting (B. Weinstock et al.), showing comparable patency rates and TLR rates with both Viabahn and bare nitinol stents. Patient enrollment was recently completed and data should soon become available. It should be noted that the Viabahn devices used in the VIBRANT trial suffer from two major drawbacks, lack of heparin bonding and no proximal edge contouring modification which may have important implication on the restenosis rates, given the fact that the primary modes of failure of the Viabahn are edge restenosis and thrombosis.

The VIPER trial compared the Viabahn endoprosthesis with PTA alone in the SFA [122]. This was a prospective, multicenter randomized study that compared 100 patients treated with PTA with 97 patients treated with stent-graft placement for stenoses or occlusions of the SFA that were 13 cm long or shorter. The 1-year primary vessel patency rate by duplex ultrasonography was 65 % with the Viabahn compared to 40 % with PTA alone.

Drug-Eluting Stents

Recent literature on sirolimus or paclitaxel drug-coated stents in the coronary arteries has shown excellent outcomes with low rates of target lesion revascularization at long-term follow-up. There have only been few published trials in the SFA. The first such randomized trial (SIROCCO-I) compared sirolimus-eluting versus bare stents (SMART, Cordis) [123], with 6-month angiographic follow-up demonstrating a statistically improved mean vessel diameter in the sirolimus group but no decreased restenosis rate. In the extension phase of the same trial (SIROCCO-II), 57 additional patients with SFA lesions were randomized to treatment with sirolimus-slow-eluting versus bare metal SMART stents [124]. Although there was a trend for inhibition of intimal hyperplasia in the sirolimus group, there were no statistically significant differences among the endpoints between the bare and drug-eluting stent groups.

A more recent multicenter randomized trial was recently concluded in which paclitaxel-eluting nitinol stent (Zilver PTX, Cook) was compared with PTA alone and bare metal stents in those who underwent stenting for suboptimal PTA outcome. The study involved 55 sites in the USA, Japan, and Germany and enrolled 479 patients. Preliminary analysis demonstrated significantly higher 12-month patency with Zilver PTX compared with bare metal Zilver (90 % vs. 73 %) [125].

The STRIDES trial is another nonrandomized study using the everolimus-eluting Dynalink stent (Abbott) and is currently underway to look primarily at 12-month in-stent restenosis rate. No preliminary data is available yet.

Biodegradable Stents

With current stent designs, one of the main problems with stenting in the SFA region seems to be related to the presence of the stent itself. As a result, the argument that stents made of absorbable, flexible materials may in fact be an ideal alternative to permanent nitinol stents in the SFA. Not only would an absorbable stent provide an ideal temporary vessel scaffolding but may also provide a useful vehicle for local delivery of pharmacological agents aimed at reducing thrombogenicity, enhancing healing, and inhibiting neointimal hyperplasia.

The demand for this technology has so far been stronger for the coronary circulation and for below-the-knee interventions where the percutaneous profile of the delivery systems necessary for these stents can be safely tolerated. Investigation of these stents in the femoropopliteal circulation has been scant. The Igaki-Tamai biodegradable peripheral stent was recently evaluated in a limited trial as part of the PERSEUS study. This device is a new knitted stent made from poly-L-lactic acid (PLLA) and is entirely biodegradable. The PERSEUS Igaki-Tamai stent trial was a prospective, nonrandomized, single-center, pilot study that recruited 45 patients with de novo lesions of the SFA (TASC types B and C). Interim results have only been published in an abstract form [126]. The primary implantation success rate was 100 % with no serious adverse events. The 6-month angiographic results revealed no reocclusions although there were nine symptomatic restenoses that were all successfully retreated, leading to an impressive assisted primary patency rate of 91 % at 9 months. It has been speculated that the restenoses seen may be related to an inflammatory reaction during the bio-absorption of the stent.

A related bioabsorbable stent design is the REVA stent that has been studied in the coronary arteries. The ReZolve Bioresorbable Coronary Stent (REVA Medical, Inc.) is a fully bioresorbable stent system, with an integral paclitaxel-eluting coating. The polymer is combined with slide-and-lock technology, a stent design that allows deployment without significant deformation of the stent structure. This is a major advantage as polymers are not as resistant to deformation as metals. A clinical coronary trial is anticipated, but no peripheral trials have been announced.

Another class of bioabsorbable stents are absorbable metallic stents. One such device has already been evaluated (AMS, Biotronik *GmbH* & Co., Switzerland). The stent material is composed of an alloy containing 90 % magnesium in combination with different rare earth elements and has been experimentally shown to be fully absorbed by the surrounding vessel wall in homogenous degradation process with no risk of particle migration or microembolism.

This device has been clinically evaluated in the infrageniculate peripheral vascular system in the AMS-INSIGHT trial (Absorbable Metal Stent Investigation in Chronic Limb Ischemia Treatment). Results from this prospective, multicenter, randomized clinical trial evaluating the AMS for the treatment of infrapopliteal lesions in patients with CLI were recently published [127]. One hundred seventeen patients with 149 lesions with chronic limb ischemia (CLI) were randomized to implantation of an AMS (60 patients), stand-alone PTA (57 patients), and PTA with "crossover" to AMS (six patients). Unfortunately, the 6-month angiographic patency was significantly lower with AMS (32 % vs. 58 %). However, the importance of this study is that it demonstrated the feasibility of this technology. The value of such a paradigm in the larger femoropopliteal vessels still needs to be evaluated.

Peri- and Postprocedural Medical Therapy

The intraprocedural use of unfractionated heparin (UFH) remains the most widely utilized and unchallenged antithrombin modality during peripheral endovascular interventions [128]. However, with the increasing complexity of modern peripheral endovascular interventions, especially in patients presenting CLI, the impact of thromboembolism and distal microembolization has become even more significant. It is becoming clear that some of the high-risk interventions will have to be performed in conjunction with distal protection devices. However, perhaps more important are the lessons learned on the importance of combined antiplatelet and direct thrombin inhibition in high-risk percutaneous coronary interventions that are quite applicable to the CLI patient population. Various combination and strategies can be used ranging from simple combination of clopidogrel pretreatment or loading with UFH or LMWH to the use of GP IIb/IIIa inhibition combination with a direct thrombin inhibitor. The combination of eptifibatide with bivalirudin has become popular in high-risk complex peripheral interventional procedures [129]. However, more conclusive randomized multicenter trials will be needed to properly evaluate these approaches, in terms of safety and cost-effectiveness.

As far as the postprocedural medical antithrombotic therapy, the regimen will depend on the class of the intervention itself, atherosclerotic disease burden, specifics of the prosthesis used, status of inflow and runoff, and the presence of hypercoagulability state. However, in general, there is strong evidence that routine antiplatelet therapy is indicated after angioplasty. Aspirin has been the mainstay, but not everyone has adequate response to aspirin [130]. The CAPRIE study indicated a benefit of treatment of clopidogrel (Plavix) for patients with PAD. The relative risk reduction of any vascular event over the use of aspirin was 24 % [131]. In patients treated with angioplasty, the effect of clopidogrel on the long-term patency of the vessel is unclear. Still, the risk appears low and the drug is probably more effective than aspirin. Since aspirin and clopidogrel work by different mechanisms of platelet inhibition, there likely is some synergy. Therefore, aggressive post-PTA treatment would include both aspirin and clopidogrel. The duration of clopidogrel therapy after PTA remains matter of debate. Routine use of warfarin is even less clear. There is no large study of Coumadin in angioplasty patients. A randomized study of aspirin versus Coumadin in 2,690 bypass grafts showed no improvement in vessel patency with Coumadin compared to aspirin alone [132]. The risks associated with Coumadin are certainly higher than with aspirin. Coumadin is reserved in our practice for post-PTA patients who are at high risk for thrombosis. Examples of this include patients with recurrent bypass thrombosis, patients with stent-graft thrombosis, and patients with a known or strongly suspected hypercoagulable state.

Conclusion

In patients with PAD, all therapeutic options should be considered as the treatment modality should be individualized based on lesion-specific characteristics as well as operator preference. Patients with minimal symptoms are best treated conservatively with progressive walking program and risk factor modification. Despite this conservative management, further therapy will be needed in at least 25 % of these patients.

Once the decision is made to intervene, a baseline noninvasive evaluation is obtained. A cross-sectional angiographic imaging modality and/or conventional angiography can then be performed. At least one-third of patients will demonstrate a lesion amenable to endovascular therapy. The appropriate intervention should be chosen based on the underlying vascular anatomy, the associated risk factors, the availability of a vein for a bypass graft, the patient's desires, and the technical expertise of the physicians involved.

PTA remains an excellent treatment tool in the femoropopliteal and tibial arteries. Use of vascular stents in the femoropopliteal system appears to be beneficial in patients with a suboptimal PTA result and long lesions (TASC C, D). Unfortunately, stents are limited by restenosis and potential fractures. Medical therapy, new generation atherectomy devices, cutting balloons, stent grafts, drug-eluting stents, excimer laser, and cryotherapy are all being investigated as means of prolonging the patency. These and other potential tools for endovascular therapy will continue to expand the role of the interventionist in the management of vascular disease.

References

1. Anderson PL, Gelijns A, Moskowitz A, et al. Understanding trends in inpatient surgical volume: vascular interventions, 1980–2000. J Vasc Surg. 2004; 39(6):1200–8.
2. Dormandy J, Heeck L, Vig S. Peripheral arterial occlusive disease: clinical data for decision making. Introduction. Semin Vasc Surg. 1999;12(2):95.
3. Bhatt DL, Hirsch AT, Ringleb PA, Hacke W, Topol EJ. Reduction in the need for hospitalization for recurrent ischemic events and bleeding with clopidogrel instead of aspirin. CAPRIE investigators. Am Heart J. 2000;140(1):67–73.
4. Anand SS, Kundi A, Eikelboom J, Yusuf S. Low rates of preventive practices in patients with peripheral vascular disease. Can J Cardiol. 1999;15(11):1259–63.
5. Criqui MH, Fronek A, Barrett-Connor E, Klauber MR, Gabriel S, Goodman D. The prevalence of peripheral arterial disease in a defined population. Circulation. 1985;71(3):510–5.
6. Kannel WB, McGee DL. Update on some epidemiologic features of intermittent claudication: the Framingham Study. J Am Geriatr Soc. 1985;33(1): 13–8.
7. McDaniel MD, Cronenwett JL. Basic data related to the natural history of intermittent claudication. Ann Vasc Surg. 1989;3(3):273–7.
8. Second European Consensus Document on chronic critical leg ischemia. Eur J Vasc Surg. 1992;6(Suppl A):1–32.
9. Second European Consensus Document on chronic critical leg ischemia. Circulation. 1991;84(4 Suppl): IV1–26.
10. Long-term mortality and its predictors in patients with critical leg ischaemia. The I.C.A.I. Group (Gruppo di Studio dell'Ischemia Cronica Critica degli Arti Inferiori). The Study Group of Critical Chronic Ischemia of the Lower Extremities. Eur J Vasc Endovasc Surg. 1997;14(2):91–5.
11. Perkins JM, Collin J, Creasy TS, Fletcher EW, Morris PJ. Exercise training versus angioplasty for stable claudication. Long and medium term results of a prospective, randomised trial. Eur J Vasc Endovasc Surg. 1996;11(4):409–13.
12. Lundgren F, Dahllöf A-G, Lundholm K, Schersten T, Volkmann R. Intermittent claudication-surgical reconstruction or physical training? A prospective randomized trial of treatment efficiency. Ann Surg. 1989; 209(3):346–55.
13. Veith FJ, Gupta SK, Wengerter KR, Rivers SP, Bakal CW. Impact of nonoperative therapy on the clinical management of peripheral arterial disease. Circulation. 1991;83(2 Suppl):I137–42.
14. Hertzer NR. The natural history of peripheral vascular disease. Implications for its management. Circulation. 1991;83(2 Suppl):I12–9.
15. Bendermacher BLW, Willigendael EM, Teijink JAW, Prins MH. Supervised exercise therapy versus non-supervised exercise therapy for intermittent claudication. Cochrane Database Syst Rev. 2006;Issue 2.
16. Mazari FA, Gulati S, Rahman MN, et al. Early outcomes from a randomized, controlled trial of supervised exercise, angioplasty, and combined therapy in intermittent claudication. Ann Vasc Surg. 2010;24(1):69–79.
17. Guidelines for percutaneous transluminal angioplasty. Standards of Practice Committee of the Society of Cardiovascular and Interventional Radiology. Radiology. 1990;177(3):619–26.
18. Hirsch AT, Haskal ZJ, Hertzer NR, et al. ACC/AHA 2005 guidelines for the management of patients With peripheral arterial disease (lower extremity, renal, mesenteric, and abdominal aortic): a collaborative report from the American Association for Vascular Surgery/Society for Vascular Surgery, Society for Cardiovascular Angiography and Interventions, Society for Vascular Medicine and Biology, Society of Interventional Radiology, and the ACC/AHA Task Force on Practice Guidelines (Writing Committee to Develop Guidelines for the Management of Patients With Peripheral Arterial Disease. J Am Coll Cardiol. 2006;47(6):e1–192. doi:10.1016/j.jacc.2006.02.024.
19. Norgren L, Hiatt WR, Dormandy JA, Nehler MR, Harris KA, Fowkes FGR. Inter-society consensus for the management of peripheral arterial disease (TASC II). Eur J Vasc Endovasc Surg. 2007;33(1, Suppl 1):S1.
20. Allie DE, Hebert CJ, Patlola RR, Ingraldi A, Walker CM. Optimal vessel sizing in peripheral vascular interventions. Treating the peripheral and infrapopliteal arteries like the LAD. Endovasc Today. 2009:34–8.
21. Saxon RR, Coffman JM, Gooding JM, Natuzzi E, Ponec DJ. Long-term results of ePTFE stent-graft versus angioplasty in the femoropopliteal artery: single center experience from a prospective, randomized trial. J Vasc Interv Radiol. 2003;14(3):303–11.
22. Wu CC, Wen SC. Cutting balloon angioplasty for resistant venous stenoses of dialysis access: immediate and patency results. Catheter Cardiovasc Interv. 2008;71(2):250–4.
23. Schroeder S, Baumbach A, Haase KK, et al. Reduction of restenosis by vessel size adapted percutaneous transluminal coronary angioplasty using intravascular ultrasound. Am J Cardiol. 1999;83(6):875–9.
24. Allie DE, Patlola RR, Ingraldi A, Hebert CJ, Walker CM. The contemporary CLI toolbox. A close look at the available devices and techniques for treating today's critical limb ischemia patients. Endovasc Today. 2009:37–50.
25. Diehm N, Shang A, Silvestro A, et al. Association of cardiovascular risk factors with pattern of lower limb atherosclerosis in 2659 patients undergoing angioplasty. Eur J Vasc Endovasc Surg. 2006;31(1): 59–63.
26. Graziani L, Silvestro A, Bertone V, et al. Vascular involvement in diabetic subjects with ischemic foot ulcer: a new morphologic categorization of disease severity. Eur J Vasc Endovasc Surg. 2007;33(4):453–60.

27. Aboyans V, Lacroix P, Criqui MH. Large and small vessels atherosclerosis: similarities and differences. Prog Cardiovasc Dis. 2007;50(2):112–25.
28. Peripheral atherectomy with the rotablator: a multicenter report. The Collaborative Rotablator Atherectomy Group (CRAG). J Vasc Surg. 1994;19(3):509–15.
29. Rabellino M, Zander T, Baldi S, et al. Clinical follow-up in endovascular treatment for TASC C-D lesions in femoro-popliteal segment. Catheter Cardiovasc Interv. 2009;73(5):701–5.
30. Bolia A, Sayers RD, Thompson MM, Bell PR. Subintimal and intraluminal recanalisation of occluded crural arteries by percutaneous balloon angioplasty. Eur J Vasc Surg. 1994;8(2):214–9.
31. Sharafuddin MJ, Hoballah J, Kresowik T, Nicholson R, Sharp W. Impact of aggressive endovascular recanalization techniques on success rate in chronic total arterial occlusions (CTOs). Vasc Endovascular Surg. 2010;44:460–7.
32. Heenan SD, Vinnicombe SJ, Buckenham TM, Belli AM. Percutaneous transluminal angioplasty by a retrograde subintimal transpopliteal approach. Clin Radiol. 1994;49(11):824–7; discussion 827–8.
33. Noory E, Rastan A, Schwarzwalder U, et al. Retrograde transpopliteal recanalization of chronic superficial femoral artery occlusion after failed re-entry during antegrade subintimal angioplasty. J Endovasc Ther. 2009;16(5):619–23.
34. Sultan S, Hynes N. Five-year Irish trial of CLI patients with TASC II type C/D lesions undergoing subintimal angioplasty or bypass surgery based on plaque echolucency. J Endovasc Ther. 2009;16(3):270–83.
35. Bolia A, Bell PR. Femoropopliteal and crural artery recanalization using subintimal angioplasty. Semin Vasc Surg. 1995;8(3):253–64.
36. Met R, Van Lienden KP, Koelemay MJ, Bipat S, Legemate DA, Reekers JA. Subintimal angioplasty for peripheral arterial occlusive disease: a systematic review. Cardiovasc Intervent Radiol. 2008;31(4):687–97.
37. Scott EC, Biuckians A, Light RE, Burgess J, Meier 3rd GH, Panneton JM. Subintimal angioplasty: our experience in the treatment of 506 infrainguinal arterial occlusions. J Vasc Surg. 2008;48(4):878–84.
38. Hayes PD, Chokkalingam A, Jones R, et al. Arterial perforation during infrainguinal lower limb angioplasty does not worsen outcome: results from 1409 patients. J Endovasc Ther. 2002;9(4):422–7.
39. Hausegger KA, Georgieva B, Portugaller H, Tauss J, Stark G. The outback catheter: a new device for true lumen re-entry after dissection during recanalization of arterial occlusions. Cardiovasc Intervent Radiol. 2004;27(1):26–30.
40. Wiesinger B, Steinkamp H, Konig C, Tepe G, Duda SH. Technical report and preliminary clinical data of a novel catheter for luminal re-entry after subintimal dissection. Invest Radiol. 2005;40(11):725–8.
41. Beschorner U, Sixt S, Schwarzwalder U, et al. Recanalization of chronic occlusions of the superficial femoral artery using the outback re-entry catheter: a single centre experience. Catheter Cardiovasc Interv. 2009;74(6):934–8.
42. Saketkhoo RR, Razavi MK, Padidar A, Kee ST, Sze DY, Dake MD. Percutaneous bypass: subintimal recanalization of peripheral occlusive disease with IVUS guided luminal re-entry. Tech Vasc Interv Radiol. 2004;7(1):23.
43. Al-Ameri H, Shin V, Mayeda GS, et al. Peripheral chronic total occlusions treated with subintimal angioplasty and a true lumen re-entry device. J Invasive Cardiol. 2009;21(9):468–72.
44. Jacobs DL, Cox DE, Motaganahalli R. Crossing chronic total occlusions of the iliac and femoral-popliteal vessels and the use of true lumen reentry devices. Perspect Vasc Surg Endovasc Ther. 2006; 18(1):31–7.
45. Boguszewski A, Torey J, Pai R, Kamalakannan D, Jefic D, Davis T. Intraluminal recanalization of SFA CTOs. Endovasc Today. 2010:33–8.
46. Heuser RR, Murarka S. The support-balloon technique for chronic total occlusion: successful recanalization of a 27-year- old occlusion. Vasc Dis Manag. 2010;7:e171–4.
47. Atmakuri SR, Lev EI, Alviar C, et al. Initial experience with a magnetic navigation system for percutaneous coronary intervention in complex coronary artery lesions. J Am Coll Cardiol. 2006;47(3):515–21.
48. Kirvaitis RJ, Heuser RR, Das TS, et al. Usefulness of optical coherent reflectometry with guided radiofrequency energy to treat chronic total occlusions in peripheral arteries (the GRIP trial). Am J Cardiol. 2004;94(8):1081–4.
49. Ramaiah V. Endovascular infrainguinal revascularization: technical tips for atherectomy device selection and procedural success. Semin Vasc Surg. 2008;21:41–9.
50. Clark TW, Groffsky JL, Soulen MC. Predictors of long-term patency after femoropopliteal angioplasty: results from the STAR registry. J Vasc Interv Radiol. 2001;12(8):923–33.
51. Abularrage CJ, Conrad MF, Hackney LA, et al. Long-term outcomes of diabetic patients undergoing endovascular infrainguinal interventions. J Vasc Surg. 2010;52(2):314–22 e1–4.
52. Adar R, Critchfield GC, Eddy DM. A confidence profile analysis of the results of femoropopliteal percutaneous transluminal angioplasty in the treatment of lower-extremity ischemia. J Vasc Surg. 1989;10(1): 57–67.
53. Johnston KW. Femoral and popliteal arteries: reanalysis of results of balloon angioplasty. Radiology. 1992;183(3):767–71.
54. Dorrucci V. Treatment of superficial femoral artery occlusive disease. J Cardiovasc Surg (Torino). 2004; 45(3):193–201.
55. Taylor Jr LM, Porter JM. Clinical and anatomic considerations for surgery in femoropopliteal disease and the results of surgery. Circulation. 1991;83(2 Suppl):163–9.
56. Veith FJ, Gupta SK, Ascer E, et al. Six-year prospective multicenter randomized comparison of autologous

saphenous vein and expanded polytetrafluoroethylene grafts in infrainguinal arterial reconstructions. J Vasc Surg. 1986;3(1):104–14.

57. Bakal CW, Sprayregen S, Scheinbaum K, Cynamon J, Veith FJ. Percutaneous transluminal angioplasty of the infrapopliteal arteries: results in 53 patients. Am J Roentgenol. 1990;154(1):171–4.
58. Brown KT, Moore ED, Getrajdman GI, Saddekni S. Infrapopliteal angioplasty: long-term follow-up. J Vasc Interv Radiol. 1993;4(1):139–44.
59. Bull PG, Mendel H, Hold M, Schlegl A, Denck H. Distal popliteal and tibioperoneal transluminal angioplasty: long-term follow-up. J Vasc Interv Radiol. 1992;3(1):45–53.
60. Horvath W, Oertl M, Haidinger D. Percutaneous transluminal angioplasty of crural arteries. Radiology. 1990;177(2):565–9.
61. Matsi PJ, Manninen HI, Suhonen MT, Pirinen AE, Soimakallio S. Chronic critical lower-limb ischemia: prospective trial of angioplasty with 1–36 months follow-up. Radiology. 1993;188(2):381–7.
62. Schwarten DE. Clinical and anatomical considerations for nonoperative therapy in tibial disease and the results of angioplasty. Circulation. 1991;83(2 Suppl):I86–90.
63. Soder HK, Manninen HI, Jaakkola P, et al. Prospective trial of infrapopliteal artery balloon angioplasty for critical limb ischemia: angiographic and clinical results. J Vasc Interv Radiol. 2000;11(8):1021–31.
64. Bradbury AW, Adam DJ, Bell J, et al. Bypass versus angioplasty in severe ischaemia of the leg (BASIL) trial: a survival prediction model to facilitate clinical decision making. J Vasc Surg. 2010;51(5 Suppl):52S–68.
65. Fogarty TJ, White RA. Biomaterials: considerations for endovascular devices. In: Back MR, editor. Peripheral endovascular interventions, vol. 4. New York: Springer; 2010. p. 141–63.
66. Shammas NW. Optimal strategy in lower extremity peripheral percutaneous interventions: an interventionalist's perspective. Vasc Dis Manag. 2009;6(2):36–40.
67. Shammas NW, Coiner D, Shammas G, Jerin M. Predictors of Provisional Stenting in Patients Undergoing Lower Extremity Arterial Interventions. Int J Angiol 2011;20:95–100.
68. Diaz ML, Urtasun F, Barberena J, Aranzadi C, Guillen-Grima F, Bilbao JI. Cryoplasty versus conventional angioplasty in femoropopliteal arterial recanalization: 3-year analysis of reintervention-free survival by treatment received. Cardiovasc Intervent Radiol. 2011;34:911–7.
69. Leon MB, Teirstein PS, Moses JW, et al. Localized intracoronary gamma-radiation therapy to inhibit the recurrence of restenosis after stenting. N Engl J Med. 2001;344(4):250–6. doi:10.1056/NEJM200101253440402.
70. Tripuraneni P, Giap H, Jani S. Endovascular brachytherapy for peripheral vascular disease. Semin Radiat Oncol. 1999;9(2):190.
71. Diamond DA, Vesely TM. The role of radiation therapy in the management of vascular restenosis. Part II. Radiation techniques and results. J Vasc Intervent Radiol. 1998;9(3):389.
72. Waksman R, Laird JR, Jurkovitz CT, et al. Intravascular radiation therapy after balloon angioplasty of narrowed femoropopliteal arteries to prevent restenosis: results of the PARIS feasibility clinical trial. J Vasc Intervent Radiol. 2001;12(8):915.
73. Schillinger M, Minar E. Advances in vascular brachy therapy over the last 10 years: focus on femoropopliteal applications. J Endovasc Ther. 2004;11(Suppl II):II-180–91. doi:10.1583/04-1298.1.
74. Wolfram RM, Budinsky AC, Pokrajac B, Pötter R, Minar E. Vascular brachytherapy with 192Ir after femoropopliteal stent implantation in high-risk patients: twelve-month follow-up results from the Vienna-5 triall. Radiology. 2005;236(1):343–51. doi:10.1148/radiol.2361040696.
75. Wohlgemuth WA, Leissner G, Wengenmair H, Bohndorf K, Kirchhof K. Endovascular brachytherapy in the femoropopliteal segment using 192Ir and 188Re. Cardiovasc Intervent Radiol. 2008;31(4):698.
76. Gage AA, Fazekas G, Riley Jr EE. Freezing injury to large blood vessels in dogs. With comments on the effect of experimental freezing of bile ducts. Surgery. 1967;61(5):748–54.
77. Laird J, Jaff MR, Biamino G, et al. Cryoplasty for the treatment of femoropopliteal arterial disease: results of a prospective, multicenter registry. J Vasc Interv Radiol. 2005;16(8):1067–73.
78. Samson RH, Showalter DP, Michael Lepore J, Nair DG, Merigliano K. CryoPlasty therapy of the superficial femoral and popliteal arteries: a reappraisal after 44 months' experience. J Vasc Surg. 2008; 48(3):634.
79. Schmieder GC, Carroll M, Panneton JM. Poor outcomes with cryoplasty for lower extremity arterial occlusive disease. J Vasc Surg. 2010;52(2):362–8.
80. Spiliopoulos S, Katsanos K, Karnabatidis D, et al. Cryoplasty versus conventional balloon angioplasty of the femoropopliteal artery in diabetic patients: long-term results from a prospective randomized single-center controlled trial. Cardiovasc Intervent Radiol. 2010;33(5):929.
81. Engelke C, Sandhu C, Morgan RA, Belli A-M. Using 6-mm cutting balloon angioplasty in patients with resistant peripheral artery stenosis: preliminary results. Am J Roentgenol. 2002;179(3):619–23.
82. Ansel GM, Sample NS, Botti CF, et al. Cutting balloon angioplasty of the popliteal and infrapopliteal vessels for symptomatic limb ischemia. Catheter Cardiovasc Interv. 2003;61:1–4.
83. Amighi J, Schillinger M, Dick P, et al. De novo superficial femoropopliteal artery lesions: peripheral cutting balloon angioplasty and restenosis rates randomizedcontrolledtrial1.Radiology.2008;247(1):267–72. doi:10.1148/radiol.2471070749.
84. Vikram R, Ross RA, Bhat R, et al. Cutting balloon angioplasty versus standard balloon angioplasty for failing infra-inguinal vein grafts: comparative study of short- and mid-term primary patency rates. Cardiovasc Intervent Radiol. 2007;30(4):607.

85. Scheinert D, Peeters P, Bosiers M, O'Sullivan G, Sultan S, Gershony G. Results of the multicenter first-in-man study of a novel scoring balloon catheter for the treatment of infra-popliteal peripheral arterial disease. Catheter Cardiovasc Interv. 2007;70(7):1034–9.
86. Tepe G, Zeller T, Albrecht T, et al. Local delivery of paclitaxel to inhibit restenosis during angioplasty of the leg. N Engl J Med. 2008;358:689–99. doi:10.1056/NEJMoa0706356.
87. Werk M, Langner S, Reinkensmeier B, et al. Inhibition of restenosis in femoropopliteal arteries: paclitaxel-coated versus uncoated balloon: femoral paclitaxel randomized pilot trial. Circulation. 2008;118(13):1358–65. doi:10.1161/CIRCULATIONAHA.107.735985.
88. Allie D, Berens E, Bramucci E, et al. Plaque excision in the peripheral vasculature. Endovasc Today. 2004;(Suppl 1):1–11.
89. Ramaiah V, Gammon R, Kiesz S, et al. Midterm outcomes from the TALON registry: treating peripherals with SilverHawk: outcomes collection. J Endovasc Ther. 2006;13(5):592–602.
90. Zeller T, Rastan A, Schwarzwalder U, et al. Midterm results after atherectomy-assisted angioplasty of below-knee arteries with use of the Silverhawk device. J Vasc Interv Radiol. 2004;15(12):1391–7.
91. Kandzari DE, Kiesz RS, Allie D, et al. Procedural and clinical outcomes with catheter-based plaque excision in critical limb ischemia. J Endovasc Ther. 2006;13(1):12–22.
92. Sixt S, Rastan A, Beschorner U, et al. Acute and long-term outcome of Silverhawk assisted atherectomy for femoro-popliteal lesions according the TASC II classification: a single-center experience. Vasa. 2010;39(3):229–36.
93. Chung SW, Sharafuddin MJ, Chigurupati R, Hoballah JJ. Midterm patency following atherectomy for infrainguinal occlusive disease: a word of caution. Ann Vasc Surg. 2008;22(3):358–65.
94. Yancey AE, Minion DJ, Rodriguez C, Patterson DE, Endean ED. Peripheral atherectomy in TransAtlantic InterSociety Consensus type C femoropopliteal lesions for limb salvage. J Vasc Surg. 2006;44(3):503.
95. Suri R, Wholey MH, Postoak D, Hagino RT, Toursarkissian B. Distal embolic protection during femoropopliteal atherectomy. Catheter Cardiovasc Interv. 2006;67(3):417–22.
96. Safian RD, Niazi K, Runyon JP, et al. Orbital atherectomy for infrapopliteal disease: device concept and outcome data for the OASIS trial. Catheter Cardiovasc Interv. 2009;73(3):406–12.
97. Belli AM, Cumberland DC, Procter AE, Welsh CL. Follow-up of conventional angioplasty versus laser thermal angioplasty for total femoropopliteal artery occlusions: results of a randomized trial. J Vasc Interv Radiol. 1991;2(4):485–8.
98. Huppert PE, Duda SH, Helber U, Karsch KR, Claussen CD. Comparison of pulsed laser-assisted angioplasty and balloon angioplasty in femoropopliteal artery occlusions. Radiology. 1992;184(2):363–7.
99. Scheinert D, Laird Jr JR, Schroder M, Steinkamp H, Balzer JO, Biamino G. Excimer laser-assisted recanalization of long, chronic superficial femoral artery occlusions. J Endovasc Ther. 2001;8(2):156–66.
100. Laird JR. Limitations of percutaneous transluminal angioplasty and stenting for the treatment of disease of the superficial femoral and popliteal arteries. J Endovasc Ther. 2006;13 Suppl 2:II30–40.
101. Serino F, Cao Y, Renzi C, et al. Excimer laser ablation in the treatment of total chronic obstructions in critical limb ischaemia in diabetic patients. Sustained efficacy of plaque recanalisation in mid-term results. Eur J Vasc Endovasc Surg. 2010;39(2):234–8.
102. Dave RM, Patlola R, Kollmeyer K, et al. Excimer laser recanalization of femoropopliteal lesions and 1-year patency: results of the CELLO registry. J Endovasc Ther. 2009;16:665–75. doi:10.1583/09-2781.1.
103. Sarkar S, Salacinski HJ, Hamilton G, Seifalian AM. The mechanical properties of infrainguinal vascular bypass grafts: their role in influencing patency. Eur J Vasc Endovasc Surg. 2006;31(6):627–36.
104. Gray BH, Sullivan TM, Childs MB, Young JR, Olin JW. High incidence of restenosis/reocclusion of stents in the percutaneous treatment of long-segment superficial femoral artery disease after suboptimal angioplasty. J Vasc Surg. 1997;25(1):74–83.
105. Saxon RR, Coffman JM, Gooding JM, Ponec DJ. Long-term patency and clinical outcome of the Viabahn stent-graft for femoropopliteal artery obstructions. J Vasc Interv Radiol. 2007;18(11):1341–9.
106. Duda SH, Bosiers M, Lammer J, et al. Sirolimus-eluting versus bare nitinol stent for obstructive superficial femoral artery disease: the SIROCCO II trial. J Vasc Interv Radiol. 2005;16(3):331–8.
107. Shah VM, Mintz GS, Apple S, Weissman NJ. Background incidence of late malapposition after bare-metal stent implantation. Circulation. 2002;106(14):1753–5. doi:10.1161/01.CIR.0000035239.90657.B1.
108. Moses JW, Carlier S, Moussa I. Lesion preparation prior to stenting. Rev Cardiovasc Med. 2004;5 Suppl 2:S16–21.
109. Sabeti S, Schillinger M, Amighi J, et al. Primary patency of femoropopliteal arteries treated with nitinol versus stainless steel self-expanding stents: propensity score-adjusted analysis. Radiology. 2004;232(2):516–21.
110. Mewissen MW. Self-expanding nitinol stents in the femoropopliteal segment: technique and mid-term results. Tech Vasc Interv Radiol. 2004;7(1):2–5.
111. Schillinger M, Sabeti S, Loewe C, et al. Balloon angioplasty versus implantation of nitinol stents in the superficial femoral artery. N Engl J Med. 2006;354(18):1879–88.
112. Krankenberg H, Schluter M, Steinkamp HJ, et al. Nitinol stent implantation versus percutaneous transluminal angioplasty in superficial femoral artery lesions up to 10 cm in length: the femoral artery stenting trial (FAST). Circulation. 2007;116(3):285–92. doi:10.1161/CIRCULATIONAHA.107.689141.

113. Laird JR, Katzen BT, Scheinert D, et al. Nitinol stent implantation versus balloon angioplasty for lesions in the superficial femoral artery and proximal popliteal artery/clinical perspective. Circ Cardiovasc Interv. 2010;3(3):267–76. doi:10.1161/CIRCINTERVENTIONS.109.903468.
114. Dick P, Wallner H, Sabeti S, et al. Balloon angioplasty versus stenting with nitinol stents in intermediate length superficial femoral artery lesions. Catheter Cardiovasc Interv. 2009;74(7):1090–5.
115. Scheinert D, Scheinert S, Sax J, et al. Prevalence and clinical impact of stent fractures after femoropopliteal stenting. J Am Coll Cardiol. 2005;45(2): 312–5. doi:10.1016/j.jacc.2004.11.026.
116. Bosiers M, Torsello G, Gissler HM, et al. Nitinol stent implantation in long superficial femoral artery lesions: 12-month results of the DURABILITY I study. J Endovasc Ther. 2009;16(3):261–9.
117. Rits J, van Herwaarden JA, Jahrome AK, Krievins D, Moll FL. The incidence of arterial stent fractures with exclusion of coronary, aortic, and non-arterial settings. Eur J Vasc Endovasc Surg. 2008;36(3): 339–45.
118. Cragg AH, Dake MD. Percutaneous femoropopliteal graft placement. J Vasc Interv Radiol. 1993;4(4): 455–63.
119. Lammer J, Dake MD, Bleyn J, et al. Peripheral arterial obstruction: prospective study of treatment with a transluminally placed self-expanding stent-graft. Radiology. 2000;217(1):95–104.
120. Deutschmann HA, Schedlbauer P, Berczi V, Portugaller H, Tauss J, Hausegger KA. Placement of Hemobahn stent-grafts in femoropopliteal arteries: early experience and midterm results in 18 patients. J Vasc Interv Radiol. 2001;12(8):943–50.
121. Kedora J, Hohmann S, Garrett W, Munschaur C, Theune B, Gable D. Randomized comparison of percutaneous Viabahn stent grafts vs. prosthetic femoral-popliteal bypass in the treatment of superficial femoral arterial occlusive disease. J Vasc Surg. 2007;45(1):10–6; discussion 16.
122. Saxon RR, Dake MD, Volgelzang RL, Katzen BT, Becker GJ. Randomized, multicenter study comparing expanded polytetrafluoroethylene-covered endoprosthesis placement with percutaneous transluminal angioplasty in the treatment of superficial femoral artery occlusive disease. J Vasc Interv Radiol. 2008; 19(6):823–32.
123. Duda SH, Pusich B, Richter G, et al. Sirolimus-eluting stents for the treatment of obstructive superficial femoral artery disease: six-month results. Circulation. 2002;106(12):1505–9.
124. Duda SH, Bosiers M, Lammer J, et al. Drug-eluting and bare nitinol stents for the treatment of atherosclerotic lesions in the superficial femoral artery: long-term results from the SIROCCO trial. J Endovasc Ther. 2006;13(6):701–10.
125. Dake MD, Scheinert D, Tepe G, et al. Nitinol Stents With Polymer-Free Paclitaxel Coating for Lesions in the Superficial Femoral and Popliteal Arteries Above the Knee: Twelve-Month Safety and Effectiveness Results From the Zilver PTX Single-Arm Clinical Study. Journal of Endovascular Therapy 2011;18: 613–623.
126. Biamino G, Schmidt A, Scheinert D. Treatment of SFA lesions with PLLA biodegradable stents: results of the PERSEUS study. J Endovasc Ther. 2005;12(Suppl (Abstracts: International Congress XVIII on Endovascular Interventions)): 1–5.
127. Bosiers M, Peeters P, D'Archambeau O, et al. AMS INSIGHT – absorbable metal stent implantation for treatment of below-the-knee critical limb ischemia: 6-month analysis. Cardiovasc Intervent Radiol. 2009;32(3):424–35.
128. Clagett GP, Sobel M, Jackson MR, Lip GYH, Tangelder M, Verhaeghe R. Antithrombotic therapy in peripheral arterial occlusive disease. The seventh ACCP conference on antithrombotic and thrombolytic therapy. Chest. 2004;126 Suppl 3:609S–26.
129. Allie DE, Hebert CJ, Lirtzman MD, et al. Combined glycoprotein IIb/IIIa and direct thrombin inhibition with eptifibatide and bivalirudin in the interventional treatment. Vasc Dis Manag. 2005; 2(6).
130. Mueller MR, Salat A, Stangl P, et al. Variable platelet response to low-dose ASA and the risk of limb deterioration in patients submitted to peripheral arterial angioplasty. Thromb Haemost. 1997;78(3):1003–7.
131. A randomised, blinded, trial of clopidogrel versus aspirin in patients at risk of ischaemic events (CAPRIE). CAPRIE Steering Committee. Lancet. 1996;348(9038):1329–39.
132. Efficacy of oral anticoagulants compared with aspirin after infrainguinal bypass surgery (The Dutch Bypass Oral Anticoagulants or Aspirin Study): a randomised trial. Lancet. 2000;355(9201): 346–51.

Part III

Venous Disease

Venous Insufficiency, Varicose Veins, and Perforators

17

Eric K. Peden and Nyla Ismail

Abstract

Venous disease affects large numbers of people in the United States. Venous disease can be due to incompetence with reflux of the deep and superficial systems, or within the superficial system itself. There are many reasons venous insufficiency develops, including pregnancy, obesity, lifestyle or job-related activities, familial/genetic factors, deep vein thrombosis, and idiopathic cases. Endoluminal treatment of venous insufficiency has rapidly gained widespread acceptance and has entered into mainstream practice. The advancement of minimally invasive techniques has enabled ambulatory clinic treatment in the majority of patients with varicose veins, getting patients back to normal activity and work more rapidly than traditional open surgical methods.

Keywords

Varicose veins • Perforator veins • Sclerotherapy • Laser ablation • Venous diseases

Venous disease affects large numbers of people in the United States, approximately 25 % of women and 15 % of men [1]. It encompasses a broad spectrum of symptoms, ranging from asymptomatic spider veins, bulging of the great saphenous vein (GSV) to leg swelling, and ulceration of the calf or ankle. Chronic venous insufficiency (CVI) implies valvular incompetence with reflux of the deep and superficial systems, or within the superficial system itself. Venous blood flow is disturbed primarily due to valvular incompetence and flows in a retrograde direction down into the leg, particularly at times of prolonged sitting or standing. There are many reasons venous insufficiency develops, including pregnancy, obesity, lifestyle or job-related activities, familial/genetic factors, deep vein thrombosis, and idiopathic cases.

CVI is defined by a number of available clinical tools including the CEAP (Clinical Etiology Anatomy Pathology) classification system, VCSS

E.K. Peden, M.D. (✉) • N. Ismail, Ph.D.
Department of Cardiovascular Surgery,
Methodist DeBakey Heart and Vascular Center,
The Methodist Hospital Research Institute,
The Methodist Hospital, 6550 Fannin St., Smith Tower,
Suite 1401, Houston, TX 77030, USA
e-mail: ekpeden@tmhs.org

J.J. Hoballah, A.B. Lumsden (eds.), *Vascular Surgery*, New Techniques in Surgery Series,
DOI 10.1007/978-1-4471-2912-7_17,

(Venous Clinical Severity Score), and a variety of quality of life (QoL) systems [2]. These tools enable standardized reporting such that different patient populations in various studies and centers can be compared in a similar fashion. Advanced CVI is used to describe patients with CEAP clinical classes 4–6, with skin changes of lipodermatosclerosis, hyperpigmentation, atrophie blanche, and healed or active venous ulcers. This group of patients represents the most challenging group to work with, but at the same time some of the most rewarding. The venous components of superficial veins, perforator veins, deep veins, and pelvic outflow frequently all require evaluation for complete treatment of this challenging patient population.

The treatment options for chronic venous insufficiency have changed dramatically over the last 10 years. The advent of minimally invasive techniques has expanded the surgical options for patients requiring treatment and has led to a proliferation of vein centers worldwide. Traditionally, venous insufficiency was treated successfully with high ligation and stripping of the greater saphenous vein. Current procedures are clinic-based with local anesthesia compared to previous surgery in a hospital operating room requiring general anesthesia. Contemporary methods utilize ablation of the vein with endoluminal techniques, rather than physical removal of the diseased veins.

The endoluminal vein treatments can be performed for both the superficial venous system of greater and small saphenous veins as well as for perforator veins. The most commonly used treatment options are radiofrequency ablation, laser ablation, and sclerotherapy (foam and liquid). These ablative techniques each use a source of energy which results in progressive fibrosis of the vessel and occlusion [3]. Radiofrequency and laser ablation use energy in the form of heat to obliterate the vein, and sclerotherapy uses a chemical that is injected directly into the vein causing injury.

Ultrasound imaging is paramount to the success of the treatment of venous disease. As a diagnostic tool, ultrasound has been found to be very versatile, accurate, and reproducible. Different venous components can be directly imaged and waveform analysis performed to determine location and degrees of obstruction and reflux. Venography has largely been replaced by ultrasound. The ablation techniques all need ultrasound imaging for diagnosis and intraprocedural guidance. Later ultrasound can also be used to evaluate the anatomic success of the treatment and check for thrombotic complications.

Tumescent anesthesia is also critical in the performance of radiofrequency and laser ablation procedures. Its use is effective at avoiding injury to both skin and nerves during treatment. It protects the perivascular tissues from the thermal energy and allows for targeted absorption by the treatment area [4]. Tumescent anesthesia enables treatment in the outpatient clinic setting and has minimal discomfort for the patient. Additionally, multiple adjunctive phlebectomies can be performed in the clinic, which previously would not have been possible without tumescence.

Superficial Veins

The focus of venous treatment historically and currently focuses on the superficial venous system. The majority of patients with advanced venous disease have valvular incompetence in their saphenous veins; however, modern ultrasound descriptions show that patients have a multisystem incompetence in the deep, superficial, and perforating veins [5, 6]. Although standard venous surgery has been focused on the superficial veins, a more complete venous evaluation may be necessary to determine the specific sites of incompetence of as well as prevent recurrence. Traditionally, the saphenofemoral reflux is thought to be responsible for most of the skin changes in venous insufficiency. Therefore, most ablation procedures are performed on the superficial venous system. Both the greater and small saphenous veins have been treated with ablation techniques.

Comparisons between percutaneous ablation techniques and conventional stripping indicate that the less invasive procedures are associated with improved outcomes. Patients who have received ablation techniques generally return to normal activities at a faster rate and report less pain as compared to patients using stripping [7, 8]. Overall, societal costs are less in the ablation group, because they can return to work sooner [8]. Recurrence from neovascularization is less common in ablation groups. In cases where stripping was associated with equivalent times for returning to work, tumescent anesthesia was used and phlebectomies were performed on the patients. Regardless of the situation, conventional stripping was linked with more pain and bruising compared to ablation techniques [9].

Techniques: Radiofrequency and Laser Ablation

Radiofrequency (RF) and laser ablation procedures use similar processes. Depending on the proposed vein segments to be treated, careful evaluation of the GSV from the saphenofemoral junction down to the knee or below the knee is performed. Size, depth, duplication, and general course of the vein are all noted. Treatment generally is isolated to above-the-knee segment to reduce the incidence of parethesias [10], although more extensive areas can be treated. Ultrasound guidance is used to access the vein percutaneously. If this is not feasible, a small incision can be made to dissect the vein or capture it with a vein hook to directly access it.

A catheter is passed up through the thigh using ultrasound or fluoroscopic guidance and guidewires if necessary. There are two types of RF catheters and several types of laser fibers with different wavelengths available from manufacturers. The final position of the catheter is placed 2 cm below the saphenofemoral junction, preferably below the junction of the inferior superficial epigastric vein within the GSV to preserve flow through the saphenofemoral junction and reduce thrombotic complications.

Perivenous tumescent anesthesia is injected to provide analgesia. Thermal ablation of the vein is painful and not possible with currently available devices without tumescent anesthesia. It also compresses the vein onto the catheter for more effective treatment and separates the catheter's thermal effects from the surrounding soft tissues, importantly the skin and saphenous nerve. The patient is placed in the Trendelenburg position either with or without external compression to increase vein wall contact. Using the manufacturer's instructions, the catheter is pulled back at a specified rate which varies by device. Ultrasound is then used to confirm an ablated appearance of the vein and patency of the common femoral vein. Color flow and Doppler signals should be absent and the saphenous vein should appear small, thickened, and minimally compressible, while the common femoral vein should be fully compressible.

Following these procedures, a compressive bandage with wraps or stockings is applied. The patient should be reevaluated in a few days with venous duplex to examine the treated vein and rule out a thrombotic complication.

Techniques: Sclerotherapy

Sclerotherapy is performed with similar techniques but with some important differences. Ultrasound guidance is necessary so that the saphenous vein can be accessed in the thigh with a short catheter. Sclerotherapy can be in a liquid or foam; however, the foam sclerotherapy results have generally been better than the liquid version in randomized trials [11, 12].

Foam sclerosant is created by mixing a gas (generally room air) in one syringe with a sclerosant in a second syringe using a stopcock. The most widely used process, also known as the Tessari method, uses ratio of 1:4, sclerosant to air [13]. The foam sclerosant modification is not FDA approved and should be discussed first with the patient. Sclerotherapy is not painful and does not require tumescence, which is a distinct advantage over the thermal ablation procedures.

Once the foam sclerosant is made, it is injected toward the saphenous junction using ultrasound guidance. Injection is stopped when the foam is close to the junction. A recent report suggests that less foam travels to the deep venous system if the injection is performed with the leg elevated

[14]. Stocking should be applied at the end of the procedure.

Comparisons of Superficial Venous Treatments

Endoluminal treatments of superficial veins have generally produced good results. Also, it has been suggested that endoluminal treatments of saphenous incompetence have decreased neovascularization and are subject to less recurrence than stripping. Although branches are left at the saphenofemoral junction with ablation which is classically ligated with high ligation, recurrence due to neovascularization is thought to be an inflammatory response related to surgical trauma at the saphenofemoral junction [7].

Direct comparisons between endoluminal techniques and stripping have been studied by several randomized trials over the last decade, but most studies are limited by small numbers of patients. The first trial to be published was the EVOLVeS trial comparing radiofrequency ablation to stripping [7]. This initial report documented early benefit of radiofrequency ablation over stripping in terms of pain, return to work, and quality of life scores. A follow-up study at 2 years demonstrated persistent obliteration of the saphenous veins, equivalent varicose vein recurrence, and continued improved quality of life scores in the ablation group [15]. Subsequent randomized trials of radiofrequency ablation compared to stripping have been performed and published with mixed results [16–18]. In Perälä's report, early failures of saphenous closure led to high recurrence rates and inferior outcomes [15]. The other studies demonstrated more rapid recovery from the ablation procedure with less complications, less pain, shorter hospital stays, earlier return to work, and improved quality of life scores [17, 18]. The varicose vein recurrence was demonstrated to be equivalent.

Laser ablation compared to stripping has been reported in three randomized trials. In the trial by Pronk, stripping was performed with tumescence and surprisingly demonstrated worse early postoperative pain in the laser group [19]. Follow-up at 1 year showed equivalent outcomes. Carradice however showed better early pain scores, improved quality of life scores, and earlier return to work with laser ablation [20]. Another randomized trial with 2-year follow-up demonstrated midterm equivalent outcomes with similar varicose vein recurrence and quality of life scores [21].

Saphenous ablation by radiofrequency compared to laser has also been studied and published. Almeida looked at early recovery from the procedure and found that radiofrequency had less pain and bruising that seemed to equalize by 4 weeks [22]. Goode and Gale likewise demonstrated improved early outcomes with radiofrequency compared to laser in terms of pain, bruising, and improvement in venous clinical severity scores (VCSS) that became equivalent by 1 month [23, 24]. Over the 1-year follow-up by Gale, there were more recanalizations in the radiofrequency group noted, leading to a more durable saphenous ablation in the laser group [24].

Several meta-analyses have been published comparing radiofrequency and laser saphenous ablation, finding that generally the success rates for laser and radiofrequency have been reported to be over 90 % with laser being slightly higher than radiofrequency [25–28].

Only a few trials of foam sclerotherapy compared to surgery have been reported with most including a saphenofemoral ligation in combination with the sclerotherapy portion. One trial comparing foam sclerotherapy alone randomized against stripping in patients with healed venous ulcerations [29]. Both groups had significant improvements in pain and swelling, and induration was equivalent.

The dreaded complication of saphenous ablation is a deep venous thrombosis. This is seen as an extension of thrombus from the saphenous vein into the common femoral vein (Fig. 17.1). Generally, the reports of these types of complication are less than 1 % [30]. There have been other reports of 16 % occurrence of thrombus in an isolated series. Paresthesia has been reported up to 15 % of the patients, but generally these symptoms are self-limited and improve with time [10].

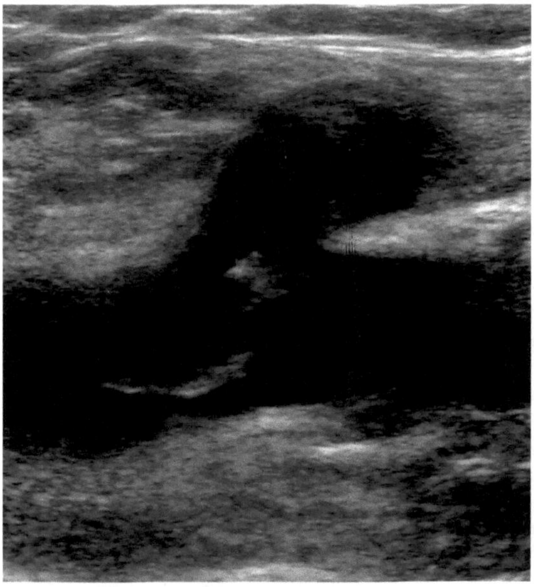

Fig. 17.1 Saphenofemoral thrombus

Comparisons between small saphenous ablation and radiofrequency and laser techniques are small in number. The occlusion rates are good (90 %), the complications have been uncommon (very few thrombus), and paresthesia rate is surprisingly low (2–7 %) [31–33].

Foam sclerotherapy has been inconsistent with reports of occlusion rates ranging from 39 to 96 % [12]. Another recent reports occlusion rates as high as 80–90 % [34]. Mixed reports of foam sclerotherapy for small versus the great saphenous veins exist.

There is some concern about the safety of foam sclerotherapy. Clearly some of the foam sclerosant travels into the deep system and system circulation. Travel into the pulmonary circulation presumably will filter most of the microbubbles, but patent foramen ovale can enable travel into the arterial system. Thousands of patients are treated worldwide, and the most commonly reported issues are transient visual disturbances [34]. Echocardiography has demonstrated bubbles visualized in the heart [14], and there have been infrequent reports of stroke and TIA [35–37]. Generally, in spite of these cases, the results are good with very few complications [38].

Iliac Vein Obstruction Syndrome

An increasingly recognized major contributor to chronic venous insufficiency is iliac vein obstruction syndrome. Described originally as May-Thurner syndrome, this condition has been well described as compression of the left common iliac vein by the right common iliac artery or a variant [39]. This compression is clearly associated with iliofemoral deep vein thrombosis, and investigation and treatment of such a lesion is paramount to successful treatment. Clinical presentation can vary widely from asymptomatic or more problematic with pain, swelling, and skin changes including ulcers. Expansive work has been published by Dr.'s Neglen and Raju among others on this topic [40–42]. Clinical suspicion about this pathological condition is raised in the presence of postthrombotic changes, pain in the leg not explained by varicosities, multiple levels of unexplained axial reflux in the deep system, and unexplained swelling. Outflow obstruction leads to increased pressure in the venous system in the leg causing progressive pathological changes of reflux and chronic venous insufficiency of widely varying degrees.

Testing with duplex ultrasound in patients with CVI should always include a comparison of the femoral waveforms between the right and left legs. Normal respiratory variation in the Doppler waveforms is expected with pulsatile waveforms in some patients. Patients with iliac vein obstruction syndrome may have blunted or continuous waveforms, and if different from the contralateral leg, this is highly suggestive (Figs. 17.2 and 17.3). Collateral flow however may be adequate such that this duplex finding is not present and a high degree of suspicion should prompt further evaluation. Magnetic resonance imaging of the venous system with time of flight image sequencing can be done of the pelvic and abdominal veins without the use of contrast and frequently yields diagnostic studies. Venography with intravascular ultrasound is the gold standard and has proven the most sensitive to the finding of compression by comparing cross-sectional area of the iliac veins at different levels (Fig. 17.4).

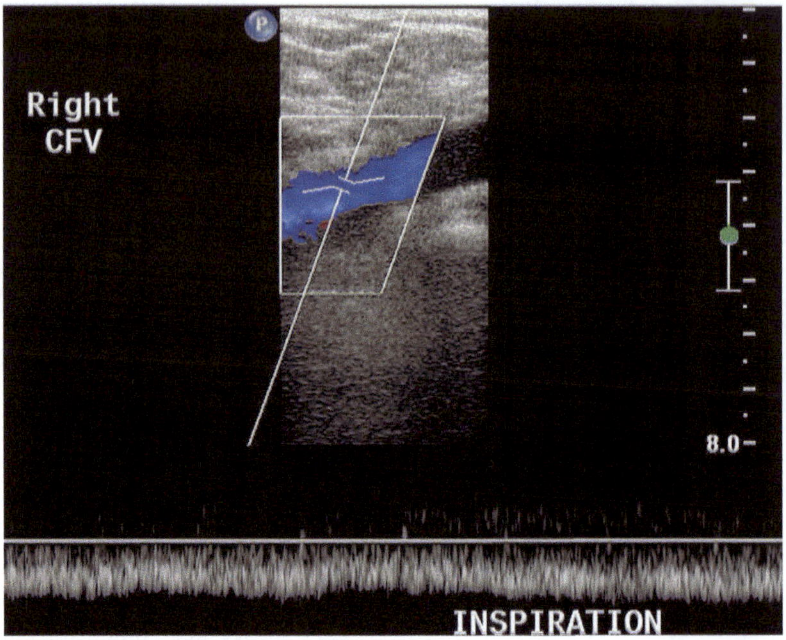

Fig. 17.2 Continuous femoral vein waveform

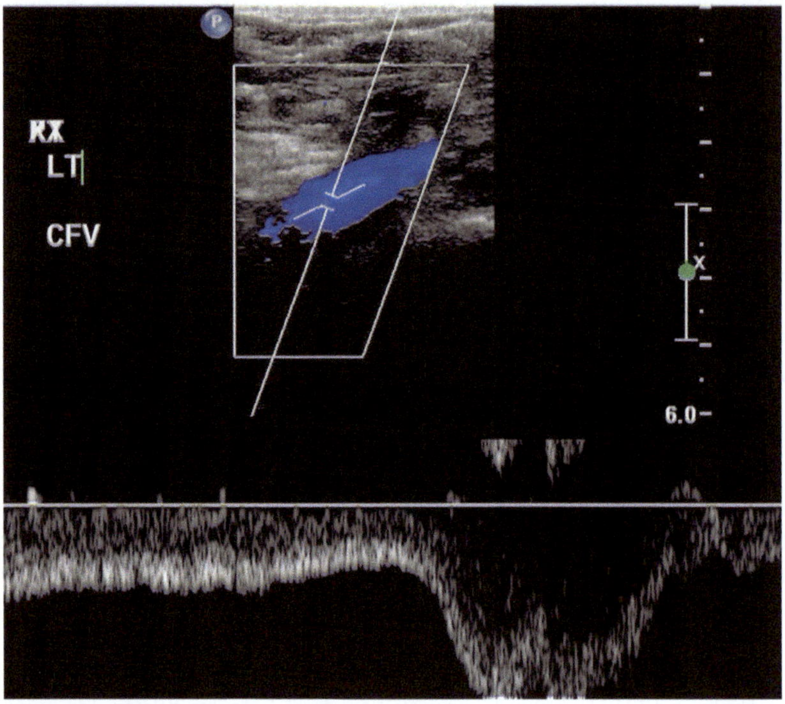

Fig. 17.3 Normal phasic femoral vein waveform

Modern treatment of iliac vein obstruction syndrome is endovascular. Angioplasty alone has been found to be far inferior to stenting. Self-expanding stents are placed with deployment of the stent ensuring adequate proximal and distal landing zones to reduce the chance of restenosis. Routinely, this requires coverage into the inferior vena cava and may require extension of the stent

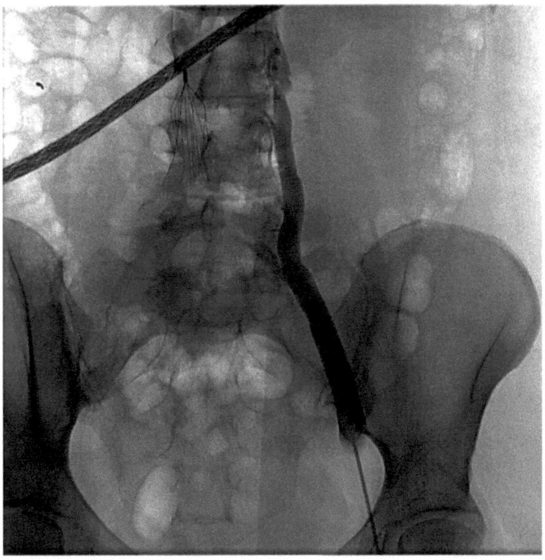

Fig. 17.4 Venogram demonstrating common iliac vein occlusion

down across the inguinal ligament into the common femoral or even femoral vein. The key to the stenting is adequate size and extent of the coverage to ensure proper flow.

Results of stenting have been reported out to 6 years with primary patency 67 %, primary assisted patency 89 %, and secondary patency 93 %. Results are considerably better for nonthrombotic cases. Clearly improved as well is that primary assisted patency is superior to secondary patency and thus all patients that have undergone iliac vein stenting should be enrolled in a surveillance program to reduce the chance of stent thrombosis. Clinically, the parameter most impacted by iliac vein stenting is pain with improvements in quality of life measurements. Swelling, ulcer healing, and venous clinical severity scores are all also reported to improve significantly after treatment.

Perforator Veins

Perforator vein treatment in the algorithm for chronic venous disease has been the subject of multiple debates and significant controversy [43, 44]. It is generally agreed upon that perforator veins do play a significant role in advanced venous disease, but benefits from their treatment are poorly studied. In addition, the appeal of perforator vein treatment has fluctuated considerably over time. Initial description of the perforator veins and the Linton procedure led to early enthusiasm but was later tempered by high wound complication rates [43]. Later endoscopic techniques led to operative procedures, but that too faded with poor results in postthrombotic limbs. Currently, the use of percutaneous techniques has caused resurgence in popularity of treating perforator veins [3].

The most current procedure, termed PAPS (percutaneous ablation perforator surgery), shows some promising results. In this trial, treatment resulted in improved venous clinical severity scores and ulcer healing [3, 45]. Also, recurrence of ulcers and perforator veins was shown to occur simultaneously establishing a link between the two symptoms [43]. Taken together, these results suggest that patients who have received perforator vein treatment alone can address some of the disease states associated with advanced venous disease and certainly suggest a role for the treatment of perforator veins in patients with advanced venous disease [46].

Techniques: Perforator Veins

Depending on the use of radiofrequency, laser, or sclerotherapy, perforator treatment techniques vary. All the treatments, however, do involve the use of ultrasound guidance to accurately visualize access to the perforator veins and to validate treatment effect. Perforator veins should demonstrate reflux across the fascial layer for greater than 0.5 s (Fig. 17.5). For radiofrequency and laser techniques, the perforator vein is accessed directly, at or preferably below the level of the fascia. For the radiofrequency perforator probe, two techniques work effectively: an over-the-wire technique and direct puncture and treatment. Preferably, a large portion of the vein is treated or two focal areas. In the clinic setting, infusion of local anesthetic around the area of the catheter prevents pain, and use of external pressure ensures good contact

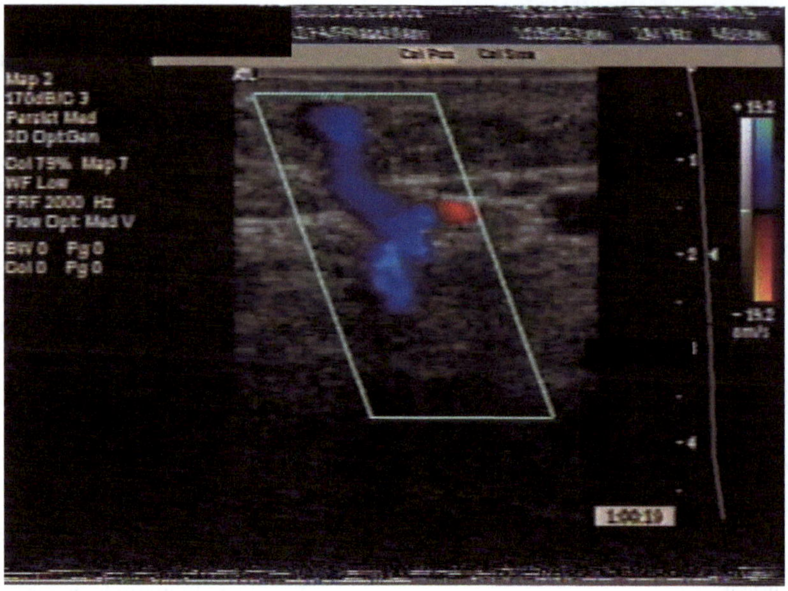

Fig. 17.5 Incompetent perforator vein

between the probe and vessel wall. The laser fiber can then be passed directly through a 21-gauge needle allowing for two to three focal treatments for 5 s each. Just as with radiofrequency, it is important to infuse local anesthetic around the catheter tip and hold external pressure. The manufacturer for radiofrequency ablation suggests a 4-min treatment, basically toggling the probe to contact each of the four walls for 1 min each. During treatment, the impedance reading on the machine can be helpful to confirm intravascular treatment. Following treatment, the vein is tested for reflux with duplex imaging, although the presence of the anesthetic can limit visualization. Generally, the perforator vein should appear shrunken and more echogenic with no color flow visualized. After completion of the procedure, compress the area for a few minutes and apply compressive bandages.

Both foam and liquid sclerotherapy have also been utilized to treat perforator veins. Direct perforator access is not mandatory and commonly a nearby varix can be accessed. Ultrasound imaging is used to visualize passage of the sclerosant into the perforator vein. Elevation of the leg is recommended and anesthetic is not required. As with radiofrequency and laser ablation, digital compression for a brief time followed by application of compressive bandaging is common.

Perforator Vein Treatment Results

Although sclerotherapy was reported for perforator vein treatment over four decades ago [47], results from perforator treatment are few and most of the information available is in the form of abstracts from national conferences. In general, the results do report high occlusion rates and few complications [3]. Occlusion rates of 75–98 % were reported with few complications; however, repeat intervention may be necessary.

Encouragingly, a report of percutaneous ablation of perforator veins with a saphenous-style radiofrequency probe has been achieved successfully [48]. In fact, 81 % of the veins showed in this study had successful ablation in a 5-year follow-up including just under half of the original patients. A recent review indicated that 90 % of perforator veins that were treated with radiofrequency were occluded in short-term follow-up [3].

Success using laser ablation of perforators is equally as promising. It has been reported that 85–100 % early closure rate with few complications is using laser ablation for perforator veins [49]. In addition, no deep venous thromboses, rare paresthesias, and a few blisters have been reported [3].

Overall, perhaps the biggest advantage of the PAPS technique is that it is reproducible. The previous, more invasive techniques of direct or endoscopic perforator ligation are very difficult to repeat. Patients with the advanced chronic venous disease often have recurrence; therefore, repeatability of the treatments becomes increasingly more important.

Conclusion

Endoluminal treatment of venous insufficiency has rapidly gained widespread acceptance and has entered into mainstream practice. The advancement of minimally invasive techniques has enabled ambulatory clinic treatment in the majority of patients with varicose veins, getting patients back to normal activity and work more rapidly than traditional open surgical methods. In addition, a more comprehensive view of the venous system including both superficial and perforator veins has achieved better results for patients with chronic venous disease. Increasing numbers of reports are being published in the literature with good results and low complication rates. As techniques continue to evolve, patients will clearly benefit from these advances in technology.

References

1. Subramonia S, Lees TA. The treatment of varicose veins. Ann R Coll Surg Engl. 2007;89:96–100.
2. Nitecki S, Kantarovsky A, Portnot I, Bass A. The contemporary treatment of varicose veins (strangle, strip, grill or poison). Isr Med Assoc J. 2006;8:411–5.
3. Elias S, Peden E. Ultrasound-guided percutaneous ablation for the treatment of perforating vein incompetence. Vascular. 2007;15(5):281–9.
4. Whiddon LL. Advances in the treatment of superficial venous insufficiency of the lower extremities. Proc (Bayl Univ Med Cent). 2007;20(2):136–9.
5. Hanrahan LM, Kechejian GJ, Cordts PR, Rodriguez AA, Araki CA, LaMorte WW, Menzoian JO. Patterns of venous insufficiency in patients with varicose veins. Arch Surg. 1991;126(6):687–90; discussion 690–1.
6. Hanrahan LM, Araki CT, Rodriguez AA, Kechejian GJ, LaMorte WW, Menzoian JO. Distribution of valvular incompetence in patients with venous stasis ulceration. J Vasc Surg. 1991;13(6):805–11; discussion 811–2.
7. Lurie F, Creton D, Eklof B, Kabnick LS, Kistner RL, Pichot O, et al. Prospective randomized study of endovenous radiofrequency obliteration (Closure) versus ligation and stripping in a selected patient population (EVOLVES study). J Vasc Surg. 2003;38:207–14.
8. Rautio T, Ohinmaa A, Perälä J, Ohtonen P, Heikkinen T, Wiik H, et al. Endovenous obliteration versus conventional stripping operation in the treatment of primary varicose veins: a randomized controlled trial with comparison of costs. J Vasc Surg. 2002;35:958–65.
9. Rasmussen LH, Bjoern L, Lawaetz M, Blemings A, Lawaetz B, Eklof B. Randomized trial comparing endovenous laser ablation of the great saphenous vein with high ligation and stripping in patients with varicose veins: short-term results. J Vasc Surg. 2007;46(2): 308–15.
10. Merchant RF, DePalma RG, Kabnick LS. Endovascular obliteration of saphenous reflux: a multicenter study. J Vasc Surg. 2002;35(6):1190–6.
11. Ouvry P, Allaert FA, Desnos P, Hamel-Desnos C. Efficacy of polidocanol foam versus liquid in sclerotherapy of the great saphenous vein: a multicentre randomised controlled trial with a 2-year follow-up. Eur J Vasc Endovasc Surg. 2008;36(3):366–70.
12. Rabe E, Otto J, Schliephake D, Pannier F. Efficacy and safety of great saphenous vein sclerotherapy using standardised polidocanol foam (ESAF): a randomised controlled multicentre clinical trial. Eur J Vasc Endovasc Surg. 2008;35(2):238–45.
13. Tessari L. Nouvelle technique d' obtention de la sclero-mousse. Phlebologie. 2000;53:129.
14. Hill D, Hamilton R, Fung T. Assessment of techniques to reduce sclerosant foam migration during ultrasound-guided sclerotherapy of the great saphenous vein. J Vasc Surg. 2008;48(4):934–9.
15. Lurie F, Creton D, Eklof B, Kabnick LS, Kistner RL, Pichot O, Sessa C, Schuller-Petrovic S. Prospective randomized study of endovenous radiofrequency obliteration (closure) versus ligation and vein stripping (EVOLVeS): two-year follow – up. Eur J Vasc Endovasc Surg. 2005;29(1):67–73.
16. Perälä J, Rautio T, Biancari F, Ohtonen P, Wiik H, Heikkinen T, Juvonen T. Radiofrequency endovenous obliteration versus stripping of the long saphenous vein in the management of primary varicose veins: 3-year outcome of a randomized study. Ann Vasc Surg. 2005;19(5):669–72.
17. Subramonia S, Lees T. Randomized clinical trial of radiofrequency ablation or conventional high ligation and stripping for great saphenous varicose veins. Br J Surg. 2010;97(3):328–36.
18. Helmy ElKaffas K, ElKashef O, ElBaz W. Great saphenous vein radiofrequency ablation versus standard stripping in the management of primary varicose veins-a randomized clinical trial. Angiology. 2011;62(1):49–54. Epub 2010 Aug 18.
19. Pronk P, Gauw SA, Mooij MC, Gaastra MT, Lawson JA, van Goethem AR, van Vlijmen-van Keulen CJ. Randomised controlled trial comparing sapheno-femoral ligation and stripping of the great saphenous vein

with endovenous laser ablation (980 nm) using local tumescent anaesthesia: one year results. Eur J Vasc Endovasc Surg. 2010;40(5):649–56.
20. Carradice D, Mekako A, Mazari FA, Samuel N, Hatfield J, Chetter IC. Randomized clinical trial of endovenous laser ablation compared with conventional surgery for great saphenous varicose veins. Br J Surg. 2011;98:501–10. doi:10.1002/bjs.7394. Epub 2011 Jan 31.
21. Rasmussen LH, Bjoern L, Lawaetz M, Lawaetz B, Blemings A, Eklöf B. Randomised clinical trial comparing endovenous laser ablation with stripping of the great saphenous vein: clinical outcomes and recurrence after 2 years. Eur J Vasc Endovasc Surg. 2010;39(5):630–5. Epub 2010 Jan 12.
22. Almeida JI, Kaufman J, Göckeritz O, Chopra P, Evans MT, Hoheim DF, Makhoul RG, Richards T, Wenzel C, Raines JK. Radiofrequency endovenous ClosureFAST versus laser ablation for the treatment of great saphenous reflux: a multicenter, single-blinded, randomized study (RECOVERY study). J Vasc Interv Radiol. 2009;20(6):752–9. Epub 2009 Apr 22.
23. Goode SD, Chowdhury A, Crockett M, Beech A, Simpson R, Richards T, Braithwaite BD. Laser and radiofrequency ablation study (LARA study): a randomized study comparing radiofrequency ablation and endovenous laser ablation (810 nm). Eur J Vasc Endovasc Surg. 2010;40(2):246–53.
24. Gale SS, Lee JN, Walsh ME, Wojnarowski DL, Comerota AJ. A randomized, controlled trial of endovenous thermal ablation using the 810-nm wavelength laser and the ClosurePLUS radiofrequency ablation methods for superficial venous insufficiency of the great saphenous vein. J Vasc Surg. 2010;52(3): 645–50. Epub 2010 Jul 17.
25. Puggioni A, Kalra M, Carmo M, Mozes G, Gloviczki P. Endovenous laser therapy and radiofrequency ablation of the great saphenous vein: analysis of early efficacy and complications. J Vasc Surg. 2005;42(3): 488–93.
26. Pannier F, Rabe E. Endovenous laser therapy and radiofrequency ablation of saphenous varicose veins. J Cardiovasc Surg (Torino). 2006;47(1):3–8.
27. Van den Bos R, Arends L, Kockaert M, Neumann M, Nijsten T. Endovenous therapies of lower extremity varicosities: a meta-analysis. J Vasc Surg. 2009;49(1): 230–9.
28. Luebke T, Brunkwall J. Systematic review and meta-analysis of endovenous radiofrequency obliteration, endovenous laser therapy, and foam sclerotherapy for primary varicosis. J Cardiovasc Surg (Torino). 2008; 49(2):213–33.
29. Figueiredo M, Araújo S, Barros Jr N, Miranda Jr F. Results of surgical treatment compared with ultrasound-guided foam sclerotherapy in patients with varicose veins: a prospective randomised study. Eur J Vasc Endovasc Surg. 2009;38(6):758–63. Epub 2009 Sep 9.
30. Hingorani AP, Ascher E, Markevich N, Schutzer RW, Kallakuri S, Hou A, Nahata S, Yorkovich W, Jacob T. Deep venous thrombosis after radiofrequency ablation of greater saphenous vein: a word of caution. J Vasc Surg. 2004;40(3):500–4.
31. Dunne J. Treatment of small saphenous vein insufficiency using endovascular radiofrequency obliteration. In: American College of Phlebology 18th congress. Marco Island; Nov 2004.
32. Gale SS et al. Early results of radiofrequency ablation of the small saphenous vein. In: 17th annual meeting of American Venous Forum. San Diego, California; 9–13 Feb 2005.
33. Kontothanassis D, Di Mitri R, Ferrari Ruffino S, Zambrini E, Camporese G, Gerard JL, Labropoulos N. Endovenous laser treatment of the small saphenous vein. J Vasc Surg. 2009;49(4):973–9.
34. Coleridge Smith P. Saphenous ablation: sclerosant or sclerofoam? Semin Vasc Surg. 2005;18(1):19–24.
35. Forlee MV, Grouden M, Moore DJ, Shanik G. Stroke after varicose vein foam injection sclerotherapy. J Vasc Surg. 2006;43(1):162–4.
36. Bush RG, Derrick M, Manjoney D. Major neurological events following foam sclerotherapy. Phlebology. 2008;23(4):189–92.
37. O'Hare JL, Earnshaw JJ. The use of foam sclerotherapy for varicose veins: a survey of the members of the Vascular Society of Great Britain and Ireland. Eur J Vasc Endovasc Surg. 2007;34(2):232–5.
38. Darke SG, Baker SJ. Ultrasound-guided foam sclerotherapy for the treatment of varicose veins. Br J Surg. 2006;93(8):969–74.
39. May R, Thurner J. The cause of predominately sinistral occurrence of thrombosis of the pelvic veins. Angiology. 1957;8:419–27.
40. Neglén P, Hollis KC, Raju S. Combined saphenous ablation and iliac stent placement for complex severe chronic venous disease. J Vasc Surg. 2006;44(4): 828–33.
41. Neglén P, Hollis KC, Olivier J, Raju S. Stenting of the venous outflow in chronic venous disease: long-term stent-related outcomes, clinical, and hemodynamic result. J Vasc Surg. 2007;46(5):979–90.
42. Raju S, Darcey R, Neglén P. Unexpected major role for venous stenting in deep reflux disease. J Vasc Surg. 2010;51(2):401–8; discussion 408. Epub 2009 Dec 14.
43. O'Donnell Jr TF. The present status of surgery of the superficial venous system in the management of venous ulcer and the evidence for the role of perforator interruption. J Vasc Surg. 2008;48(4):1044–52.
44. Meissner MH. "I enjoyed your talk, but…": evidence-based medicine and the scientific foundation of the American Venous Forum. J Vasc Surg. 2009;49(1): 244–8.
45. Bergan JJ. Perforating veins. In: Bergan JJ, Goldman MP, editors. Varicose veins and telangiectasias: diagnosis and treatment. St. Louis: Quality Medical Publishing; 1993.

46. Masuda EM, Kessler DM, Lurie F, Puggioni A, Kistner RL, Eklof B. The effect of ultrasound-guided sclerotherapy of incompetent perforator veins on venous clinical severity and disability scores. J Vasc Surg. 2006;43(3):551–6; discussion 556–7.
47. Hobbs JT. Surgery and sclerotherapy in the treatment of varicose veins, a random trial. Arch Surg. 1974;109: 793–6.
48. Bacon JL, Dinneen AJ, Marsh P, Holdstock JM, Price BA, Whiteley MS. Five-year results of incompetent perforator vein closure using TRans-Luminal Occlusion of Perforator. Phlebology. 2009;24(2): 74–8.
49. Fegan WG. Continuous compression technique of injection varicose veins. Lancet. 1963;2:109–12.

Deep Venous Thrombosis

18

Hossam F. El-Sayed

Abstract

Acute DVT is a common disease with potentially life-threatening consequences and long-term life-altering complications. It imposes huge economic burden on the society. The disease is difficult to diagnose because of the lack of sensitivity and specificity of its clinical manifestations. Diagnostic algorithms are needed for safe and effective diagnosis. The treatment is standard anticoagulation therapy which reduces significantly the mortality risk and recurrence of the disease but does a much poorer job when it comes to the long-term morbidity of the disease. Active management of acute DVT, especially proximal iliofemoral DVT, using catheter-directed thrombolysis with or without mechanical thrombectomy modalities is gaining momentum and may prove to be the standard therapy of the future as it adds to the standard therapy the significant reduction of the long-term morbidity specifically postthrombotic syndrome.

Keywords

Venous • Vein • Thrombectomy • Thrombolysis • Percutaneous Thrombosis • Deep

Introduction

Venous thromboembolism (VTE) is a common disorder and is comprised of two different but related clinical syndromes, deep vein thrombosis (DVT) and pulmonary embolism (PE). VTE is actually the third most common cardiovascular pathology after coronary artery disease and stroke [1].

VTE has annual incidence rates varying from 1 case per 10,000 in young adults to 1 per 100 in the elderly [2, 3]. The total number of new cases in the USA each year is more than 275,000. This is responsible for a cost of treatment of estimated 2.5 billion dollars per year [4]. VTE is an important cause of morbidity and mortality, particularly in hospitalized patients. PE is the cause of death or a major contributing factor in up to 16 %

H.F. El-Sayed, M.D., Ph.D., RVT
Division of Vascular Surgery,
Department of Cardiovascular Surgery,
Weil Cornell Medical College, The Methodist Hospital,
6550 Fannin St., Smith Tower, Suite 1401,
Houston, TX 77030, USA
e-mail: hfelsayed@tmhs.org

J.J. Hoballah, A.B. Lumsden (eds.), *Vascular Surgery*, New Techniques in Surgery Series,
DOI 10.1007/978-1-4471-2912-7_18, © Springer-Verlag London 2012

of patients who die in the hospital. However, in some series, the diagnosis of PE is suspected before death in less than one-third of patients. It is therefore important to have a high index of suspicion for the presence of VTE and to initiate appropriate diagnostic tests and therapy [5].

It is also a significant source of long-term morbidity secondary to postthrombotic syndrome (PTS), due to chronic venous insufficiency secondary to DVT and its sequelae. It is estimated that the cumulative incidence of PTS changes at 1, 2, and 5 years are 17, 23, and 28 %, respectively. The incidence of severe skin changes including venous ulceration is between 2.6 % at 1 year and 9.3 % at 5 years [6].

Pathophysiology

Etiology

In 1860, Rudolf Virchow described the famous triad of factors that are still considered the main factors in the pathogenesis of venous thrombosis, i.e., damage to the vein, slowing of the venous flow, and changes in the blood leading to an increased tendency to form clots (hypercoagulability). When DVT occurs in the setting of recognized risk factor, it is often defined as secondary, whereas that occurring in the absence of recognizable risk factors is termed primary or idiopathic [7]. The risk factor associated with acute DVT is summarized in Table 18.1.

Table 18.1 Risk factors for acute deep venous thrombosis and pulmonary embolism

Risk factors for DVT or PE	Odds ratio	95 % Confidence interval
Hospitalization		
With recent surgery	21.72	9.44–49.93
Without recent surgery	7.98	4.49–14.18
Trauma	12.69	4.06–39.66
Malignant neoplasm		
With chemotherapy	6.53	2.11–20.23
Without chemotherapy	4.05	1.93–8.52
Previous central venous catheter or pacemaker	5.55	1.57–19.59
Previous superficial vein thrombosis	4.32	1.76–10.61
Neurologic disease with extremity paresis	3.04	1.25–7.38
Varicose veins		
Age 45 years	4.19	1.56–11.30
Age 60 years	1.93	1.03–3.61
Age 75 years	0.88	0.55–1.43
Congestive heart failure		
Thromboembolism not categorized as a cause of death at postmortem examination	9.64	2.44–38.10
Thromboembolism categorized as a cause of death at postmortem examination	1.36	0.69–2.68

Adapted from Heit et al. [8]

Many contributing factors are associated and predispose to acute DVT, the details of which are beyond the scope of this book. Immobilization, prolonged travel particularly the "economy-class syndrome" which occurs in people who sit in a cramped position during extended aircraft flights, is a well-recognized predisposing factor. History of previous venous thromboembolism, malignancy, and recent surgery are considered high on the list of risk factors for acute DVT. Inherited thrombophilia with its different variants including factor V Leiden mutation, prothrombin gene mutation, and protein C and S deficiency, just to name a few, is also a major risk factor especially of primary DVT. Acquired thrombophilia syndromes like lupus anticoagulants and anticardiolipin antibodies are also important risk factors. Pregnancy and the use of oral contraceptive pills have long been recognized as higher risk factors for the development of DVT in female population. Also, anatomical compression of the veins especially the left common iliac vein (May-Thurner syndrome) is a congenital risk factor for acute DVT of the left iliofemoral vein segment, which is five times as common as right iliofemoral DVT [9]. The syndrome occurs due to the compression of the left common iliac vein by the right common iliac artery that crosses in front of the vein pinching it against the sacrum. In the upper extremity, primary upper extremity DVT due to compression at the thoracic outlet (Paget-Schroetter syndrome) is another variant of vein compression syndrome [10].

Pathogenesis

The development of the acute thrombus starts at an area of stasis like the soleal veins or at the base of a valve cusp facing the valve sinus. It occurs due to disturbance of the balance between thrombosis and thrombolysis due to the variety of risk factors involved. Once the process starts, there is upregulation of the adhesion molecules P-selectin and E-selectin and thereby promotion of leukocyte interactions. This sets the stage for inflammatory amplification of the thrombotic process [11]. Physiologic clot formation is balanced by a constant process of thrombolysis to prevent pathologic thrombosis. Plasmin is the main fibrinolytic enzyme, with its substrate being fibrin, fibrinogen, and other coagulation factors. The primary inhibitor of plasminogen activators is plasminogen activator inhibitor-1 (PAI-1). PAI-1 secretion is enhanced during the acute thrombosis process and may be a factor in suppressing fibrinolysis and thus promoting the process of thrombosis [12].

Natural History

The relative balance between organization, thrombolysis, propagation, recanalization, and rethrombosis determines the outcome of human acute DVT. Venous duplex ultrasound which permits individual venous segments to be observed over time has documented that recanalization does occur in most patients after an episode of acute DVT. Van Ramshorst and associates found that most recanalizations occur within the first 6 weeks, with flow reestablished in 87 % of cases [13]. Killewich and colleagues reported a linear decrease in thrombus load, and by 24–36 weeks, only 26 % of the original thrombus remained [14]. However, recanalization may continue albeit at a slower rate for months to years after the acute event [15]. Rethrombosis has also been reported in the affected segments. The incidence of recurrent thrombosis is 5.2 % of those who were treated with standard anticoagulation for 3 months compared with 47 % in those who were inadequately treated [16, 17].

Complications

Pulmonary Embolism (PE)

This is the most devastating complication of acute DVT. With that said, the majority of these incidents are clinically silent. Recent studies have shown that in patients with symptomatic acute DVT of the lower extremity, 50–80 % develop asymptomatic PE. It was also found that symptomatic PE complicates up to 17 % of patients with proximal upper extremity acute DVT [18]. Patients with symptomatic PE have 18 times the mortality rate compared to patients with acute DVT alone [18]. Patients who survive the acute PE event are still at risk of development of chronic thromboembolic pulmonary hypertension (CTEPH). Recent data have suggested that CTEPH occurs more often than previously suspected, with the disorder developing in 3.8 % of patients after surviving acute PE. The most common symptom in those patients is progressive exertional dyspnea with worsening right ventricular failure, edema, chest pain, light-headedness, and syncope developing as the disease progresses [19].

Postthrombotic Syndrome (PTS)

This is a group of clinical manifestations in patients who have history of acute DVT due to ambulatory venous hypertension in their affected limbs. It is the most common late complication of acute DVT and is responsible for a greater degree of chronic socioeconomic and quality of life morbidity. The cause of ambulatory venous hypertension is a combination of venous reflux secondary to valvular incompetence and residual luminal obstruction [20, 21]. The manifestations of PTS range from painful, swollen, heavy leg, and venous claudication to the most severe end of the spectrum of venous ulceration [22]. PTS is a relatively common and highly significant sequel of acute DVT. Eighty percent of symptomatic acute DVTs are above the knee (proximal), with a cumulative incidence of PTS of 50 % at 2 years post DVT [23]. Severe PTS is reported in 50 % of those cases and leg ulceration is present up to 10 % of patients. Recent research has shown that quality of life among patients with PTS is poorer than that among patients of similar age with other chronic conditions such as arthritis, chronic lung disease, or diabetes. Severe PTS leads to such a poor quality of life that is comparable to experiencing angina, cancer, or congestive heart failure [24].

Diagnosis

When approaching a patient with suspected DVT of the lower extremity, it is important to appreciate that only a minority of the patients actually have the disease and will require anticoagulation. False positive clinical signs occur in up to 50 % of patients. It is also important to remember only 40 % of patients with venous thrombosis have any clinical signs of the disorder. For those reasons, it is important to use validated algorithms to evaluate patients with suspected DVT, along with objective testing to establish the diagnosis. Given the potential risks associated with proximal lower extremity DVT that is not treated (e.g., fatal pulmonary embolism) and the potential risk of anticoagulating a patient who does not have a DVT (e.g., fatal bleeding), accurate diagnosis is essential.

Symptoms of acute DVT classically include unilateral swelling, pain, and discoloration of the involved extremity. A complete thrombosis history including age of onset, location of prior thromboses, and results of objective studies documenting thrombotic episodes in the patient as well as any family members should be obtained. The presence of family history or previous thrombosis attacks strongly suggests the presence of a hereditary defect and/or increased probability of an acute DVT attack [25]. History of potential risk factors should be extensively obtained from these patients again to evaluate their probability of having a new acute DVT.

On clinical exam, typical manifestations include unilateral limb swelling and edema. Warmth, tenderness, and erythema can also be present. Tenderness over the major veins in the thigh can be present. The limb involved can be swollen, painful, and blanched, a condition that has been termed as phlegmasia alba dolens. Investigators originally believed that the blanching was due to spasm and compromise of arterial flow, but recent evidence recognized that cutaneous edema is responsible. If the extent of thrombosis is extensive with impeding the venous return of the affected extremity, limb loss may occur due to cessation of arterial flow. The clinical picture is termed phlegmasia cerulea dolens, or painful blue leg. With the loss of sensory and motor function, venous gangrene is likely unless venous outflow of the limb is restored.

As mentioned, because the clinical picture is both of low sensitivity and specificity, confirmatory objective tests are needed to rule in or out the possibility of DVT.

Contrast Venography (CV)

This was historically the gold standard for diagnosis of acute DVT. It is performed by injecting a contrast material directly into the venous system through the dorsal foot veins while the superficial veins are occluded at the ankle by a tourniquet. A defect in the venous column is diagnostic. The test is invasive, inconvenient to the patient, and expensive and can be a cause of acute DVT by itself [26]. Venography is currently only used when noninvasive testing is not clinically feasible or the results are equivocal.

Duplex Examination

This has replaced the contrast venography as the diagnostic standard in the USA. The test is simple, noninvasive with little inconvenience to the patient, and associated with a high sensitivity and specificity of 96 and 100 %, respectively, and a negative predictive value of 98–99 % which means that a negative test essentially excludes the diagnosis of acute DVT [27]. The test depends on using the Doppler to evaluate the flow characteristics in the vein as an indirect evidence of venous obstruction. It also combines that with B-mode (two-dimensional) ultrasound to evaluate areas with suspected thrombosis to evaluate compressibility as a direct evidence of filling defects inside the vein and also characterizing the venous thrombus. Chronic thrombi have greater echogenicity, heterogeneity, and an irregular surface. The addition of color-flow Doppler scanning has also improved the sensitivity and specificity of ultrasound scanning when used as a screening test in asymptomatic patients even when used for distal veins.

MRV, CTV, and Isotope Scanning

Magnetic resonance venography (MRV) utilizes the ability of magnetic resonance to distinguish stationary from moving signals. MRV is less expensive than CV. On the other hand, it was found to have a sensitivity and specificity of 100 and 96 %, respectively, and was found to be as accurate as CV in detecting acute DVT. It is considered complementary to duplex ultrasound when the results are equivocal especially detecting DVT of the iliac veins above the inguinal ligament, an area that is difficult to evaluate using duplex ultrasound [28].

CT scan is increasingly used for the diagnosis of PE, and the addition of computed tomographic venography (CTV) makes it a single test to evaluate for both PE and DVT. Although CTV may have clinical utility in patients with PE and thus higher pretest probability of DVT, its precise role is not yet defined. The results of studies to date may be biased because of patient selection. Additionally, the cost to the patient may be as much as six times higher than that of duplex scanning, and the CTV involves additional radiation exposure [29].

Isotope scanning for acute DVT has been approved utilizing technetium 99m and apcitide that binds to glycoprotein IIb/IIIa receptor on activated platelets and is specific for acute thrombosis. Although the role of this modality shows promise as a diagnostic evaluation of acute DVT, it still remains to be defined in clinical practice.

D-Dimer

These are products of the degradation of cross-linked fibrin by plasmin. They can be detected by monoclonal antibodies that can differentiate the degradation products of fibrin from fibrinogen. The test is extremely sensitive with a sensitivity approaching 97 %. However, these measurements are nonspecific with a specificity as low as 35 % [30]. The sensitivity for isolated calf vein thrombosis is 2–8 % lower than that for proximal-vein thrombosis [31]. The sensitivity of the test is also lower when the interval between thrombosis and testing exceeds 2–3 weeks and with the use of anticoagulants. D-dimer measurements have a little diagnostic utility in inpatients as it is less sensitive with a false-negative rate of up to 29 % and a very low specificity especially those who are morbidly obese, bedridden, older than 60 years, and with malignant disease.

The clinical utility of D-dimer depends on its negative predictive value (NPV) in that particular clinical setting. According to Baye's theorem, the NPV of a particular diagnostic test depends on the prevalence of the disease in the population tested. The prevalence of a disease in a certain population is expressed as pretest probability of the presence of that disease. In simple terms, in a population of low prevalence (pretest probability) of acute DVT, a negative D-dimer test essentially excludes acute DVT. However, if the pretest probability of acute DVT is high, the negative D-dimer test cannot exclude acute DVT.

Multiple scoring systems are available to determine the pretest probability of acute DVT in the outpatient settings. Factors used in those scoring systems include the presence of risk factors of DVT, the presence of objective clinical signs as factors raising the pretest probability of acute DVT, and the presence of possible alternate diagnoses which lower the pretest probability [32].

Diagnostic Strategy

Although duplex ultrasound is extremely accurate in diagnosing acute DVT, its overuse in the evaluation of patients with suspected acute DVT imposes intense burden on the hospital resources specifically the vascular lab. For that reason, diagnostic strategies have been developed in an attempt to be more efficient in utilizing these resources and reduce cost. As mentioned above, the suspicion of acute DVT in hospitalized patients requires confirmatory testing, usually duplex ultrasound, due to the high pretest probability of the disease in that population.

The situation is different in the outpatient setting where the prevalence of the disease and hence the pretest probability are much lower. In those patients, the first step is to stratify their pretest probability for the presence of acute DVT using one of the available risk stratification scores, commonly the Wells score (Table 18.2). This is based on the presence of risk factors of acute DVT, objective clinical signs of acute DVT, and the possibility of alternative diagnosis. Patients are classified into low, intermediate, or high pretest probability of acute DVT. Patients with low and intermediate probability are exposed to D-dimer testing. In case it is negative, that essentially excludes the diagnosis of acute DVT in the low-probability and intermediate-probability patients, which require no further duplex ultrasound testing as in those patients the negative predictive value of the test approaches 100 %. On the other hand, patients with high pretest probability for DVT will require duplex ultrasound, as the negative predictive value of D-dimer in those patients is around 85 %. In other words, the false-negative rate of 15 % is unacceptably high if we rely on a negative D-dimer test. In case of low- and intermediate-pretest-probability patients, the presence of a positive D-dimer testing requires confirmation duplex ultrasound. The use of these strategies has been tested in multiple studies that showed the safety and efficacy of adopting them. Schutgens and associates evaluated such a combined diagnostic approach in 812 patients with the use of ultrasound reserved for patients with high pretest probability score and abnormal D-dimer result. The incidence of venous thromboembolism during the 3 months of follow-up was only 0.6 % with a low or moderate pretest probability and normal D-dimer result (NPV 99 %) [35]. Because 23–50 % of outpatients can be stratified into the low-pretest-probability group, this approach significantly reduces resource utilization. The total number of ultrasound examinations required for outpatient referrals with suspicion of acute DVT was reduced by 29 % [35].

Table 18.2 Pretest probability of deep vein thrombosis (Wells score)

Clinical feature	Score
Active cancer (treatment ongoing or within the previous 6 months or palliative)	1
Paralysis, paresis, or recent plaster immobilization of the lower extremities	1
Recently bedridden for more than 3 days or major surgery, within 4 weeks	1
Localized tenderness along the distribution of the deep venous system	1
Entire leg swollen	1
Calf swelling by more than 3 cm when compared to the asymptomatic leg (measured below tibial tuberosity)	1
Pitting edema (greater in the symptomatic leg)	1
Collateral superficial veins (nonvaricose)	1
Alternative diagnosis as likely or more likely than that of deep venous thrombosis	−2
Score	
High probability	3 or greater
Moderate probability	1 or 2
Low probability	0 or less
Modification	
This clinical model has been modified to take one other clinical feature into account: a previously documented deep vein thrombosis (DVT) is given the score of 1. Using this modified scoring system, DVT is either likely or unlikely, as follows:	
DVT likely	2 or greater
DVT unlikely	1 or less

Adapted from Wells et al. [33, 34]

Table 18.3 Goals of therapy on acute DVT

Goals
1. Prevent extension of DVT
2. Prevent pulmonary embolism
3. Relieve pain and swelling in extremity
4. Prevent postthrombotic syndrome
5. Prevent recurrent thrombosis

Treatment

The therapeutic goals of treatment of acute DVT of the lower extremity include prevention of clot extension and possible resultant PE and the relief of lower extremity pain and swelling as a consequence of venous obstruction. The long-term goals include prevention of recurrent thrombosis and the preservation of venous valvular function and patency to prevent the development of PTS (Table 18.3) [36].

The contemporary management of acute lower extremity DVT includes three alternatives:

- Standard anticoagulation therapy alone
- The use of thrombolytic therapy in conjunction with anticoagulation
- Endovenous thrombectomy using devices designed to mechanically remove the thrombus combined with thrombolytic therapy (the term pharmacomechanical thrombectomy) in addition to anticoagulation

Standard anticoagulation therapy represents the backbone of any treatment regimen. Anticoagulation achieves mainly the first two objectives of therapy including prevention of clot extension and prevention of PE [37]. To a lesser extent, anticoagulation helps in alleviating the symptoms of DVT including extremity pain and swelling. It is also important in prevention of recurrence of DVT and PE [37]. However, anticoagulation alone has no direct thrombolytic effect and is ineffective in restoring venous patency, especially in patients with extensive proximal DVT. Spontaneous thrombus regression occurs in <50 %, and complete clot resolution occurs in <5 % of cases treated with anticoagulation therapy alone [38, 39].

Thrombus removal using thrombolytic therapy with or without thrombectomy offers the potential to rapidly clear the thrombus from the obstructed venous segments with resultant rapid symptomatic relief of the patient as well as preserving the valvular function reducing the chances of subsequent obstruction and reflux and hence PTS. There is mounting evidence to suggest that thrombus removal or early thrombus resolution after acute DVT is associated with improved outcomes [40]. Experimental observations of acute DVT in the canine models also demonstrated that thrombolytic therapy resulted in less thrombus and more preservation of valve competence immediately and at 4 weeks after therapy compared with placebo [41, 42].

Improved clinical outcomes were observed as reviewed by Comerota and Aldridge of 13 studies comparing thrombolytic therapy versus anticoagulation alone. In this review, complete or significant lysis was observed in only 4 % of patients in the anticoagulation arm compared to 45 % of patients with thrombolysis therapy. Successful lysis in long-term follow-up was associated with less incidence of PTS and improved venous function [38]. A Cochrane review compared thrombolysis with standard anticoagulation across 12 randomized controlled trials comprising 700 patients. The majority of these studies included only patients treated with systemic thrombolysis. Clot lysis was seen more frequently in early and late follow-up. The incidence of PTS was reduced significantly (relative risk, 0.66; 95 % CI, 0.47–0.94) [43]. A 50 % reduction in the formation of lower limb ulcers was demonstrated. In addition, multiple institutional case series and RCTs reported the use of catheter directed thrombolysis (CDT) and mechanical thrombectomy (Table 18.4). Although there is considerable variation in the design and combination of therapies used, all convey the message that venous patency can often be restored in the short and long term with catheter-delivered therapy. In addition, significant improvement in quality of life has also been demonstrated [1]. Unfortunately, larger randomized studies are required to

Table 18.4 Summary of previous trials investigating the role of catheter-delivered therapy for DVT

Study (year)	Design	Limbs treated	Pathology	Arms	Agent	Short-term patency	Long-term patency
Bjarnason et al. (1997)	Institution series	87	Acute iliofemoral DVT	CDT (87) ± angioplasty ± stent ± PMT	Urokinase	Immediate: 69 (79 %); iliac, 86 %; femoral	1 year: iliac, 63 % primary, 78 % secondary; femoral, 40 % primary, 51 % secondary
Mewissen et al. (1999)	National registry data	303	Acute and chronic suprapopliteal	CDT	Urokinase	Immediate: grade III in 96 (31 %), II in 162 (52 %), I in 54 (17 %)	1 year: 181 (60 %)
Gandini et al. (1999)	Institution series	8	Iliocaval thrombosis	PMT	None	Immediate: 6 (75 %)	2 years: 6 (75 %)
Elsharawy et al. (2002)	Single blind RCT	35	Iliofemoral DVT <10 days	CDT + (18), anticoagulation alone (17)	Streptokinase	1 week: CDT, 11 (61 %); control, 0 (0 %)	6 months: CDT, 2 (13 %); control, 2 (12 %)
Jackson et al. (2005)	Institution series	28	Acute supra popliteal DVT (4 had symptoms >14 days)	CDT ± stenting ± PMT		Immediate: 5 (18 %) complete lysis, 20 (72 %) partial	1 year: 22 (80 %)
Lin et al. (2006)	Retrospective comparison of CDT and PMT	98	Acute symptomatic lower limb DVT	CDT (46), PMT (52)		CDT: 32 (75 %) complete, 14 (25 %) partial; PMT: 39 (75 %) complete, 13 (25 %) (primary assisted)	1 year: CDT, 29 (64 %); PMT, 35 (68 %)
Protack et al. (2007)	Institution series	69	Lower extremity DVT	CDT (27), PMT (12), both (30)		Immediate: grade III in 46 (67 %), II in 19 (26 %), I in 4 (6 %)	2 years: 57 (83 %) freedom from rethrombosis
Rao et al. (2009)	Institution series	43	Symptomatic iliofemoral DVT (19, >14 days)	CDT + PMT	r-TPA	Immediate: grade III, III lysis in 41 (95 %)	Not reported

Shi et al. (2009)	Institution series	16	Massive lower limb DVT	CDT + PMT + IVC filter	Urokinase	Immediate: grade III and III lysis in 14 (89 %), I in 2 (11 %)	Follow-up:[a] 12 (75 %)
Baekgaard et al. (2009)	Institution series	103	DVT <14 days, open distal popliteal vein	CDT + stockings (103) + stent (57)	r-TPA	1 week: 95/103 (92 %)	6 years: 84 (82 %) mean follow-up 50 months
Enden et al. (2009)	Open multicenter RCT: short-term report	103	Iliofemoral DVT <21 days and symptoms	CDT + anticoagulation (50), anticoagulation alone (53)	r-TPA	Immediate: grade III in 24, II in 20 for CDT group	6 months: 32 (64 %) of CDT group vs. 19 (36 %) of control

Adapted from Patterson et al. [1]

All patients were treated postprocedure with standard anticoagulation unless otherwise stated. Grade III lysis, complete; grade II lysis, 50–90 %; grade I lysis, <50 %

[a]Timing not available

establish definitive recommendations for care. Currently, two large trials are underway that will randomize patients with acute DVT to catheter-directed venous thrombolysis versus anticoagulation alone [44, 45].

Standard Therapy

The standard therapy for acute DVT of the lower extremities has not changed for the past decades. It includes anticoagulation, which constitutes the backbone of therapy in addition to compression therapy. The benefit of anticoagulation in the treatment of acute DVT was first demonstrated in 1960 [46] and confirmed by randomized clinical trials [47, 48].

Historically, the standard therapy included starting the patient on unfractionated heparin in the hospital usually using intravenous infusion with the goal of therapy is an activated partial thromboplastin time ratio (aPTT) that is 1.5–2.5 of the normal. Heparin is usually given simultaneously with warfarin and is overlapped with warfarin for a minimum of 4–5 days until the international normalized ratio (INR) has been within the therapeutic range (2.0–3.0) for two consecutive days [49]. This overlap is required because, during the first few days of warfarin therapy, prolongation of the INR mainly reflects depression of factor VII, which has a half-life of only 5–7 h. Thus, although the extrinsic coagulation pathway is suppressed, the intrinsic coagulation pathway that does not require factor VII remains intact during this early period. Warfarin is continued then for a total duration of 3–6 months to prevent recurrent thrombosis [17].

With that said, there have been several points of controversy regarding that regimen:

- What anticoagulants to use with the introduction of low molecular weight (LMW) heparin
- What the duration of therapy is using warfarin
- Activity after diagnosis of acute DVT

The introduction of LMW heparin in the 1980s revolutionized the early treatment of venous thromboembolism by simplifying dosing and administration [47]. LMW heparin was found to have several advantages over unfractionated heparin [50]:

- Greater bioavailability when given by subcutaneous injection.
- Duration of anticoagulant effect is greater, permitting once or twice daily administration.
- Anticoagulant response is highly correlated with body weight permitting administration of a fixed dose.
- Laboratory monitoring is not necessary.
- Lower risk of heparin-induced thrombocytopenia.

Subcutaneous, unmonitored LMW heparin was compared with continuous intravenous heparin for the treatment of proximal venous thrombosis in a number of clinical trials. LMW heparin, given once or twice daily, is at least as effective and as safe as and may be superior to unfractionated heparin in patients with proximal venous thrombosis. LMW heparin was found to have greater inhibition of in vivo thrombin generation [51], higher rates of thrombus regression, and lower rates of recurrent venous thromboembolism, major bleeding, and mortality [52–55]. LMW heparin is also more feasible for use in an outpatient setting without loss of efficacy thus avoiding hospitalization associated with the use of unfractionated heparin [56, 57]. For these benefits of LMW heparin over unfractionated heparin, it is recommended that clinicians use LMW heparin over unfractionated heparin for the initiation of therapy of acute deep venous thrombosis [58].

As mentioned before, after the initial treatment using both heparin and warfarin, the duration of therapy continues for 3–6 months. The aim of prolonged therapy is to reduce the risk of recurrent thrombosis. Warfarin was found to be extremely effective in this situation reducing the risk of recurrent thrombosis from 47 to 2 % [17, 59]. Attempts to decrease the duration of treatment with warfarin to 4 weeks or 6 weeks have resulted in higher rates of recurrent venous thromboembolism (VTE) in comparison with the standard 3–6 months regimen [60, 61]. For patients with VTE and a reversible or time-limited risk factor (e.g., trauma, surgery), treatment should continue for a minimum of 3 months. Treatment for longer than 6 months is not necessary, since the risk of recurrence in such patients is <3 % [58, 62]. For those patients with a continuing risk factor that is potentially reversible (e.g., prolonged immobilization), long-term warfarin therapy should be continued until the risk factor is reversed. In patients with unprovoked (idiopathic) proximal VTE and patients with recurrent VTE after completion of therapy, the 2008 American College of Chest Physicians (ACCP) guidelines have given a strong recommendation for indefinite treatment [48].

Interventional Therapy

The interventional therapy for acute DVT includes thrombolysis with or without mechanical thrombectomy, which is always in addition to the standard anticoagulation therapy. It is gratifying that the 8th ACCP Consensus Committee on Antithrombotic Therapy for Venous Thromboembolic Disease has made definitive recommendations regarding treatment strategies for thrombus removal in patients with DVT [48]. In the recommendations, patients with acute iliofemoral DVT who are appropriate risk candidates should preferentially be treated with catheter-directed thrombolysis (CDT) (grade 2B). The committee also recognized the importance of correcting underlying venous lesions after successful CDT and that pharmacomechanical techniques might be preferable to CDT alone to shorten treatment time if resources are available. They also recommended operative venous thrombectomy if catheter-based interventions are not available in such setting. If neither catheter-based techniques nor venous thrombectomy is available to patients with extensive venous thrombosis, systemic thrombolytic therapy is recommended (grade 2C) for good-risk patients at low risk of bleeding. It is to be remembered that all interventional therapy modalities are more effective dealing with acute DVT of less than 2 weeks duration and that the older the clot gets, the less effective those modalities are in clearing the thrombus [63].

Thrombolytic Therapy

There is currently no consensus regarding to the ideal thrombolytic agent to be used. The basic mechanism of thrombolytic therapy is the activation of fibrin-bound plasminogen to form the active enzyme plasmin, which dissolves the clot [64]. Streptokinase was the first agent to be used as a thrombolytic therapy. Later, urokinase and plasminogen activators became available. There are claims of varying degrees of efficacy and potential for complications [64, 65]. However, a retrospective review has been performed to compare the various thrombolytic agents used in the treatment of DVT. Grunwald and Hofmann reported that urokinase and the plasminogen activators were essentially equal in terms of efficacy and complication rates [66]. Catheter-directed thrombolysis (CDT) delivers the thrombolytic agent locally into the thrombus using infusion catheter placed within the thrombus. It has emerged as the superior method of thrombolysis. CDT addresses many of the limitations imposed by systemic thrombolysis such as unpredictability of thrombo-ablative effect and high risk for hemorrhagic complications [67]. Intra-thrombus delivery protects thrombolytic agents from neutralization by circulating antiplasmin such as plasminogen activator inhibitor (PAI-1) and allows dissolution of the thrombus in smaller distal vessels that are otherwise not accessible to systemic thrombolysis [68]. This technique also has the potential to accelerate thrombolysis and reduce the overall dose needed and the duration of thrombolytic infusion, thus increasing the likelihood of successful outcome and a reduction in bleeding complications [36].

In this technique, access of the deep venous system is acquired through the posterior tibial vein in the distal leg or the popliteal vein in the popliteal fossa aided by the use of duplex ultrasound guidance. After placement of a short sheath, a standard 0.035-in. wire is passed

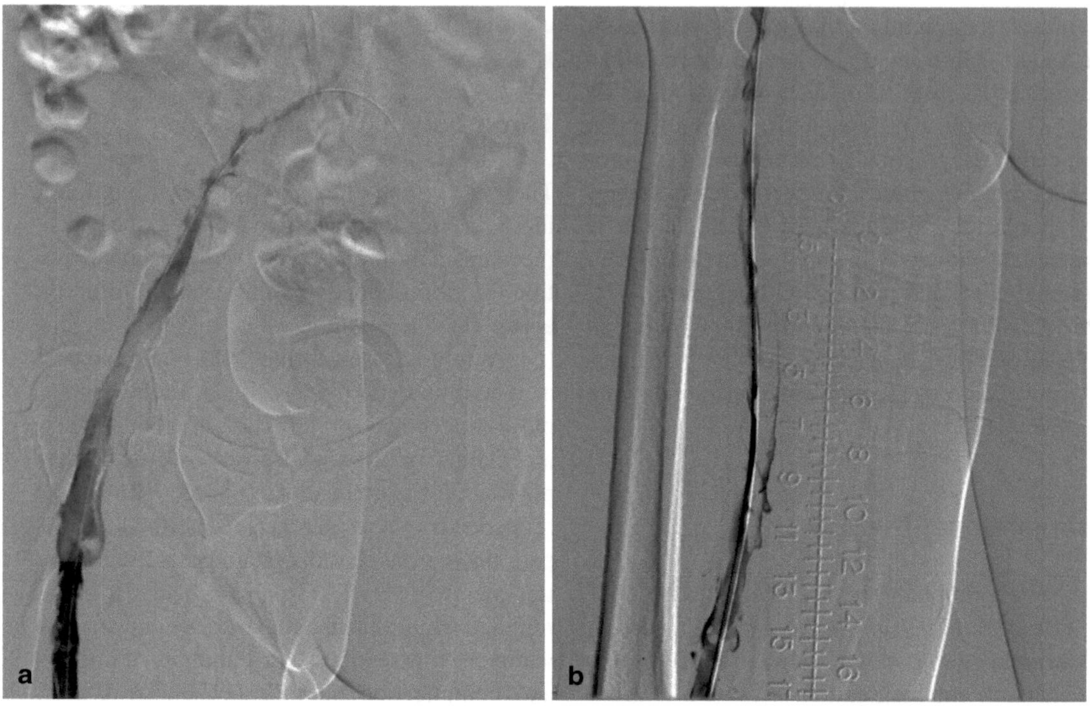

Fig. 18.1 Acute left iliofemoral DVT in a patient with May-Thurner syndrome (patient is in the prone position). (**a**) The acute iliac vein thrombosis. (**b**) Acute femoral vein thrombosis

proximally into the affected proximal iliofemoral segment. An infusion catheter is then passed over the wire and left in place for the infusion of the thrombolytic agent (Fig. 18.1). Nowadays, recombinant tissue plasminogen activator (r-tPA) is the usual thrombolytic agent used for CDT. The usual dose is 1–2 mg/h for overnight thrombolysis. The patient is taken back to the angiography suite where a repeat venogram is performed. If there is still significant residual thrombus present, another round of infusion thrombolysis is performed overnight. The National Venous Registry is the largest report to date of patients treated with lytic therapy for acute DVT using CDT [69]. In the group of patients with acute first-time iliofemoral DVT, 65 % had complete clot resolution. Patients, who had more complete clot resolution with CDT, had more preservation of their valvular function and better QoL scores. Also, patients in whom CDT failed to clear the thrombus had outcomes similar to those treated with anticoagulation alone [69].

Percutaneous Mechanical Thrombectomy

Percutaneous mechanical thrombectomy has emerged as an important tool in the armamentarium for the management of acute DVT, particularly in patients when pharmacologic thrombolysis is contraindicated. Multiple devices have been developed for percutaneous thrombectomy with or without adjunctive thrombolysis [70–73].

Pharmacomechanical Thrombolysis

Combining percutaneous mechanical thrombectomy with CDT, also known as pharmacomechanical thrombectomy (PMT), has the potential to achieve more complete clot removal as well as decrease the dose and duration of thrombolytic therapy than either therapy alone [36]. It has been studied recently with comparable or better success rates compared with CDT but with the added benefit of a shorter hospital and intensive care stay and decreased costs [45, 72, 74]. Multiple devices have been on the market and are used in conjunction with CDT. The most commonly used devices available currently are:

AngioJet® Rheolytic Thrombectomy System (Possis Medical, Minneapolis, MN) (Fig. 18.2)

This is an approved device by the US Food and Drug Administration for the treatment of DVT. This device is composed of a catheter that uses high-pressure jets that push saline back from the tip at 10,000 PSI. This action in combination with strategically placed juxtaposed side holes relies on Bernoulli's effect to create a low-pressure zone during the mechanical disruption of the thrombus. The catheter infuses normal saline through an infusion port while simultaneously suctioning through the effluent port. Microscopic particles of thrombus debris as well as other blood products are removed. If the effluent port is clamped, then the infusion port can act as mechanical "pulse spray," whereby the clot can be laced with a thrombolytic drug that is preloaded in the system. After lacing the thrombus with intermittent initiation of the pulse spray containing thrombolytic drug, a 15–20-min pause is used to allow the thrombolytic action to take effect. The effluent port is then unclamped, and only normal saline is used to perform standard AngioJet® thrombectomy. There are multiple 6-F catheters that come with the system with different lengths and for use in different diameter vessels [75].

Trellis-8® (Bacchus Vascular, Santa Clara, CA) (Isolated Segmental Pharmacomechanical Thrombolysis) (Fig. 18.3)

The device is approved by the US Food and Drug Administration for the specific treatment of DVT. This is a hybrid catheter that isolates the thrombosed vein segment between two occluding balloons. The thrombolytic agent is infused into the thrombus between the occluding balloons. A dispersion wire is inserted into the catheter shaft assuming a spiral configuration, that, when activated, spins at 1,500 rpm. After 15–20 min of dwell time, the liquefied and particulate thrombus is then aspirated. The proximal occluding balloon is designed to prevent PE. Isolation of the thrombolytic agent to the thrombosed segment has the theoretical advantage of reducing the systemic effect of thrombolysis and hence the risk of bleeding. The catheter requires an 8-F sheath and traverses over a 0.035-in. guidewire. Catheter lengths are 80 and 120 cm, and treatment zones between balloons can be 10, 15, or 30 cm [36].

EKOS EndoWave® (EKOS Corporation, Bothell, WA) (Ultrasound-Accelerated Thrombolysis) (Fig. 18.4)

This device relies on the use of low-energy, high-frequency ultrasound (2 MHz) to alter the

a

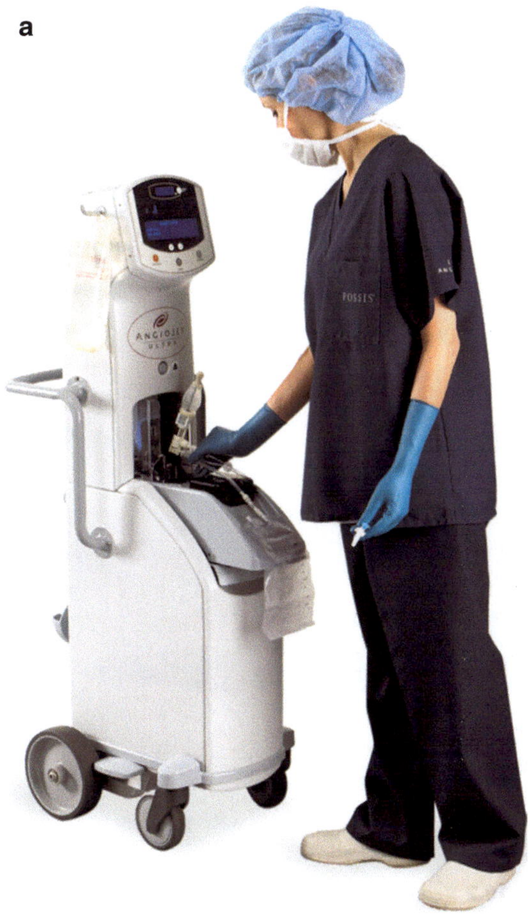

Fig. 18.2 AngioJet® Rheolytic Thrombectomy System (**a**, **b**, and **c**)

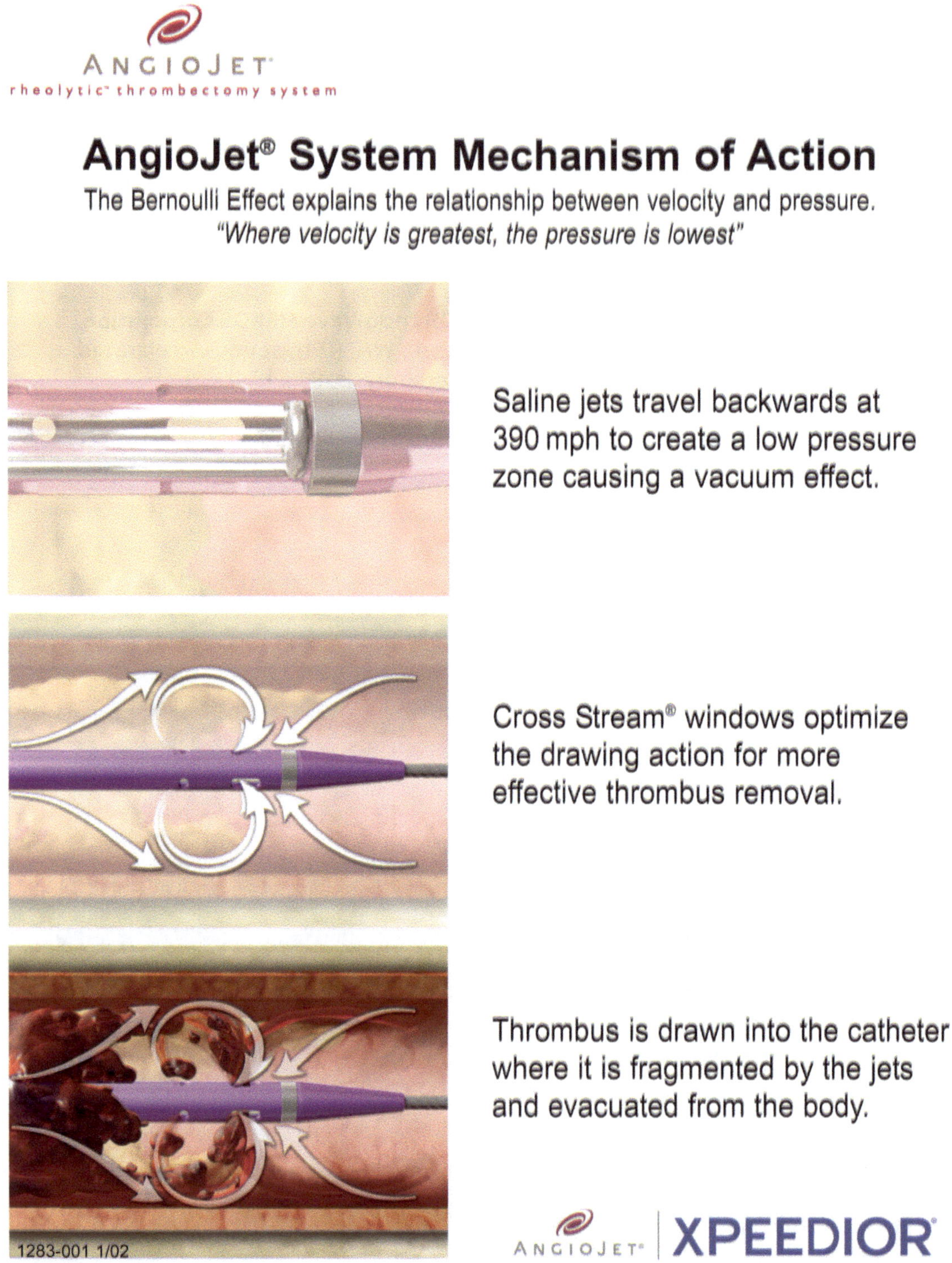

Fig. 18.2 (continued)

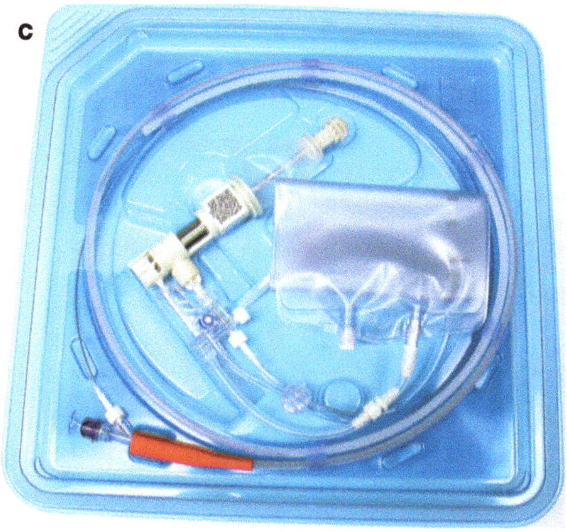

Fig. 18.2 (continued)

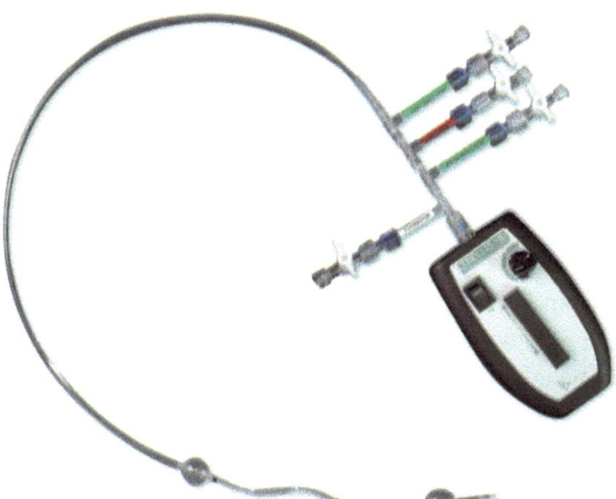

Fig. 18.3 Trellis peripheral infusion system

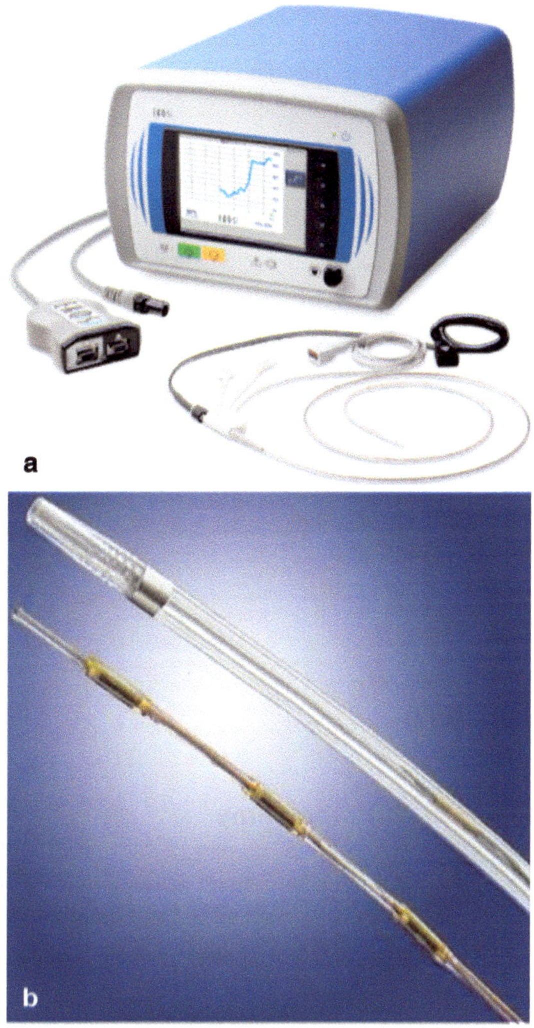

Fig. 18.4 The EKOS ultrasound-accelerated thrombolysis system. (**a**) The EkoSonic Control Unit. (**b**) The EKOS infusion catheter and ultrasound wire

thrombus structure and allow the thrombolytic drug to be more effective. The EKOS EndoWave® catheter does not mechanically fragment the thrombus; rather, it reversibly increases its permeability. Multiple lengths to apply simultaneous ultrasound energy and infusion are available and vary from 6 to 50 cm. The 5.2-F catheter has 4 lm. The central lumen takes the 0.035-in. ultrasound wire and also uses that same lumen with an expanded area to carry the central coolant using normal saline. Three other lumens placed on the outer core of the catheter in a triangular configuration carry the drug for delivery to the thrombus. In each of these 3 lm reside thermocouples to monitor changes in temperature-flow patterns. The EKOS EndoWave® primarily affects fibrin strands. Braaten et al. demonstrated a 44 % reduction in diameter of fibrin strands. This effect translated into 65 % more individual strands being exposed. Furthermore, the ultrasound did not cause any fibrin strand breakage. These structural changes potentially increase the number of plasminogen receptor sites [75–77].

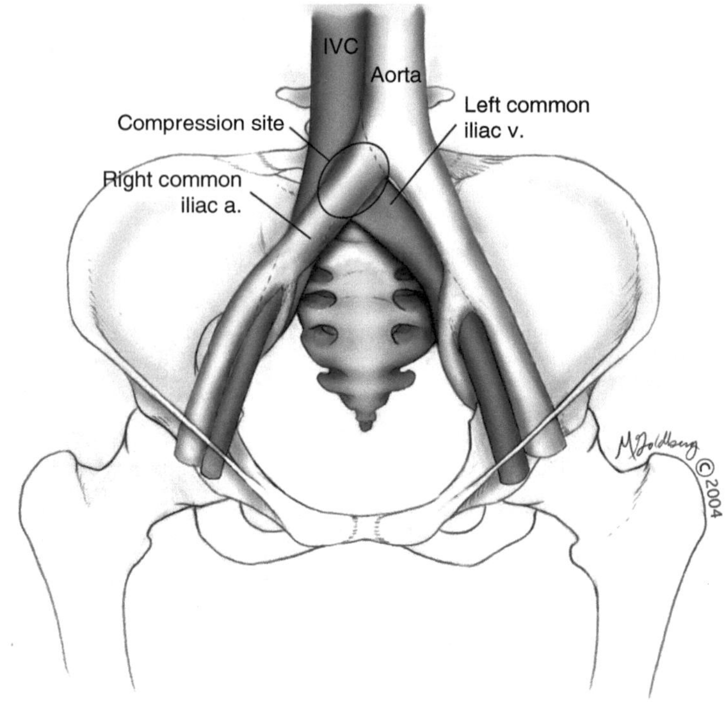

Fig. 18.5 Anatomic basis of May-Thurner syndrome. The right common iliac artery compresses the proximal left common iliac vein

Aspiration Thrombectomy

This is a technique where there is a dynamic withdrawal of the aspiration wide-bore catheter or sheath while maintaining negative pressure using a syringe, i.e., an aspiration catheter is introduced into the thrombus-filled vein through a second sheath and is withdrawn or pulled back through the thrombus-filled vein while negative pressure is applied and maintained using a syringe. Using this technique, a large thrombus can be remodeled because of the more powerful negative pressure, allowing for a more effective aspiration thrombectomy or can be an adjunct to using the other pharmacomechanical thrombectomy methods. Although being a simple technique, nothing much is reported in the literature about its use. Recently, Oguzkurt et al. [78] and Kwon et al. [73] have reported using this technique with excellent results.

Theoretically, during the interventional therapy for acute DVT, patients are exposed to the risk of possible PE. The need for IVC filters during endovascular management of an extensive DVT has been debated. Pulmonary embolization consisting of small fragments is common during CDT and PMT. However, the vast majority of these events are asymptomatic and of little clinical consequence to the patient [79]. However, in the presence of a free-floating IVC thrombus or in patients with limited cardiopulmonary reserve who are unlikely to tolerate minor embolic events, IVC filtration may be appropriate with the use of permanent or temporary filters [73].

After completion of the CDT or PMT, completion venogram should be performed for the evaluation of any culprit lesions that may have been the cause of the acute DVT. A typical example of that is the May-Thurner syndrome where there is proximal stenosis of the left common iliac vein due to compression by the right common iliac artery. The treatment of such lesions is instrumental in successful therapy of the acute DVT and in the prevention of recurrent venous thromboembolism (VTE) [75] (Figs. 18.5 and 18.6).

Several technical points are important to remember that make endovenous interventions significantly different from intra-arterial interventions. Recognition of these differences is important to achieve the desired successful results

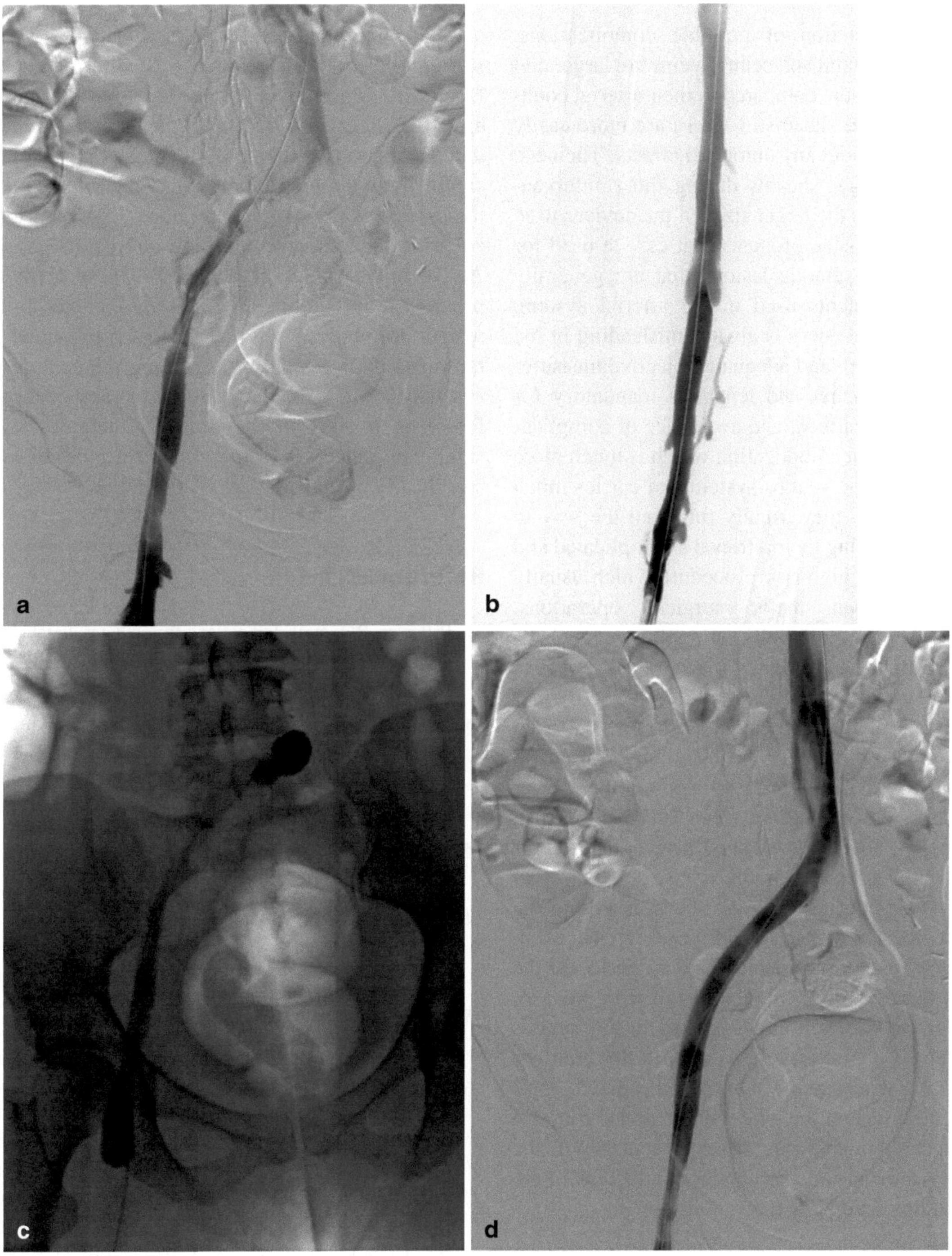

Fig. 18.6 Clinical case of May-Thurner syndrome with pharmacomechanical thrombectomy for acute iliofemoral DVT. This is the same case in Fig. 18.1 during therapy. The patient is in the prone position that is why the images appear flipped. (**a**) Iliac vein post overnight thrombolysis using the EKOS system. There is still residual obstruction at the proximal left common iliac vein. (**b**) The femoral vein is completely cleaned by using only overnight thrombolysis using the EKOS system. (**c**) The Trellis system in place for pharmacomechanical thrombolysis of the iliac vein system. Note the stenosis of the proximal left common iliac vein as evidenced by the indentation of the proximal device balloon. (**d**) The left iliac vein system is completely patent with unrestricted flow after stenting of the left common iliac vein using Wallstent® (Boston Scientific)

and the reduction of possible complications. Because the axial and central veins are larger and lower in pressure compared to their arterial counterparts, larger sheaths (8–12 F) are more easily tolerated without any untoward effects. The need for these larger sheaths during those interventions is due to the larger sizes of the devices used and the large size of stents that can be used for treatment of stenotic lesions that are generally larger than stents used in the arterial system. Sizing these devices is always misleading in the venous system, and adequate objective measurement of diameter and length is mandatory for successful treatment and avoidance of complications like stent embolization which is much more common in the venous system and carries much higher risk as they usually travel all the way to the heart making their retrieval a complicated and an extremely high-risk procedure which usually required open major surgical operations. Measurement by visually estimating or "eyeballing" should be absolutely discouraged. Because of the venous wall being more fragile and thinner than that of the arteries, caution must be taken when performing power injection of contrast. Typically the pressure settings on the power injector should range between 200 and 400 psi. Also, end-hole catheters should never be used for power injection as these can cause perforation of large veins during contrast injection. Along the same lines, caution should be exercised using guidewires as it is much easier to perforate the vein during wire manipulations than in the arterial tree. Also, retrograde access in the venous system is possible as the valves do not interfere with the wire passage. On the other hand, antegrade passage of the wire will be hindered by the valves, although during cases of acute DVT, the valves are wide open secondary to the bulk of the thrombus occupying the venous lumen.

Summary

Acute DVT is a common disease with potentially life-threatening consequences and long-term life-altering complications. It imposes huge economic burden on the society. The disease is difficult to diagnose because of the lack of sensitivity and specificity of its clinical manifestations. Diagnostic algorithms are needed for safe and effective diagnosis. The treatment is standard anticoagulation therapy which reduces significantly the mortality risk and recurrence of the disease but does a much poorer job when it comes to the long-term morbidity of the disease. Active management of acute DVT, especially proximal iliofemoral DVT, using catheter-directed thrombolysis with or without mechanical thrombectomy modalities is gaining momentum and may prove to be the standard therapy of the future as it adds to the standard therapy the significant reduction of the long-term morbidity specifically postthrombotic syndrome.

References

1. Patterson BO, et al. Indications for catheter-directed thrombolysis in the management of acute proximal deep venous thrombosis. Arterioscler Thromb Vasc Biol. 2010;30(4):669–74.
2. Anderson Jr FA, et al. A population-based perspective of the hospital incidence and case-fatality rates of deep vein thrombosis and pulmonary embolism. The Worcester DVT Study. Arch Intern Med. 1991;151(5):933–8.
3. Nordstrom M, et al. A prospective study of the incidence of deep-vein thrombosis within a defined urban population. J Intern Med. 1992;232(2):155–60.
4. Hull RD, Pineo GF, Raskob GE. The economic impact of treating deep vein thrombosis with low-molecular-weight heparin: outcome of therapy and health economy aspects. Haemostasis. 1998;28 Suppl 3:8–16.
5. Turpie AG, Chin BS, Lip GY. Venous thromboembolism: pathophysiology, clinical features, and prevention. BMJ. 2002;325(7369):887–90.
6. Prandoni P, et al. The long-term clinical course of acute deep venous thrombosis. Ann Intern Med. 1996;125(1):1–7.
7. Kakkar VV, et al. Natural history of postoperative deep-vein thrombosis. Lancet. 1969;2(7614):230–2.
8. Heit JA, Silverstein MD, Mohr DN, et al. Risk factors for deep vein thrombosis and pulmonary embolism: Population-based case–control study. Arch Intern Med. 2000;160:809.
9. May R, Thurner J. The cause of the predominantly sinistral occurrence of thrombosis of the pelvic veins. Angiology. 1957;8(5):419–27.
10. Shebel ND, Marin A. Effort thrombosis (Paget-Schroetter syndrome) in active young adults: current concepts in diagnosis and treatment. J Vasc Nurs. 2006;24(4):116–26.

11. Wakefield TW, Myers DD, Henke PK. Mechanisms of venous thrombosis and resolution. Arterioscler Thromb Vasc Biol. 2008;28(3):387–91.
12. Esmon CT. Inflammation and thrombosis. J Thromb Haemost. 2003;1(7):1343–8.
13. van Ramshorst B, et al. Thrombus regression in deep venous thrombosis. Quantification of spontaneous thrombolysis with duplex scanning. Circulation. 1992;86(2):414–9.
14. Killewich LA, et al. Regression of proximal deep venous thrombosis is associated with fibrinolytic enhancement. J Vasc Surg. 1997;26(5):861–8.
15. Prandoni P, et al. A simple ultrasound approach for detection of recurrent proximal-vein thrombosis. Circulation. 1993;88(4 Pt 1):1730–5.
16. Hull RD, et al. Continuous intravenous heparin compared with intermittent subcutaneous heparin in the initial treatment of proximal-vein thrombosis. N Engl J Med. 1986;315(18):1109–14.
17. Hull R, et al. Warfarin sodium versus low-dose heparin in the long-term treatment of venous thrombosis. N Engl J Med. 1979;301(16):855–8.
18. Hingorani A, et al. Upper extremity versus lower extremity deep venous thrombosis. Am J Surg. 1997; 174(2):214–7.
19. Pengo V, et al. Incidence of chronic thromboembolic pulmonary hypertension after pulmonary embolism. N Engl J Med. 2004;350(22):2257–64.
20. Comerota AJ, Gravett MH. Iliofemoral venous thrombosis. J Vasc Surg. 2007;46(5):1065–76.
21. Rao AS, et al. Pharmacomechanical thrombectomy for iliofemoral deep vein thrombosis: an alternative in patients with contraindications to thrombolysis. J Vasc Surg. 2009;50(5):1092–8.
22. Kahn SR, et al. Definition of post-thrombotic syndrome of the leg for use in clinical investigations: a recommendation for standardization. J Thromb Haemost. 2009;7(5):879–83.
23. Prandoni P, et al. Below-knee elastic compression stockings to prevent the post-thrombotic syndrome: a randomized, controlled trial. Ann Intern Med. 2004; 141(4):249–56.
24. Kahn SR, et al. Determinants of health-related quality of life during the 2 years following deep vein thrombosis. J Thromb Haemost. 2008;6(7):1105–12.
25. Bezemer ID, et al. The value of family history as a risk indicator for venous thrombosis. Arch Intern Med. 2009;169(6):610–5.
26. Bettmann MA, et al. Contrast venography of the leg: diagnostic efficacy, tolerance, and complication rates with ionic and nonionic contrast media. Radiology. 1987;165(1):113–6.
27. Mattos MA, et al. Color-flow duplex scanning for the surveillance and diagnosis of acute deep venous thrombosis. J Vasc Surg. 1992;15(2):366–75; discussion 375–6.
28. Butty S, et al. Body MR venography. Radiol Clin North Am. 2002;40(4):899–919.
29. Peterson DA, et al. Computed tomographic venography is specific but not sensitive for diagnosis of acute lower-extremity deep venous thrombosis in patients with suspected pulmonary embolus. J Vasc Surg. 2001;34(5):798–804.
30. Kelly J, Hunt BJ. Role of D-dimers in diagnosis of venous thromboembolism. Lancet. 2002;359(9305):456–8.
31. van der Graaf F, et al. Exclusion of deep venous thrombosis with D-dimer testing – comparison of 13 D-dimer methods in 99 outpatients suspected of deep venous thrombosis using venography as reference standard. Thromb Haemost. 2000;83(2):191–8.
32. Wells PS, et al. Accuracy of clinical assessment of deep-vein thrombosis. Lancet. 1995;345(8961):1326–30.
33. Wells PS, Anderson DR, Bormanis J, et al. Value of assessment of pretest probability of deep-vein thrombosis in clinical management. Lancet. 1997;350:1795.
34. Wells PS, Anderson DR, Rodger M, et al. Evaluation of D-Dimer in the diagnosis of suspected deep-vein thrombosis. N Eng J Med. 2003;349:1227.
35. Schutgens RE, et al. Combination of a normal D-dimer concentration and a non-high pretest clinical probability score is a safe strategy to exclude deep venous thrombosis. Circulation. 2003;107(4):593–7.
36. Kiernan TJ, et al. Current status of pharmacological thrombolytic therapy and mechanical thrombectomy for the treatment of acute deep venous thrombosis. Cardiovasc Hematol Agents Med Chem. 2009;7(1):12–8.
37. Buller HR, et al. Antithrombotic therapy for venous thromboembolic disease: the seventh ACCP conference on antithrombotic and thrombolytic therapy. Chest. 2004;126(3 suppl):401S–28.
38. Comerota AJ, Aldridge SC. Thrombolytic therapy for deep venous thrombosis: a clinical review. Can J Surg. 1993;36(4):359–64.
39. Killewich LA, et al. Spontaneous lysis of deep venous thrombi: rate and outcome. J Vasc Surg. 1989;9(1): 89–97.
40. Augustinos P, Ouriel K. Invasive approaches to treatment of venous thromboembolism. Circulation. 2004;110(9 suppl 1):I27–34.
41. Rhodes JM, et al. Thrombolysis for experimental deep venous thrombosis maintains valvular competence and vasoreactivity. J Vasc Surg. 2000;31(6):1193–205.
42. Cho JS, et al. Effects of thrombolysis and venous thrombectomy on valvular competence, thrombogenicity, venous wall morphology, and function. J Vasc Surg. 1998;28(5):787–99.
43. Watson L, Armon M. Thrombolysis for acute deep venous thrombosis. Cochrane Database Syst Rev. 2007; Art No. CD002783.
44. Vedantham S. Catheter-directed thrombolysis for deep vein thrombosis. Curr Opin Hematol. 2010;17(5): 464–8.
45. Enden T, et al. Catheter-directed Venous Thrombolysis in acute iliofemoral vein thrombosis – the CaVenT study: rationale and design of a multicenter, randomized, controlled, clinical trial (NCT00251771). Am Heart J. 2007;154(5):808–14.
46. Barritt DW, Jordan SC. Anticoagulant drugs in the treatment of pulmonary embolism. A controlled trial. Lancet. 1960;1(7138):1309–12.

47. Hirsh J, Bates SM. Clinical trials that have influenced the treatment of venous thromboembolism: a historical perspective. Ann Intern Med. 2001;134(5):409–17.
48. Kearon C, et al. Antithrombotic therapy for venous thromboembolic disease: American College of Chest Physicians evidence-based clinical practice guidelines (8th edition). Chest. 2008;133(6 suppl):454S–545.
49. Ansell J, et al. Pharmacology and management of the vitamin K antagonists: American College of Chest Physicians evidence-based clinical practice guidelines (8th edition). Chest. 2008;133(6 suppl):160S–98.
50. Weitz JI. Low-molecular-weight heparins. N Engl J Med. 1997;337(10):688–98.
51. Kakkar VV, et al. Randomized trial of different regimens of heparins and in vivo thrombin generation in acute deep vein thrombosis. Blood. 2002;99(6):1965–70.
52. Lensing AW, et al. Treatment of deep venous thrombosis with low-molecular-weight heparins. A meta-analysis. Arch Intern Med. 1995;155(6):601–7.
53. Siragusa S, et al. Low-molecular-weight heparins and unfractionated heparin in the treatment of patients with acute venous thromboembolism: results of a meta-analysis. Am J Med. 1996;100(3):269–77.
54. Merli G, et al. Subcutaneous enoxaparin once or twice daily compared with intravenous unfractionated heparin for treatment of venous thromboembolic disease. Ann Intern Med. 2001;134(3):191–202.
55. Breddin HK, et al. Effects of a low-molecular-weight heparin on thrombus regression and recurrent thromboembolism in patients with deep-vein thrombosis. N Engl J Med. 2001;344(9):626–31.
56. Koopman MM, et al. Treatment of venous thrombosis with intravenous unfractionated heparin administered in the hospital as compared with subcutaneous low-molecular-weight heparin administered at home. The Tasman Study Group. N Engl J Med. 1996;334(11): 682–7.
57. Dunn A, et al. Effect of intravenous heparin administration on duration of hospitalization. Mayo Clin Proc. 2004;79(2):159–63.
58. Snow V, et al. Management of venous thromboembolism: a clinical practice guideline from the American College of Physicians and the American Academy of Family Physicians. Ann Intern Med. 2007;146(3): 204–10.
59. Hull R, et al. Adjusted subcutaneous heparin versus warfarin sodium in the long-term treatment of venous thrombosis. N Engl J Med. 1982;306(4):189–94.
60. Research Committee of the British Thoracic Society. Optimum duration of anticoagulation for deep-vein thrombosis and pulmonary embolism. Lancet. 1992;340(8824):873–6.
61. Schulman S, et al. A comparison of six weeks with six months of oral anticoagulant therapy after a first episode of venous thromboembolism. Duration of Anticoagulation Trial Study Group. N Engl J Med. 1995;332(25):1661–5.
62. Baglin T, et al. Incidence of recurrent venous thromboembolism in relation to clinical and thrombophilic risk factors: prospective cohort study. Lancet. 2003;362(9383):523–6.
63. Daniels LB, et al. Relation of duration of symptoms with response to thrombolytic therapy in pulmonary embolism. Am J Cardiol. 1997;80(2):184–8.
64. Kiernan TJ, Gersh BJ. Thrombolysis in acute myocardial infarction: current status. Med Clin North Am. 2007;91(4):617–37; x.
65. Schweizer J, et al. Comparative results of thrombolysis treatment with rt-PA and urokinase: a pilot study. Vasa. 1998;27(3):167–71.
66. Grunwald MR, Hofmann LV. Comparison of urokinase, alteplase, and reteplase for catheter-directed thrombolysis of deep venous thrombosis. J Vasc Interv Radiol. 2004;15(4):347–52.
67. Janssen MC, et al. Local and systemic thrombolytic therapy for acute deep venous thrombosis. Neth J Med. 2005;63(3):81–90.
68. Comerota AJ, Paolini D. Treatment of acute iliofemoral deep venous thrombosis: a strategy of thrombus removal. Eur J Vasc Endovasc Surg. 2007;33(3): 351–60; discussion 361–2.
69. Mewissen MW, et al. Catheter-directed thrombolysis for lower extremity deep venous thrombosis: report of a national multicenter registry. Radiology. 1999; 211(1):39–49.
70. Greenberg RK, et al. Mechanical versus chemical thrombolysis: an in vitro differentiation of thrombolytic mechanisms. J Vasc Interv Radiol. 2000; 11(2 Pt 1):199–205.
71. Sharafuddin MJ, Hicks ME. Current status of percutaneous mechanical thrombectomy. Part II. Devices and mechanisms of action. J Vasc Interv Radiol. 1998; 9(1 Pt 1):15–31.
72. Lee KH, et al. Mechanical thrombectomy of acute iliofemoral deep vein thrombosis with use of an Arrow-Trerotola percutaneous thrombectomy device. J Vasc Interv Radiol. 2006;17(3):487–95.
73. Kwon SH, et al. Percutaneous aspiration thrombectomy for the treatment of acute lower extremity deep vein thrombosis: is thrombolysis needed? Clin Radiol. 2009;64(5):484–90.
74. Vedantham S, et al. Pharmacomechanical thrombolysis and early stent placement for iliofemoral deep vein thrombosis. J Vasc Interv Radiol. 2004;15(6):565–74.
75. McLafferty RB. Endovascular management of deep venous thrombosis. Perspect Vasc Surg Endovasc Ther. 2008;20(1):87–91.
76. Parikh S, et al. Ultrasound-accelerated thrombolysis for the treatment of deep vein thrombosis: initial clinical experience. J Vasc Interv Radiol. 2008;19(4): 521–8.
77. Braaten JV, Goss RA, Francis CW. Ultrasound reversibly disaggregates fibrin fibers. Thromb Haemost. 1997;78(3):1063–8.
78. Oguzkurt L, Tercan F, Ozkan U. Manual aspiration thrombectomy with stent placement: rapid and effective treatment for phlegmasia cerulea dolens with impending venous gangrene. Cardiovasc Intervent Radiol. 2008;31(1):205–8.
79. Sharafuddin MJ, et al. Endovascular management of venous thrombotic and occlusive diseases of the lower extremities. J Vasc Interv Radiol. 2003;14(4):405–23.

19 Retrievable Inferior Vena Cava Filters

Joseph J. Naoum

Abstract

Venous thromboembolisms constitute a significant cause of death among the critically ill patients, multiple injured trauma patients, patients undergoing lower extremity catheter-related venous thrombolysis for DVT, selected orthopedic, bariatric, and pregnant patients. The use of retrievable inferior vena cava filters can have the advantage of preventing a fatal pulmonary embolus in those patients at inherent risk without the long-term morbidity associated with its continued presence. Careful patient selection and technique can ensure proper placement and successful retrieval. In addition, a stringent patient follow-up can translate into higher retrieval rates.

Keywords

Inferior vena cava filter • Retrievable filter • Deep vein thrombosis Pulmonary embolus • Venous thromboembolisms

Introduction

Hospitalized patients are at risk for developing deep vein thrombosis (DVT), and without appropriate thromboprophylaxis, the incidence of DVT can vary between 10 and 60 % [1]. Thromboprophylaxis involves the use of low-dose unfractionated heparin (LDUH), low-molecular-weight heparin (LMWH), sequential compression devices (SCD), and early ambulation. Venous thromboembolism (VTE) or pulmonary embolus (PE) can be unpredictable, have a sudden onset, and carry a significant morbidity and mortality. It is a feared complication.

The American College of Chest Physicians (ACCP) current guidelines recommend the placement of an inferior vena cava filter (IVCF) in patients with documented VTE or PE and a contraindication to anticoagulation, complications of bleeding as a result of anticoagulation, failure of

J.J. Naoum, M.D., FACS
Division of Vascular Surgery,
DeBakey Heart and Vascular Center,
Weill-Cornell Medical College,
Cardiovascular Surgery Associates,
The Methodist Hospital,
6550 Fannin St. Suite 1401, Houston,
TX 77030, USA
e-mail: joseph.naoum@umcrh.com

J.J. Hoballah, A.B. Lumsden (eds.), *Vascular Surgery*, New Techniques in Surgery Series,
DOI 10.1007/978-1-4471-2912-7_19, © Springer-Verlag London 2012

anticoagulation, or VTE despite therapeutic anticoagulation [2]. In addition to these guidelines, the Eastern Association for the Surgery of Trauma (EAST) recommends that the prophylactic use of IVC filters be considered in patients who are at increased risk of bleeding complications and thus with a contraindication to anticoagulation and patients with injury patterns that will result in a prolonged period of immobility such as those with closed head injury, spinal cord injury with paraplegia, complex pelvic fractures, and multiple long bone fractures [3]. Prophylactic indications for IVCF placement have been further expanded to include selected high-risk patients with risk factors for VTE such as patients undergoing bariatric surgery, orthopedic procedures, or with a previous history of DVT or PE, and during catheter-directed treatment of DVT.

In a study Decousus and associates [4] randomized 400 patients with proximal deep vein thrombosis who were at risk for PE. Two hundred patients had an IVCF placed, while the remainder 200 patients did not. A PE occurred during the first 12 days after randomization in 4.8 % of patients who did not receive an IVCF compared to 1.1 % of patients who had an IVCF implanted. They demonstrated that implanted filters significantly reduced the occurrence of both symptomatic and asymptomatic PE. Follow-up at 2 and 8 years showed that the rate for recurrent DVT was 20.8 and 35.7 % in patients with the permanent filter compared to 11.6 and 27.5 % in patients without filter, respectively. This suggests that an IVCF has mostly a short-term benefit with complications occurring late. Therefore, filters that can be retrieved and are not permanent may have an advantage in the prevention of PE without the increased risk of DVT in the long term. In addition, the contraindication to anticoagulation or increased risk for VTE can be temporary, and a retrievable IVCF (rIVCF) can serve as an effective prevention against PE during that specific period. These findings have encouraged the development and use of retrievable over permanent filters.

The use of retrievable filters can be considered when there is a definable endpoint for retrieval, or if the need for retrieval is uncertain and a permanent need is possible [5]. In general, filters should not be placed in patients who do not have a direct access route to the IVC, have a chronically thrombosed IVC, are bacteremic, have septic emboli, or have IVC diameters that exceed the filter's manufactured specifications [6]. Pregnant women should understand the risks involved if and when fluoroscopy is used during filter placement. Filter retrieval is not suggested when there is a trapped thrombus burden greater than 25 % of the filter's volume, there is filter incorporation into the wall of the vena cava [7] or strut penetration of the vena cava wall [8], or if the patient remains at risk for ongoing VTE.

Table 19.1 Common retrievable filters used in the United States

Filter type	Material	IVC diameter (MM)	MRI conditional[a]	Retrieval window (days)
OptEase	Nitinol	≤30	Yes	23
Celect	Conichrome	≤30	Yes	365[b]
Eclipse	Nitinol	≤28	Yes	300
Option	Nitinol	≤30	Yes	175
ALN	Stainless steel	≤28	Yes	No limit

[a]Conditions specific for each device as detailed in the instructions for use (IFU)
[b]Predicted

Retrievable Filters

Important properties of an ideal retrievable filter include (1) a low profile for percutaneous placement and ease of deployment, (2) precise placement and fixation without migration, (3) proper self-centering alignment without tilt in the IVC, (4) the ability to trap clot effectively and prevent PE, (5) ease of retrieval over a wide window of time, (6) low associated fracture and complication rate, (7) MRI compatibility, and (8) low cost.

The most common retrievable filters used in the USA have undergone improvements and changes in the past decade (Table 19.1). The OptEase filter (Cordis Endovascular, Warren, NJ) has a symmetrical nitinol double basket design that offers a dual layer filtration and is MRI conditional. It is designed to accommodate IVC diameters ≤ 30 mm and its anchors allow it to resist migration. It can be delivered from a femoral or jugular/subclavian vein approach. It has a caudal hook for retrieval using a snare through a femoral vein approach. It is recommended for retrieval up to 23 days post implantation. The Celect filter (Cook, Bloomington, IN) is a conichrome single cone design that is MRI conditional. It can be delivered from a femoral or jugular/subclavian vein approach. It is designed to accommodate IVC diameters ≤ 30 mm and has a strut design that self-centers the filter within the IVC. The filter's anchors allow it to resist migration. It has a cephalad hook for retrieval using a snare through an internal jugular (IJ) vein approach. It has a predicted 89 % probability of retrieval at 365 days. The Eclipse filter (Bard Peripheral Vascular, Tempe, AZ) has an electropolished nitinol cone design that provides two levels of filtration and is MRI conditional. It can be delivered from a femoral or jugular/subclavian vein approach. Its nitinol design allows it to elastically deform while its anchors allow the filter to resist migration. It is designed to accommodate IVC diameters ≤ 28 mm with a caval-centering design. At its cephalad apex, it has a central nitinol sleeve with a hook for retrieval using a snare or a Recovery Cone (Bard Peripheral Vascular, Tempe, AZ) via an IJ approach. It is recommended for retrieval out to 300 days after implantation. The Option filter (Manufactured by Rex Medical, Conshohocken, PA and distributed by Angiotech, Gainesville, FL) has nitinol struts arising from a central apical location and is MRI conditional. It can be delivered from a femoral or jugular approach using a separate delivery system for each. Small and larger retention anchor hooks allow the filter to resist migration. It is designed to accommodate IVC diameters up to 30 mm. A retrieval hook is centrally located at its cranial apex for filter retrieval with a snare via an IJ approach. The ALN filter (Aln International, Inc., Chicago, IL) is a stainless steel conical-shaped filter that is MRI conditional. It can be delivered from a femoral, IJ, or upper extremity approach using the designated kit delivery system. This filter has three centering legs and six retention hooks that allow the filter to resist migration. Retrieval is recommended with the specifically designed Pincer removal kit (Aln International, Inc., Chicago, IL) from a jugular vein approach.

Expanded Use of rIVCF

Trauma

Trauma patients with multiple bone injuries, those with spinal cord or closed head injury, intracranial or cerebral hemorrhage, or intra-abdominal solid organ injury pose a problem for the common measures of thromboprophylaxis especially when anticoagulation cannot be used or SCDs cannot be applied. It has been reported that among trauma patients, the incidence of PE and DVT can be as high as 20.3 and 65 %, respectively [9]. In addition, approximately 65 of trauma patients develop a PE within the first 24 h of admission [10]. Hoff and colleagues [11] placed an IVCF in selected high-risk patients after blunt trauma. Seventy-four percent of patients had at least one orthopedic injury, approximately half had a pelvic fracture, an equal number was limited to bed rest or spinal precaution, 91 % had a contraindication to pharmacologic prophylaxis, and 31 % had injuries that precluded the use of SCDs. Half the patients had the filter retrieved without complications. In a study of severely injured military trauma patients, rIVCFs were placed for PE prophylaxis in 32 % patients and for therapeutic VTE prevention in 68 % of patients. Retrieval was not attempted in 63 % of patients for a persistent indication for IVCF. Failure to retrieve the filter occurred only in 2.8 % of patients while 15 % were lost to follow-up. The authors concluded that rIVCFs can be safely used with minimal low-term morbidity; however, they acknowledged that better follow-up can improve retrieval rate [12]. Smoot and associates [13] also reviewed the use of rIVCF in 140 trauma patients over a 4-year period. Filters were successfully removed in 61 % of patients with a technical success rate of 97 %. However, as described before, a significant number of trauma patients were also lost to follow-up. In addition, this study pointed out that IVCFs are not infallible with a PE observed in 3 % of patients. In general, these studies show that the use of rIVCF in high-risk trauma patients offers a versatile option for the prevention of VTE and PE.

Orthopedic Surgery

Austin and associates [14] recommend the use of IVCF in orthopedic patients with confirmed PE, proximal DVT in the perioperative period, or a medical contraindication to anticoagulation. Their recommendations were based on their study of 95 joint arthroplasty patients who received an IVCF that was effective in preventing a fatal PE. In a survey by the American Association of Hip and Knee Surgeons (AAHKS), 25 % of surgeons used IVCF in the management of high-risk patients undergoing total hip and knee arthroplasty [15]. These patients have a recognized high risk for the development of VTE, and IVCF has been shown to be efficacious in the prevention of PE [16, 17]. Of interest, patients with orthopedic injuries and pelvic fractures are very likely to have their filters retrieved [11].

Bariatric Surgery

There are several, well-established patient factors that significantly increase the risk of DVT and VTE after bariatric surgery. These patient factors include advanced age, previous history of VTE, immobilization, BMI $\geq$ 55 kg/m^2, venous stasis disease, hypercoagulable states, estrogen medication, and the dysregulation of proteins involved in the coagulation and fibrinolytic pathways [18, 19]. Overall, the incidence of VTE after bariatric surgery varies from 1 to 3 % [18]. Although a fatal PE after bariatric surgery is rare, it is the leading cause of 30-day mortality. Interestingly, in patients who die after Roux-en-Y gastric bypass, half die due to technical complications, whereas the other half die of complications of their obesity. Clinically, only 20 % of patients were suspected to have a PE; yet at autopsy, 80 % of patients had a PE [20]. Morbidly obese patients undergoing Roux-en-Y gastric bypass have an unexpectedly high rate of clinically silent pulmonary emboli contributing to an increase in morbidity and mortality.

We reviewed our clinical data in patients at high risk for PE who underwent placement of a rIVCF prior to gastric bypass for morbid obesity during an 18-month period. The indications for prophylactic rIVCF placement included a history of DVT (71 %), hypercoagulable state (43 %), and PE (14 %). Half of the patients had more than one risk factor. The average body mass index at the time of filter placement was 51 ± 10.8. The retrieval of the IVCF was successful in all attempted patients after an average of 148 ± 63 days and following a weight loss of approximately 82 ± 31 lb. There were no complications related to filter placement or retrieval. One patient developed a recurrent DVT in the extremity contralateral to the IVCF placement access site. There were no PEs and no deaths [21].

Vaziri and colleagues [18] observed a 21 % incidence of recurrent DVT, 15 % incidence of thrombus in the IVCF, and no PE in a group of patients who had an IVCF placed during bariatric surgery and who had a previous history of VTE. They concluded that concurrent IVCF placement is safe, feasible, and an effective preventative measure in high-risk morbidly obese patients. Based on their observation, they recommend the use of rIVCFs in conjunction with standard VTE prophylaxis for patients with a history of VTE undergoing bariatric surgery.

Catheter-Directed Treatment of DVT

Deep venous thrombosis occurs in large-diameter veins; thus, the thrombus burden and VTE potential during pharmacological or catheter-directed thrombolysis (CDT) and mechanical thrombectomy can be great especially if the more proximal veins are involved. Percutaneous maneuvers in these thrombus-burdened veins can lead to the release of clot and debris which can migrate to the pulmonary vasculature. Théry and associates [22] observed that VTE was captured by tempo-

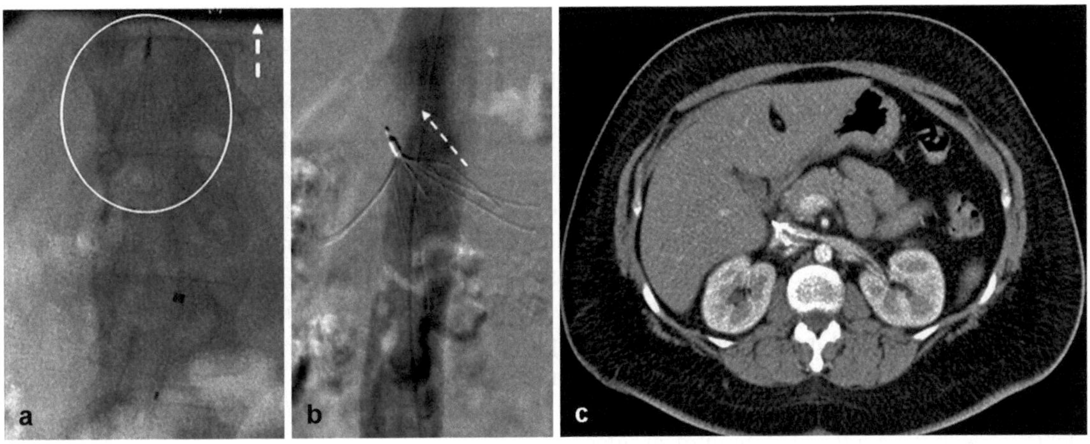

Fig. 19.1 IVCF tilt during pregnancy. (**a**) Initial IVCF position at the time of placement in the suprarenal IVC. (**b**) IVCF position at the time of retrieval 6 weeks after delivery via C-section. The rIVCF has migrated in a caudal direction with some struts seen in the renal veins. (**c**) Computed tomography showing the rIVCF within the IVC and left renal vein. The *white arrows* indicate the direction of the filter's apex

rary IVCF in 29–33 % of patients following 24 h of systemic thrombolysis. Kölbel and colleagues [23] reviewed their 12-year experience of CDT and mechanical thrombectomy during the treatment of acute iliocaval thrombosis. Visible emboli trapped within the rIVCF were found in 58 and 43 % of patients, respectively. Yet, none developed a clinical symptomatic PE or a complication related to the placement or retrieval of the rIVCF. The authors concluded that thrombus embolization is common during treatment and that the placement of a rIVCF during therapy can prevent both silent and symptomatic PE.

Pregnancy

Pregnant women with DVT or a history of VTE are managed with conventional LMWH anticoagulation for the duration of pregnancy. However, therapeutic pharmacologic anticoagulation must be stopped to avoid bleeding complications during delivery. The rationale is that rIVCF can offer protection against VTE and PE during the window in which anticoagulation is halted. In pregnancy, the recommendation is to place an IVCF in the suprarenal location to avoid compression by the gravid uterus. Intravascular volume changes during pregnancy, the dynamic physiologic variability of the caval diameter, the forces exerted during uterine contraction, the intra-abdominal pressure changes during vaginal delivery, or the manipulations that occur during C-section can alter the caliber or diameter of the cava and lead to IVCF tilt in 5.3–16 % of patients (Fig. 19.1), migration, or device fracture in 2.7 % of cases [24–26]. In a study by Seshadri and colleagues [27], 92 % of women had successful removal of the rIVCF when clot was not found trapped within the filter.

Filter Placement

Typically, the procedure is performed in an angiographic suite or operating room with fluoroscopic guidance. We recommend using a duplex ultrasound to interrogate the target vein and achieve precise percutaneous access with a 22-gauge needle and a micropuncture 4-Fr system. When possible, the right femoral vein approach is preferred. Anatomically, it offers a shorter and straighter access to the IVC. Commonly, a marking pigtail catheter is used to perform an IVC venogram to determine the size of the IVC and to delineate the origin of the renal veins. A variety of rIVCFs can be placed depending on physician's preference and diameter of the IVC. The author prefers to advance the dilator and introducer sheath over a 0.035-in. starter wire of choice; however, in the obese patient, he has found that a super stiff 0.035-in. wire allows for improved push ability through the subcutaneous tissues. Filters should be deployed following the standard manufacturer's instructions for use. Following filter insertion, a completion IVC venogram can be performed.

Patients who cannot receive intravenous contrast due to allergy or renal insufficiency and who are pregnant and the use of angiography is not necessarily recommended, IVCF placement can be achieved with the guidance of an intravascular ultrasound (IVUS). Intravascular ultrasound provides real-time endoluminal characteristics and very accurate sizing of the IVC. Briefly, a double ipsilateral femoral venous access can be achieved as described above, one for the IVUS and the other for the filter access. Alternatively, a single puncture with placement of a large enough sheath that can accommodate both the IVUS and the filter delivery system can be used. In addition, the femoral vein contralateral to the IVUS access site can be cannulated for filter delivery and placement when possible. It is important to identify the following anatomic landmarks to ensure the proper intended location for filter placement either in the infrarenal or suprarenal IVC before delivery: (1) right atrium, (2) renal veins, (3) iliac vein confluence, and (4) IVC diameter. The filter is deployed using real-time IVUS imaging.

There is another group of patients in whom transportation to an endovascular suite or operating room is accompanied by inherent risks usually due to severe respiratory failure, hemodynamic instability, or severity of injury. These patients can benefit from bedside rIVCF placement. The above technique using IVUS can be particularly useful. Aidinian and associates [28] reviewed their experience of IVUS-guided bedside IVCF placed in military patients with complex injuries. The authors reported a 93 % success rate and one technical complication of filter misplacement in the common iliac vein as a result of misidentification of the venous anatomy. Similarly, others have shown that using IVUS guidance, rIVCF can be safely and accurately placed at bedside in 93.1 and 97.2 % of multiple trauma and critically ill patients, respectively. Misplacement was also into the iliac vein or in relation to the renal veins [5, 29]. Based on their experience, Killingsworth and associates [5] have implemented an algorithm for IVUS-guided bedside IVCF placement. Instead of IVUS, transabdominal ultrasound-guided bedside IVCF placement has also been described with a failure rate between 2 and 15 % [30, 31].

Filter Retrieval

It is important to establish if there is any thrombus burden within the rIVCF prior to removal. This can be imaged with a CT scan using intravenous contrast. Alternatively, when filter removal is intended, a pigtail catheter should be placed at the confluence of the iliac veins and an IVC venogram performed to delineate any clots within the device. Filters should be removed according to the manufacturer's guidelines which usually require the capture or snare of the filter apex or hook (Fig. 19.2).

Failure of intended retrieval is most commonly the result of filter tilt in which the apex comes in close proximity or contact with the IVC wall. Balloon-assisted removal [32] of tilted rIVCF involves the use of a large angioplasty balloon inflated below nominal pressure to free the apex and guide it toward the IVC center line for capture or snare (Fig. 19.3). Alternatively, another technique the author has used involves gaining opposite access through both the IJ and femoral vein. A large 12- to 14-Fr sheath is placed through the access site intended for retrieval in order to accommodate the wires and the retrieval device or snare. Stiff wires are guided past the filter on the side of the tilt and snared at either end as "body floss." Applying tension on the wires can mobilize the filter away from the IVC wall and allow capture (Fig. 19.4). Another technique also involves the dual access described above. Instead, a wire is looped around the filter apex and snared

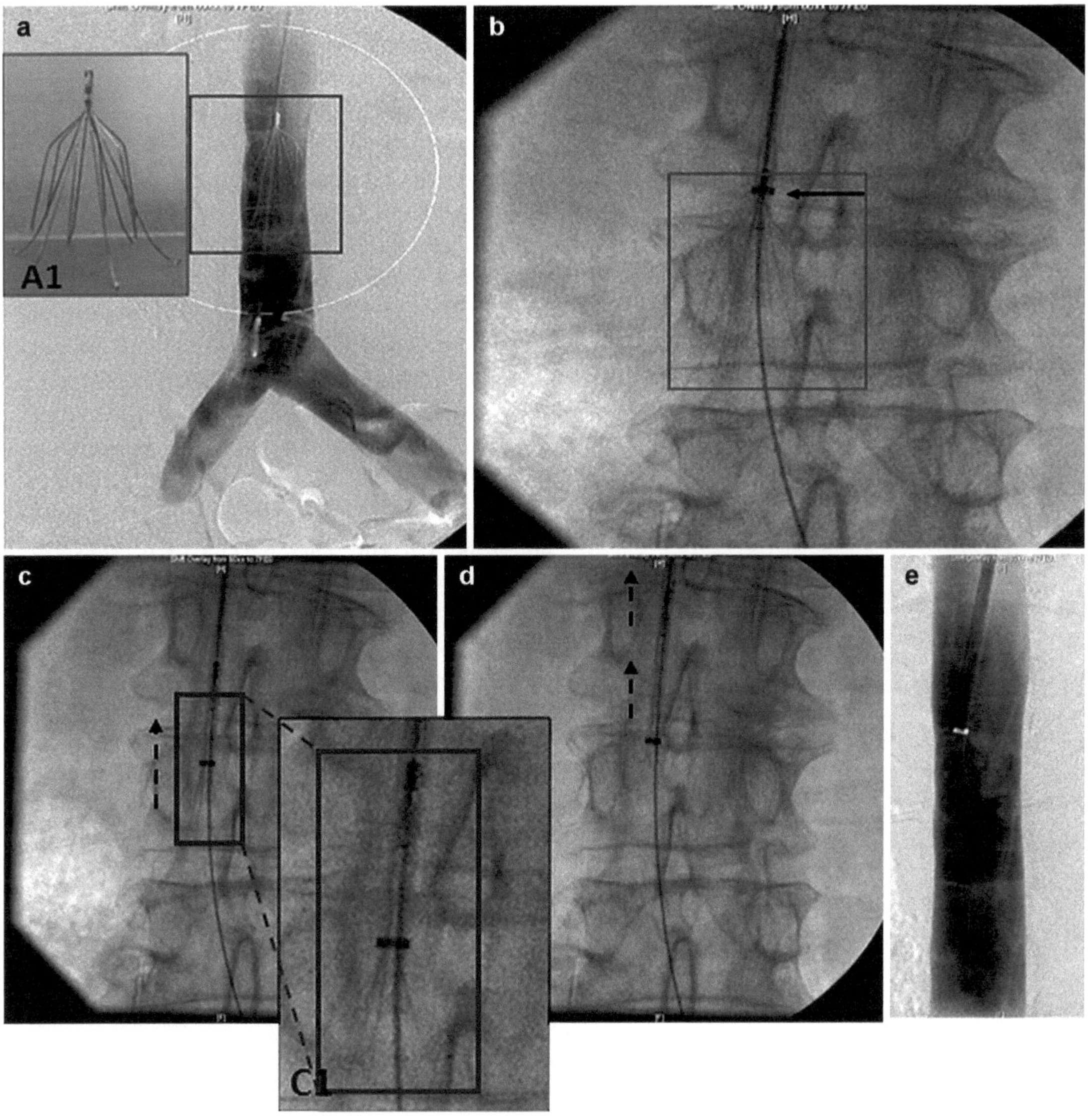

Fig. 19.2 Retrieval of an IVCF. (**a**) IVC venogram through a pigtail catheter placed at the confluence of the iliac veins. Trapped clots are not observed within the filter. (**a1**) Eclipse rIVCF. (**b**) Captured rIVCF with the Recovery Cone (*solid arrow*). (**c** and **c1**) rIVCF collapse and early retrieval into the sheath. (**d**) Filter completely retrieved into the sheath (*dotted arrows* show the direction of retrieval). (**e**) Completion IVC venogram showing contrast in the IVC without defects or extravasation

back into the sheath and out. The sheath is then advanced over the wire loop until enough tension is placed to allow displacement of the filter's apex away from the IVC wall and toward the midline where it can be captured through the venous access from the opposite end (Fig. 19.5). Van Ha and colleagues [33] demonstrated that modified techniques are useful in difficult retrievals when conventional maneuvers fail. After removal of the filter, an IVC venogram is performed to evaluate the IVC for defects, tears, or extravasation of contrast in case of perforation.

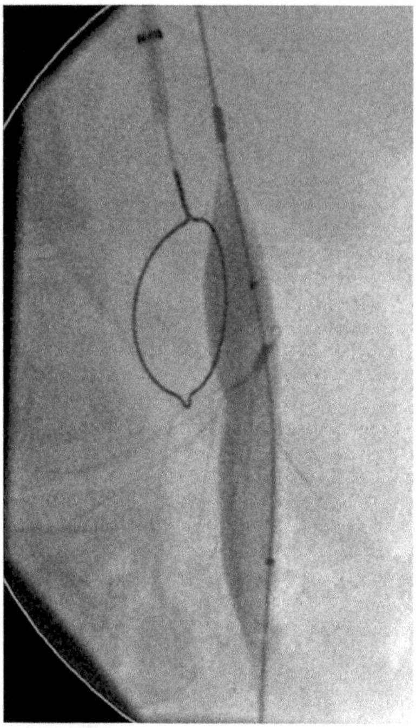
Fig. 19.3 Balloon-assisted snare of a tilted rIVCF

Complications

As any procedure, placement and retrieval of IVCFs is not devoid of potential complications. Therefore, the benefit of placing and removing the filter must be balanced against other alternatives. Some of these complications are described. Inadvertent arterial puncture or initial access complications can be minimized with the use of ultrasound-guided venous puncture and the use of a micropuncture kit as described previously. Access site hematomas can still occur. The migration rate of new generation filters is approximately 0.3 % [17]. Misplacement is a technical complication that needs to be identified promptly and corrected. The risks of DVT as it relates to the presence of an IVC filter were previously addressed in this chapter. Occlusion of the filter can occur as a result of device thrombogenicity or extension of the thrombus from the underlying DVT. It becomes a catch 22 when the filter is

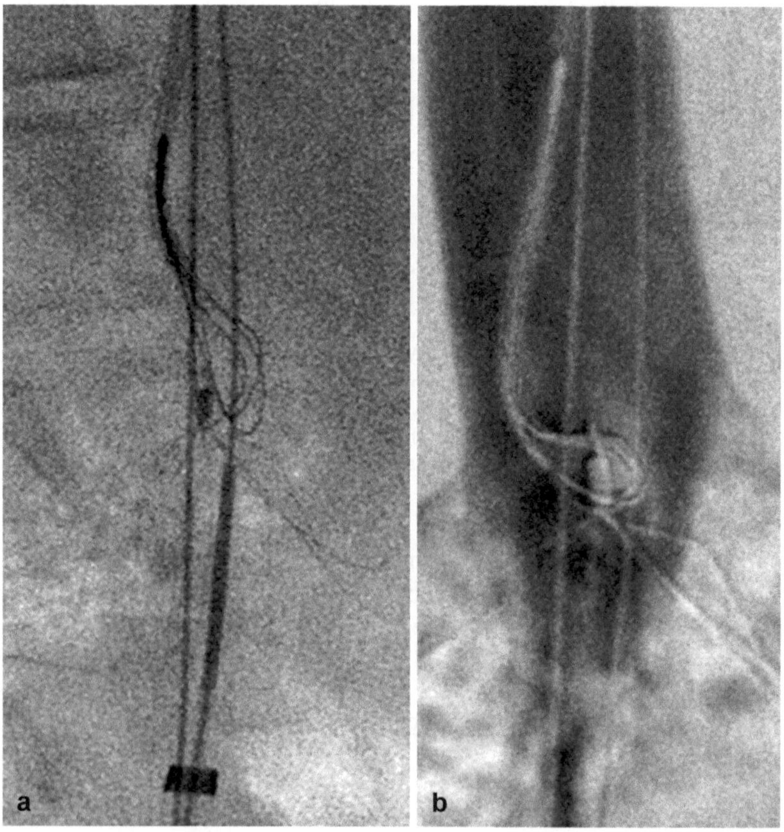

Fig. 19.4 Dual wire technique aligns the filter to allow capture with a snare

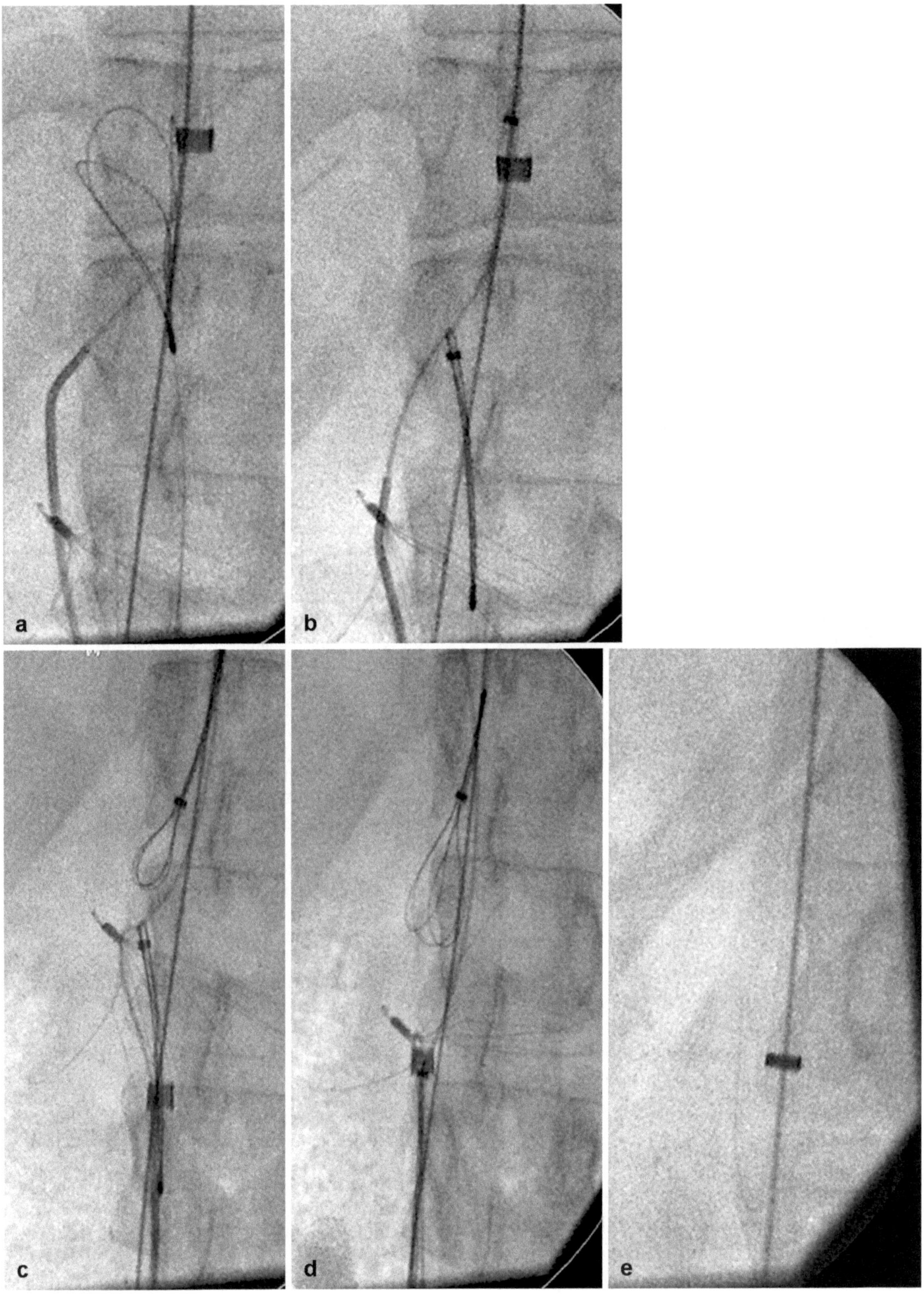

Fig. 19.5 (**a–c**) A wire is looped around the filter apex and snared back into the sheath and out. (**d, e**) The sheath is advanced over the wire loop until enough tension is placed to push the filter's apex and hook away from the IVC wall and toward the midline where it is retrieved using a snare

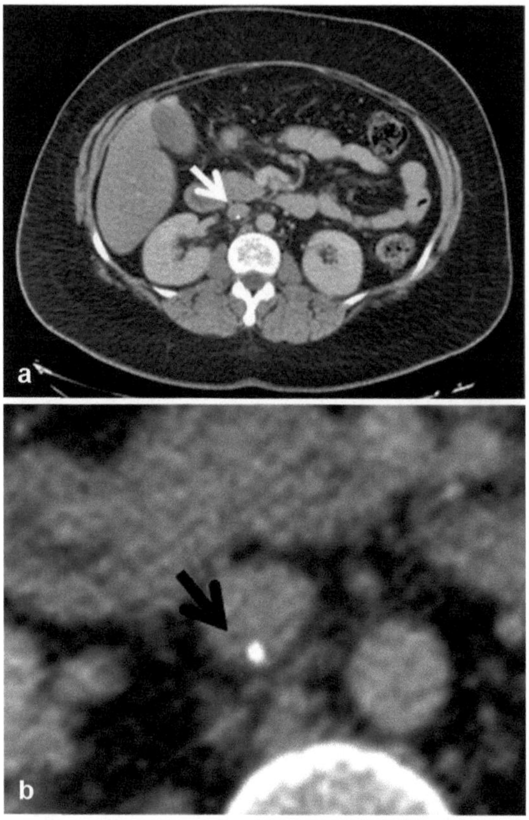

Fig. 19.6 (**a**) Retained broken rIVCF nitinol strut in the IVC. (**b**) Magnified view of the same

capable of preventing VTE and PE, but in the process it can contribute to IVC occlusion from the clot burden. Tilting or angulation can prevent successful retrieval. Filter fracture or retained fracture strut after retrieval can also occur (Fig. 19.6). Yet, with proper patient selection and experience with different devices and techniques, the process of rIVCF placement and retrieval can be efficacious and associated with a low risk and complication rate.

Conclusions

Venous thromboembolism constitutes a significant cause of death among the critically ill, multiple injured, and at-risk surgical patients. Retrievable IVCF plays an important role in the prevention of fatal PE. Proper filter and patient selection along with meticulous technique during implantation and retrieval is accompanied by successful results with minimal comorbidity. Patient follow-up is paramount to ensure higher retrieval rates.

References

1. Zhan C, Miller MR. Excess length of stay, charges, and mortality attributable to medical injuries during hospitalization. JAMA. 2003;290:1868–74.
2. Geerts WH, Bergqvist D, Pineo GF, et al. Prevention of venous thromboembolism: American college of chest physicians evidence – based clinical practice guidelines (8th edition). Chest. 2008;133:381S–453.
3. Roger FB, Cipolle M, Velmahos G, et al. Practice management guidelines for the prevention of venous thromboembolism in trauma patients: the EAST practice management guidelines work group. J Trauma. 2002;53(1):142–64.
4. Decousus H, Leizorovics A, Parent F, et al. A clinical trial of vena caval filters in the prevention of pulmonary embolism in patients with proximal deep-vein thrombosis. N Engl J Med. 1998;338:409–15.
5. Killingsworth CD, Taylor SM, Patterson MA, et al. Prospective implementation of an algorithm for bedside intravascular ultrasound-guided filter placement in critically ill patients. J Vasc Surg. 2010;51:1215–21.
6. Baerlocher M, Noble J. IVC filters: an introduction to a simple concept turned clinical. Univ Toronto Med J. 2004;81(3):239–42.
7. Mission JF, Kerlan RK, Tan JH, Fang MC. Rates and predictors of plans for inferior vena cava filter retrieval in hospitalized patients. J Gen Intern Med. 2010; 25(4):321–5.
8. Berczi V, Bottomley JR, Thomas SM, Taneja S, Gaines PA, Cleveland TJ. Long-term retrievability of IVC filters: should we abandon permanent devices? Cardiovasc Intervent Radiol. 2007;30:820–7.
9. Sevitt S, Gallagher N. Venous thrombosis and pulmonary embolism: a clinicopathological study in injured and burned patients. Br J Surg. 1961;48:475–89.
10. Owings JT, Kraut E, Battistella F, et al. Timing of the occurrence of pulmonary embolism in trauma patients. Arch Surg. 1997;132(8):862–7.
11. Hoff WS, Hoey BA, Wainwright GA, et al. Early experience with retrievable inferior vena cava filters in high-risk trauma patients. J Am Coll Surg. 2004; 199(6):869–74.
12. Johnson ON, Gillespie DL, Aidinian G, et al. The use of retrievable inferior vena cava filters in severely injured military trauma patients. J Vasc Surg. 2009; 49:410–6.
13. Smoot RL, Kock CA, Heller SF, et al. Inferior vena cava filters in trauma patients: efficacy, morbidity, and retrievability. J Trauma. 2010;68(4):899–903.
14. Austin MS, Parvizi J, Grossman S, et al. The inferior vena cava filter is effective in preventing fatal pulmo-

nary embolus after hip and knee arthroplasties. J Arthroplasty. 2007;22(3):343–8.
15. Mesko JW, Brand RA, Iorio R, et al. Venous thromboembolic disease management patterns in total hip arthroplasty and total knee arthroplasty patients. J Arthroplasty. 2001;16(6):679–88.
16. Imberti D, Prisco D. Retrievable vena cava filters: key considerations. Thromb Res. 2008;122:442–9.
17. Hann CL, Streiff MB. The role of vena caval filters in the management of venous thromboembolism. Blood Rev. 2005;19:179–202.
18. Vaziri K, Bhanot P, Hungness ES, et al. Retrievable inferior vena cava filters in high-risk patients undergoing bariatric surgery. Surg Endosc. 2009;23:2203–7.
19. Ahima RS, Flier JS. Adipose tissue as an endocrine organ. Trends Endocrinol Metab. 2000;11:327–32.
20. Judy Melinek J, et al. Autopsy findings following gastric bypass surgery for morbid obesity. Arch Pathol Lab Med. 2002;126:1091–5.
21. Naoum JJ, Peden EK, Davies MG. Retrievable IVC filter placement for prophylaxis against PE in high-risk patients prior to gastric bypass surgery. Society for Vascular Medicine, Cleveland, Apr 2010.
22. Thery C, Bauchart JJ, Lesenne M, et al. Predictive factors of effectiveness of streptokinase in deep venous thrombosis. Am J Cardiol. 1992;69:117–22.
23. Kolbel T, Alhadad A, Acosta S, et al. Thrombus embolization into IVC filters during catheter-directed thrombolysis for proximal deep venous thrombosis. J Endovasc Ther. 2008;15:605–13.
24. Streiff MB. Vena cava filters: a review for intensive care specialist. J Intensive Care Med. 2003;18:59–79.
25. Kumar BC, Chakraverty S, Zealley I. Failed retrieval of potentially retrievable IVC filters: a report of two cases. Cardiovasc Intervent Radiol. 2006;29:126–7.
26. Wiky S, Doenz F, Meuwly J, et al. Clinical experience with retrievable Gunther Tulip vena cava filters. J Endovasc Ther. 2003;10:994–1000.
27. Seshadri T, Tran H, Lau KK, et al. Ins and outs of inferior vena cava filters in venous thromboembolisms: the experience at Monash Medical Centre and review of the published reports. Intern Med J. 2008; 38:38–43.
28. Aidinian G, Fox CJ, White PW, et al. Intravascular ultrasound – guided inferior vena cava filter placement in the military multitrauma patients: a single-center experience. Vasc Endovascular Surg. 2009; 43(5):497–501.
29. Rosenthal D, Kochupura PV, Wellons ED, et al. Gunther tulip and celect IVC filters in multiple-trauma patients. J Endovasc Ther. 2009;16:494–9.
30. Amankwah KS, Seymour K, Costanza M, et al. Transabdominal duplex ultrasonography for bedside inferior vena cava filter placement: examples, technique, and review. Vasc Endovascular Surg. 2009; 43(4):379–84.
31. Sato DT, Robinson KD, Gregory RT, et al. Duplex directed caval filter insertion in multi-trauma and critically ill patients. Ann Vasc Surg. 1999;69(8): 365–71.
32. Lynch FC. Balloon-assisted removal of tilted inferior vena cava filters embedded tips. J Vasc Interv Radiol. 2009;20(9):1210–4.
33. Van Ha TG, Vinokur O, Lorenz J, et al. Techniques used for difficult retrievals of the Gunther Tulip inferior vena cava filter: experience in 32 patients. J Vasc Interv Radiol. 2009;20(1):92–9.

Part IV

Miscellaneous

First Rib Resection and Thoracoscopic Cervical Sympathectomy

20

Mohammad Bashir, Joss Dean Fernandez, Kalpaj Parekh, and Mark Iannettoni

Abstract

Idiopathic hyperhidrosis (excessive sweating) is a common benign condition that may cause a patient significant social, emotional, and professional distress. By definition, hyperhidrosis is the secretion of sweat in amounts greater than physiologically needed for thermoregulation. Diagnosis consists of focal, visible, excessive sweating of at least 6 months duration without apparent cause with at least two of the following criteria:

Bilateral and relatively symmetric
Impairs daily activities
At least one episode per week
Onset before age 25
Family history of idiopathic hyperhidrosis
Focal sweating stops during sleep

Hyperhidrosis is commonly localized to the palm, soles, and axillae. Palmar hyperhidrosis may result in social embarrassment and may affect the patient's ability to handle equipment that requires a gripping. There is evidence for a genetic component to hyperhidrosis. Eccrine glands are innervated by the sympathetic nervous system. In patients with idiopathic hyperhidrosis, the sweat glands are normal. The cause of hyperhidrosis appears to be an exaggerated central response to normal emotional stress. The differential of sweating is broad but includes infectious causes, lymphoma, autonomic dysreflexia, hyperthyroidism, carcinoid syndrome, pheochromocytoma, and perimenopausal hot flashes. These should be considered especially if symptoms occur at night or are associated with flushing.

Keywords

Surgery • Vascular surgery • Rib resection • Sympathectomy • Complications

M. Bashir, M.D. • J.D. Fernandez, M.D.
K. Parekh, M.D. (✉) • M. Iannettoni, M.D.
Cardiothoracic Surgery,
University of Iowa Hospitals and Clinics,
Iowa City, IA, USA
e-mail: kalpaj-parekh@uiowa.edu

J.J. Hoballah, A.B. Lumsden (eds.), *Vascular Surgery*, New Techniques in Surgery Series,
DOI 10.1007/978-1-4471-2912-7_20, © Springer-Verlag London 2012

Thoracoscopic Sympathectomy

Diagnosis and Clinical Evaluation

Idiopathic hyperhidrosis (excessive sweating) is a common benign condition that may cause a patient significant social, emotional, and professional distress. By definition, hyperhidrosis is the secretion of sweat in amounts greater than physiologically needed for thermoregulation [1]. Diagnosis consists of focal, visible, excessive sweating of at least 6 months duration without apparent cause with at least two of the following criteria:

Bilateral and relatively symmetric
Impairs daily activities
At least one episode per week
Onset before age 25
Family history of idiopathic hyperhidrosis
Focal sweating stops during sleep

Hyperhidrosis is commonly localized to the palm, soles, and axillae. Palmar hyperhidrosis may result in social embarrassment and may affect the patient's ability to handle equipment that requires a gripping. There is evidence for a genetic component to hyperhidrosis [2]. Eccrine glands are innervated by the sympathetic nervous system. In patients with idiopathic hyperhidrosis, the sweat glands are normal. The cause of hyperhidrosis appears to be an exaggerated central response to normal emotional stress. The differential of sweating is broad but includes infectious causes, lymphoma, autonomic dysreflexia, hyperthyroidism, carcinoid syndrome, pheochromocytoma, and perimenopausal hot flashes. These should be considered especially if symptoms occur at night or are associated with flushing.

Medical Management

Most commercially available over-the-counter antiperspirants contain a low-dose metal salt (usually aluminum) that physically obstructs the opening of sweat gland ducts. These over-the-counter products are only successful in treating patients with very mild symptoms. Antiperspirants such as 20 % aluminum chloride in ethanol (Drysol) or 6.25 % aluminum tetrachloride (Xerac) may provide adequate therapy for patients with mild symptoms. Antiperspirants have a rapid onset of action but not as durable [3]. Antiperspirants are normally applied at night, with onset of action occurring as early as 48 h. Use of these solutions is often associated with skin irritation especially within the axillae. Iontophoresis is the process of introducing ionized substance into the skin using a direct current. For hyperhidrosis, the patient's hands are submerged in tap water while a direct current is applied. Decreased pH due to an increase in H^+ ions during tap water iontophoresis may contribute to eccrine gland dysfunction. Treatments may be administered at home [4]. Small randomized trials have demonstrated an 81 % reduction in sweating [5]. This therapy can be time consuming, taking 20–30 min a day. With time, treatments may be reduced to three times a week. Botulinum toxin A blocks the release of neuronal acetylcholine from the presynaptic junction of autonomic neurons. Multiple injections (10–30) are required especially on the hands. Randomized trials have demonstrated 82 % efficacy up to 16 weeks when treating axillary hyperhidrosis [6].

Surgical Management

The concept behind sympathectomy for treatment of hyperhidrosis is the interruption of sympathetic innervation to the sweat glands. Sympathetic outflow is responsible for sensory-motor innervation to the thoracic viscera. The motor supply to the organs also supplies the sweat glands of the skin in the axilla and upper extremity.

Indications for Surgery

Patients considered for surgery are those with primary hyperhidrosis and severe symptoms affecting their daily lives, making social work interaction embarrassing. Patients with palmer, axillary, plantar, and craniofacial sweating have all been described to benefit from sympathectomy with different success rates [7, 8]. In general, plantar hyperhidrosis is not an indication for thoracoscopic sympathectomy. Nevertheless, some patients report improvement in plantar hyperhidrosis after the procedure. Most patients present after trying medical therapies without success or only transient relief. We consider thoracic sympathectomy to be the treatment of choice for this pathophysiologic condition. This procedure also has been described in all age groups including adolescents with excellent results [9].

Surgical Anatomy

The sympathetic chain is located longitudinally in the retropleural region overlying the rib heads at their articulation with the transverse process of the vertebral body. The inferior cervical and T1 ganglia fuse to form the stellate ganglion; it is in the apicoposterior location often covered by fatty tissue. T1 root mainly supplies the head and neck region, whereas most of the innervation to the hand originates in the T2 ganglion and partly from the T3 ganglia. The axillary region is supplied by the T4 and T5 ganglia of the sympathetic chain. The nerve of Kuntz arises from the postganglionic fibers of T2 and T3 which bypass the stellate ganglion and carry sympathetic fibers to the inferior portion of the brachial plexus. Identification of the ganglion levels is guided by the appropriate rib levels. The second ganglion is situated at the lower edge of the second rib within the second intercostal space.

Technique

This technique requires general anesthesia with double-lumen endotracheal intubation. The patient is placed in the lateral decubitus position. We elect to do this and reposition the patient for the contralateral side, as this provides the most optimal visualization. Alternatively, the patient can be positioned in the sitting position with both arms extended and supported. We prefer not to use this position so that potential injuries due to positioning are avoided. Potentially, a single lumen tube can be used, but this would require carbon dioxide insufflation to improve visualization. Pressure above 15 mmHg should be avoided as this is associated with hemodynamic instability and should be used with extreme caution. The thoracic cavity is approached via one 5-mm incision in the midaxillary line, in the mammary fold. Two additional 5-mm ports are placed in the second and third intercostal spaces in the axillary hair line, and the lung is collapsed (see Fig. 20.1). The sympathetic chain is then identified running over the rib heads, and the overlying pleura is excised; dissection is carried using hook electrocautery. It is very important to locate the level of the intended resection prior to opening the pleura. This is done as above according to the rib levels. Care must be taken to avoid injury to nearby intercostal vessels during dissection. This is achieved by opening the pleura on top of the rib and starting the plane of dissection that way (see Fig. 20.2). After circumferential dissection of the chain, attention is turned to ablation, and this could be achieved using different methods. In 2007, a randomized study by Inan et al. looked at outcomes of different techniques used to ablate

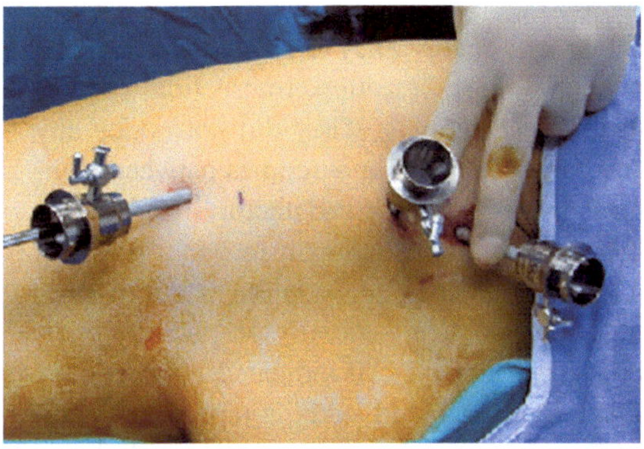

Fig. 20.1 Port placement during thoracoscopic sympathectomy

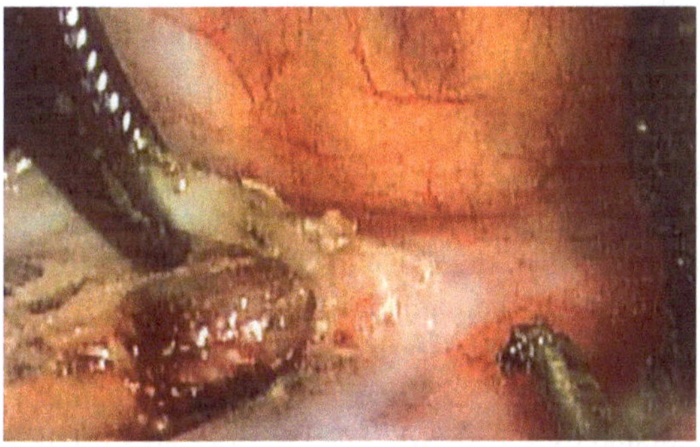

Fig. 20.2 The parietal fascia has been incised, and the sympathetic chain is grasped as it is excised

the thoracic chain. They divided their patients into four groups: resection, transection, cautery ablation, and clipping. They did not notice any significant difference in outcomes between techniques and all achieved satisfactory results [10]. We prefer to resect the chain in our institution. An important question also is the extent of ablation. In our practice, generally for palmar hyperhidrosis, excision of T2 is indicated and adequate. A randomized blinded study comparing T2 versus T2 and T3 ablation for palmar hyperhidrosis was performed by Katara et al. in 2007. They did not find any difference in symptomatic relief or recurrence with a mean follow-up period of 23 months [11], while for axillary hyperhidrosis, most will take T2 along with T3 and frequently T4 ganglion as well [12]. The use of electrocautery above the T2 level is avoided not to injure the T1 ganglion and cause Horner's syndrome. Also identification of the nerve of Kuntz or any accessory fibers and their ablation is important to avoid recurrence. After resection, the air is evacuated from the chest using a small catheter and the lung is inflated by anesthesia. The incisions are closed and the patient extubated. This procedure is done as an outpatient procedure with follow-up in clinic in 1–2 weeks.

Complications

Early Complications

Pneumothorax is the most common early complication and is seen in up to 75 % of patients [13]. Chest tube is rarely required, and most are treated conservatively. Patients who might need a chest tube are those with history of prior surgery or adhesions [8]. Other complications that have been reported include subcutaneous emphysema, injury to subclavian artery, and chylothorax [14]. In the same series, Gossot et al. reported a 5.3 % incidence of significant (300–600 ml) intraoperative bleeding [14]. Rebound sweating is a temporary recurrence of sweating that occurs in 31 % of patients [15]. Horner's syndrome is seen in less than 1 % of patients. Wait et al. found in their series that this was associated with sympathectomy more compared to sympathotomy [8].

Late Complications

The commonest long-term complication is compensatory sweating. The incidence of compensatory sweating varies considerably in the literature and is reported to be up to 62 % [8]. However, most of these were reported as mild symptoms with only 6 % reported as severe or bothersome. It is also reported as high as 89 % in the literature with 35 % of the patients severely affected by it [16]. The severity and presence is higher in patients who undergo lower level sympathectomy involving T2-T4 for axillary hyperhidrosis compared to patients who undergo only T2 ablation for palmer hyperhidrosis. Inclusion of T5 in the sympathectomy or sympathotomy results in more severe compensatory sweating [8]. In a prospective study where patients had two different approaches for ablation (resection versus transection) on either side, none of the patients could appreciate any difference in regard to compensatory sweating [17]. Another long-term complication is gustatory sweating, and the reason for this is still obscure. The incidence varies from 38 to 50 % in the literature and is particularly related to spicy foods or foods with acidity like oranges or apples [18]. Of note, there has been some reports regarding disturbances in cardiac rhythm both intraoperatively, postoperatively, and long-term bradycardia [19]. While more and more patients undergo this procedure, there will be more reported complications, and evidence will emerge, leading to more patient awareness regarding those side effects.

Results

In our experience, thoracoscopic sympathectomy is very effective in treating hyperhidrosis especially in the palmar and axillary region. This is confirmed by multiple studies in the literature with long-term follow-up. The attractiveness of this procedure is the lack of major morbidity compared to the open approach. Also, better visualization is achieved by the thoracoscopic approach compared to the open one.

Recently (2010), Wait et al. reported their results in 322 patients with different indications.

They found that the region most responsive for sympathectomy was palmar followed by craniofacial, axillary, and plantar. In general, patient satisfaction was up to 93.8 % in all groups [8]. Similar results are confirmed by other studies with range of satisfaction, even up to 6 years of follow-up, as high as 90 % [20]. The main reason for long-term dissatisfaction with the results of the procedure is related to compensatory sweating [21]. Recurrence of symptoms is very rare in our experience and as reported in the literature. This was attributed to the use of transection rather than resection without significant difference as reported by Assalia et al. in 2007 [17].

First Rib Resection

Diagnosis and Clinical Evaluation

Neurogenic

The neurologic signs and symptoms that result for neurogenic thoracic outlet syndrome range from vague intermittent paresthesias with provocation to muscle atrophy. The diagnosis is often difficult and confounded by psychiatric disorders or secondary gain as in workers' compensation. No single test may lead to diagnosis, but instead a constellation of signs and symptoms will rule out other causes and may direct treatment. Physical therapy should be sought early to address postural abnormalities and muscle imbalance. Evaluation should include potential distal sites of nerve entrapment at the elbow, forearm, and wrist.

Patients typically complain of paresthesias along the medial border, a T1 distribution, of the forearm and hand. They may describe discomfort along the shoulder girdle that radiates into the upper arm. Symptoms are worsened by activity of the upper extremity especially with elevation over head or carrying objectives with the arms in the dependent position. Symptoms of neurogenic thoracic outlet syndrome are chronic and insidious; though not infrequently patients may report an antecedent injury.

The cervical spine should be completely examined including passive and active range of motion. Cervical spine nerve impingement can be screened using the Spurling's test. Axial compression on the patient's head which is extended and laterally flexed may solicit symptoms radiating down the extremity. A positive Spurling's test indicated cervical radiculopathy. Rotator cuff tendinitis is assessed with active shoulder range of movement, palpating the insertion of the rotator cuff on the greater tuberosity. This does not exclude concomitant thoracic outlet syndrome.

Chest radiographs are required for all patients to identify bone abnormalities such as cervical ribs, prior fractures, or degenerative changes. Cervical ribs can be found in 1 % of the population and are associated with 6–11 % of patients with thoracic outlet syndrome [22]. Cervical spine radiographs may provide additional information. Computed tomography is of less utility in the diagnosis of thoracic outlet syndrome [23]. This modality should be reserved for patients that have associated findings of lymphadenopathy, trauma, or lung mass. Magnetic resonance imaging (MRI) may provide information concerning the shoulder girdle and may rule out rotator cuff tear. Impingement of the brachial plexus may be visualized especially with provocative maneuvers in severe cases using MRI [24].

The purpose of provocative test is to elicit the symptoms of thoracic outlet syndrome by compressing the clavicular costal space. Most provocative tests rely on compression of the axillary artery and, therefore, may not be reliable as an indicator of neurogenic thoracic outlet syndrome. There are four maneuvers that may be included in the evaluation of patient complaining of thoracic outlet syndrome type symptoms. Combining these tests with pressure in the supraclavicular fossa may increase the diagnostic yield.

Adson's maneuver: The patient's arm is down by the side, and the head is turned toward symptomatic side. While the patient inhales and performs a Valsalva, the radial pulse is monitored.

Halsted maneuver: The patient stands with the shoulders backward and downward in a military posture. The radial pulse is again monitored.

Wright's maneuver: Involves shoulder hyperabduction to 180° with the elbows flexed, again monitoring the radial pulse.

Roos' test: Involves rapid opening and closing of the hand for 3 min while the arm is abducted at 90° and externally rotated with the elbow flexed at 90°. Reproduction of the patient's symptoms is considered a positive test.

Tinel's sign involves eliciting paresthesias at the site of nerve compression by applying 4–6 taps with the examiner's digit. The sensation of tingling is a positive sign. The test may be performed over the supraclavicular fossa. Pain or tenderness is not considered a positive sign.

Somatosensory evoked potentials (SSEPs) allow for proximal testing of the brachial plexus. Results have been mixed with some investigators demonstrating 74 % of thoracic outlet patients with an abnormal SSEP [25]. While others have not found these measurements to be useful [26], nerve conduction velocities are useful in determining distal points of compression. Conduction studies have not been universally accepted as standard criteria for the diagnosis of thoracic outlet syndrome. Normal values using the Krusen-Caldwell technique are:

>72 m/s across thoracic outlet
>55 m/s across elbow
>59 m/s across forearm
>2.5 m/s across wrist

The location of a conduction delay may isolate the location of the nerve compression [27]. Distal sites of compression are commonplace in patients with thoracic outlet syndrome. In a review of 50 patients with TOS, more than 50 % of patients had clinical evidence of carpal and cubital tunnel syndrome [23]. The double-crush concept presumes that a single area of compression may not be sufficient to cause a clinical syndrome. The entire upper extremity should be evaluated for nerve compression.

Venous

The syndrome of venous thoracic outlet obstruction resulting in acute subclavian thrombosis is termed Paget-Schroetter syndrome and is also referred to as effort thrombosis. This syndrome typically manifests as sudden onset of arm swelling in a young healthy individual. A history of recent new or strenuous exercise involving the upper extremities may sometimes be elucidated. Compression of the subclavian vein occurs between the first rib and either hypertrophic or abnormal scalene tendon attachments. Chronic compression of the vein can cause perivenous fibrosis, which may lead to venous obstruction. In some, a hypercoagulable state may be a contributing factor [28].

Diagnosis requires suspicion in a young patient presenting with acute upper extremity edema. Physical exam will reveal venous engorgement and cyanosis. Pulses are often exaggerated due to venous hypertension. Elevation of the limb may reduce the severity of the symptoms. Although, traditionally, venography was used to diagnose subclavian vein, this is often reserved for therapeutic treatments that are often preceded by noninvasive sonographic studies. Ultrasound finding includes non-compressibility, enlargement of the diameter of the vein, hypoechoic material within the vein, and lack of Doppler flow. The ability to compress the subclavian vein itself is limited by the clavicle and chest wall.

Once the diagnosis is made, chest radiography may help determine any bone abnormalities. While venography may direct thrombolytic therapy, it is seldom used as a diagnostic tool alone. Computed tomography or MRI may be used in patients where other etiologies of venous obstruction are being considered.

Arterial

The arterial thoracic outlet syndrome is the rarest form of thoracic outlet syndrome occurring in only 1 %. Patients with arterial thoracic outlet syndrome are often young and healthy with a history of vigorous arm activity. Symptoms include digital ischemia, upper extremity claudication, pallor, paresthesia, and pain in the hand and are the result of subclavian stenosis and embolization. Hand symptoms can mimic Raynaud's syndrome, often delaying diagnosis. Chronic compression of the subclavian artery may lead to fibrosis and stenosis. Poststenotic dilatation and chronic trauma may lead to subclavian aneurysm formation. Mural thrombus may embolize resulting in hand symptoms. A bruit may be auscultated in the supraclavicular fossa. Provocative maneuvers may demonstrate loss of radial pulse, though not a specific finding. Arterial compression with provocative maneuvers produces a decrease in palpable arterial pulses in up to 60 % of healthy, asymptomatic individuals [29]. Arterial thoracic outlet syndrome may also occur concomitantly with the neurogenic form and should be considered in all cases. With a liberal use of arterial imaging, an 82 % rate of arterial pathology in patients treated for thoracic outlet syndrome with known bone abnormalities may be found [30]. Initial evaluation should include bilateral blood pressure measurements. Ultrasound duplex may reveal underlying stenosis or aneurysm. Arteriography is useful during the planning of intervention. Concomitant subclavian artery stent grafting and first rib resection have been described as a successful strategy [31]. Stenting of the subclavian artery without decompression of the thoracic outlet is worth mentioning only to be condemned.

Conservative Management

Nonoperative management is considered to be the initial management, especially in patients with neurogenic symptoms. This holds true in the absence of the rare progressive neurological and vascular pathology related to the syndrome [32, 33]. The approach to the patient should start with modification of aggravating positions and postures. Activities that require heavy lifting, vibrating tools, repetitive motion, and elevation of the limb should be avoided. At night, patients are encouraged to develop sleeping habits with arms on the sides. Education cannot be overemphasized in the symptomatic patient. Physical therapy that addresses postural abnormalities, neural mobility, and muscle imbalance relieves the symptoms in most patients [33]. The success of physical therapy depends on dealing with the brachial plexus nerve compression and muscle imbalance in the cervicoscapular region. Typically, treatment begins with postural correction with stretching exercises to regain normal muscle length. This is followed by strengthening exercises to maintain the new posture. Also, pain and edema relief is very important, and exercises to help with that should be included [34]. Most programs concentrate on neck and shoulder muscle with graded restoration of scapula control [32]. Heat therapy before exercise and icing after is recommended. Conservative treatment has to continue for 4–6 months before surgery is considered in most cases [35]. Once patient starts therapy, he should continue in a stepwise fashion with progression of difficulty. If symptoms recur during treatment, patient should step down on the exercise program to easier exercises.

Other deconditioning factors such as obesity, poor respiratory function, and breast hypertrophy should be addressed. Lindgren et al. published in 1997 their experience after therapy with 119 patients and a follow-up period of 2 years. Eighty-eight percent of patients were satisfied with the outcome of their therapy, and the same number followed through with their exercise throughout the follow-up period [36].

Indications for Surgery

Symptomatic patients unresponsive to postural and positional modalities including physical therapy are candidates for operative decompression. The symptomatic patient includes patient with neurogenic, arterial, or venous symptoms. It is contemplated that patients with effort vein thrombosis should be considered for surgery after the initial episode without any other modality applied. In those patients, immediate thrombolytic therapy followed by early surgical decompression has been shown to be safe and effective while significantly decreasing the duration of disability suffered by patients [37].

Surgical Anatomy

The thoracic cavity communicates with the root of the neck through an opening called the thoracic inlet; however, clinicians call it the thoracic outlet since neurovascular structures emerge from the thorax to enter the neck and upper limbs. It is also called the cervicoaxillary canal. It is the space where compression occurs, resulting in the symptomatic patient. It is divided by the first rib into a proximal space that contains the scalene triangle and the costoclavicular space and a distal space that is basically the axilla. The proximal space is the critical space. In particular, the scalene triangle (which is located between the anterior scalene muscle, middle scalene muscle, and the first rib inferiorly) contains the brachial plexus and the subclavian artery. Both scalene muscles insert on to the first rib. The subclavian vein is anterior to this triangle. Also, it is important to note the presence of the phrenic nerve on the anterior surface of the anterior scalene muscle and the long thoracic nerve on the posterior surface of the middle scalene. The brachial plexus in the scalene triangle consists of the nerve roots (C5-T1) and the three trunks (upper, middle, and lower). It is surrounded by the axillary sheath which includes the artery as well. Sibson's fascia is a thickening of connective tissue that covers the lung apex, extending from the first rib to the transverse process of the C7 which is in close proximity to the thoracic duct on the left side.

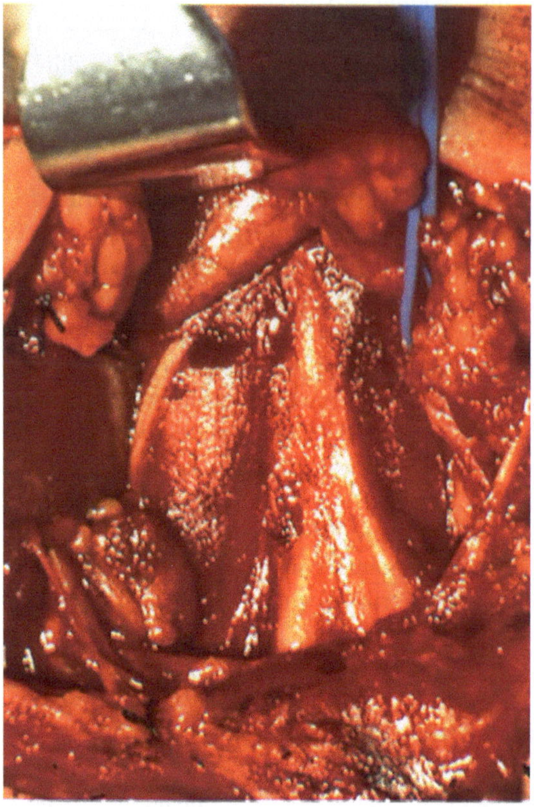

Fig. 20.3 After retracting the fat pad, the brachial plexus is visible; the phrenic nerve is seen overlying the anterior scalene muscle (Reprinted with permission from Pearson and Patterson [38])

Technique

Supraclavicular

The supraclavicular surgical approach has the advantages of direct access to the brachial plexus for neurolysis and the cervical ribs for resection. The patient is positioned in the supine position with a roll between the scapulas and the head extended and slightly rotated to the contralateral side. Avoidance of long-acting paralytics and the use of a nerve stimulator are helpful adjuncts. An incision is made parallel and 1–2 cm above the clavicle. The platysma muscle is divided along the incision. The supraclavicular nerves below the platysmas are spared and mobilized to avoid paresthesia of the area. The omohyoid is divided and the supraclavicular fat pad is elevated laterally. The most lateral portion of the sternocleidomastoid muscle is divided. The phrenic nerve is identified on the anterior surface of the anterior scalene muscle traveling lateral to medial (Fig. 20.3). With minimal handling of the phrenic nerve, the anterior scalene is divided sharply at its insertion on to the first rib. The long thoracic nerve is located on the posterior aspect or within the middle scalene muscle. Care should be taken when sharply detaching the broad fibrous middle scalene attachment to the first rib insertion. The subclavian artery is identified along with the thyrocervical trunk. Traction using vessel loop may facilitate dissection of the artery. The brachial plexus upper, middle, and lower trunks are mobilized with sharp dissection. Fibrous bands of Sibson's fascia are excised. The first rib is then divided using rib shears. The anterior half of the first rib is removed using rongeurs to the level of its insertion onto the manubrium. The

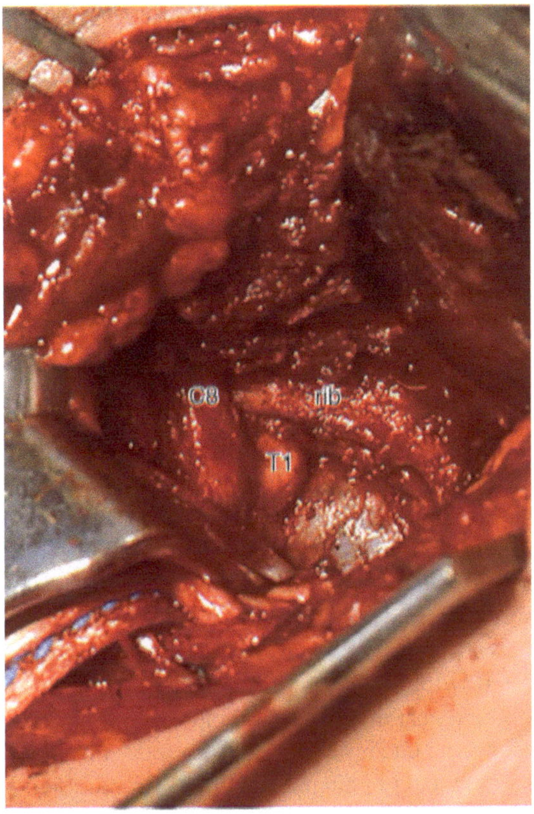

Fig. 20.4 Careful dissection will reveal the C8 root which passes above and the T1 root which passes below the first rib (Reprinted with permission from Pearson and Patterson [38])

posterior half of the first rib is removed in similar fashion to the transverse process. Care must be taken to not injure the C8 root which passes above and the T1 root which passes below the first rib as shown in Fig. 20.4. The pleural dome may be opened to allow drainage into the chest and prevent any hematoma formation in the neck. A Jackson-Pratt® small drain is placed through a counter incision. The sternocleidomastoid is re-approximated along with the platysma and skin.

This is the approach preferred by the authors as it allows direct visualization of the nerves and allows adequate neurolysis of the brachial plexus. By extending the incision medially and dividing the manubrium as described by Grunenwald et al., it provides excellent exposure of the subclavian vessels for venolysis and roof patch angioplasty in cases of Paget-Schroetter syndrome [39, 40].

Transaxillary

The transaxillary approach was first reported by Roos and popularized by Urschel and Razzuk [41, 42]. The advantages of this approach include a cosmetic incision and direct access to the peripheral subclavian vein. Accessing and performing complete neurolysis of the brachial plexus may be compromised by this approach. The patient is placed in a decubitus position, with the ipsilateral arm draped in to the field to allow manipulation throughout the case. The traction is applied to the ipsilateral arm either by an apparatus or an assistant. Hyperextension should be avoided to prevent brachial injury. The incision for the transaxillary approach is located below the axillary hairline, transversely between the pectoralis major muscle anteriorly and the latissimus dorsi muscle posteriorly. Dissection is carried down to the chest wall. Superiorly along the chest wall, the first rib is identified. The brachial artery may be palpated and identified along with the nerve as they exit the thoracic outlet. The first rib is dissected using a periosteal elevator until the anterior scalene muscle is identified. The vein and artery are protected by a right-angle clamp around the anterior scalene muscle. The anterior scalene is divided at its insertion on the first rib. The pleural surface of the first rib is freed, avoiding a defect in the pleural and associated pneumothorax. A section of first rib is then removed. The anterior portion of the rib is removed by dividing the costoclavicular ligament. The anterior portion of the first rib is removed to the level of the manubrium. The posterior portion of the first rib requires careful dissection of the middle scalene and the intimately associated C8-T1 brachial plexus roots. Removal of the posterior portion of the rib often requires reduction with rongeurs until the transverse process is reached. Once the rib is removed, accessory adhesions may be freed from the inferior surface of the brachial plexus. The vein may be exposed more meticulously. In the case of venous thoracic outlet syndrome, vein patch angioplasty is possible from this location.

Thoracoscopic

Thoracoscopic first rib resection has been reported in the literature without widespread use. We do not perform this procedure; however, it has been described by Ohtsuka et al. in 1999 [43]. This involves placing the patient in the lateral decubitus position and double-lumen intubation. It also involves special endoscopic instruments (endoscopic drill, endoscopic elevators, and rongeurs). Three 10-mm incisions are used, one lower for the camera port and two higher placed in the third intercostal space and the fifth intercostal space, for the use of working instruments. The pleura is incised over the first rib and the intercostal muscles detached. The vein, artery, and brachial plexus are identified. They are freed from the first rib using blunt dissection with elevators. Then the endoscopic drill is used to transect the rib while protecting the neurovascular structures by placing the elevator behind the rib. The scalene muscles are taken off the first rib by removing both the bone and periosteal tissue from the muscle attachments. The rib is removed through a port, and then the resected ends are trimmed using a rongeur. The area is irrigated, no drain is left, and the incisions closed [43]. This technology has not been utilized in a widespread fashion, and long-term results or outcomes have not been compared to other standard open procedures. Thus, further studies and experience with this technique are needed. Recommendation for using this procedure cannot be made at this time.

Complications

In general, the surgical approach to treatment of thoracic outlet syndrome is safe as reported by most series. Complications are mostly related to injury to surrounding structures and long-term pain and sensory issues. The more significant injuries are those to major neurovascular structures; however, they are infrequent and the more common injuries are to the smaller diameter nerves such as long thoracic and phrenic nerve [33]. Incidence is reported as high as 11 %; however, most of those cases were temporary resolving in few months [44]. Also, injury to the sensory nerves, intercostal brachial nerve in the transaxillary approach and supraclavicular nerve in the supraclavicular approach, is reported by most patients which could be temporary or permanent.

Pneumothorax is another potential complication with violation of the pleura that might require evacuation [45]. Thoracic duct injuries are also reported and should be suspected with pleural effusion and draining wounds [37].

Postoperative hematoma could lead to compression of the nerve structures leading to injury; some people advocate opening the pleura to prevent this complication [33].

Long-term pain complaints are common, and this could be related to scar tissue, poor post-op physical therapy, or even poor patient selection. Patients presenting with neurogenic symptoms to begin with might require secondary intervention like repeating physical therapy, Botox injections for chemo-denervation, and muscle relaxation and/or pain management referral more often compared to other presentations [45]. Even sympathectomy has been described for postoperative causalgia in very rare cases [37]. So patient selection and correct diagnosis cannot be overemphasized.

Recurrence of thoracic outlet syndrome could be related to inadequate resection of the first rib [46].

Results

The lack of randomized control trials and the variety of treatment methodologies make analysis of the data difficult. The use of combined thrombolysis followed by decompression of the thoracic outlet is likely the best approach. This may result in 87 % symptom relief in long-term follow-up [47]. This was despite a 64 % reocclusion rate. There is no role for stenting of the venous obstruction without decompression of the thoracic outlet [48]. External compression of the stent and repetitive motions within the area may lead to stent fracture or restenosis.

References

1. Hornberger J, et al. Recognition, diagnosis, and treatment of primary focal hyperhidrosis. J Am Acad Dermatol. 2004;51(2):274–86.
2. Ro KM, et al. Palmar hyperhidrosis: evidence of genetic transmission. J Vasc Surg. 2002;35(2):382–6.
3. Goh CL. Aluminum chloride hexahydrate versus palmar hyperhidrosis. Evaporimeter assessment. Int J Dermatol. 1990;29(5):368–70.
4. Holzle E, Alberti N. Long-term efficacy and side effects of tap water iontophoresis of palmoplantar hyperhidrosis – the usefulness of home therapy. Dermatologica. 1987;175(3):126–35.
5. Dahl JC, Glent-Madsen L. Treatment of hyperhidrosis manuum by tap water iontophoresis. Acta Derm Venereol. 1989;69(4):346–8.
6. Naumann M, Lowe NJ. Botulinum toxin type A in treatment of bilateral primary axillary hyperhidrosis: randomised, parallel group, double blind, placebo controlled trial. BMJ. 2001;323(7313):596–9.
7. Vorkamp T, et al. Hyperhidrosis: evolving concepts and a comprehensive review. Surgeon. 2010;8(5):287–92.
8. Wait SD, et al. Thoracoscopic sympathectomy for hyperhidrosis: analysis of 642 procedures with special attention to Horner's syndrome and compensatory hyperhidrosis. Neurosurgery. 2010;67(3):652–6; discussion 656–7.
9. Wait SD, et al. Biportal thoracoscopic sympathectomy for palmar hyperhidrosis in adolescents. J Neurosurg Pediatr. 2010;6(2):183–7.
10. Inan K, et al. Thoracic endoscopic surgery for hyperhidrosis: comparison of different techniques. Thorac Cardiovasc Surg. 2008;56(4):210–3.
11. Katara AN, et al. Comparing T2 and T2-T3 ablation in thoracoscopic sympathectomy for palmar hyperhidrosis: a randomized control trial. Surg Endosc. 2007;21(10):1768–71.
12. Baumgartner FJ, Toh Y. Severe hyperhidrosis: clinical features and current thoracoscopic surgical management. Ann Thorac Surg. 2003;76(6):1878–83.
13. Ojimba TA, Cameron AE. Drawbacks of endoscopic thoracic sympathectomy. Br J Surg. 2004;91(3):264–9.
14. Gossot D, et al. Early complications of thoracic endoscopic sympathectomy: a prospective study of 940 procedures. Ann Thorac Surg. 2001;71(4):1116–9.
15. Asking B, Svartholm E. Degeneration activity: a transient effect following sympathectomy for hyperhidrosis. Eur J Surg Suppl. 1994;572:41–2.
16. Licht PB, Pilegaard HK. Severity of compensatory sweating after thoracoscopic sympathectomy. Ann Thorac Surg. 2004;78(2):427–31.
17. Assalia A, et al. Thoracoscopic sympathectomy for primary palmar hyperhidrosis: resection versus transection – a prospective trial. World J Surg. 2007;31(10):1976–9; discussion 1980–1.
18. Herbst F, et al. Endoscopic thoracic sympathectomy for primary hyperhidrosis of the upper limbs. A critical analysis and long-term results of 480 operations. Ann Surg. 1994;220(1):86–90.
19. Dumont P. Side effects and complications of surgery for hyperhidrosis. Thorac Surg Clin. 2008;18(2):193–207.
20. Dumont P, Denoyer A, Robin P. Long-term results of thoracoscopic sympathectomy for hyperhidrosis. Ann Thorac Surg. 2004;78(5):1801–7.
21. Bachmann K, et al. Thoracoscopic sympathectomy for palmar and axillary hyperhidrosis: four-year outcome and quality of life after bilateral 5-mm dual port approach. Surg Endosc. 2009;23(7):1587–93.
22. Sanders RJ, Haug CE. Thoracic outlet syndrome: a common sequela of neck injuries, vol. xx. Philadelphia: Lippincott; 1991. 348 p.
23. Novak CB, Mackinnon SE, Patterson GA. Evaluation of patients with thoracic outlet syndrome. J Hand Surg Am. 1993;18(2):292–9.
24. Aralasmak A, et al. MR imaging findings in brachial plexopathy with thoracic outlet syndrome. AJNR Am J Neuroradiol. 2010;31(3):410–7.
25. Machleder HI, et al. Somatosensory evoked potentials in the assessment of thoracic outlet compression syndrome. J Vasc Surg. 1987;6(2):177–84.
26. Komanetsky RM, et al. Somatosensory evoked potentials fail to diagnose thoracic outlet syndrome. J Hand Surg Am. 1996;21(4):662–6.
27. Caldwell JW, Crane CR, Krusen EM. Nerve conduction studies: an aid in the diagnosis of the thoracic outlet syndrome. South Med J. 1971;64(2):210–2.
28. Flinterman LE, et al. Current perspective of venous thrombosis in the upper extremity. J Thromb Haemost. 2008;6(8):1262–6.
29. Gergoudis R, Barnes RW. Thoracic outlet arterial compression: prevalence in normal persons. Angiology. 1980;31(8):538–41.
30. Criado E, Berguer R, Greenfield L. The spectrum of arterial compression at the thoracic outlet. J Vasc Surg. 2010;52(2):406–11.
31. Malliet C, et al. Endovascular stent-graft and first rib resection for thoracic outlet syndrome complicated by an aneurysm of the subclavian artery. Acta Chir Belg. 2005;105(2):194–7.
32. Watson LA, Pizzari T, Balster S. Thoracic outlet syndrome part 2: conservative management of thoracic outlet. Man Ther. 2010;15(4):305–14.
33. Mackinnon SE, Novak CB. Thoracic outlet syndrome. Curr Probl Surg. 2002;39(11):1070–145.
34. Crosby CA, Wehbe MA. Conservative treatment for thoracic outlet syndrome. Hand Clin. 2004;20(1):43–9, vi.
35. Kenny RA, et al. Thoracic outlet syndrome: a useful exercise treatment option. Am J Surg. 1993;165(2):282–4.
36. Lindgren KA. Conservative treatment of thoracic outlet syndrome: a 2-year follow-up. Arch Phys Med Rehabil. 1997;78(4):373–8.

37. Barkhordarian S. First rib resection in thoracic outlet syndrome. J Hand Surg Am. 2007;32(4):565–70.
38. Pearson FG, Patterson GA. Pearson's thoracic and esophageal surgery. 3rd ed. Philadelphia: Churchill Livingstone/Elsevier; 2008.
39. Grunenwald D, Spaggiari L. Transmanubrial osteomuscular sparing approach for apical chest tumors. Ann Thorac Surg. 1997;63(2):563–6.
40. Molina JE, Hunter DW, Dietz CA. Protocols for Paget-Schroetter syndrome and late treatment of chronic subclavian vein obstruction. Ann Thorac Surg. 2009;87(2):416–22.
41. Roos DB. Transaxillary approach for first rib resection to relieve thoracic outlet syndrome. Ann Surg. 1966;163(3):354–8.
42. Urschel Jr HC, Razzuk MA. Neurovascular compression in the thoracic outlet: changing management over 50 years. Ann Surg. 1998;228(4):609–17.
43. Ohtsuka T, Wolf RK, Dunsker SB. Port-access first-rib resection. Surg Endosc. 1999;13(9):940–2.
44. Sharp WJ, et al. Long-term follow-up and patient satisfaction after surgery for thoracic outlet syndrome. Ann Vasc Surg. 2001;15(1):32–6.
45. Chang DC, et al. Surgical intervention for thoracic outlet syndrome improves patient's quality of life. J Vasc Surg. 2009;49(3):630–5; discussion 635–7.
46. Mingoli A, et al. Long-term outcome after transaxillary approach for thoracic outlet syndrome. Surgery. 1995;118(5):840–4.
47. Machleder HI. Thrombolytic therapy and surgery for primary axillosubclavian vein thrombosis: current approach. Semin Vasc Surg. 1996;9(1):46–9.
48. Lee JT, et al. Long-term thrombotic recurrence after nonoperative management of Paget-Schroetter syndrome. J Vasc Surg. 2006;43(6):1236–43.

Hemodialysis Access Creation and Maintenance

21

William C. Jennings and Sidney M. Glazer

Abstract

Approximately 350,000 Americans with end-stage renal disease receive hemodialysis therapy with annual Medicare costs over $23 billion.

Individuals with an arterial venous fistula (AVF) have lower mortality, morbidity, and costs when compared to patients with central catheters and grafts. AVF rates have increased dramatically over the last several years. Ultrasound evaluation is important for both preoperative access planning and in postoperative management. Vascular access options and techniques have expanded significantly. Endovascular techniques for access maturation and maintenance have become established as the preferred method of intervention when necessary.

This chapter reviews the many established and new options for hemodialysis vascular access in addition to the diagnosis and treatment of associated complications and issues of long-term maintenance.

Keywords

Arterial venous fistula • AV fistula • AVF • Proximal radial artery Transposition • Steal syndrome • Central venous occlusion • Arterial venous graft • Surveillance • Monitoring • Vascular access • Intervention Angioplasty

Introduction

An arterial venous fistula (AVF) is the recommended permanent vascular access for hemodialysis (HD) by the National Kidney Foundation Kidney Disease Outcomes Quality Initiative (KDOQI), the National Vascular Access Improvement Initiative (Fistula First), and the Society for Vascular Surgery [1–3]. Patients undergoing HD with AVF access have lower mortality rates in addition to fewer complications

W.C. Jennings, M.D., FACS (✉)
Department of Surgery,
University of Oklahoma College of Medicine, Tulsa,
4502 E. 41st Street, Tulsa, OK 74135, USA
e-mail: william-jennings@ouhsc.edu

S.M. Glazer, M.D., FACS
Department of Surgery, University of California, Irvine,
101 The City Drive South, Pavilion III, Orange,
CA 92868-3298, USA
e-mail: sglazer@uci.edu

J.J. Hoballah, A.B. Lumsden (eds.), *Vascular Surgery*, New Techniques in Surgery Series,
DOI 10.1007/978-1-4471-2912-7_21,

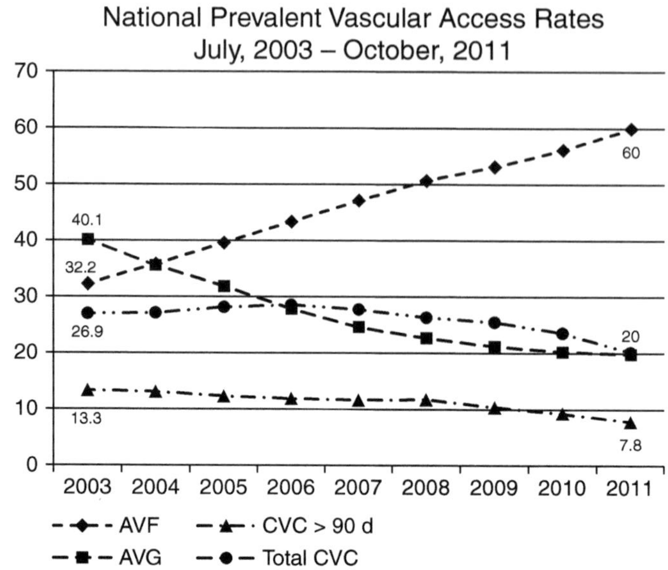

Fig. 21.1 Data shown from the [2]. Vascular access reported for patients in the United States. *AVF* arteriovenous fistula, *AVG* arteriovenous graft, *CVC > 90d* catheter present >90 days, *total CVC* all patients with catheter access

and hospitalizations, leading to lower overall costs when compared to individuals with central vein catheters (CVC) or arteriovenous grafts (AVG) [4–8]. Individuals with autogenous access have lower circulating levels of inflammatory mediators such as serum C-reactive protein, tumor necrosis factor, and others, when compared to patients with CVCs or AVGs [9, 10]. The United States population is both expanding and aging with anticipated increasing need for HD services [11, 12]. The number of patients new to HD increased 9.8 % yearly from 1996 to 2003. After accounting for population growth, the rate of dialysis initiation increased by 57 % during this time period [13, 14]. However, since 2003, the increasing incidence of patients starting HD has slowed to 3.6 % in 2009 compared to 2008. Prevalence of dialysis patients at the end of 2009 was 398,861. The mean age and percentage with diabetes for prevalent HD patients are expected to continue increasing in future years [15].

Despite the general consensus that permanent vascular access is superior to CVC-based dialysis, approximately 80 % of new HD patients start dialysis with a catheter. Total CVC use in the United States hemodialysis population has slowly decreased since 2006, although the percentage is higher than many other developed countries (Fig. 21.1) [16–18]. CVC-based HD access places patients at increased risk for complications such as infection, central venous stenosis or occlusion, mechanical catheter dysfunction, thrombosis, and worse subsequent AVF outcomes [1, 2, 19–21]. The higher infection rate associated with a CVC leads to more procedures and increased morbidity and mortality risk compared to individuals receiving dialysis by an AVG or AVF [1, 19–23]. Bradbury et al. reported conversion to a permanent access (AVF or AVG) from a CVC was associated with a lower adjusted mortality hazard ratio of 0.69 (95 % confidence interval, 0.55–0.85). These findings were persistent across demographic groups and facilities. Vascular access conversion to a CVC from an AVG or AVF was associated with an adjusted mortality hazard ratio of 1.81 (95 % confidence interval, 1.22–2.68) [24]. When CVC access is necessary, a right internal jugular vein tunneled catheter has the lowest complication rate. Subclavian vein catheter placement should be avoided when at all possible due to the high rate of subsequent central venous stenosis and occlusion. The availability of ultrasound guidance for placement of CVCs is important, improving placement safety and catheter function [25].

Total Medicare costs rose 7 % in 2007 to $410 billion. CKD affects an estimated 27 million Americans, consuming more than 24 % of current Medicare costs [11]. At the current rate of increase, Medicare costs for CKD are expected to double by the year 2030 [11]. End-stage renal disease (ESRD) Medicare costs increased 6.1 % in 2007 to $23.9 billion involving more than 430,000 patients [16]. Foley and Collins analyzing the 2006 United States Renal Data System (USRDS) Annual Data Report found Medicare costs for patients with ESRD increased 57 % between 1999 and 2004 [26]. Dialysis access plays an important role in these costs. Almost 20 % of the total spending for hemodialysis is involved in vascular access with up to 50 % of hospitalization costs for ESRD in the first year of HD related to access issues [14]. CVCs not only have the greatest health risks for dialysis access, they also have a major cost impact [27]. Among the prevalent hemodialysis population, the most common access-related event is placement of a new CVC, with 0.65 catheter events per year in 2006 for those already using a CVC, 0.24 for those with an AVG, and 0.12 for those with an AVF [16].

AVGs are intermediate in mortality, morbidity, and are associated with higher costs, while AVFs demonstrate the best profile [19]. Medicare costs in 2007 expressed as per person per year for ESRD patients with AVF vascular access were about $60,000, 18–25 % lower than those for patients with a CVC or AVG. Per person per year access event costs were $7,451, $5,960, and $3,194 for individuals with an AVG, CVC, or AVF, respectively [16]. While AVF rates have increased dramatically in the United States during the last several years, improving AVF maturation rates and continuing to decrease the use of CVCs remain important opportunities for dialysis access improvement [2, 8, 17, 22] (Fig. 21.1). The 2009 Annual Renal Data System Report found that infectious hospitalization rates in the hemodialysis population have declined for two successive years, suggesting that complications associated with catheters may be starting to decline [16].

Several systematic and thorough reviews for vascular access options are available including clinical guidelines from the National Kidney Foundation, Fistula First, the Society for Vascular Surgery, and others [1–3, 28]. Most access procedures are accomplished with local anesthesia and sedation or by regional block in an outpatient setting. Autogenous assess operations and interventional procedures generally do not require prophylactic antibiotics [29, 30]. Several authors have reported success in maintaining autogenous vascular access in most or all patients [31–33].

Ultrasound and Contrast Vessel Mapping

Preoperative Planning and Evaluating Postoperative Maturation and Dysfunction

Ultrasound (US) vessel mapping before access creation and postoperatively to evaluate maturation are key elements in planning a successful vascular access as well as increasing the number of functional AVFs established [3, 34, 35]. Direct US examination by the operating surgeon yields the most useful information in our opinion [36, 37]. Venous imaging is accomplished with the patient lying with the back elevated 30°, in a comfortably warm room, and having an arm tourniquet in place. Higher probe frequency and shallow focal depth settings allow excellent imaging for access planning with direct real-time observation of the outflow vein(s) size and compliance, with detection of subtle areas of stenosis, especially at puncture and tributary sites. Accurate venous imaging requires simple interface of the probe with the skin surface through the US gel. The examiner must avoid applying probe pressure to the extremity as even the lightest compression may obscure superficial veins. Arterial imaging evaluates vessel size, calcific disease and flow volume. We also use US briefly just prior to vascular access operations, confirming the surgical plan and mapping the incision site(s) along with key vascular anatomy. The vasodilatation produced by supraclavicular brachial plexus block in the study by Schenk allowed a more distal fistula to be created than planned in 37 % of patients without increasing the failure rate [38].

Preoperative venography is preferred for vessel mapping by some surgeons and generally needed to evaluate the central venous system in patients with a history of multiple central venous catheters, pacemakers, or physical findings suggesting central venous stenosis or obstruction. In patients approaching dialysis, the use of ≤20 ml of contrast which is diluted 1–3× to increase volume is considered a very low risk to remaining renal function [39, 40]. Central venous stenosis is not an absolute contraindication to AVF construction if other options are not available. Arm swelling may not develop, and percutaneous angioplasty is often successful if symptoms arise. Even an occluded central venous lesion with well-developed collateral veins may support a moderately low-flow functional AVF without significant swelling [41].

During the surgical follow-up period and after access maturation, ultrasound evaluation adds important information to physical examination for the vascular access patient, particularly for those patients with AVFs. Ultrasound examination allows evaluation of vein location, size, depth, and AVF flow volume, in addition to mapping the course and marking the optimal AVF cannulation sites prior to use.

Investigation of a nonmaturing, dysfunctional, or steal-related access problems is greatly enhanced by US evaluation in concert with information from the dialysis unit, clinical history, and physical examination. We expect initial cannulation for AVFs in 4–6 weeks and most AVGs in 2–4 weeks. US is important in selecting those patients where initial AVF cannulation is expected to be successful or those where a brief period of continued observation is warranted. Prolonged periods of observation for nonmaturing AVFs should be avoided. US confirms the need for a prompt fistulogram in these patients and guides the interventionalist in planning the procedure [42]. Recent reports suggest US may be used alone for successful access angioplasty imaging in selected patients, without the need for intravenous contrast or fluoroscopy [43]. Physical examination of a dysfunctional access (discussed elsewhere in this chapter) is enhanced by US findings, guiding and selecting the intervention required. Analysis and treatment of steal syndrome is substantially aided by reliable access flow measurement available with most US units.

Radiocephalic Arteriovenous Fistulas

A radiocephalic AVF (RC-AVF) remains the recommended first choice for dialysis access [1–3]. Even in a discussion of new concepts in vascular surgery, this original autogenous dialysis access deserves mention. The first dialysis access AVF was created in 1965 by Kenneth C. Apell at the Veteran's Administration Hospital in Bronx, New York in collaboration with James Cimino and others [44]. It quickly became the gold standard for dialysis access. However, in recent years, the role for RC-AVFs has been the subject of debate with several authors reporting that RC-AVFs often thrombose or fail to mature, leading to frustration among patients, their nephrologists, and surgeons [45–47]. In a review of the author's (WCJ) experience with radiocephalic AVF, >95% functional cumulative patency rate was reported after 2 years follow-up [48]. This success was attributed to careful patient selection, ultrasound mapping, and follow-up with prompt interventions for those fistulas that fail to mature or develop subsequent dysfunction. Angioplasty of calcified forearm arteries can salvage some dysfunctional fistulas [49]. The anastomosis may be end to side, or if a side-to-side configuration is chosen, the distal vein segment should be ligated, directing all access flow into the targeted vein for cannulation and to minimize the risk of hand swelling. A recent report by Shenoy et al. found that the side-to-side anastomosis with ligation of the distal vein to minimize vein twisting reduced overall fistula failure from 40.3 to 16.7% [50]. One of the authors (SMG) utilizes greater mobilization of the radial artery, minimizing the amount of vein dissection. Adjacent venous tributaries may be ligated through the same incision, especially perforating veins that would otherwise diminish blood flow in the planned outflow vein targeted for cannulation.

We feel the key to successful RC-AVF construction is in selecting individuals where good outcomes can be anticipated by preoperative evaluation. These individuals must have a normal arterial examination and an intact palmer arch.

Normal radial artery flow is 20–30 ml/min, and this must increase to 5–600 ml/min within 4–6 weeks. A small and/or calcific and noncompliant radial artery will not support a mature and functional AVF nor maintain adequate flow for AVG patency. Of equal importance is a distensible cephalic or median antebrachial vein, without narrowing throughout the forearm by both physical and ultrasound examinations. A radial artery internal diameter ³ 2.0 mm is generally recommended and the outflow vein should be ³ 2.5 mm for successful RC-AVF construction (48). Both inflow and outflow criteria must be clearly assured to avoid unacceptable failure rates. This selective approach may appropriately exclude up to 90% of patients from RC-AVFs. Ultrasound examination is particularly important in identifying individuals not suited for RC-AVFs and aids in identifying a more suitable proximal autogenous access location. Simply "exploring the wrist" and constructing an AVF with poor vessels leads to prolonged catheter use, additional procedures, and eventual access failure and abandonment.

Antecubital and Bidirectional Flow Arteriovenous Fistulas

The RC-AVF remains our first choice for dialysis access when feasible; however, our most common operation is an AVF constructed in the antecubital fossa, utilizing the proximal radial artery (PRA) for inflow when possible [51–54]. This operation is generally performed through a longitudinal incision just below the crease of the elbow. The lateral antebrachial cutaneous nerve is usually located just lateral to the deep communicating (perforating) vein but may course medial to it. The radial artery is easily mobilized and offers adequate inflow with lower risk of steal syndrome. PRA-AVFs generally have a lower flow rate potential than brachial artery fistulas. When the brachial artery is used for inflow, care should be taken to limit the anastomosis length to <75% of the diameter of the brachial artery to minimize the risk of steal syndrome [55]. The antecubital location offers many options for AVF construction. This site is generally the confluence of the deep communicating (perforating) vein, median cephalic, median cubital, and median antebrachial veins (Fig. 21.2). The PRA assumes a more anterior position at this location and is easily mobilized for AVF construction. Direct inflow into the upper cephalic vein is available through the median cephalic vein with an anastomosis to the PRA or brachial artery (Fig. 21.3a). The deep communicating vein or the median cubital vein may offer a convenient end-to-side anastomosis for inflow into the upper arm cephalic or retrograde flow into the median antebrachial vein (Fig. 21.3b). The end-to-side configuration is particularly helpful in obese individuals where the inflow vessel may be substantially deeper. The deep communicating vein is continuous with the radial vein adjacent to the PRA and may be incorporated into a convenient branch patch anastomosis (Fig. 21.4). If the deep communicating vein is not used for an AVF anastomosis, it should be ligated to avoid flow into the deep veins instead of the targeted superficial system. The median cubital vein is continuous with the basilic vein and may offer an outflow option for a primary or staged transposition. If not used as the targeted outflow vein, the median

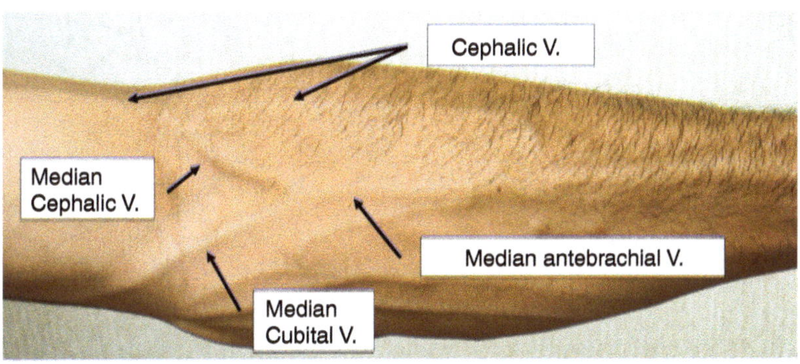

Fig. 21.2 Forearm superficial venous anatomy

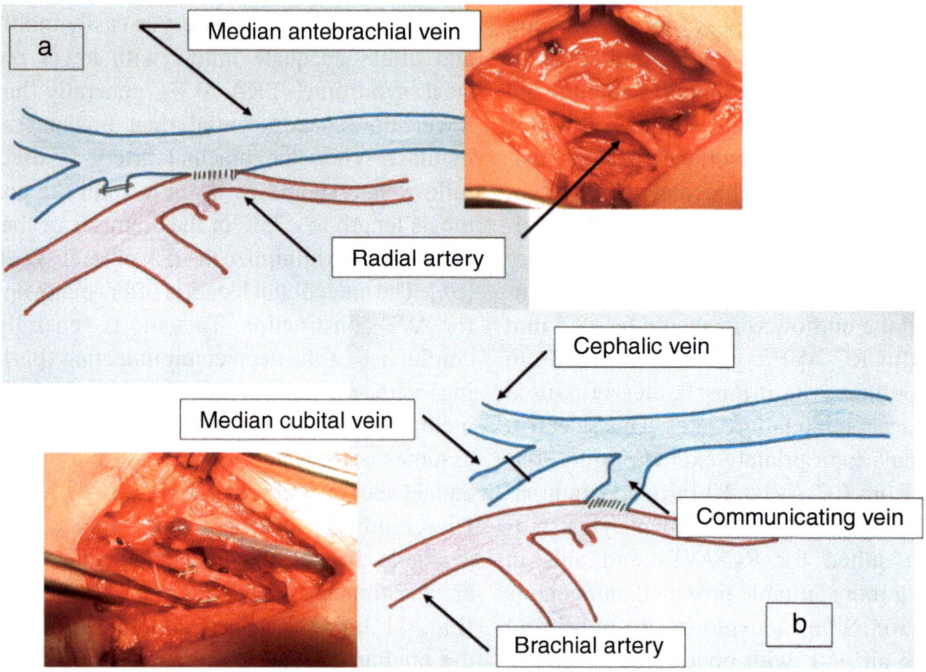

Fig. 21.3 Proximal radial artery inflow arteriovenous fistulas (PRA-AVF). (**a**) Side-to-side anastomosis and (**b**) end-to-side anastomosis. Photos with corresponding schematic images show bidirectional vascular access flow (*dashed lines*). Severe arterial occlusive disease may uncommonly involve the PRA. Creating the anastomosis at the bifurcation of the brachial artery, proximal to the recurrent radial artery (muscular branch), will gain adequate inflow in these patients (From Jennings [52]. Copyright © (2006) American Medical Association. All rights reserved)

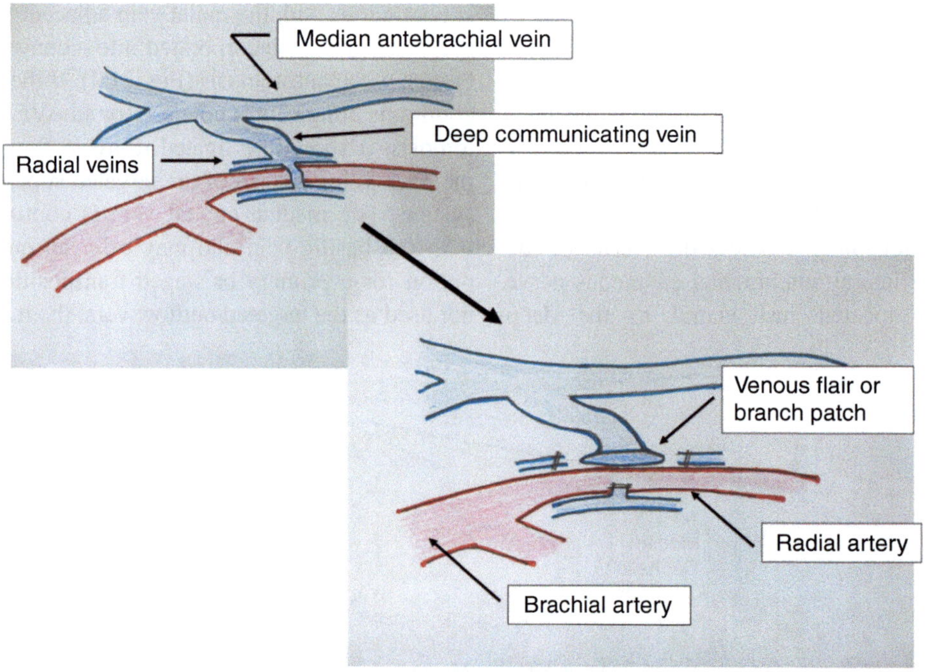

Fig. 21.4 Schematic image of an end-to-side PRA-AVF showing the deep communicating (perforating) vein as it joins one of the paired radial venae comitantes. The divided radial vein branch is incorporated into the communicating vein, creating a broad flair or branch patch for the anastomosis to the artery

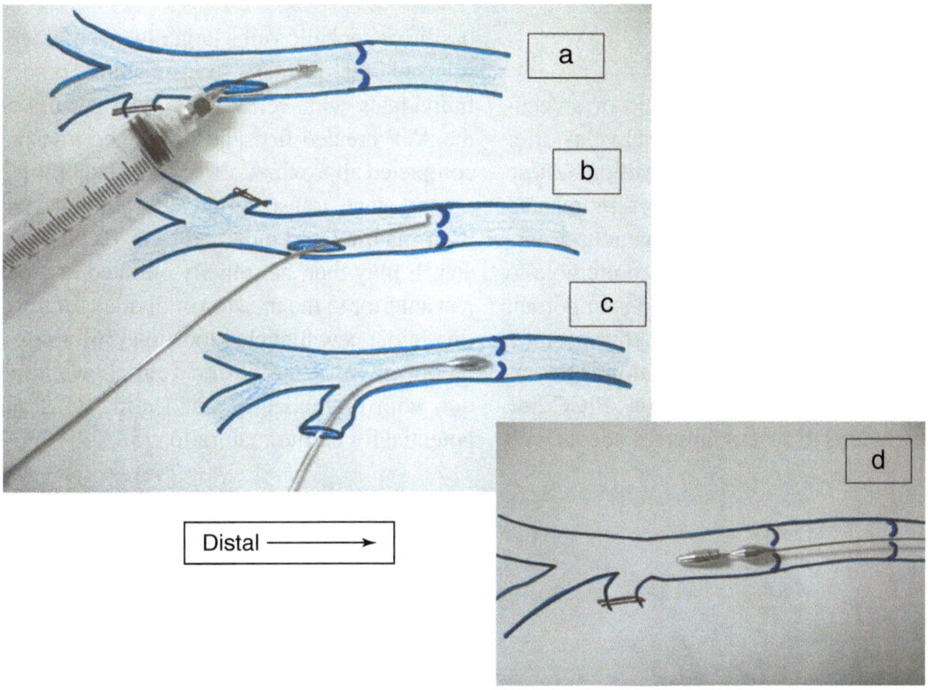

Fig. 21.5 Schematic images of methods for disrupting venous valves are shown, gaining retrograde AVF flow. (**a**) Titis needle, (**b**) antegrade valvulotome, or (**c**) vessel probe may be passed through the venous opening for the planned AVF anastomosis. (**d**) In situ retrograde valvulotome passed from a small vein at the wrist

cubital vein should also be ligated or restricted to avoid competitive AVF outflow resulting in non-maturation of the planned access. This outflow planning concept should be emphasized. It is critically important for prompt access maturation that access outflow be directed to the veins targeted for cannulation and outflow veins not part of the AVF circuit are ligated.

Bidirectional flow is possible in many antecubital fistulas and may be established by disrupting the initial valve(s) using a valvulotome, probe, or other instrument through the valve leaflets under direct vision through the venotomy prior to constructing the AVF anastomosis [46]. Bidirectional flow may be helpful in several situations. These include not only the potential for dialysis sites to develop by retrograde flow into the forearm but also improvement in flow to maintain patency in marginal fistulas and offering sites for intervention if needed. Smaller veins may develop over time should the forearm site occlude with the potential for uninterrupted dialysis access without catheter placement should other outflow braches become occluded.

Figure 21.5 shows methods for disrupting venous valves, gaining retrograde AVF flow. Interrupting the first valve may be all that is necessary and confirmed by ease of irrigation distally. The initial valve is often quite close to the venotomy, and if located at the anastomotic site, the leaflets should be excised. Any tributary in the area that is planned for ligation can be opened first and serve as an entry point for valve disruption. A self-centering valvulotome may also be passed through a small vein at the wrist after the anastomosis has been completed (Fig. 21.5d). Forearm cannulation becomes possible in about 65% of patients with bidirectional AVF flow established. Sites in the distal one-third of the forearm may mature but tend to develop stenosis because of the reverse taper of the veins or from previous venipunctures and intravenous catheters. However, the basilic vein is the recipient of most of the distal runoff and may have matured if a revision becomes necessary. Significant venous hypertension with the retrograde fistula is uncommon but can be treated by ligating offending communicating or superficial veins as necessary.

Transposition AV Fistulas

For individuals where a radiocephalic or antecubital direct AVF is not feasible, several veins offer the outflow opportunity for transposition. These include the basilic, brachial, cephalic, femoral, and saphenous veins [56–60]. An autogenous transposition vascular access is generally preferable to placing an AVG [61]. US examination is important to confirm feasibility and plan the transposition procedure in addition to detecting anatomic anomalies or short stenotic segments such as PICC line sites that might lead to access failure. Patients with basilic or cephalic veins larger than 4 mm are often selected for primary transposition procedures. Individuals with veins 2.5–4 mm generally have the AVF created first and the staged transposition completed approximately 4 weeks later [56]. At the second-stage transposition, the outflow vein will have matured and enlarged to 6–10 mm in diameter. It may then be reliably elevated to a position just anterior to the incision or divided for transposition into a new tunneled location [56]. Endoscopic mobilization of the basilic vein allows transposition with dramatically smaller incisions and the potential for earlier maturation [58, 59] (Fig. 21.6).

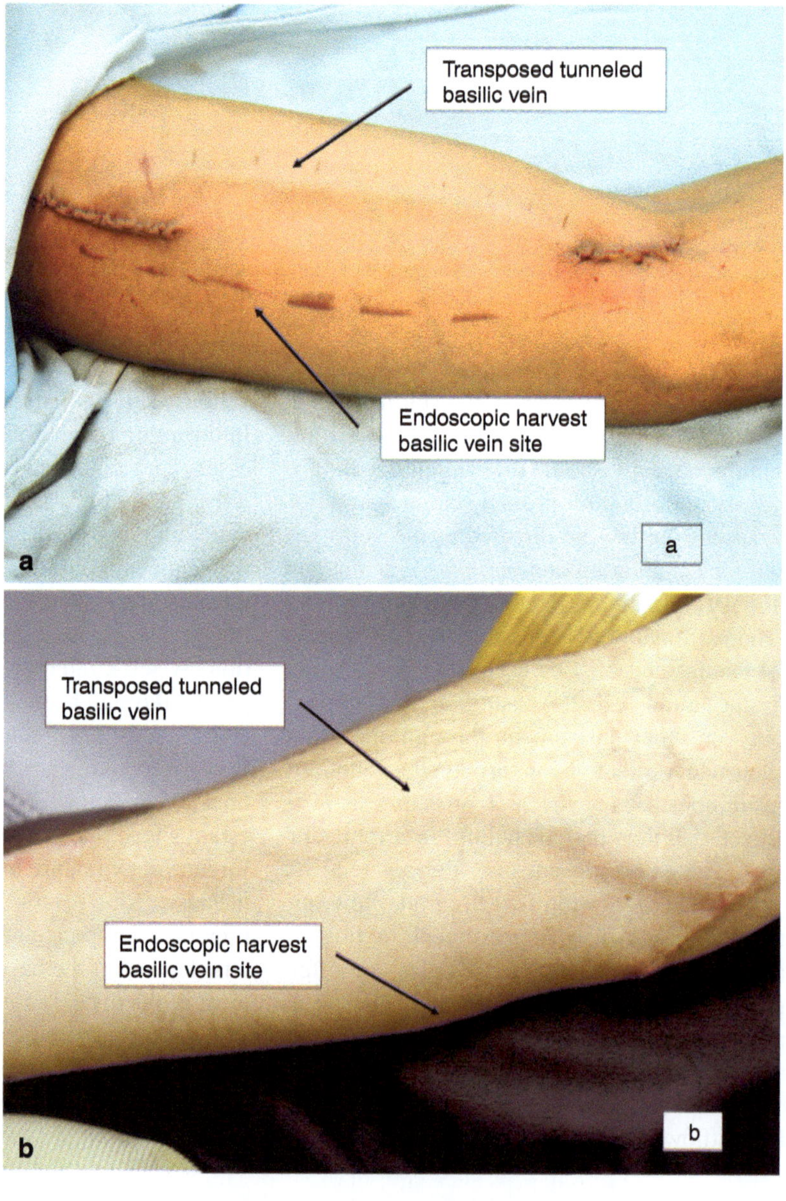

Fig. 21.6 (**a**, **b**) Endoscopic harvest and tunneled transposition AVFs of the arm and forearm basilic veins

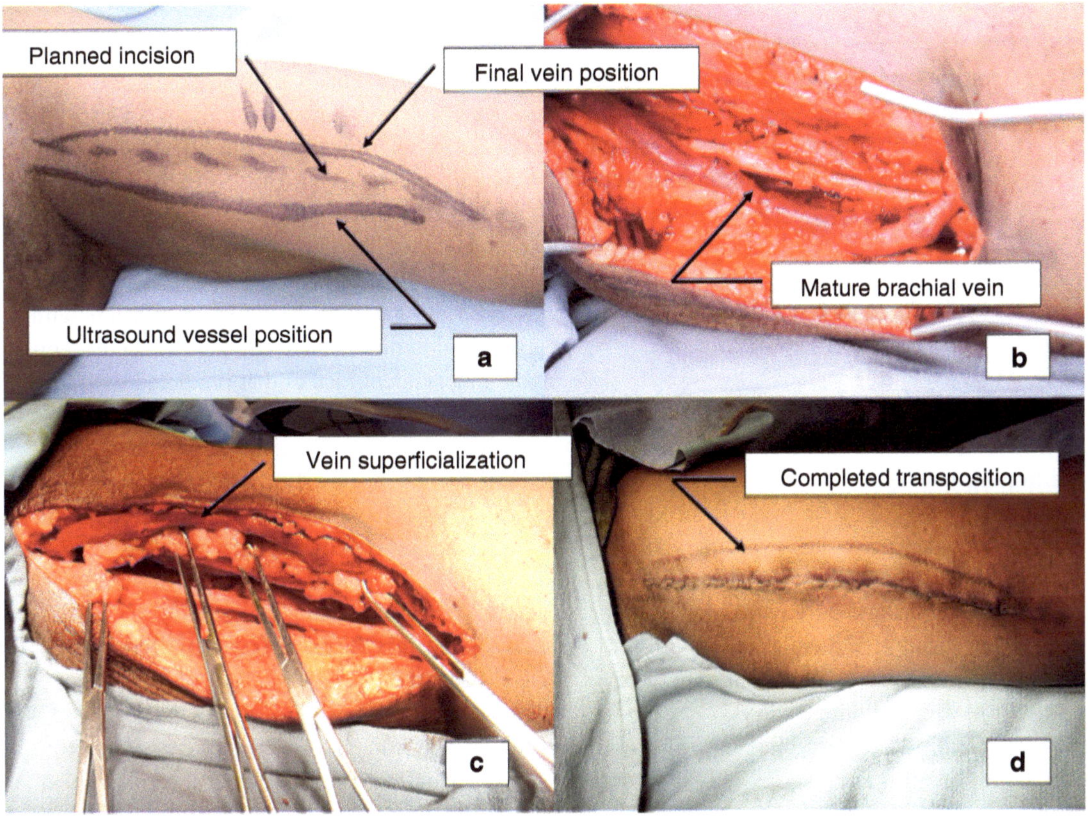

Fig. 21.7 (**a–d**) The second stage of a brachial vein transposition is shown. Arterial inflow was provided by a first-stage proximal radial artery to radial vein AVF created 4 weeks prior to this operation. (**a**) Preoperative ultrasound vessel mapping aids in planning the procedure. (**b**) The mature brachial vein is exposed. (**c**) The brachial vein AVF is superficialized to an anterior position. (**d**) The completed staged AVF transposition

Almost all brachial vein transpositions should be done as staged procedures [57] (Fig. 21.7). We use the proximal radial artery for inflow in the first-stage AVF when possible. Forearm basilic vein transpositions are attractive procedures and appropriate when ultrasound mapping suggests adequate size and a compliant conduit together with adequate arterial inflow. One of the authors (SMG) has used the ulnar artery and forearm basilic vein for AVF access without transposition, the patient flexing the elbow for cannulation. Transposition procedures achieve the new superficial and accessible vein location by tunneling the vein (Fig. 21.6). Superficialization or elevation procedures refer to repositioning the vein under the skin just anterior to the incision, without the need to divide the vein and construct a new anastomosis (Fig. 21.7). We prefer vein tunneling when possible. However, limited vein length found with many staged brachial vein transpositions and some basilic veins will require superficialization with a narrow skin flap created anterior to the incision, avoiding cannulation through the surgical scar. Alternatively, a concave skin incision is made with a straight tunnel anterior to the bed of the vein. Both techniques require care to avoid rotation, kinking, or acute angulation as the vein is repositioned from its native location.

We find the great saphenous vein (GSV) to be generally less distensible and compliant than other veins and require a 6-mm minimum diameter for use as a transposition or translocation. The GSV can be wrapped around a 24-F chest tube to create an 8-mm-diameter spiral vein graft, but the suturing is long and tedious. Femoral vein transposition AVFs have been found to offer reliable vascular access; however, they are a major undertaking [62]. Care must be taken to avoid steal syndrome as outlined by Gradman et al. [62, 63]. The anastomosis should be limited in size and in accordance with the dimensions of the inflow artery [55]. This operation carries increased morbidity and requires hospitalization and general anesthetic [62–64].

Hemodialysis Access for Older Patients

The United States population aged 65 and over is expected to double by 2035 with more than 70 million people aged 65 years or older [65]. Chronic kidney disease and dialysis needs are increasing in older individuals and at a higher rate than for the nonelderly population [66, 67]. Many authors report autogenous access in older individuals is feasible and reliable [31, 68–74]. Other investigators found less than satisfactory results with AVFs and suggest AVGs should be used more often in the elderly patient [75, 76]. A recent review of 461 autogenous access operations in patients older than 65 years of age found a 94 % functional patency rate at 2-year follow-up [74]. For those elderly individuals in need of permanent dialysis access, constructing a relatively lower flow PRA-AVF and planning a single outflow vessel such as the upper arm cephalic vein for earliest possible maturation may be the best initial choice [72, 74]. The upper arm cephalic vein is often larger, and in elderly patients with thin and fragile forearm skin and soft tissue, targeting this AVF conduit into the upper arm will likely help meet the goal of prompt and successful cannulation.

Debate continues as to the appropriate treatment for the more elderly and frail patients with ESRD in considering dialysis therapy and mode of vascular access. Expected survival times may affect dialysis decisions in these fragile patients. Peritoneal dialysis has generally been considered a poor option for these individuals. However, hemodialysis also substantially impacts their quality of life. Both CVCs and permanent vascular access have potential risks for access morbidity and cardiac complications. The answer to "What is the best medical care for fragile, elderly ESRD patients?" is not clear [77, 78]. It might be "best medical care without dialysis," and if dialysis is elected, then possible CVC vascular access may be appropriate for the relatively small subgroup of extremely frail and elderly patients with short life expectancy. A clinical scoring system devised by Couchoud et al. was able to predict 6-month prognosis in older patients when starting dialysis [79]. The system was used as a tool to facilitate discussion with patients and families faced with these difficult decisions. Independent factors that predicted mortality at 6 months were low BMI, diabetes, congestive heart failure (Stages III–IV), peripheral vascular disease (Stages III–IV), dysrhythmia, active malignancy, severe behavioral disorder, impaired mobility, and unplanned dialysis [79].

Hemodialysis Access for Children and Adolescents

Although peritoneal dialysis is often the first choice for children with ESRD, the majority of pediatric patients in the United States are maintained on hemodialysis [80]. Autogenous access has been increasingly recognized as not only feasible but accompanied by high success rates for these children [37, 51, 81–83]. The same sequence of access operation options from the adult literature works well in children. As in adults, a radiocephalic AVF is our first choice but may not be feasible. Antecubital AVFs using the PRA when possible offer reliable long-term permanent access. Transposition AVFs using the basilic vein in addition to the femoral and brachial veins have been used successfully by several authors, both as primary and staged procedures [81, 84].

Using an interrupted as opposed to running suture technique for access creation may be important in smaller children, allowing the anastomosis to enlarge as the patient grows. An interrupted suture anastomosis might also result in later enlargement of the AVF with the potential for later development of a high-flow access and steal syndrome or cardiac issues. Using a RC-AVF or PRA-AVF should minimize this risk. Interventional options with balloon angioplasty are less commonly needed in children but appear to be equally effective with those in adults. Bourquelot et al. have emphasized microvascular techniques and reported their extensive experience with successful autogenous access even in very small children [85].

Obesity: Functional Hemodialysis Access

The percentage of overweight and obese individuals in the United States is increasing dramatically [86]. Obesity in the hemodialysis patient often makes the permanent vascular access options more challenging due to outflow vein depth. Fistula First suggests venous outflow cannulation sites should be within 6 mm of the skin level for reliable access [2]. For obese individuals, this cannulation depth recommendation may be accomplished through vein elevation, transposition, or translocation [87–89]. However, these operations require outflow vein length be expended both to gain the superficial position required for cannulation and then return of the vein to the deeper arterial inflow level. We prefer a relatively new procedure, lipectomy, excising the subcutaneous tissue overlying the AVF outflow vein [90, 91]. We have found lipectomy to be successful in allowing prompt and reliable cannulation of autogenous access in obese individuals. The operation is relatively simple and has been described in both the forearm and the upper arm [90, 91] (Fig. 21.8). The lipectomy procedure is appealing because the venous conduit is left undisturbed in its native path and venous side branches are left intact, possibly adding to access longevity if central venous or cephalic arch occlusion/stenosis later compromises the major outflow channel. We generally perform the lipectomy as a staged procedure 3–4 weeks after the AVF is created. Utilizing two and occasional three transverse incisions over the targeted veins is the preferred technical approach. Planning the operation and incision sites is aided by US examination by the operating surgeon. A drain may or may not be necessary, and access cannulation is generally allowed at 3–4 weeks. Liposuction is another option that may become more common in the future for gaining reliable AVF cannulation sites in obese patients [92].

Novel Approaches to Vascular Access Creation

Extending Vein Length for Transposition AVFs

We have constructed successful AVF transpositions combining segments of brachial and basilic veins or utilizing both brachial veins [93]. These procedures have all been constructed as staged transpositions with a proximal radial artery-brachial vein inflow as the first stage in most patients. After the planned first-stage AVF has matured over a 4–6-week period, US examination during the follow-up period generally demonstrates a single outflow vein that is enlarged throughout the length of the upper arm. This targeted brachial or basilic vein becomes suitable for a later staged transposition. We rarely discover that the proximal portion of the targeted outflow vein fails to enlarge. In these patients, a proximal basilic vein segment or both brachial veins have usually matured. Ultrasound was critical in identifying these opportunities to use these large parallel vein segments with an end-to-end anastomosis, gaining the needed additional length for superficialization or tunneling. Both brachial veins may mature and may be mobilized throughout their length. This technique has been particularly helpful in obese individuals. Arm swelling has not been a problem with brachial vein AVFs unless central venous occlusion or stenosis is present, as with any access. Even then, many patients remain free of arm swelling with adequate venous return through collateral veins.

Using Abandoned AVF Mature Vein Conduits

Rarely an AVF is abandoned or ligated due to arm swelling secondary to noncorrectable central venous occlusion with venous hypertension, acute bleeding, or other issues. These AVF outflow veins (often cephalic veins) may be well matured and are often lengthy and quite tortuous. The mature veins may offer an ideal conduit for translocation to the contralateral arm or lower

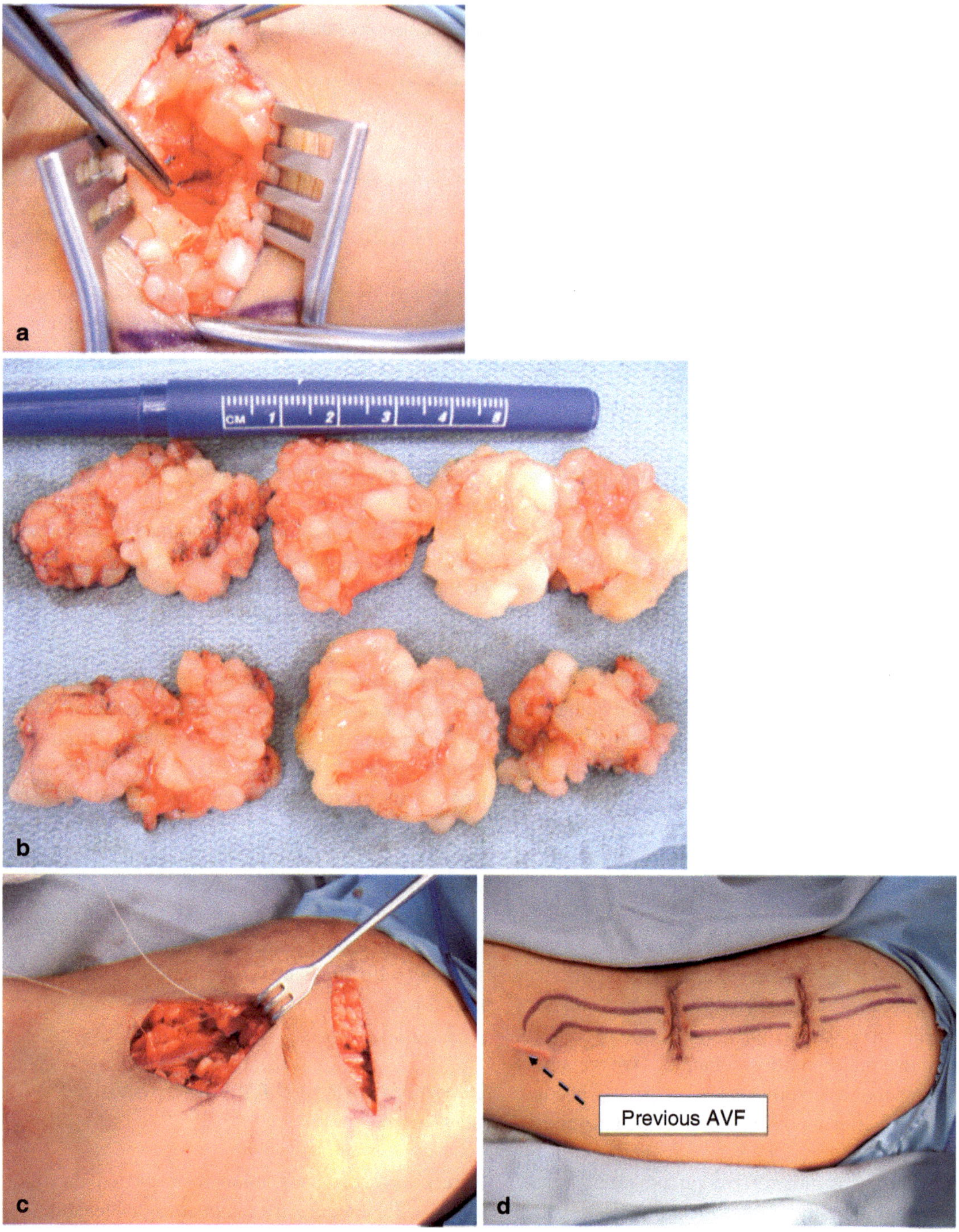

Fig. 21.8 Lipectomy technique: (**a**) The distended cephalic vein is exposed by opening the superficial investing fascia longitudinally. (**b**) Adipose tissue specimens excised in segments. (**c**) After lipectomy, deep dermal tissue is sutured to the opened superficial investing fascia. (**d**) The completed lipectomy procedure (From Barnard et al. [91]. © Copyright Elsevier)

extremity. These veins offer surprising length when mobilized in addition to the well-developed and mature vein wall. After the AVF translocation to the opposite arm or lower extremity, cannulation is usually possible within a few weeks.

Antecubital AVFs with Only Retrograde Venous Outflow

Occasionally, patients will have an adequate median antebrachial vein in the mid forearm; however, vessels at the wrist are not adequate for a successful radiocephalic AV fistula. The vein at the wrist may be too small or the radial artery at the wrist is inadequate for a simple fistula, or both. If an adequate upper arm cephalic vein is not present, these individuals will require a transposition procedure. The surgeon may avoid more extensive procedures and utilize the forearm vein by constructing a reverse flow AVF, creating a proximal radial artery AVF and disrupting the venous valves, allowing forearm access sites to develop [52]. A valvulotome may be utilized if disruption of the initial venous valve is not sufficient to establish retrograde flow as described in the bidirectional flow discussion in this chapter. AVF outflow will be through multiple side channels into the deep venous system and medially into the basilic venous system. The dialysis staff should be instructed for cannulation that the access flow is retrograde and venous return is directed toward the hand. Arm swelling is rare in these individuals unless central venous occlusion is present. If swelling develops a fistulogram with appropriate outflow angioplasty generally resolves the problem. Rarely a large branch into the dorsum of the hand is ligated or occluded by coil insertion.

Proximalization of AVF Inflow in Patients at High Risk for Steal Syndrome

Patients who have severe peripheral vascular disease are at high risk for steal syndrome after creation of a permanent access. Those individuals often have failed access in the opposite or same extremity with a history of ligation for previous steal syndrome; some have amputations, a history of tissue loss, or disability due to ischemia. These patients are usually diabetic, and physical examination confirms significant peripheral vascular disease with lack of distal pulses. Ultrasound may show adequate venous outflow system for autogenous access creation. However, noncompliant and heavily calcified brachial and distal arterial systems are present suggesting a high risk for developing steal syndrome if a new access is constructed. Arteriography in these individuals confirms distal noncorrectable arterial occlusive disease and relatively normal axillary arteries. We have successfully used primary AVF inflow proximalization, creating a functional vascular access and avoiding steal syndrome in these patients at high risk for hand ischemia [94]. The axillary artery inflow procedures utilized either a reversed flow basilic vein transposition with valvulotomy, a reversed basilic vein, a cephalic vein harvested from the forearm and placed in a loop configuration to the axillary artery, or a translocated reversed saphenous vein. In thin patients, a short loop basilic vein AVF based on the proximal brachial or axillary artery can be created without the need to use retrograde AVF outflow. The transposed upper arm cephalic vein can also be looped into the axilla for inflow. In all of these instances, the axillary or proximal brachial artery was used for inflow. This more proximal inflow location has a dramatically larger artery that is relatively free of calcific disease and allows an anastomosis that will not result in steal syndrome following access creation.

Axillary artery inflow with retrograde venous outflow AVFs for high-steal-risk patients works on the established principle of proximalization for the successful treatment of steal syndrome [95] utilizing a significantly larger and compliant artery, relatively free of occlusive disease and avoiding an AVF anastomosis to a small and diseased brachial artery.

Novel Graft Configurations

While we advocate autogenous access in every patient if possible and secondary fistulas whenever feasible, some individuals may require graft placement. For patients with unreconstructable central vein obstruction, an arterial-arterial graft has been reported [96]. The axillary artery can be divided below the clavicle allowing placement of a loop interposition expanded polytetrafluoroethylene (ePTFE) graft. Blood flows of about 250 ml/min can be obtained on dialysis. Higher flows may be obtained when the femoral artery is used, but the risk of serious complications is much higher. For those able to tolerate major thoracic surgery, a subclavian vein to right atrium bypass graft through a sternotomy or right third intercostal space incision has been described when there is a working access upstream to CV occlusion [97]. An axillary-femoral vein ringed graft for decompression of an upper extremity access with venous outflow obstruction has also been successful.

In the unusual situation when an AVF is not feasible in either the forearm or in the arm and antecubital vein AVG outflow options have been exhausted, external ringed or intrawall reinforced graft may be used across the elbow to superficial and deep veins. We emphasize that these potential outflow veins offer an opportunity for an autogenous primary or staged transposition for many surgeons. Rather than starting with a brachial artery to axillary vein graft in the arm, a loop forearm graft can use venous outflow, and possibly arterial inflow, from the distal arm. This preserves proximal vein sites for future use. Results with midthigh arterial and venous anastomoses using lateral thigh graft tunneling were reported to have equivalent outcomes to the traditional loop from the groin vessels, while complications were less severe and the potential to revise to a more proximal outflow site with subsequent procedures were preserved [98]. Use of the iliac vessels through a retroperitoneal approach allows positioning of a loop graft configuration onto the abdominal wall for cannulation when other options are not available.

Secondary Arteriovenous Fistulas

Converting Arteriovenous Grafts to Autogenous Access

AVFs created following failure or repeated interventions of existing AVGs have been termed secondary fistulas (SAVF) [1, 2, 99]. KDOQI Guidelines and Fistula First recommend that each patient be reevaluated for conversion to an AVF after failure of an AVG. Patients with forearm AVGs should have a plan in place for SAVF construction if the AVG requires repeated intervention. Patients with an established forearm AVG may have a mature outflow vein available for creating the new SAVF. US imaging identifies access options and aids in planning the conversion operation. When the established AVG outflow conduit into the upper arm is the cephalic vein, immediate cannulation is usually available, avoiding the need for CVC placement. It is important to avoid use of the upper arm for graft revisions or another AVG when the forearm AVG fails. If the established AVG outflow is a basilic or brachial vein requiring, in effect, a "staged" transposition of this mature vein, then a CVC will be required for a brief period. The absence of arm swelling prior to the AVG failure argues that the central venous system is free of significant obstruction or that adequate collateralization has developed to support the access. Even patients with failed or failing upper arm AVGs will likely have opportunities for new AVFs in the contralateral or even in the ipsilateral arm when carefully evaluated with US and contrast venous mapping (Fig. 21.9).

New Grafts and Devices

It soon became apparent after the creation of the distal radiocephalic fistula that some patients would not have suitable vessels for a direct AVF. This problem only worsened as patient comorbidities increased, routinely including diabetes, obesity, peripheral vascular disease, and the very elderly. Since the introduction of ePTFE grafts in the mid-1970s, many new devices and grafts have entered the market, but most found limited use or have been withdrawn.

In the late 1970s, stainless steel and then polypropylene tubes known as Sparks' mandrels were implanted in the patient's subcutaneous tissue to create collagen tubes for HD access. Some of the lesions from that experience are

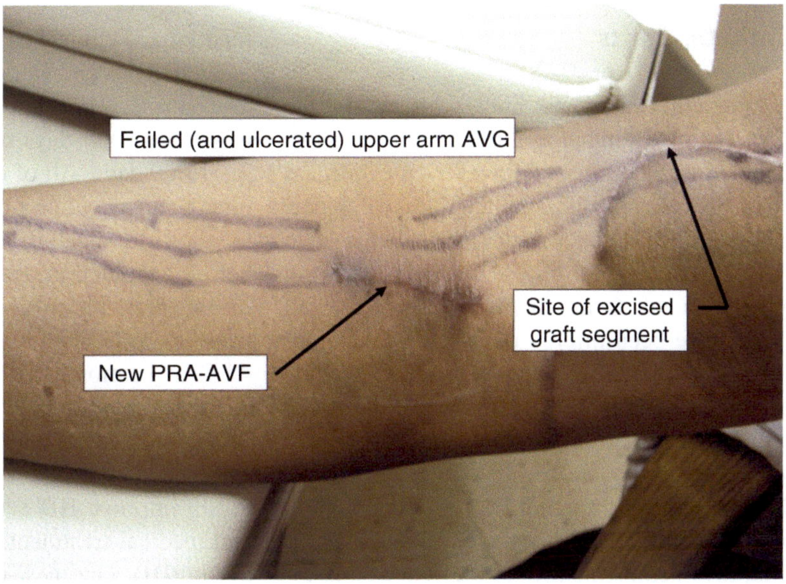

Fig. 21.9 Conversion of an eroded AV graft to secondary arteriovenous fistula using the proximal radial artery (*PRA*) for inflow (From Slayden et al. [99]. © Copyright John Wiley & Sons, Inc)

being applied today in the development of tissue-engineered vascular conduits for dialysis access. In the 1980s, the Bentley DiaTAP button (American Bentley, Irvine, CA., USA) and the Hemasite (Renal Systems, Minneapolis, Minn., USA) offered the hope of needleless immediate access to circulation through an exteriorized cap. Complications such as bleeding and infection caused those efforts to fail. In the late 1990s, the LifeSite (Vasca, Inc., Tewksbury, MA, USA) and Dialock (Biolink Corp., Norwell, MA, USA) systems combined subcutaneous port(s) with tunneled catheter(s) to reduce catheter-related bacteremia (CRB). While they appeared to reduce infection rates somewhat, technical problems with port placement and infection limited their popularity, and they are now off the market. In this decade, antiseptic prophylactic catheter lock solutions are demonstrating considerable success at reducing CRB. A high-dose citrate compound was removed by the FDA after a reported death, but others look promising in ongoing clinical trials.

Numerous biologic and synthetic graft variations have been developed since the initial use of ePTFE. However, standard ePTFE outcomes are generally viewed as the gold standard, and no large prospective randomized controlled trials (RCT) with new grafts have been done comparing the two.

Biologic Grafts

The first nonautologous biologic graft, a glutaraldehyde-treated bovine carotid artery, was used in 1970. Degeneration with aneurysm formation and a tendency to disintegrate when infected decreased its popularity. The graft processing was changed to improve these problems, and this collagen tube continues to be sold today as the Artegraft®* (Artegraft, Inc., North Brunswick, NJ, USA*) with improved results [100]. The bovine mesenteric vein graft marketed as Procol®* (Hancock Jaffe Laboratories, Irvine, CA, USA*) was shown to have a lower infection rate and required fewer interventions than PTFE in a nonrandomized study [101]. It has a significantly higher cost than ePTFE and has been used when repeated thromboses or infection occurs with an ePTFE graft. Cryopreserved femoral vein allografts are also available and may be used when a graft must be placed into a contaminated field or in vascular access reconstruction after removal of an infected graft. Decellularized bovine ureter has been used for HD access, but primary patency rates were disappointing.

Synthetic Grafts

The polyether urethane urea graft offers the advantage of cannulation after 24 h to avoid or minimize catheter use. However, its stiffness makes it technically challenging to place. Patencies and infection risk are no better than ePTFE. Many variations in the manufacturing and design of 6-mm-diameter standard wall ePTFE have been offered by several companies in hope of improving outcomes. These include differing graft wall porosity, multilayering of the graft to increase strength, stepped or tapering to reduce steal risk, thick wall, thin wall, stretch, adding external or internal wall support rings to reduce kinking and compression, hooded grafts to improve hemodynamics at the venous anastomosis, internal carbon or heparin coating to improve patency, external gel coating to reduce seroma and make tunneling easier, and a clear polyethylene sheath to reduce friction during tunneling. Some of these changes have been combined in a single graft. A penetrating U-shaped clip has been purported to speed construction of an interrupted anastomosis, although the device has not been widely adopted. A large retrospective study did show improved patency using an interrupted nonpenetrating clip versus a running-sutured anastomosis [102]. A small vessel single-fire anastomotic device has also been developed. While small studies often show a benefit for some of these variations in grafts, devices, or surgical techniques, no large RCTs have been done.

The HeRO® (Hemodialysis Reliable Outflow) (Hemosphere, Inc., Minneapolis, Minn., USA*) device, known originally as the GraftCath, was approved by the FDA as a graft in 2008. It is intended for those patients who are approaching or have become catheter dependent due to noncorrectable central venous obstruction. A 6-mm-diameter ePTFE graft with inflow from the brachial artery in the arm is connected near the deltopectoral groove to a 5-mm internal diameter nitinol-reinforced silicone catheter using a titanium connector. The radiopaque tip is positioned in the right atrium usually by way of the internal jugular vein. The device has also been placed through the subclavian or femoral veins. A nonrandomized clinical trial compared HeRO to tunneled dialysis catheter (TDC) and AVG literature as controls. The HeRO-related bacteremia rate was 0.70/1,000 days compared to TDC rate of 2.3/1,000 days. All of the HeRO-related bacteremias occurred while a bridging TDC was in place to allow for healing of the ePTFE component before cannulation. HeRO primary patency at a mean follow-up of 8.6 months was 38.9 % compared to AVG literature of 58 % at 6 months and 42 % at 12 months. HeRO secondary patency at 8.6 months was 72.2 % compared to AVG of 76 % at 6 months and 65 % at 12 months [103].

Clinical and basic science research is continuing to improve HD access including new grafts and medical treatments to reduce intimal hyperplasia (IH). One new graft recreates the natural swirling movement of blood, while another recent graft has incorporated a flow diffuser or double outflow channel at the venous anastomosis with both reporting improved hemodynamics. Clinical trials are ongoing with a gelatin wrap impregnated with allogenic aortic endothelial cells to reduce IH. Injection of antimetabolites to reduce cell division and local gene therapy to produce vasodilation are being studied [104]. Advances have come slowly in the last 40 years since ePTFE grafts, and AVFs remain the best options for the vast majority of patients at this time.

Vascular Access Monitoring and Surveillance

Monitoring

The NKF-KDOQI guidelines define monitoring as "the evaluation of the vascular access by means of physical examination (inspection, palpation, and auscultation) to detect physical signs that suggest the presence of dysfunction [1]." It is recommended to be done at least monthly. While it is usually assigned to the dialysis nurse, dialysis coordinator, or nephrologist, the surgeon knows the construction of the access best and should participate in patient follow-up during access maturation and maintenance. The surgeon's physical examination (PE) is particularly useful at the 4–6-week postoperative maturation visit. The recording of baseline findings when the surgeon releases the patient to start cannulation is especially important since later changes from that baseline exam are often diagnostic of a specific problem. In a study reviewing the role of vascular access PE by Beathard, 91.7 % of patients sent for angiography on the basis of a PE were found to have >50 % venous outflow stenosis [105]. A study with only AVG patients found a sensitivity of 57 % and specificity of 89 % in predicting venous anastomotic stenosis with PE [106]. It takes only moments for an experienced examiner to perform a normal vascular access examination, requires no equipment other than a stethoscope, and is easily repeated. The HD access is a circuit that begins at the left ventricle and ends at the right atrium. Changes in physiology and disease states such as hypertension, congestive heart failure, and peripheral arterial disease will affect the examination of the access. The PE findings should relate to the variable characteristics of arterial inflow, the access conduit, and venous outflow. Changes in examination are a reflection of energy, pressure, and flow reductions proceeding from artery to vein along the access. Every bruit and thrill results in a downstream drop in energy, pressure, and flow [107]. Since the PE of native fistulas and grafts is somewhat different, they will be discussed separately starting with fistulas.

Inspection

Fistulas should not appear pulsatile and should, at least partially, collapse with extremity elevation. If this is not the case, venous outflow obstruction should be suspected. If there is an anastomosis to the brachial artery more than 4-mm long, the high inflow will prevent collapse, but it should soften with elevation. Infection is rare in autogenous accesses. However, cellulitis or focal abscess may develop, particularly at cannulation sites. Aneurysms should be noted, and the size recorded. Friable overlying skin or ulceration requires prompt attention, especially with any history of bleeding. Pale or cyanotic finger nails or inability to move the fingers well may be an indication of clinically important steal. Extremity swelling or collateral veins at the shoulder may indicate central vein disease.

Palpation

There should be a strong thrill throughout systole and diastole in the perianastomotic area. If there is a pulse at the anastomosis, severe stenosis is likely present somewhere in the venous outflow portion of the circuit. In radiocephalic AVFs at the wrist, two-thirds of stenoses occur in the vein within 4 cm of the anastomosis. A localized thrill away from the anastomosis indicates a stenosis. It is critical to remember that the proximal radial artery or brachial artery anastomoses are too deep to palpate. Feeling a thrill superficial to such fistulas does not exclude at least moderate stenosis within 2 cm of the anastomosis. If a stenosis is suspected, a normal access flow measurement is reassuring. Adding elevation of the extremity to the examination often helps pinpoint the site of stenosis. When elevating an extremity with a high-grade stenosis in the vein, the transition point between dilated and collapsed veins indicates the site of stenosis. While still elevated, the rate of refilling of the vein when it is compressed downstream gives an estimate of the amount of inflow and severity of the stenosis. For veins that do not collapse with elevation because of large inflow, downstream compression should still cause the vein to dilate more. If it does not enlarge at all, outflow obstruction is likely. Large accessory veins sometimes delay or prevent maturation by draining blood from the main channel. They can be located by occluding the outflow vein every 2 cm starting just downstream to the anastomosis. The occluding finger will feel a pulse until it moves beyond a large accessory vein. Direction of flow in an access can be determined by occluding the conduit and feeling which side becomes pulsatile. Sometimes, a thrill is palpated over the infraclavicular fossa indicating a terminal cephalic arch or central vein stenosis.

Auscultation

A low-pitched, continuous bruit throughout systole and diastole is normal at the anastomosis. The higher the pitch and the shorter the bruit, the greater the stenosis predicted. The bruit normally becomes lower in pitch and softer the further from the anastomosis. A localized high-pitched bruit away from the anastomosis indicates a stenosis at that point. A "thumping sound" or no diastolic bruit suggests very low access flow and impending occlusion.

Grafts

The PE of synthetic grafts is somewhat more difficult to interpret because of the stiff wall (low compliance), higher flows, gradual pressure drop across the entire length, and the lack of branches. However, the same techniques and physiologic approach are used as with a native fistula. A record of the baseline exam by the surgeon when the patient is released to start cannulations is again essential, because changes are much more important than an isolated exam. For example, if the patient started with a thrill and bruit throughout systole and diastole at the anastomosis and returns in 3 months with a pulsatile anastomosis and bruit in systole and only ½ of diastole, high-grade stenosis at the venous anastomosis is very likely. Grafts should dilate slightly when occluded downstream unless there is a high-grade stenosis in the outflow vein. Grafts tend not to collapse with elevation, except for pseudoaneurysms, but should become softer. If thrills are present at both arterial and venous anastomoses and in the mid graft, significant stenosis is very unlikely [108]. High graft flow is associated with a forearm graft without a pulse at the venous anastomosis and a thrill in the distal part of the arm or especially in the axilla [109].

The vascular access examiner will gain confidence with increasing experience and by correlating patient outcomes and imaging results with physical findings. Quoting Dr. Gerald Beathard, "…we often ignore an effective technique that is literally at the tip of our fingers. The patient's access has a lot to say if we will listen" [105].

Surveillance

The NKF-KDOQI defines surveillance as "the periodic evaluation of the vascular access by means of tests which may involve special instrumentation and for which an abnormal test result suggests the presence of dysfunction" [1]. At least monthly testing is advised. Recommended methods are intra-access flow measurements with trend analysis, directly measured or derived static venous or arterial segment dialysis pressure ratios, and duplex ultrasound with flow measurement and/or imaging. Access flows <600 ml/min in grafts or <400–500 ml/min in fistulas are abnormal and are associated with an increased risk of thrombosis. Static venous segment pressure ratio >0.5 in grafts or fistulas or an arterial segment static pressure ratio >0.75 in grafts is also abnormal. A key element of surveillance is a commitment to access intervention based on predetermined surveillance threshold values with the premise that a treatable lesion will be discovered and the patient will benefit from the interventional testing and procedure [110, 111]. In general, one does not respond to a single abnormal surveillance flow or pressure ratio measurement. Trend analysis and associated abnormal physical or clinical findings increase the power to detect dysfunction.

We conclude that monitoring by physical examination of the vascular access is generally felt to be helpful in predicting access dysfunction prior to access failure, although it is difficult to analyze in a prospective randomized fashion [105, 112]. Surveillance has not, as yet, been persuasively shown to extend functional vascular access life for AVGs or AVFs, although some investigators report fewer thrombotic events. A study in children found a reduction in access-related costs [113–117]. Paulson et al. point out that there are no convincing large prospective randomized controlled studies for access surveillance. In addition, multiple interventions may worsen local inflammatory processes and stimulate restenosis, possibly making access life shorter in some patients [104]. The group concludes, "…there is a consensus that physical examination combined with good clinical judgment is essential to the management of vascular accesses [116]".

We feel that vascular access monitoring is useful and appropriate based on physical findings and routinely available dialysis parameters. Each dialysis site should have a designated access leader/teacher conducting and recording regular examinations and evaluations. The responsible examiner might be a physician, nurse, physician assistant, or dialysis coordinator. Abnormal findings and trends may suggest a fistulogram with intervention as indicated. Patients can and should also be involved and educated about these problems. Each dialysis unit should incorporate monitoring and decide individually if surveillance works best for their patients while we await definitive studies.

The Swollen Arm Associated with Vascular Access

Central and Proximal Venous Stenosis and Occlusion

Central vein (CV) or proximal venous stenosis and complete occlusion are generally associated with long-term and/or multiple dialysis catheters [17]. Although patients may be asymptomatic with venous outflow provided by multiple large collateral vessels, elevated vascular access outflow pressure often causes significant symptoms such as pain and swelling in the affected extremity that may extend into the head, neck, and chest wall or breast. Specific diagnosis and treatment with contrast imaging and angioplasty with or without stent placement is often successful; however, these lesions tend to recur [118, 119]. Access ligation may be necessary in some patients, although establishing a new permanent access in another extremity for these individuals is often difficult. Even finding alternative catheter sites may be challenging. Surgical bypass of these central venous lesions is a major undertaking, particularly in this group of patients, but has been reported in selected patients [120–122].

We find balloon angioplasty to be successful in most patients and reserve stenting for those individuals with recurrent lesions every 3 months or resistant lesions that demonstrate significant elastic recoil after treatment. When stenting is necessary, there is accumulating evidence that covered stents reduce recurrent stenosis rates compared to bare stents. In the study by Anaya-Ayala, covered stents in the CVs achieved primary, primary assisted, and secondary patencies of 56, 86, and 100 % at 12 months, respectively [123]. For patients with severe symptoms where percutaneous angioplasty was not possible, we have recently successfully utilized a proximal banding procedure developed for access-related steal syndrome by Miller [124–126]. We found both access flow and pressure were decreased in the venous outflow tract. Short-term outcomes in these patients have been excellent with access preservation and relief of symptoms. This option might be considered prior to major surgical bypass operations for individuals where CV angioplasty and stenting has failed. In some patients, where more conservative options have failed, excision of the mature venous conduit and translocation to the thigh as an autogenous access option may be a better solution than a thigh graft.

Dialysis Access-Associated Steal Syndrome and Cardiac Risk Associated with High-Flow Permanent Vascular Access

The best method of dealing with dialysis-associated steal syndrome (DASS) is to avoid it when possible by minimizing the risk of occurrence. Potentially lower inflow access options to consider include constructing RC-AVFs or PRA-AVFs when feasible and limiting the size of the anastomosis in relation to the native brachial artery diameter when inflow is required at that site. AVGs carry greater risk of DASS than AVFs because of higher initial flow with the former [127]. In addition, peritoneal dialysis might be considered for patients at high risk for DASS.

As many as 2 % of radial and 9 % of brachial artery-based hemodialysis access patients may require some form of intervention for DASS [127]. Physical examination plus segmental blood pressures, access flow measurements, pulse volume recordings, finger pressures, digital/brachial indices, and pulse oximetry supine and with the

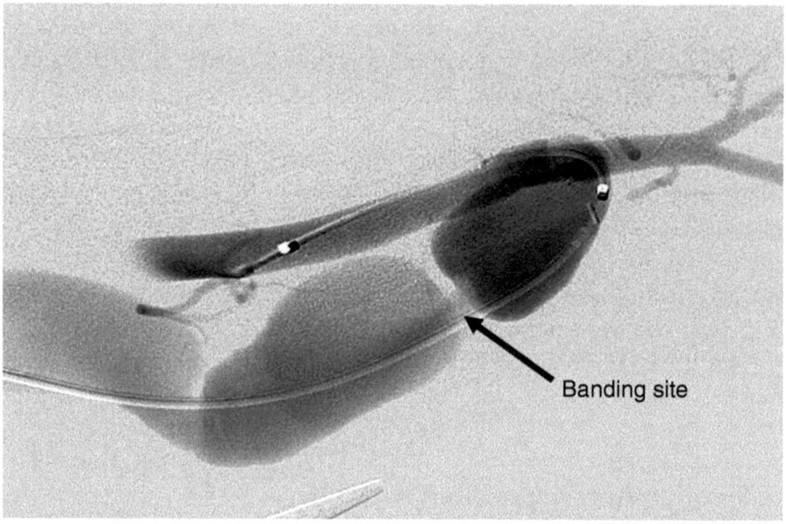

Fig. 21.10 Completion arteriogram after MILLER banding using real-time US flow monitoring [110]. The angioplasty catheter has been deflated and advanced into the brachial artery for the completion contrast injection but was centered at the banding site as the restricting sutures were tied over the inflated 4-mm angioplasty balloon. Distal arterial flow was not visualized prebanding and is now present

limb elevated are important elements of successful evaluation and treatment planning for severely symptomatic steal syndrome. DASS remains a clinical diagnosis. Symptoms occur at variable finger pressures and may develop at higher levels in the upper than lower extremity [128]. Arteriography is recommended once the decision is made on clinical grounds that invasive treatment is necessary. A complete study from the aortic arch to finger tips is desirable to determine the optimal procedure. In addition, up to 20 % of these patients are found to have a proximal correctable inflow lesion that is treated at the time of arteriography.

DASS may be associated with a high (>1,200 ml/min), moderate (800–1,200 ml/min), or low (<800 ml/min) flow vascular access. Higher-flow AVFs may become a more recognized problem with recent studies demonstrating the effects on pulmonary artery pressure and cardiac output in individuals with permanent vascular access [77]. Many reports and references are available outlining evaluation and treatment of DASS [1, 2, 55, 127, 129]. Patients with mild symptoms of numbness but without motor deficit, constant pain, ulceration, or threatened tissue loss may be monitored without intervention. When symptoms or physical findings require intervention, sacrifice of the access by ligation or coil occlusion may be necessary in critical situations, but access-preserving procedures for symptomatic patients are recommended. Procedures to maintain a functioning access include traditional surgical banding (flow restriction), bypass revision to distal arterial inflow (RUDI), simple conversion of the anastomosis from brachial to radial artery, and more [125, 130–132]. Banding as a flow limiting option was often felt to be unreliable in the past, because it was usually done without objective measurement of flow and pressure. This situation was greatly improved by Miller et al. in his report of a precise banding technique using an angioplasty balloon as the banding dowel [125, 126]. This simple procedure is often accomplished in the angiogram suite. We have utilized this technique with success and find it particularly helpful in high access flow situations using real-time access flow monitoring with ultrasound (Fig. 21.10). Access flow volume measurements may lead to a discovery of DASS with a low- or moderate-flow fistula caused by severe distal peripheral vascular disease with high resistance in the arterial bed. Banding may not offer a good solution to this problem, and we do not recommend it. Distal revascularization and interval ligation (DRIL) has been the gold standard for treatment of steal syndrome since first described by Schanzer et al. in 1988 [133]. However, it has been replaced in our practice with inflow proximalization [95]. We use inflow proximalization for DASS patients with low or moderate access flow fistula and severe distal vascular disease and in patients with a threatened distal extremity. This procedure hemodynamically offers nearly the same benefit as DRIL procedure without ligation of the brachial artery. The access is maintained, usually with improved flow characteristics. However, inflow for the access is relocated to the larger and more compliant axillary artery. We find this combination of precision banding for high-flow fistulas and proximalization procedures for severely threatened limbs and low-flow fistulas to allow treatment for essentially all DASS patients without access ligation. The surgeon and interventionalist's collaboration and working knowledge of all options offers the best opportunity for resolution of the patient's symptoms with the least invasive operative or interventional procedure while maximizing the likelihood of access salvage. Peritoneal dialysis may be an appropriate choice for some patients at high risk for steal syndrome. In 2007, the rate of ESRD incidence was 20.8 per million population for peritoneal dialysis in the United States, while the prevalent peritoneal dialysis population remained stable [15]. Peritoneal dialysis may be underutilized and offers reliable dialysis with significantly lower cost than hemodialysis options. Dr. Jack Work has often described peritoneal dialysis access as "the good catheter," bringing attention to this overlooked option for CVC reduction [134].

Vascular Access Aneurysms

Vascular access aneurysms are relatively common and most require no specific therapy other than careful selection of cannulation sites. Etiologies are most often use of cannulation site by inspection (area or cluster puncture), outflow obstruction, high access flow, and infection. These issues should be addressed to limit progression and at the time of repair. Patients developing access aneurysms should have a thorough physical examination of the access, as outlined previously in the chapter, making careful note of increased pulsatility downstream to the aneurysm, overlying skin condition, and condition of cannulation sites. Areas of skin thinning or effacement, ulceration, cellulitis, or a history of spontaneous bleeding at cannulation sites require urgent surgical evaluation. If the skin over the aneurysm is soft and freely movable (elevates easily between the examiner's thumb and index finger), there is no imminent danger of bleeding. Access flow measurements are helpful in the evaluation and treatment planning. These patients should be evaluated with a fistulogram for possible cephalic arch or central venous outflow obstruction and the lesions corrected by angioplasty if present. Patients with smaller and stable AVF aneurysmal dilations, where skin condition is good and adequate soft tissue overlying the enlarged venous segment is present, may be safely cannulated around of base. Establishing buttonhole (same site) cannulation may aid in preservation of these fistulas. AVG aneurysms are uniformly false aneurysms. Repair generally involves vascular bypass and decompressing the aneurysm with a new graft segment. Debridement of the old graft is necessary only if it is infected. Even small and stable AVG aneurysms should not be used as cannulation sites. Preferred access sites should be outlined with a marker and suggested cannulation sites located for the dialysis staff.

In patients where a large AVF aneurysm has developed or if there are changes in skin condition requiring intervention, we recommend resection or aneurysmorrhaphy. This may require only excision of the anterior wall of the aneurysm(s) in an elliptical fashion with a linear closure of the vein, closing the soft tissue and skin in separate layers. Use of a sterile tourniquet simplifies the process. We prefer not to place a covered stent in a cannulation region. Although controversial, stent placement in noncannulation sites for recurrent and resistant stenosis, particularly in central venous sites, has been successful in access salvage [135]. However, placing covered stents in AVF aneurysms that will eventually or immediately become cannulation sites introduces a foreign body that is now surrounded by a large resolving thrombus in the stented aneurysm segment, placing that region at risk for eventual infection. Patients presenting with acute bleeding, where skin condition has deteriorated overlying a false aneurysm, should undergo immediate repair, as these sites are at risk for another episode of hemorrhage. Stenting of these lesions should be avoided. With ulceration and recurrent skin breakdown associated with repeated cannulation and cellulitis, these sites may be secondarily infected, placing the new foreign body stent at risk.

When an aneurysm requires elective surgical intervention, the distal (usually cephalic) vein is mature and often tortuous. This outflow vein may be mobilized to gain adequate length for a direct end-to-end anastomosis after resection of the aneurysm. If ultrasound examination shows thrombus in the aneurysm, a partially closed straight vascular clamp should be placed obliquely on the outflow vein before circumferential dissection of the aneurysm to avoid pulmonary embolism. Injection of local anesthetic or normal saline helps to separate the skin from the aneurysm wall, making dissection easier. Small areas of scarred and densely adherent skin overlying the aneurysm(s) are often left in place during dissection and excised during the aneurysmorrhaphy. Primarily repairing the mature vein or false aneurysm may be accomplished with continuous vascular suture or utilizing a stapling device, as outlined by Pierce et al. [136]. We have used staplers for aneurysm repair and found it to be satisfactory although not superior to suture repair. We utilize a 10-mm catheter as a dowel with the stapler technique to ensure an adequate lumen is maintained as the stapler is applied. The revised vein should be placed in a new tunnel if possible, rather than the original bed to lessen the risk of hematoma around the vein. In order to avoid use of a catheter, repair of the entire conduit may be staged. Some have recommended placement of a Dacron® or metal mesh around the reconstructed vein to reduce recurrence, but we have not found this necessary.

Cannulation

While surgeons do not generally cannulate the vascular access they create, it is still important for them to understand what is involved. Approximately 300 punctures a year are performed on each access with three times a week dialysis. The three cannulation techniques in use are the rope ladder, site by inspection (area puncture), and constant site (buttonhole). Rope ladder had been the traditional recommended method. The analogy is to a climbing rope with knots placed equidistant along its length. The punctures are spread equidistant along the cannulation zone. This limits the skin and vessel or graft damage in any one area to decrease aneurysm formation, stenosis, and infection. Site by inspection or area (cluster) puncture is discouraged but remains relatively common with facility staff because it is the easiest to perform. It involves choosing two small areas in the cannulation zone and utilizing these limited regions exclusively. This method leads to a higher incidence of aneurysms, adjacent stenosis, infection, and bleeding. The constant site method or buttonhole uses cannulation sites repeatedly through the same two to three holes with the same angle of entry. A reliable pathway is created allowing eventual conversion to the noncutting buttonhole needle [137]. Experience has shown the buttonhole technique to markedly reduce aneurysm formation and the accompanying stenosis. AVFs with very short cannulation zones can be used. Training and attention to detail, especially as it relates to scab management to prevent infection, are critical to success with this technique. We recommend establishing three buttonhole sites and rotating use. Fistula First recommends buttonhole as the cannulation method of choice for AVFs. It is not recommended for grafts at this time. On average, it takes about 2 weeks using a standard sharp needle and the same cannulator to establish the site. After the site is mature, the dull buttonhole needle is used, and other cannulators can do the puncture. Simpler techniques to establish a mature site are in development. Many patients report less pain, although this is not universal.

With AVF cannulation, the standard needle cuts elastic tissue and smooth muscle with every pass through the vessel. The clot that fills the hole is eventually replaced by weaker and less flexible fibrous tissue. Repeated punctures in close proximity lead to aneurysm development and thinning of overlying skin. Hemodynamic changes brought on by the aneurysm may lead to intimal hyperplasia and stenosis [138]. With grafts, repeated punctures in a small area lead to disintegration of the anterior wall and phagocytosis of small graft fragments and pseudoaneurysm formation.

Most units have a standard protocol for using a new AVF or graft. Grafts are generally easier to cannulate. They have a uniform size and depth. Wall edges can be easily felt. Fistulas vary in size, depth, course, and wall strength. Fistulas are initially cannulated with a 17-gauge arterial draw needle and connection to a catheter for venous return if present. If not, both 17-gauge needles are placed in the AVF at first use. Over the course of 2–3 weeks, pump speed and needle size are increased to 300–450 ml/min and 15 gauge, respectively. A tourniquet should always be used with cannulation to reduce the risk of back wall puncture. Infiltration hematoma not only delays use of the access but often leads to fistula stenosis. Some units have established a rating system for staff so that only the most qualified cannulators can start using new fistulas.

While there is general agreement that grafts can be cannulated 2–4 weeks after placement and sooner with some grafts designed for earlier puncture, there is a wide range for first fistula cannulation. Data from the Dialysis Outcomes and Practice Patterns Study (DOPPS) showed median time in Japan is 25 days, Germany 42 days, the UK 96 days, and the USA 98 days. There was no evidence of decreased long-term fistula survival as long as cannulation was not started <14 days after surgical creation [139]. Brescia et al. reported in 1966 using the distal radiocephalic fistula the day after it was created in their young male patients with chronic glomerulonephritis. Recent evidence indicates fistula blood flow is already >600 ml/min by 2–3 weeks in fistulas that are going to mature. KDOQI established the rule of 6's for a mature AVF that is ready for cannulation. It should have a diameter of 6 mm, depth of <6 mm, blood flow of at least 600 ml/min, and be at least 6 weeks after surgery [1]. Others have reported 95 % maturation rate if the diameter was at least 4 mm and the flow at least 500 ml/min [140]. We recommend a maturation evaluation by the surgeon at a month after fistula creation using physical examination and usually duplex ultrasound. The best areas for puncture are marked on the arm, longitudinal ultrasound images of the fistula are given to the patient for the facility staff, and a digital photograph of the marked extremity may be emailed to the facility and placed in the patient's chart. A study of cannulation complications by Van Loon et al. in the Netherlands found 51 % of patients had a miscannulation during the first three dialysis sessions [141]. Ongoing communication between facility staff and the surgeon is necessary for optimal outcomes.

Percutaneous Techniques for Access Maturation and Salvage

Our goal for initial AVF cannulation is generally 4–6 weeks after access construction, because it has been shown that fistula flow and vein size should be adequate by that time [142]. If the access fails to mature in this time period, a fistulogram is obtained with intervention as indicated. A Dialysis Access Consortium Study found that 60 % of fistulas in the trial were not ready for use by 5 months after creation [143]. However, the intervention rate was very low in this study, and the percentage of failed AVFs was well above the current national mean [144, 145]. Interventional procedures are key aspects of successful AVF maturation and maintenance for many patients. These less invasive techniques have become common, offering both diagnosis and treatment for a dysfunctional vascular access. A recent study looked at primary balloon angioplasty for small-caliber veins with diameter <3 mm during surgery and serial balloon angioplasty maturation (BAM) of the segment to be cannulated using 2–3-mm larger balloons every 2 weeks to enlarge forearm veins to 8-mm diameter and arm veins to 12–16 mm. Such dilations not only speed maturation but may avoid the need for superficialization. "Overall, 47 of 55 patients (85.4 %) obtained a working AVF at the initial site, and 53 (96.3 %) received working AVFs. All fistulas were functioning at 90 days after the final

BAM [146]." Other innovative interventional procedures include rerouting through a collateral vein when the main channel is no longer usable or insertion of a percutaneous stent, bridging to an adjacent outflow vein. Angioplasty rates for HD access continue to rise, reaching 0.4 and 0.95 events per patient year for those with a fistula or graft, respectively in 2006. These rates were 2.6 and 1.9 times greater than in 1998 [16]. Radiologists, surgeons, interventional nephrologists, and interventional cardiologists all perform these procedures. Functional AVFs with problems noted during dialysis monitoring such as poor inflow, recirculation, prolonged post cannulation bleeding, or high venous pressures require evaluation with physical examination, ultrasound, and a fistulogram. Fluoroscopic imaging with the option of balloon angioplasty offers the opportunity for AVF maturation into a functional dialysis access and salvage of a dysfunctional or thrombosed AVF or AVG [1, 2, 147, 148]. Individual treatment options and technical success are linked to multiple factors such as underlying medical and vascular disease, inflow stenosis, condition of the access conduit, outflow availability, and physician training and skill. As opposed to arterial angioplasty, higher-pressure balloons, sometimes up to 30 atm, may be needed to open stenosis in these veins. Vessel recoil 15 min post procedure and recurrent intimal hyperplasia within 3 months remain unresolved issues. Cutting balloons, cryoplasty, lasers, coated stents, and other devices as well as medications are being studied to determine their utility in this area. Techniques for declotting grafts are well established with about 90 % initial success rate using pharmacomechanical methods. However, declotting fistulas is more difficult and methods are still evolving with initial success rates of 65–90 % being reported. Thromboaspiration through a large sheath is used successfully by some physicians. Others use a variety of mechanical wall contact or noncontact devices with or without thrombolytic agents. Thrombus burden is usually <5 ml in a graft, but very large fistulas can have 50 ml of clot or more. Use of a downstream temporary occlusion balloon or other device to prevent pulmonary embolus should be considered. Surgical revision is favored by some surgeons for those patients with a very large clot burden. Consensus for prophylactic use of balloon angioplasty of >50 % stenosis found with surveillance and particularly stent deployment has not been established [116, 135]. Multiple stent devices are available; none have emerged as uniquely superior. Stent placement in AVF cannulation zones is controversial, and we surgically revise these segments if possible. Similarly, stent placement electively for an aneurysm in cannulation regions should be avoided if feasible. Stent placement within AVGs is less controversial. However, the extended life of the graft is modest. Placing a stent through an AVG venous outflow anastomosis uses critical vein length that should be reserved in most cases, for a secondary AVF construction [99]. A recent study showed reduced recurrent venous anastomotic stenosis with grafts when a covered stent was placed in this location as opposed to angioplasty alone, achieving a 6-month treatment area primary patency of 51 % and access circuit primary patency of 38 % versus 23 % and 20 %, respectively, for balloon angioplasty alone [149]. However, another prospective, randomized multicenter clinical trial found angioplasty alone achieved a 6-month treatment area primary patency of 40.5 % and access circuit primary patency of 36.3% [150]. Larger studies are pending. Covered stents placed within a recurrent or resistant central venous stenosis are being used more frequently as discussed previously, but larger and longer-term studies are needed to define their role [135]. The proper size of the angioplasty and deployed stent are important elements of success. Successful access intervention with balloon angioplasty using only US imaging and avoiding the use of contrast has recently been reported [43].

Our recommended approach of aggressive intervention to achieve prompt AVF maturation and to correct any subsequent dysfunction will result in early fistulograms and balloon angioplasty as indicated. This will lead to lower primary patency rates but higher assisted and cumulative (secondary) patency rates. Figure 21.11 shows data from a review of over 900 consecutive AVF vascular access operations

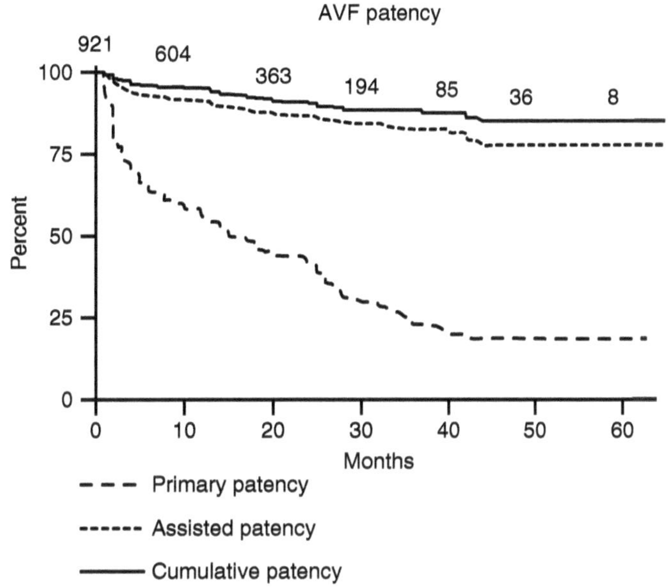

Fig. 21.11 Arteriovenous fistula (*AVF*) patency (Adapted from: Jennings and Broughan [32]. © Copyright John Wiley & Sons, Inc)

by one of the authors (WCJ). No grafts were used during this study period. Primary, primary assisted, and cumulative (secondary) patency were 55.8, 91.3, and 95.2 % at 12 months and 41.8, 86.6, and 90.6 % at 24 months, respectively [32]. Of the 57 AVFs that failed and were not salvaged, 28 patients later had a successful AVF at another site, while others were converted to PD or were transplanted, further reducing CVC usage.

Conclusions

The use of ultrasound for both preoperative vessel mapping and postoperative management has played a key role in increasing the number of patients with AVFs, in addition to improving access maturation and salvage. Options for AVF creation and techniques have expanded significantly. Endovascular techniques to aid maturation and maintenance of the vascular access have become established as the preferred method of intervention when necessary. Research continues into the development of better conduit materials, prevention of intimal hyperplasia, and many other challenging areas of hemodialysis access to improve patient outcomes. Although not the topic of this chapter, peritoneal dialysis is the appropriate choice for some patients, especially if hemodialysis access options are poor.

References

1. National Kidney Foundation clinical practice guidelines for vascular access. Am J Kidney Dis. 2006; 48(Suppl 1):S176–247.
2. Fistula first: national vascular access improvement initiative. http://www.fistulafirst.org/. Cited 10 Jan 2012.
3. Sidawy AN, Spergel LM, Besarab A, et al. The Society for Vascular Surgery: clinical practice guidelines for the surgical placement and maintenance of arteriovenous hemodialysis access. J Vasc Surg. 2008;48(5 suppl):2S–5.
4. Dhingra RK, Young EW, Hulbert-Shearon TE, Leavey SF, Port RK. Type of vascular access and mortality in U.S. hemodialysis patients. Kidney Int. 2001;60(4): 1443–51.
5. Young E. Vascular access. Current practice and practical aspects of management, ASN renal week 2000. Toronto: ASN; 2000. p. 377–85.
6. Ascher E, Gade P, Hingorani A, et al. Changes in the practice of angioaccess surgery: impact of dialysis outcome and quality initiative recommendations. J Vasc Surg. 2000;31(1 Pt 1):84–92. Erratum in: J Vasc Surg 2000 Apr; 31(4):818.
7. Eggers P, Milam R. Trends in vascular access procedures and expenditures in Medicare's ESRD program.

In: Henry ML, editor. Vascular access for hemodialysis-VII. Chicago: Gore; 2001. p. 133–43.
8. Perera GB, Mueller MP, Kubaska SM, Wilson SE, Lawrence PF, Fujitani RM. Superiority of autogenous arteriovenous hemodialysis access: maintenance of function with fewer secondary interventions. Ann Vasc Surg. 2004;18(1):66–73. Epub 2004 Jan 20.
9. Goldstein SL, Ikizler TA, Zappitelli M, Silverstein DM, Ayus JC. Non-infected hemodialysis catheters are associated with increased inflammation compared to arteriovenous fistulas. Kidney Int. 2009;76(10):1063–9. Epub 2009 Aug 12.
10. Anderson SG, Jennings WC. Elevated TNF levels in serum from dialysis patients using arteriovenous grafts or catheters compared to arteriovenous fistulas for vascular access. Poster/abstract: Southwestern surgical congress, Tucson, 21–24 Mar 2010.
11. US Renal Data System, USRDS. Annual data report: atlas of chronic kidney disease and end-stage renal disease in the United States. Bethesda: National Institutes of Health, National Institute of Diabetes and Digestive and Kidney Diseases; 2008.
12. National Institute on Aging [Internet] Bethesda; 2009 Dec 10. Press release, Dramatic changes in U.S. aging highlighted in new census, NIH report, Impact of Baby Boomers Anticipated; 2006. http://www.nia.nih.gov/NewsAndEvents/PressReleases/PR2006030965PlusReport.htm. Accessed 6 Oct 2010.
13. Kurella M, Covinsky KE, Collins AJ, Chertow GM. Octogenarians and nonagenarians starting dialysis in the United States. Ann Intern Med. 2007;146:177–83.
14. Añel RL, Yevzlin AS, Ivanovich P. Vascular access and patient outcomes in hemodialysis: questions answered in recent literature. Artif Organs. 2003; 27(3):237–41.
15. U S Renal Data System, USRDS. Annual data report. Atlas of chronic kidney disease and end-stage renal disease in the United States. Bethesda: National Institutes of Health, National Institutes of Diabetes and Digestive and Kidney Diseases; 2011.
16. U S Renal Data System, USRDS. Annual data report. Atlas of chronic kidney disease and end-stage renal disease in the United States. Bethesda: National Institutes of Health, National Institutes of Diabetes and Digestive and Kidney Diseases; 2009.
17. Spergel LM. Reducing tunneled hemodialysis catheter morbidity. Has the fistula first breakthrough initiative caused an increase in catheter prevalence? Semin Dial. 2008;21(6):550–2.
18. Ethier J, Mendelssohn DC, Elder SJ, et al. Vascular access use and outcomes: an international perspective from the dialysis outcomes and practice patterns study. Nephrol Dial Transplant. 2008;23:3219–26.
19. Xue JL, Dahl D, Ebben JP, Collins AJ. The association of initial hemodialysis access type with mortality outcomes in elderly Medicare ESRD patients. Am J Kidney Dis. 2003;42(5):1013–9.
20. Polkinghorne KR, McDonald SP, Atkins RC, Kerr PG. Vascular access and all-cause mortality: a propensity score analysis. J Am Soc Nephrol. 2004;15:477–86.
21. Port FK, Pisoni RL, Bommer J, et al. Improving outcomes for dialysis patients in the international Dialysis Outcomes and Practice Patterns Study. Clin J Am Soc Nephrol. 2006;1:246–55.
22. Vazquez MA. Vascular access for dialysis: recent lessons and new insights. Curr Opin Nephrol Hypertens. 2009;18(2):116–21.
23. Maya ID, Allon M. Vascular access: core curriculum 2008. Am J Kidney Dis. 2008;51:702–8.
24. Bradbury BD, Chen F, Furniss A, Pisoni RL, Keen M, Mapes D, Krishnan M. Conversion of vascular access type among incident hemodialysis patients: description and association with mortality. Am J Kidney Dis. 2009;53(5):804–14.
25. Vaux EC, Shail R, Rabindranath KS. Ultrasound use for the placement of haemodialysis catheters (review). Cochrane Database Syst Rev. 201X, Issue X. Art. No: CD005279. doi: 10.1002/14651858.CD005279.pubX.
26. Foley RN, Collins AJ. End-stage renal disease in the United States: an update from the United States Renal Data System. J Am Soc Nephrol. 2007;18(10):2644–8. Epub 2007 Jul 26.
27. Schon D, Blume SW, Niebauer K, et al. Increasing the use of arteriovenous fistula in hemodialysis: economic benefits and economic barriers. Clin J Am Soc Nephrol. 2007;2:268–76.
28. Spergel LM, Ravani P, Asif A, Roy-Chaudhury P, Besarab A. Autogenous arteriovenous fistula options. J Nephrol. 2007;20(3):288–98.
29. Lewis CG, Wells MK, Jennings WC. Avoidance of prophylactic antibiotics in creation of native arteriovenous fistulas. Dial Transplant. 2003;32(5):306–8.
30. Salman L, Asif A. Antibiotic prophylaxis: is it needed for dialysis access procedures? Semin Dial. 2009;22(3):297–9.
31. Konner K, Hulbert-Shearon TE, Roys EC, Port FK. Tailoring the initial vascular access for dialysis patients. Kidney Int. 2002;62:329–38.
32. Jennings WC, Broughan TA. Arteriovenous fistulas in a complex vascular access referral practice. Semin Dial. 2009;22(2):213–8.
33. Dalman RL, Harris EJ. Transition to all-autogenous hemodialysis access: the role of preoperative vein mapping. Ann Vasc Surg. 2002;16:624–30.
34. Malovrh M. Noninvasive evaluation of vessels by duplex sonsography prior to construction of AV fistulae for hemodialysis. Nephrol Dial Transplant. 1998;12:125–9.
35. Ascher E, Gade P, Hingorani A, Mazzariol F, Gunduz Y, Fodera M, et al. Changes in the practice of angioaccess surgery: impact of dialysis outcome and quality initiative recommendations. J Vasc Surg. 2000;31(1 Pt 1):84–92.
36. Parmley MC, Broughan TA, Jennings WC. Vascular ultrasonography prior to dialysis access surgery. Am J Surg. 2002;184(6):568–72.
37. Gradman WS, Lerner G, Mentser M, Rodriguez H, Kamil ES. Experience with autogenous arteriovenous access for hemodialysis in children and adolescents. Ann Vasc Surg. 2005;19(5):609–12.

38. Schenk III WG. Improving dialysis access: regional anesthesia improves arteriovenous fistula prevalence. Am Surg. 2010;76(9):938–42.
39. Hyland K, Cohen RM, Kwak A, et al. Preoperative mapping venography in patients who require hemodialysis access: imaging findings and contribution to management. J Vasc Interv Radiol. 2008;19(7):1027–33.
40. Asif A, Cherla G, Merrill D, et al. Venous mapping using venography and the risk of radiocontrast-induced nephropathy. Semin Dial. 2005;18(3):239–42.
41. Jennings WC, Taubman K. Alternative autogenous arteriovenous hemodialysis access options. Semin Vasc Surg. 2011;24(2):72–81.
42. ACR practice guideline for the performance of vascular ultrasound for postoperative assessment of dialysis access. http://www.acr.org/SecondaryMainMenuCategories/quality_safety/guidelines/us/us_postoperative_dialysis.aspx. Accessed 20 Aug 2010.
43. Fox D, Amador F, Clarke D, Velez M, Cruz J, Labropoulos N, Ryan M, Gelman L. Duplex guided dialysis access interventions can be performed safely in the office setting: techniques and early results. Eur J Vasc Endovasc Surg. 2011;42(6):833–41.
44. Brescia MJ, Cimino JE, Appell K, Hurwich BJ. Chronic hemodialysis using venipuncture and a surgically created arteriovenousfistula. N Engl J Med. 1966;275:1089–92.
45. Tordoir JH, Rooyens P, Dammers R, et al. Prospective evaluation of failure modes in autogenous radiocephalic wrist access for haemodialysis. Nephrol Dial Transplant. 2003;18:378–83.
46. Biuckians A, Scott EC, Meier GH, et al. The natural history of autologous fistulas as first-time dialysis access in the KDOQI era. J Vasc Surg. 2008;47: 415–21.
47. Davidson I, Gallieni M, Saxena R, Dolmatch B. A patient centered decision making dialysis access algorithm. J Vasc Access. 2007;8:59–68.
48. Jennings WC, Kindred MG, Broughan TA. Creating radiocephalic arteriovenous fistulas: technical and functional success. J Am Coll Surg. 2009;208(3):419–25. Epub 2009 Jan 21.
49. Raynaud A, Novelli L, Bourquelot P, et al. Low-flow maturation failure of distal accesses: treatment by angioplasty of forearm arteries. J Vasc Surg. 2009;49(4):995–9.
50. Bharat A, Jaenicle M, Shenoy S. A novel technique of vascular anastomosis to prevent juxta-anastomotic stenosis following arteriovenous fistula creation. J Vasc Surg. 2012;55(1):274–80.
51. Jennings WC, Turman MA, Taubman KE. Arteriovenous fistulas for hemodialysis access in children and adolescents using the proximal radial artery inflow site. J Pediatr Surg. 2009;44(7): 1377–81.
52. Jennings WC. Creating arteriovenous fistulas in 132 consecutive patients: exploiting the proximal radial artery arteriovenous fistula: reliable, safe and simple forearm and upper arm hemodialysis access. Arch Surg. 2006;141(1):27–32; discussion 32.
53. Bruns SD, Jennings WC. Proximal radial artery as inflow site for native arteriovenous fistula. J Am Coll Surg. 2003;197:58–63.
54. Miller R, Taubman K, Jennings WC. Proximal radial artery and bidirectional flow arteriovenous fistulas for hemodialysis access, vascular access for hemodialysis XII symposium, Las Vegas, 12–14 May 2010. J Vas Access 2010.
55. Wixon CL, Hughes JD, Mills JL. Understanding strategies for the treatment of ischemic steal syndrome after hemodialysis access. J Am Coll Surg. 2000;191(3):301–10.
56. Arroyo MR, Sideman MJ, Spergel L, Jennings WC. Primary and staged transposition arteriovenous fistulas. J Vasc Surg. 2008;47(6):1279–83.
57. Jennings WC, Sideman MJ, Taubman KE, Broughan TA. Brachial vein transposition arteriovenous fistulas for hemodialysis access. J Vasc Surg. 2009;50(5):1121–5; discussion 1125–6. Epub 2009 Sep 26.31.
58. Paul EM, Sideman MJ, Rhoden DH, Jennings WC. Endoscopic basilic vein transposition for hemodialysis access. J Vasc Surg. 2010;51(6):1451–6. Epub 2010 Mar 20.
59. Jennings WC, Dorsey KW, Alder JD. Vascular surgery: minimally invasive basilic vein arteriovenous fistula transposition for hemodialysis vascular access. In: James ST, Yao MD, William H, Pearce MD, Mark Eskandari MD, editors. People's Medical Publishing House—USA, Ltd., Vascular surgery 2011.
60. Roberts JK, Sideman MJ, Jennings WC. The difficult hemodialysis access extremity: proximal radial arteriovenous fistulas and the role of angioscopy and valvulotomes. Am J Surg. 2005;190(6):869–73.
61. Keuter XH, De Smet AA, Kessels AG, van der Sande FM, Welten RJ, Tordoir JH. A randomized multicenter study of the outcome of brachial-basilic arteriovenous fistula and prosthetic brachial-antecubital forearm loop as vascular access for hemodialysis. J Vasc Surg. 2008;47(2):395–401. Epub 2007 Dec 26.
62. Gradman WS, Laub J, Cohen W. Femoral vein transposition for arteriovenous hemodialysis access: improved patient selection and intraoperative measures reduce postoperative ischemia. J Vasc Surg. 2005;41(2):279–84.
63. Gradman WS, Cohen W, Haji-Aghaii M. Arteriovenous fistula construction in the thigh with transposed superficial femoral vein: our initial experience. J Vasc Surg. 2001;33(5):968–75.
64. Hazinedaro lua SM, Tüzünera A, Aylib D, Demirera S, Dumanc N, Yerdela MA. Femoral vein transposition versus femoral loop grafts for hemodialysis: a prospective evaluation. Transplant Proc. 2004;36(1): 65–7.
65. National Institute on Aging [Internet] Bethesda, MD; 2009 Dec 10. Press release, Dramatic changes in U.S. aging highlighted in new census, NIH report, Impact of Baby Boomers Anticipated; 2006. [Cited 8 Jun 2010]. http://www.nia.nih.gov/NewsAndEvents/PressReleases/PR2006030965PlusReport.htm. Accessed 06 Aug 2010.

66. Tattersall J. Dialysis in the over-80s. Age Ageing. 2005;34(2):100–1.
67. Collins AJ, Kasiske B, Herzog C, Chavers B, Foley R, Gilbertson D, et al. Excerpts from the United States renal data system 2006 annual data report. Am J Kidney Dis. 2007;49(1 suppl 1):A6–7. S1–296.
68. Ekbal NJ, Swift PA, Chalisey A, Steele M, Makanjuola D, Chemla E. Hemodialysis access-related survival and morbidity in an elderly population in South West Thames, UK. Hemodial Int. 2008;12 suppl 2:S15–9.
69. Persic V, Ponikvar R, Buturovic-Ponikvar J. Preoperative ultrasonographic mapping of blood vessels before arteriovenous fistula construction in elderly patients with end-stage renal disease. Ther Apher Dial. 2009;13(4):334–9.
70. Berardinelli L, Vegeto A. Lessons from 494 permanent accesses in 348 haemodialysis patients older than 65 years of age: 29 years of experience. Nephrol Dial Transplant. 1998;13 suppl 7:73–7.
71. Lok CE, Oliver MJ, Su J, Bhola C, Hannigan N, Jassal SV. Arteriovenous fistula outcomes in the era of the elderly dialysis population. Kidney Int. 2005;67(6): 2462–9.
72. Lazarides MK, Georgiadis GS, Antoniou GA, Staramos DN. A meta-analysis of dialysis access outcome in elderly patients. J Vasc Surg. 2007;45(2): 420–6.
73. Ridao-Cano N, Polo JR, Polo J, Pérez-García R, Sanchez M, Gómez-Campderá FJ. Vascular access for dialysis in the elderly. Blood Purif. 2002;20(6): 563–8.
74. Jennings WC, Landis L, Taubman KE, Parker DE. Creating functional autogenous vascular access in older patients. J Vasc Surg. 2011;53(3):713–9.
75. Chan MR, Sanchez RJ, Young HN, Yevzlin AS. Vascular access outcomes in the elderly hemodialysis population: a USRDS study. Semin Dial. 2007;20(6): 606–10.
76. Richardson 2nd AI, Leake A, Schmieder GC, Biuckians A, Stokes GK, Panneton JM, et al. Should fistulas really be first in the elderly patient? J Vasc Access. 2009;10(3):199–202.
77. Beigi AA, Sadeghi AM, Khosravi AR, Karami M, Masoudpour H. Effects of the arteriovenous fistula on pulmonary artery pressure and cardiac output in patients with chronic renal failure. J Vasc Access. 2009;10(3):160–6.
78. Yong DS, Kwok AO, Wong DM, Suen MH, Chen WT, Tse DM. Symptom burden and quality of life in end-stage renal disease: a study of 179 patients on dialysis and palliative care. Palliat Med. 2009;23(2):111–9.
79. Couchoud C, Labeeuw M, Moranne O, Allot V, Esnault V, Frimat L, et al. A clinical score to predict 6-month prognosis in elderly patients starting dialysis for end-stage renal disease. Nephrol Dial Transplant. 2009;24(5):1553–61.
80. Chand DH, Valentini RP, Kamil ES. Hemodialysis vascular access options in pediatrics: considerations for patients and practitioners. Pediatr Nephrol. 2009;24(6):1121–8. Epub 2008 Apr 8.
81. Kim AC, McLean S, Swearingen AM, Graziano KD, Hirschi RB. Two-stage basilic vein transposition-a new approach for pediatric dialysis access. J Pediatr Surg. 2010;45(1):177–84; discussion 184.
82. Tannuri U, Tannuri AC, Watanabe A. Arteriovenous fistula for chronic hemodialysis in pediatric candidates for renal transplantation: technical details and refinements. Pediatr Transplant. 2009;13(3):360–4. Epub 2008 Sep 10.
83. Chand DH, Bednarz D, Eagleton M, Krajewski L. A vascular access team can increase AV fistula creation in pediatric ESRD patients: a single center experience. Semin Dial. 2009;22(6):679–83.
84. Haricharan RN, Aprahamian CJ, Morgan TL, Harmon CM, Barnhart DC. Intermediate-term patency of upper arm arteriovenous fistulae for hemodialysis access in children. J Pediatr Surg. 2008;43(1):147–51.
85. Bourquelot P. Vascular access in children: the importance of microsurgery for creation of autologous arteriovenous fistulae. Eur J Vasc Endovasc Surg. 2006;32(6):696–700. Epub 2006 Jun 6.
86. Wang Y, Beydoun MA, Liang L, Caballero B, Kumanyika SK. Will all Americans become overweight or obese? Estimating the progression and cost of the US obesity epidemic. Obesity (Silver Spring). 2008;16(10):2323–30. Epub 2008 Jul 24.
87. Stoikes N, Nezakatgoo N, Fischer P, et al. Salvage of inaccessible arteriovenous fistulas in obese patients: a review of 132 brachiocephalic fistulas. Am Surg. 2009;75(8):705–9; discussion 709.
88. Cull DL, Taylor SM, Carsten CG, et al. The fistula elevation procedure: a valuable technique for maximizing arteriovenous fistula utilization. Ann Vasc Surg. 2002;16(1):84–8. Epub 2002 Jan 16.
89. Weyde W, Krajewska M, Letachowicz W, et al. Obesity is not an obstacle for successful autogenous arteriovenous fistula creation in haemodialysis. Nephrol Dial Transplant. 2008;23(4):1318–22. Epub 2007 Oct 23.
90. Bourquelot P, Tawakol JB, Gaudric J, et al. Lipectomy as a new approach to secondary procedure superficialization of direct autogenous forearm radial-cephalic arteriovenous accesses for hemodialysis. J Vasc Surg. 2009;50(2):369–74, 374.e1.
91. Barnard KJ, Taubman KE, Jennings WC. Accessible autogenous vascular access for hemodialysis in obese individuals using lipectomy. Am J Surg. 2010;200(6): 798–802.
92. Ochoa DA, Mitchell RE, Jennings WC. Liposuction over a shielded arteriovenous fistula for hemodialysis access maturation. J Vasc Access. 2010;11(1):69–71.
93. Jennings WC, Howard CA, Lee FS, McMurray D. Extending outflow brachial vein length for transposition arteriovenous fistulas. J Vasc Access. 2011;12: 377–80.
94. Jennings WC, Brown RE, Ruiz C. Primary arteriovenous fistula inflow proximalization for patients at

high risk for dialysis access-associated ischemic steal syndrome. J Vasc Surg. 2011;54(2):554–8.
95. Zanow J, Kruger U, Scholz H. Proximalization of the arterial inflow: a new technique to treat access-related ischemia. J Vasc Surg. 2006;43(6):1216–21; discussion 1221.
96. Zanow J, Kruger U, Petzold M, Petzold K, Miller H, Scholz H. Arterioarterial prosthetic loop: a new approach for hemodialysis access. J Vasc Surg. 2005;41:1007–12.
97. El-Sabrout RA, Duncan JM. Right atrial bypass grafting for central venous obstruction associated with dialysis access: another treatment option. J Vasc Surg. 1999;29:472–8.
98. Scott JD, Cull DL, Kalbaugh CA, Carsten CG, et al. The mid-thigh loop arteriovenous graft: patient selection, technique, and results. Am Surg. 2006;72:825–8.
99. Slayden GC, Spergel L, Jennings WC. Secondary arteriovenous fistulas: converting prosthetic AV grafts to autogenous dialysis access. Semin Dial. 2008;21(5):474–82. Epub 2008 Jun 20.
100. Kennealey PT, Elias N, Hertl M, et al. A prospective, randomized comparison of bovine carotid artery and expanded polytetrafluoroethylene for permanent hemodialysis vascular access. J Vasc Surg. 2011; 53(6):1640–8.
101. Katzman HE, Glickman MH, Schild AF, Fujitani RM, Lawson JH. Multicenter evaluation of the bovine mesenteric vein bioprostheses for hemodialysis access in patients with an earlier failed prosthetic graft. J Am Coll Surg. 2005;201:223–30.
102. Shenoy S, Miller A, Petersen F, Kirsch WM, et al. A multicenter study of permanent hemodialysis access patency: beneficial effect of clipped vascular anastomotic technique. J Vasc Surg. 2003;38: 229–35.
103. Katzman HE, McLafferty RB, Ross JR, Glickman MH, Peden EK, Lawson JH. Initial experience and outcome of a new hemodialysis access device for catheter-dependent patients. J Vasc Surg. 2009;50: 600–7.
104. Lee T, Roy-Chaudhury P. Advances and new frontiers in the pathophysiology of venous neointimal hyperplasia and dialysis access stenosis. Adv Chronic Kidney Dis. 2009;16(5):329–38. Volume 16, issue 5, pages 329–338.
105. Beathard GA. Physical examination of the dialysis vascular access. Semin Dial. 1998;11:231–6.
106. Leon C, Orozco-Vargas LC, Krishnamurthy G, et al. Accuracy of physical examination in the detection of arteriovenous graft stenosis. Semin Dial. 2008;21:85–8.
107. Gelbfish GA. Clinical surveillance and monitoring of arteriovenous access for hemodialysis. Tech Vasc Interv Radiol. 2008;11:156–66.
108. Terrotola SO, Scheel PJ, Powe NR, et al. Screening for dialysis access graft malfunction: comparison of physical examination with US. J Vasc Interv Radiol. 1996;7:15–20.
109. Agarwal R, McDougal G. Buzz in the axilla: a new physical sign in hemodialysis forearm graft evaluation. Am J Kidney Dis. 2001;38:853–7.
110. Besarab A, Asif A, Roy-Chaudhury P, Spergel LM, Ravani P. The native arteriovenous fistula in 2007. Surveillance and monitoring. J Nephrol. 2007;20(6): 656–67.
111. Campos R, Riella MC. Challenge for the interventional nephrologist: monitoring the arteriovenous fistula. Contrib Nephrol. 2008;161:12–22.
112. Campos RP, Chula DC, Perreto S, Riella MC, Nasciemento MM. Accuracy of physical examination and intra-access pressure in the detection of stenosis in hemodialysis arteriovenous fistula. Semin Dial. 2008;21(3):269–73. Epub 2008 Feb 1.
113. Ram SJ, Nassar R, Work J, Abreo K, Dossabhoy NR, Paulson WD. Risk of hemodialysis graft thrombosis: analysis of monthly flow surveillance. Am J Kidney Dis. 2008;52:930–8.
114. Tessitore N, Bedogna V, Gammaro L, Lipari G, Poli A, Baggio E, Firpo M, Morana G, Mansueto G, Maschio G. Diagnostic accuracy of ultrasound dilution access blood flow measurement in detecting stenosis and predicting thrombosis in native forearm arteriovenous fistulae for hemodialysis. Am J Kidney Dis. 2003;42(2):331–41.
115. Allon M, Robbin ML. Hemodialysis vascular access monitoring: current concepts. Hemodial Int. 2009;13:153–62.
116. Paulson WD et al. A controversial CMS mandate for hemodialysis vascular access surveillance. Nephrol News Issues. September 3, 2009.
117. Goldstein SL, Allsteadt A, Smith CM, Currier H. Proactive monitoring of pediatric hemodialysis vascular access: effects of ultrasound dilution on thrombosis rates. Kidney Int. 2002;62(1):272–5.
118. Agarwal AK, Patel BM, Haddad NJ. Central vein stenosis: a nephrologist's perspective. Semin Dial. 2007;20(1):53–62.
119. Oderich GS, Treiman GS, Schneider P, Bhirangi K. Stent placement for treatment of central and peripheral venous obstruction: a long-term multi-institutional experience. J Vasc Surg. 2000;32(4):760–9.
120. Suliman A, Greenburg JI, Angle N. Surgical bypass of symptomatic central venous obstruction for arteriovenous fistula salvage in hemodialysis patients. Ann Vasc Surg. 2008;22(2):203–9.
121. Kalra M, Gloviczki P, Andrews JC, et al. Open surgical and endovascular treatment of superior vena cava syndrome caused by nonmalignant disease. J Vasc Surg. 2003;38(2):215–23.
122. Myers JL, Mukherjee D. Bypass graft to the contralateral internal jugular vein for outflow obstruction of a functioning hemodialysis access fistula. J Vasc Surg. 2000;32:818–20.
123. Anaya-Ayala JE, Smolock CJ, Colvard BD, et al. Efficacy of covered stent placement for central venous occlusive disease in hemodialysis patients. J Vasc Surg. 2011;54(3):754–9.

124. Jennings WC, Miller GA, Coburn ZM, Howard CA, Lawless MA. Vascular access flow reduction for arteriovenous fistula salvage in symptomatic patients with central venous occlusion. J Vasc Access. 2012;13:157–62.
125. Miller GA, Goel N, Friedman A, Khariton A, Jotwani MC, Savransky Y, et al. The MILLER banding procedure is an effective method for treating dialysis-associated steal syndrome. Kidney Int. 2010;77:359–66.
126. Goel N, Miller GA, Jotwani MC, Licht J, Schur I, Arnold WP. Minimally invasive limited ligation endoluminal-assisted revision (MILLER) for treatment of dialysis access-associated steal syndrome. Kidney Int. 2006;70(4):765–70.
127. van Hoek F, Scheltinga MR, Kouwenberg I, Moret KE, Beerenhout CH, Tordoir JH. Steal in hemodialysis patients depends on type of vascular access. Eur J Vasc Endovasc Surg. 2006;32(6):710–7. Epub 2006 Jul 26.
128. Scali ST, Huber TS. Treatment strategies for access-related hand ischemia. Semin Vasc Surg. 2011;24: 128–36.
129. Gradman WS, Pozrikidis C. Analysis of options for mitigating hemodialysis access-related steal phenomena. Ann Vasc Surg. 2004;18(1):59–65. Epub 2004 Jan 12.
130. Ehsan O, Bhattacharya D, Darwish A, Al-khaffaf H. 'Extension technique': a modified technique for brachio-cephalic fistula to prevent dialysis access-associated steal syndrome. Eur J Vasc Endovasc Surg. 2005;29(3):324–7.
131. Beecher B, Taubman K, Jennings WC. Simple and durable resolution of steal syndrome by conversion of brachial artery arteriovenous fistulas to proximal radial artery inflow. J Vasc Access. 2010;11(4):352–5.
132. Miller GA, Khariton K, Kardos SV, Koh E, Goel N, Khariton A. Flow interruption of the distal radial artery: treatment for finger ischemia in a matured radiocephalic AVF. J Vasc Access. 2008;9(1):58–63.
133. Schanzer H, Schwartz M, Harrington E, Haimov M. Treatment of ischemia due to "steal" by arteriovenous fistula with distal artery ligation and revascularization. J Vasc Surg. 1988;7(6):770–3.
134. Fistula first comprehensive fistula construction and management program for surgeons: how to make fistulas that work; 2010. http://www.hdcn.com/symp/10ff/10ff.htm. Accessed 10 Jan 2012.
135. Salman L, Asif A. Stent graft for nephrologists: concerns and consensus. Clin J Am Soc Nephrol. 2010;5:1347–52.
136. Pierce GE, Thomas JH, Fenton JR. Novel repair of venous aneurysms secondary to arteriovenous dialysis fistulae. Vasc Endovascular Surg. 2007;41(1):55–60.
137. Twardowski ZJ. Constant site (buttonhole) method of needle insertion for hemodialysis. Dial Transplant. 1995;24:559–76.
138. Kronung G. Plastic deformation of cimino fistula by repeated puncture. Dial Transplant. 1984;13: 635–6.
139. Rayner HC, Pisoni RL, Gillespie BW, Goodkin DA, et al. Creation, cannulation and survival of arteriovenous fistulae: data from the dialysis outcomes and practice patterns study. Kidney Int. 2003;63:323–30.
140. Robbin ML, Chamberlain NE, Lockhart ME, et al. Hemodialysis arteriovenous fistula maturity: US evaluation. Radiology. 2002;225:59–64.
141. Van Loon MM, Kessels AGH, Van Der Sande FM, Tordoir JHM. Cannulation and vascular access-related complications in hemodialysis: factors determining successful cannulation. Hemodial Int. 2009;13:498–504.
142. Asif A, Roy-Chaudhury P, Beathard GA. Early arteriovenous fistula failure: a logical proposal for when and how to intervene. Clin J Am Soc Nephrol. 2006; 1:332–9.
143. Dember LM, Beck GJ, Allon M, et al. Effect of clopidogrel on early failure of arteriovenous fistulas for hemodialysis: a randomized controlled trial. JAMA. 2008;299(18):2164–71.
144. Hentschel DM, Atif A. Effect of clopidogrel of arteriovenous fistulas for dialysis. JAMA. 2008;300(14): 1647–8.
145. Lynch JR, Wasse H, Armistead NC, McClellan WM. Achieving the goal of the fistula first breakthrough initiative for prevalent maintenance hemodialysis patients. Am J Kidney Dis. 2011;57:79–89.
146. De Marco Garcia LP, Davila-Santini LR, Feng Q, Calderin J, Krishnasastry KV, Panetta TF. Primary balloon angioplasty plus balloon angioplasty maturation to upgrade small-caliber veins (<3 mm) for arteriovenous fistulas. J Vasc Surg. 2010;52:139–44.
147. Beathard GA, Arnold P, Jackson J, Litchfield T. Physician operators forum of RMS lifeline. Aggressive treatment of early fistula failure. Kidney Int. 2003;64(4):1487–94.
148. Turmel-Rodrigues L, Mouton A, Birmelé B, Billaux L, Ammar N, Grézard O, et al. Salvage of immature forearm fistulas for haemodialysis by interventional radiology. Nephrol Dial Transplant. 2001;16(12): 2365–71.
149. Haskal ZJ, Trerotola S, Dolmatch B, Schuman E, Altman S, et al. Stent graft versus balloon angioplasty for failing dialysis-access grafts. N Engl J Med. 2010;362:494–503.
150. Vesely TM, Siegel JB. Use of the peripheral cutting balloon to treat hemodialysis-related stenoses. J Vasc Interv Radiol. 2005;16(12):1593–603.

New Oral Anticoagulants in Surgery 22

Jihane Abou Rahal, Zaher K. Otrock,
Joseph E. Maakaron, and Ali Taher

Abstract

For over 50 years, the only available oral anticoagulants for the treatment and prevention of thromboembolic diseases have been vitamin K antagonists (VKA) such as warfarin. Although highly effective, VKAs have many disadvantages: they have a narrow therapeutic range with a subsequent need for frequent monitoring, a >10-fold interindividual variation in dose–response, and numerous interactions with drugs and food. Thus, antithrombotics have been developed, and they emerged to circumvent these problems and limitations.

Keywords

Oral anticoagulants • Dabigatran • Rivaroxaban • Apixaban • Venous thromboembolic disease

For over 50 years, the only available oral anticoagulants for the treatment and prevention of thromboembolic diseases have been vitamin K antagonists (VKA) such as warfarin. Although highly effective, VKAs have many disadvantages: they have a narrow therapeutic range with a subsequent need for frequent monitoring, a >10-fold interindividual variation in dose–response, and numerous interactions with drugs and food [1]. Thus, antithrombotics have been developed, and they emerged to circumvent these problems and limitations.

Recently, three new oral anticoagulants, namely, dabigatran, rivaroxaban, and apixaban, have been approved for the prevention of venous thromboembolic events. They offer the advantages of having stable pharmacokinetic and pharmacodynamic

J. Abou Rahal • J.E. Maakaron • A. Taher (✉)
Department of Internal Medicine,
American University of Beirut Medical Center,
Beirut, Lebanon

Z.K. Otrock
Department of Pathology and Laboratory Medicine,
American University of Beirut Medical Center,
Beirut, Lebanon

J.J. Hoballah, A.B. Lumsden (eds.), *Vascular Surgery*, New Techniques in Surgery Series,
DOI 10.1007/978-1-4471-2912-7_22, © Springer-Verlag London 2012

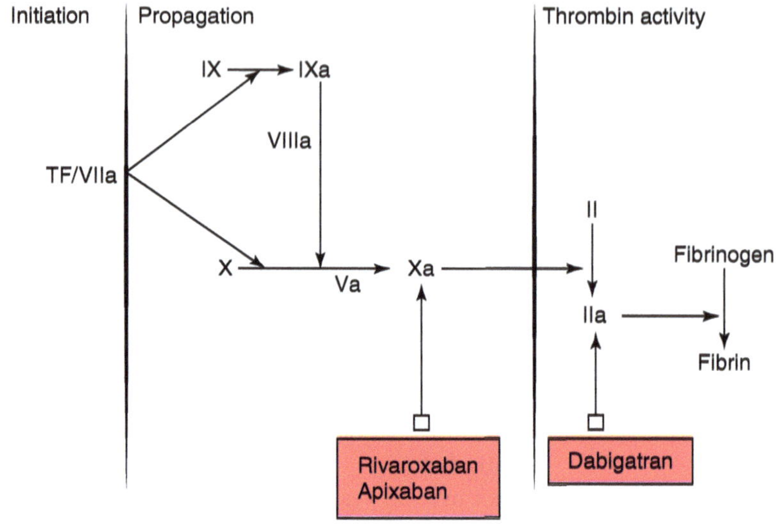

Fig. 22.1 Site of action of the new oral anticoagulants

properties: a wide therapeutic window, little interindividual variability, and minimal food and drug interaction. As a result, they do not require monitoring [2].

This chapter discusses each of these three drugs, including their properties and approved applications to the surgical field as well as current guidelines and recommendations for their use.

Overview

Patients undergoing major surgery have a high risk of developing postoperative venous thromboembolism (VTE). Venous thrombi are intravascular deposits composed of fibrin and blood cells and contain relatively few platelets. They develop as a result of alteration in blood flow, vascular endothelial injury, and activation of the coagulation pathway. Anticoagulants are the keystone in preventing and treating this complication. In hospitalized patients not receiving thromboprophylaxis, the absolute risk of developing deep vein thrombosis ranges between 15 and 60 % with procedures such as orthopedic, general, urologic, or gynecologic surgeries [3]. Several agents have been traditionally used for the prevention and treatment of VTE in the perioperative period. These include unfractionated and low molecular weight heparin (LMWH) and fondaparinux, given subcutaneously or parenterally, and the oral warfarin. These anticoagulants are multi-targeted in that they act on several factors of the coagulation cascade [4]. In contrast, the new oral drugs were developed to target single factors critical to the coagulation process (see Fig. 22.1). They block the initiation and propagation of the coagulation cascade or attenuate fibrin formation by impeding prothrombin. Based on the step they inhibit, these mono-targeted oral anticoagulants can be divided into two categories [3]:

- Direct inhibitors of activated factor Xa such as rivaroxaban and apixaban: target the propagation of the coagulation cascade as factor Xa at the beginning of the common coagulation pathway.
- Direct thrombin (factor IIa) inhibitors such as dabigatran: inhibit thrombin by binding directly to its active site. As a result, they prevent this procoagulant from converting fibrinogen to fibrin and from activating factors V, VIII, XI, and XIII [5].

Dabigatran Etexilate

Dabigatran etexilate is an oral prodrug with 6 % bioavailability and is rapidly and completely converted by plasma esterases to dabigatran. Dabigatran is a concentration-dependent, competitive, selective, reversible direct thrombin inhibitor [6]. As a direct inhibitor, it does not need a cofactor to inhibit thrombin, as opposed to indirect inhibitors like heparin that bind to antithrombin before acting on thrombin or factor Xa. When thrombin is trapped in clots, it is somewhat protected from heparin but accessible to direct thrombin inhibitor [7].

The plasma concentration of dabigatran takes about 2 h to reach its peak levels, and it has a half-life of 12–17 h after repeated dosing. Approximately 35 % of the circulating drug is bound to plasma proteins (see Table 22.1). Elimination is mainly through the kidneys that excrete about 80 % of the drug unchanged. Studies have shown that moderately severe liver dysfunction or Child-Pugh B has little effect on the drug pharmacodynamics [6].

Table 22.1 Comparison of the pharmacological properties of new oral anticoagulants

	Dabigatran	Rivaroxaban	Apixaban
Target	Thrombin	Factor Xa	Factor Xa
Bioavailability	6 %	80 %	50–80 %
Tmax (h)	2	2.5–4	1–3
Half-life (h)	12–17	6–7	8–15
% Protein binding	35	95	87
CYP metabolism	0	30	15
Main elimination	Renal (80 %)	Renal (60 %), fecal (40 %)	E!iJliSi.!Y and fecal (75 %)

The absorption of dabigatran is reduced with decreased gastrointestinal motility and gastric acidity. A slower absorption can, therefore, be observed with high fat and caloric food, when taken concomitantly with proton pump inhibitors, or in the early postoperative period. Known drug–drug interactions include interaction with P-gp-related drugs such as amiodarone, verapamil, quinidine, and ketoconazole (P-gp inhibitors). The manufacturer advises caution with the P-gp inducers rifampin and St. John's wort as they may decrease the maximum concentration of the drug [7] (see Table 22.2).

Dabigatran etexilate has been approved in many countries for the prevention of VTE after total hip or knee replacement surgeries [8]. It has also been approved in the USA and Canada for the prevention of strokes or systemic emboli in nonvalvular atrial fibrillation patients [7]. Dosing for VTE prevention is 150 mg or 220 mg once daily, to be started 1–4 h postoperatively at half the dose once (i.e., 75 or 110 mg) before continuing with the full recommended dosage on day 2 [5, 7] (see Table 22.3). The drug is still under

Table 22.2 Significant drug–drug interactions with new oral anticoagulants

Dabigatran	P-glycoprotein	Inhibitors	Amiodarone
			Verapamil
			Quinidine
			Ketoconazole
		Inducers	Rifampin
			St. John's wort
Rivaroxaban	CYP3A4	Inhibitors of both pathways	Azole antimycotics
			HIV Protease inhibitors
	P-glycoprotein	Strong CYP3 inhibitors	Clarithromycin
			Erythromycin
		Strong CYP3 inducers	Rifampin
			St. John's wort
			Carbamazepine
			Phenytoin
			Phenobarbital
Apixaban	CYP3A4	Inhibitor	Ketoconazole
			Ritonavir

Table 22.3 Surgical indications and associated dosage of new oral anticoagulants

	Surgical indication	Dosage
Dabigatran	Postoperative thromboprophylaxis in total knee or hip arthroplasty	Day of surgery: 110 mg (1–4 h post-surgery)
		Following day (and ongoing): 220 mg once daily
Rivaroxaban	Postoperative thromboprophylaxis in total hip or knee replacement surgery	Day of surgery: 10 mg (6–10 h post-surgery)
		Following day (and ongoing): 10 mg once daily
Apixaban	Postoperative thromboprophylaxis in total knee or hip arthroplasty	Day of surgery: 2.5 mg twice daily (12–24 h post-surgery)
		Following day (and ongoing): 2.5 mg twice daily

evaluation for the treatment and secondary prevention of venous thromboembolic disease.

One of the major advantages of new oral anticoagulants is the fact that they do not require laboratory monitoring. This stems from the drug's predictable pharmacological profile. Furthermore, based on currently available evidence, it seems unlikely that routine monitoring using anticoagulant tests provides any clinical benefit. Nevertheless, they may be of interest in patients needing emergent procedures, those who develop bleeding or thrombosis while on dabigatran, or in cases of overdose. In these instances, a normal TCT (thrombin clotting time) rules out the presence of dabigatran. PT and aPTT are relatively insensitive in measuring the anticoagulant effect. The most sensitive test seems to be the ECT (ecarin clotting time) that shows a linear dose–response relation to the drug [9]. Unfortunately, this test is not readily available in laboratories. However, clinical studies have evaluated fixed dose of dabigatran and recommend standard doses for most patients. Despite little evidence available yet, it seems logical to consider lower doses in elderly patients especially with impaired renal function. The European Medicines Agency (EMA) recommends a 220-mg daily dose for VTE prophylaxis, to be reduced to 150 mg if patients are >75 years of age, have altered kidney function (creatinine clearance between 30 and 50 mL/min), or in those receiving amiodarone or verapamil [10].

The risk of major bleeding in patients receiving dabigatran is similar to that associated with prophylactic enoxaparin. It is reported to range between 0.6 and 2 % and is dose-dependent, affecting the surgical wound in around 90 % of cases [11]. Unlike ximelagatran, a direct thrombin inhibitor that was withdrawn from the market due to unacceptable liver toxicity, dabigatran intake was not associated with liver dysfunction. Aside from bleeding, the major side effect of dabigatran was dyspepsia [12].

There is no sufficient data on when to stop the drug before an elective procedure although extrapolation from the half-life indicates that after 24 h of stopping the dabigatran, the plasma level drops to 25 %. The new anticoagulant has no antidote yet, and the management of life-threatening bleeding remains empirical. Early administration of charcoal possibly decreases its absorption. Moreover, studies on animal models suggest that administration of factor VIIa or prothrombin complexes may counteract high levels of dabigatran. Hemodialysis removes 60 % of the drug in 2 h [6].

Rivaroxaban

Rivaroxaban acts as a selective, competitive, and reversible direct inhibitor of factor Xa. The small molecule can inhibit factor Xa both when the factor is free or bound to the prothombinase complex and clot-associated. Around 95 % of the drug is protein bound mostly to albumin in the blood [13]; it has a bioavailability of 80 % and reaches maximal plasma concentration after 2.5–4 h, with a half-life of 6–7 h (see Table 22.1) [5]. Its elimination is through the kidneys and feces after two-third is metabolized in the liver [5, 13].

Known drug interactions include azole antimycotics, HIV protease inhibitors, clarithromycin, erythromycin (increase the plasma concentration of rivaroxaban), as well as rifampin, phenytoin, carbamazepine, phenobarbital, and St John's wort (decrease its plasma concentration) (see Table 22.2) [14].

Because of its predictable pharmacologic properties, only one dose can be given to all patients regardless of age, gender, or body weight. Monitoring is neither required routinely nor for dose adjustment. There is no laboratory test validated for the monitoring of rivaroxaban activity. Indeed although PT and aPTT show a linear concentration-dependent response, they should not be used to assess the level of anticoagulation as the increase in clotting time varies greatly, depending on the thromboplastin reagent used for the test [15].

Rivaroxaban has been approved in many countries (Canada, USA, and Europe) for pharmacological prophylaxis against VTE in patients undergoing total hip and knee replacement surgery at a dose of 10 mg once daily (see Table 22.3) [5, 7]. The regimen is started about 6–10 h postoperatively. It is not approved for pregnant and breast-feeding women, children younger than 18 years, patients with severe renal insufficiency or hepatic disease with coagulopathy, and finally in subjects receiving azole antimycotics and HIV protease inhibitors. The data collected showed that rivaroxaban was more efficient in preventing DVT as compared to LMWH (enoxaparin) but may cause increased bleeding [16]. However, the safety evidence was of moderate quality, thus carrying some level of uncertainty which necessitates long-term follow-up [7].

Rivaroxaban has not been associated with increased risk of bleeding when compared to enoxaparin. It should be noted, however, that the trials did not take into account bleeding at the surgical site when accounting for number of bleedings for both rivaroxaban and LMWH [7]. It was not associated with liver toxicity. No antidote is available to antagonize the effect of rivaroxaban [5]. As the drug is highly protein bound, dialysis has little role in cases of bleeding or overdose. Studies on rats have shown reversal of drug effect with high doses of prothrombin concentrate complex. In addition, an antidote has been recently suggested in the form of an inactive recombinant factor Xa with a high affinity to rivaroxaban. Although experimental results are promising, clinical application and availability of the antidote are still far from reality [7].

Apixaban

Apixaban is a selective, reversible, direct factor Xa inhibitor that binds to the active site of factor Xa without the need of antithrombin [17–19]. Similar to rivaroxaban, it can act on both circulating factor Xa and to factor Xa when bound within the prothrombinase complex as well. Oral bioavailability ranges between 50 and 80 % [5, 18]; time to maximal plasma concentration is between 1 and 3 h [2, 5] and the half-life of the drug is 8–15 h [2, 5, 20] (see Table 22.1). The drug is metabolized by CYP3A4 in the liver and eliminated in the feces (75 %) and by the kidneys (25 %) [2, 5]. Ketoconazole and ritonavir (potent inhibitors of CYP3A4) are contraindicated with apixaban because they raise its plasma levels (see Table 22.2) [21]. As mentioned previously with other new oral anticoagulants, laboratory monitoring is not recommended routinely or for dose adjustment [3]. The drug has minimal effect on PT and aPTT [2].

Apixaban is currently approved by the European Commission for the prevention of VTE in patients undergoing scheduled hip or knee replacement surgeries. It was found to have similar rate of major and clinically relevant bleeding as enoxaparin, against which it was compared in clinical trials [17, 22]. The dose used for thromboprophylaxis is 2.5 mg twice daily to be started 12–24 h after surgery (see Table 22.3). Apixaban is currently under evaluation for treatment of VTE in the Amplify clinical trials [19].

As apixaban is eliminated mainly through the feces and/or biliary tract, it is less likely to accumulate or to require dose adjustment in case of renal dysfunction [19, 23]. In different phase III clinical studies, the rate of bleeding ranged from less frequent to equal to that observed with enoxaparin when both were used for thromboprophylaxis, thus exhibiting a good safety profile [22]. As with other new oral anticoagulants, there is currently no antidote for apixaban.

Guidelines

The latest ACCP (American College of Chest Physicians) guidelines, published in February 2012, have included the new oral anticoagulants in many of their recommendations.

In Orthopedic Surgery

- One of the following: Apixaban, rivaroxaban, dabigatran, LMWH, fondaparinux, low-dose unfractionated heparin (LDUH), VKA, aspirin (all grade 1B), or intermittent pneumatic compression device (IPCD) (grade 1C) is recommended as antithrombotic prophylaxis for a duration of 1–14 days in patients undergoing total hip replacement (THA) or total knee replacement (TKR) [24].
- Among the suggested drugs, it is recommended to use LMWH in preference.

The reasons ACCP provides for recommending LMWH over the new oral anticoagulants include lack of long-term safety data for all three drugs and the possibility of increased bleeding with rivaroxaban.

In the event patients undergoing major orthopedic surgeries decline or are uncooperative with injections or an IPCD, recommendations favor the use of apixaban or dabigatran (and if both are not available, then rivaroxaban or VKA) rather than alternative prophylaxis.

In Nonorthopedic Surgery

- The ACCP does not recommend the use of the new oral anticoagulants in nonorthopedic surgery for the prevention of VTE [25].

Therapy of VTE Disease

- In non-oncologic patients with pulmonary embolism or lower extremity DVT, VKA is recommended over LMWH for prolonged therapy. If VKA therapy is not available, then LMWH is preferred over dabigatran and rivaroxaban (Grade 2C) [26].

Note that there is currently only one completed study respectively for each of dabigatran and rivaroxaban assessing their use in the treatment of VTE. Although the results of these studies showed comparable efficacy and safety to VKA, the trials suffer from serious imprecision in the outcome measurement and lack of long-term follow-up [27].

Keep in Mind

Thus far, the results of trials testing the new oral anticoagulants have been encouraging from the standpoint of efficacy and safety. The advent of new blood thinners promises a new era in the prevention and treatment of VTE. Although these new drugs provide solutions to many of the old anticoagulant problems, it is doubtful they represent the ideal agent. More studies are needed to assess their full potential and, more importantly, to address many unanswered questions concerning potential drawbacks. Dabigatran, which is renally cleared, does not have a studied, recommended, adjusted dose (see Table 22.4). This is especially pertinent, given that the vast majority of the patients enrolled in the trials while studying the pharmacokinetics and the risk of bleeding associated with dabigatran etexilate were middle-aged subjects with a renal clearance higher than 50 ml/min. On the other hand, real-life patients needing the anticoagulants will include a big proportion of elderly with decreased renal function, putting these patients at risk of accumulating the drug and increasing the risk of bleeding [27]. Rivaroxaban, also eliminated through the kidneys, has not been studied in patients with damaged kidney function and is contraindicated in this population, thus limiting its clinical application in a big chunk of patients at risk of VTE.

Post-marketing studies will provide greatly valuable information about the risks of these drugs. It is likely that in the outpatient setting, subjects will be less compliant, a risk exacerbated by dyspepsia in the case of dabigatran. A more accurate estimate of the efficacy and safety will hopefully be available to us in the near future, allowing a more precise comparison with available anticoagulants. Still more data is needed to

Table 22.4 Factors affecting concentration of new oral anticoagulants

	Dabigatran	Rivaroxaban	Apixaban
Renal insufficiency:			
Moderate (CrCI 30–50 ml/in) – Mild (50–80 m/min)	Recommended dose: 75 mg × 2 taken OD	No dose adjustment needed	No data available
	Limited clinical experience		
Severe (CrCI <30 ml/min)	Contraindicated	Caution with CrCI 15–29 m/min	No data available
		Not recommended with CrCI <15 m/min	
Extreme of weights	Very little experience	No dose adjustment	No data available
	No adjustment necessary needed		
	Close clinical surveillance		
Age older >75 years	Recommended dose 75 mg × 2 once per day	No dose adjustment needed	No data available

OD daily, *CrCl* creatinine clearance

address the issue of whether extremes of weights and age affect the drug properties. Finally, it is particularly important for surgical patients to have more information regarding surgical site bleeding. Although factor Xa inhibitors (rivaroxaban and apixaban) have been approved for thromboprophylaxis in orthopedic surgeries, after trials reported bleeding rates were equivalent to those associated with LMWH (enoxaparin), it is worth noting that the bleeding evaluated in those trials did not include surgical site bleeding. Post-marketing safety issues will hopefully address this point and provide us with a more accurate portrayal of these drugs' adverse events and safety.

Conclusion

Oral direct factor Xa and thrombin inhibitors offer many advantages that range from their immediate onset of action to their wide therapeutic index, few drug interactions, and fixed dosage with little interindividual variability without the need for monitoring. Possible shortcomings of these drugs include the risk of poor compliance (overdosing or underdosing) that is difficult to pick up by a physician as routine laboratory monitoring is not needed. Further data is needed to assess the role of these new agents in surgery, whether for acute illness or general and particularly oncologic surgeries where vomiting may affect the optimal absorption and activity of the drugs.

Dabigatran, apixaban, and rivaroxaban, with their predictable pharmacological profile, have a number of promising features. However, their full therapeutic potential as well as their drawbacks need further assessment and are likely to grow clearer as the results of many studies currently under trial become available to us.

References

1. Lassen MR. Recent developments in the use of oral anticoagulants. Expert Opin Pharmacother. 2009;11: 1769–81.
2. Galanis T, Thomson L, Palladino M, Merli G. New oral anticoagulants. J Thromb Thrombolysis. 2011;31:310–20.
3. Merli G, Spyropoulos AC, Caprini JA. Use of emerging oral anticoagulants in clinical practice: translating results from clinical trials to orthopedic and general surgical patient populations. Ann Surg. 2009;250:219–28.
4. Hirsh J. Current anticoagulant therapy – unmet clinical needs. Thromb Res. 2003;109 Suppl 1:1S–8.
5. Bauer KA. Recent progress in anticoagulant therapy: oral direct inhibitors of thrombin and factor Xa. J Thromb Haemost. 2011;9 Suppl 1:12S–9.
6. Stangier J, Clemens A. Pharmacology, pharmacokinetics, and pharmacodynamics of dabigatran etexilate, an oral direct thrombin inhibitor. Clin Appl Thromb Hemost. 2009;15 Suppl 1:9S–16.
7. Ageno W, Gallus AS, Wittkowsky A, Crowther M, Hylek EM, Palareti G. Oral anticoagulant therapy: Antithrombotic Therapy and Prevention of Thrombosis, 9th ed: American College of Chest Physicians Evidence-Based Clinical Practice Guidelines. Chest. 2012;141 Suppl 2:44S–88.

8. Kendoff D, Perka C, Fritsche HM, Gehrke T, Hube R. Oral thromboprophylaxis following total hip or knee replacement: review and multicentre experience with dabigatran etexilate. Open Orthop J. 2011;5:395–9.
9. van Ryn J, Stangier J, Haertter S, et al. Dabigatran etexilate–a novel, reversible, oral direct thrombin inhibitor: interpretation of coagulation assays and reversal of anticoagulant activity. Thromb Haemost. 2010;103:1116–27.
10. Dahl OE, Kurth AA, Rosencher N, Noack H, Clemens A, Eriksson BI. Thromboprophylaxis with dabigatran etexilate in patients over seventy-five years of age with moderate renal impairment undergoing or knee replacement. Int Orthop. 2012;36:741–8.
11. Oldgren J, Budaj A, Granger CB. Dabigatran vs. placebo in patients with acute coronary syndromes on dual antiplatelet therapy: a randomized, double-blind, phase II trial. Eur Heart J. 2011;32:2781–9.
12. Bendel SD, Bona R, Baker WL. Dabigatran: an oral direct thrombin inhibitor for use in atrial fibrillation. Adv Ther. 2011;28:460–72.
13. Gulseth MP, Michaud J, Nutescu EA. Rivaroxaban: an oral direct inhibitor of factor Xa. Am J Health Syst Pharm. 2008;65:1520–9.
14. Nutescu E, Chuatrisorn I, Hellenbart E. Drug and dietary interactions of warfarin and novel oral anticoagulants: an update. J Thromb Thrombolysis. 2011;31:326–43.
15. Samama MM, Guinet C. Laboratory assessment of new anticoagulants. Clin Chem Lab Med. 2011;49:761–72.
16. Turpie AG, Lassen MR, Davidson BL, et al. Rivaroxaban versus enoxaparin for thromboprophylaxis after total knee arthroplasty (RECORD4): a randomised trial. Lancet. 2009;373:1673–80.
17. Van Es J, Eerenberg ES, Kamphuisen PW, Buller HR. How to prevent, treat, and overcome current clinical challenges of VTE. J Thromb Haemost. 2011;9 Suppl 1:265S–74.
18. Samama CM, Godier A. Perioperative deep vein thrombosis prevention: what works, what does not work and does it improve outcome? Curr Opin Anaesthesiol. 2011;24:166–70.
19. Jiménez D, Yusen RD, Ramacciotti E. Apixaban: an oral direct factor-xa inhibitor. Adv Ther. 2012;29:187–201.
20. Wong PC, Pinto DJ, Zhang D. Preclinical discovery of apixaban, a direct and orally bioavailable factor Xa inhibitor. J Thromb Thrombolysis. 2011;31: 478–92.
21. Weitz JI, Eikelboom JW, Samama MM. New antithrombotic drugs: Antithrombotic Therapy and Prevention of Thrombosis, 9th ed: American College of Chest Physicians Evidence-Based Clinical Practice Guidelines. Chest. 2012;141 Suppl 2:120S–51.
22. Huang J, Cao Y, Liao C, Wu L, Gao F. Apixaban versus enoxaparin in patients with total knee arthroplasty. A meta-analysis of randomised trials. Thromb Haemost. 2011;105:245–53.
23. Huo MH. New oral anticoagulants in venous thromboembolism prophylaxis in orthopaedic patients: Are they really better? Thromb Haemost. 2011;106: 45–57.
24. Falck-Ytter Y, Francis CW, Johanson NA, Curley C, Dahl OE, Schulman S, Ortel TL, Pauker SG, Colwell Jr CW. Prevention of VTE in orthopedic surgery patients: Antithrombotic Therapy and Prevention of Thrombosis, 9th ed: American College of Chest Physicians Evidence-Based Clinical Practice Guidelines. Chest. 2012;141 Suppl 2:278S–325.
25. Gould MK, Garcia DA, Wren SM, Karanicolas PJ, Arcelus JI, Heit JA, Samama CM. Prevention of VTE in nonorthopedic surgical patients: Antithrombotic Therapy and Prevention of Thrombosis, 9th ed: American College of Chest Physicians Evidence-Based Clinical Practice Guidelines. Chest. 2012;141 Suppl 2:227S–77.
26. Kearon C, Akl EA, Comerota AJ, Prandoni P, Bounameaux H, Goldhaber SZ, Nelson ME, Wells PS, Gould MK, Dentali F, Crowther M, Kahn SR. Antithrombotic therapy for VTE disease: Antithrombotic Therapy and Prevention of Thrombosis, 9th ed: American College of Chest Physicians Evidence-Based Clinical Practice Guidelines. Chest. 2012;141 Suppl 2:419S–94.
27. Prandoni P, Taher A. Insights from the dabigatran versus warfarin trial in patients with venous thromboembolism (the RE-COVER trial). Expert Opin Pharmacother. 2010;11 Suppl 6:1035S–7.

Index

J.J. Hoballah, A.B. Lumsden (eds.), *Vascular Surgery*, New Techniques in Surgery Series,
DOI 10.1007/978-1-4471-2912-7, © Springer-Verlag London 2012

J

K

L

M

N

O

P

MIX
Papier aus verantwortungsvollen Quellen
Paper from responsible sources
FSC® C105338

If you have any concerns about our products,
you can contact us on
ProductSafety@springernature.com

In case Publisher is established outside the EU,
the EU authorized representative is:
Springer Nature Customer Service Center GmbH
Europaplatz 3, 69115 Heidelberg, Germany

Printed by Libri Plureos GmbH
in Hamburg, Germany